The Battle For Our Lives

Our Immune System's War Against The Microbes That Aim To Invade Us

By Daniel Keays

LIBRARY OF CONGRESS CATALOGING-IN-PUBLICATION DATA

Names: Keays, Daniel, author.

Title: The battle for our lives : our immune system's war against the microbes that aim to invade us / by Daniel Keays.

Description: First edition. | San Diego, California : Daniel Keays, [2023] | Includes bibliographical references.

Identifiers: ISBN: 979-8-218-30230-6 (paperback) | 979-8-218-30231-3 (eBook) | LCCN: 2023920204

Subjects: LCSH: Immune system. | Pathogenic microorganisms. | Immune response--Regulation. | Antibiotics. | Vaccines. | Medicine--History. | Infection--Prevention. | Communicable diseases--Prevention. | Diseases--Causes and theories of causation. | Germ theory of disease. | BISAC: MEDICAL / Infectious Diseases. | MEDICAL / Immunology. | MEDICAL / Microbiology. | MEDICAL / History.

Classification: LCC: QR181 .K43 2023 | DDC: 616.07/9--dc23

Printed in the USA

FIRST EDITION

This book is for educational purposes only. This book does not replace the advice of a medical professional. Consult your physician before making medical decisions.
The information in this book was correct at the time of publication. The author does not assume any liability for loss or damage caused by errors or omissions.

Cover: Natalie Narbonne (Original Book Cover Designs)

JMJ

For My Beloved Family,
With All My Love and Heartfelt Gratitude.
Semper Pater amat vos.

DJK

Contents

Introduction
Our Innermost Secrets

In the late 1860s, a major snowstorm struck the Midwest of the United States. While most inhabitants hunkered down in their homes, one unfortunate woman was outside, became disoriented, and couldn't get to shelter. They found her body face-down in the snow a couple of days later.

A recently recovered local newspaper revealed a story about the unfortunate incident. The woman lived alone on a small farm just outside of town. She had moved to the area a few years before with her husband, who had passed away a short time before. The newspaper described her as "an elderly woman, aged 47."

Elderly? Age 47? That may come as a shock to us in the 21st century, but such was the state of affairs in the United States just a hundred and fifty years ago. If you were a woman born in 1850, your life expectancy was 40 years. Just 38 if you were male. The numbers are skewed since infant and childhood mortality was much higher than today. Still, if you lived to be 20 back then, your life expectancy from that point on was age 60. The average age of death in 1900 was 47. People living into their 70s were somewhat rare.

Things have changed. The reasons are many and varied, but one clear contribution to increasing the longevity and quality of our lives has been greater control of infectious diseases, with advances in sanitation, vaccination, and antibiotics, in that order. When did you last walk out of your house worrying about getting diphtheria, smallpox, or typhoid? Before the 1940s, a simple scratch could get infected, fester, and lead to a fatal case of "blood poisoning," more appropriately called sepsis. Tuberculosis used to be rampant. Malaria was once common in the United States. Rabies was not uncommon and 100% fatal. Babies often died of whooping cough. The list goes on and on. Humans were subject to an almost inevitable fatal collision with infectious diseases.

Gradually, science and technology advanced our understanding and control of many of the worst diseases. Change came haltingly, often accompanied by contentious disputes, but over time the benefits of appropriate measures became so apparent that they are now firmly ingrained in the population's psyche.

In fact, in the late 1960s, things went a little too far the other way. William Stewart, U.S. Surgeon General, is reported to have testified before Congress with words to the effect that "we can close the book on infectious diseases." In fairness to Dr. Stewart, his testimony was an attempt to divert some federal funding from infectious diseases to other areas like cancer and heart disease, and he may have been given to some hyperbole. Still, his sentiments reflected the general feeling of the time. Polio had just been conquered, smallpox was nearly extinct, and vaccines protective against diseases like measles, mumps, and rubella were becoming common. Typhoid, cholera, and dysentery were rare in the developed world. And, perhaps most impressive of all, new antibiotics were coming to market almost monthly. A girl born in 1900 had a life expectancy of 51 years. For one born in 1950, it was 72. A friend specializing in infectious diseases began his training in the early 1970s. Colleagues not so good-naturedly ridiculed him for entering a "dying field." Yes, sir, infectious diseases were soon to be relegated to the dustbin of history.

In retrospect, the thought of conquering nature seems like such hubris. We can mitigate some of its effects, alter a minor portion of it to suit our needs, and sometimes temporarily avoid its realities. But change it? No. Biological systems progress unceasingly and without remorse. Infectious organisms are incredibly adaptable and fluid and will continue to confound our best efforts to confront them. The best we can hope for is some respite. Microbes constantly mutate, seeking the critical factor that will enable them to fill a niche.

Popular opinion has it that all microbes are all bad all the time. But, in reality, they are an indispensable part of us. The most prominent ingredient by weight in human breast milk are chemicals called oligosaccharides. Curiously, humans can't digest oligosaccharides. They pass through us like cellulose. But some bacteria digest them readily, to our benefit and theirs.

So right from the start, nature has provided us with the means to cultivate a luxuriant flora of microorganisms within our bowels.

The vermiform appendix was long thought to be the most useless bodily tissue, probably just some holdover from prehistoric times. But recent theory suggests that it is a little sack of reserve bacteria. Given its location at the entrance to the large intestine, it is perfectly positioned to supply us with the right kind of microorganisms if natural diseases like cholera or dysentery disrupt our normal intestinal flora.

Many people have learned the hard way the value of our natural microbiota. "Good" bacteria protect us from harmful ones by being firmly established in a spot where the pathogens would like to attack. Some make natural antimicrobial substances that inhibit the "bad" bacteria. But when we take an antibiotic, it doesn't distinguish the good from the bad and kills bacteria indiscriminately. After taking an antibiotic, women sometimes get a vaginal yeast infection because the yeast, resistant to common antibiotics, now has a bacteria-free area to colonize, the normal bacterial flora of the region having been eliminated. Diarrhea is a not uncommon side effect of antibiotic use because the normal state of bacterial interaction with the cells lining our bowel has become disrupted.

Not only do our friendly bacteria help us to keep away the potentially harmful ones, but they are also indispensable in developing and maintaining our immune system.

We are immersed in and surrounded by microorganisms. Bacteria are all over us, in our mouth, intestinal tract, skin, and vagina. So how come we're not all dead? After all, once we die, it only takes a few hours before microbes start to have their way with us, and we begin to decompose. To our benefit, there is a barrier between our bodies and the bugs, and it is very effective. It's our immune system.

When we study anatomy or physiology in school, we often discuss each area separately. This week we'll talk about the bones. Next week it's the muscles. Then the heart and circulatory system, etc. When we get to the immune system, we sometimes regard it as a stand-alone entity, with each part going about its business as if in a vacuum. But to fully comprehend the wonder and magnificence of the immune system, we must see it as the integrative, interactive marvel it is. It consists of a panoply of cells, chemical signals, primary and backup systems, and memory methods, some of which we are born with, called innate, and some of which we acquire throughout life. The immune system is not only in charge of our protection from infectious agents, but it interacts with numerous other cellular systems to ensure the proper function of every bodily system.

There are several different types of cells in the immune system, each with a specific purpose. The skin is a crucial member, serving as a barrier. There are cells in the blood and tissues, including macrophages, neutrophils, and a wide array of lymphocytes, with interesting names like T-helper, T-killer, natural killer, and B cells. Each has several types and sub-types. A mysterious and perplexing number of chemical signals and agents are produced to guide the system and allow it to carry out and fine-tune its mission. The complexity of the immune system is astonishing, and it is remarkably effective.

The immune system is not unique to humans or mammals. All animals, including the most primitive and least complex, have a form of immunity to protect them from parasites and invaders. Many of these systems have been passed along through the ages to make their way to us, albeit with many modifications. The entire process evolved to make us completely immune to all types of bacteria and viruses. If that's the case, then how come we still get sick? Microbes grow and evolve as well. Suppose our immune system has a cell or chemical to counteract a particular microbe. In that case, the microbe can undergo a mutation or acquire genetic coding to produce a different chemical or structure, allowing it to neutralize or circumvent the immune system's defense. Then the immune cells must adapt to the new virulence factor of the microbe. Once that happens, the microbe can mutate and come at us again. And on and on. It's a continual cat-and-mouse game, with the bugs mutating to evade the immune response and the immune system adapting to meet the new challenge. We'll never be completely free of infectious diseases.

The pandemic of the early 2020s caused by the previously relatively innocuous Coronavirus virus incontestably illustrates the point. Viral mutations, stifled immune responses, and altered viral interactions led to the introduction of a strain of virus previously unknown. Ramifications continue unabated.

A properly functioning immune system is essential for freedom from infectious diseases and other conditions. Immune cells and chemical agents are directly responsible for inflammation, which is involved in conditions such as diabetes, heart disease, various intestinal disorders, arthritis, etc. Sometimes, the immune system goes awry, causing a severe condition known as autoimmune disease, where the body, in a sense, attacks itself.

Understanding an infectious disease requires us to understand the actions of the immune system as well as the invasive properties of the microbe. It's a fascinating tale of attack, intrigue, and deception. We're just beginning to understand the mysteries.

Words to Remember

Apoptosis.   The cells of our body have a self-destruct feature. When something goes wrong inside the cell, a series of chemical reactions is initiated, resulting in the cell's death. Apoptosis is one of those odd words that can be pronounced correctly in two different ways. We can say either a-POP-ta-sis or apo-TOE-sis. It comes from the Greek, meaning a falling away, such as a leaf falling from a tree during autumn. Apoptosis suggests an orderly process in keeping with nature, not a traumatic one.

White Blood Cells.   If we place a blood specimen in a test tube, then spin the tube in a centrifuge for a short time, it will separate into three distinct layers. At the bottom is a large dark red section of red blood cells. A straw-colored fluid at the top is a little greater volume than the bottom red blood cell portion. It is known as serum if the blood is allowed to clot before centrifuging. It is known as plasma if the blood is kept from clotting (anti-coagulated).

Between the two prominent layers is a narrow band of off-white or dull yellow made up of white blood cells and platelets. Because of its color, buff, it is called the buffy coat.

All red blood cells are the same. Not so the white blood cells, which are naturally divided into groups. The most common ones are granulocytes, lymphocytes, and macrophages. Each type is further divided into more groups, each having a different function. Some white blood cells stay in the bloodstream; others exit and function outside the circulation. The white blood cells are critical in keeping us safe from infectious diseases.

Antibody.   We acquire proteins in our body that have a critical function: to seek out and attach themselves to an invading microbe. The proteins don't bind randomly to just any microbe. They attach very selectively to a specific microbe, and to a minute, unique part of it. These proteins are called antibodies. By adhering to the invading microbe, whether a virus, bacterium, fungus, parasite, or toxin, the antibody can inhibit the invader's activity and act in concert with the body's defense cells to help eliminate it. The part of the microbe or toxin that initiates the formation of antibodies is called an antigen, short for "antibody generator." The small, specific part of the antigen the antibody attaches to is called an epitope.

Most antibodies are not innate but are produced by our immune cells after encountering a foreign invader. The foreign material needn't be harmful, just different from the materials of our own body.

Antibodies are part of the immune system, so the proteins are given the term "immuno." They look sorta, kinda, like a globe, so they are called "globulins." The full chemical name is immunoglobulin, often abbreviated Ig. There are four major types of antibodies; each assigned a capital letter designation. Each has a unique role. About five days after the first encounter with the invader, IgM is the first antibody released. IgG is a more specific antibody released a couple of weeks later. IgA is a secretory antibody, released to areas outside the bloodstream, like into the bowel and saliva. IgE specializes in attacking parasites.

Receptor. On the surface of most of the cells of our body are a plethora of tiny appendages, lining the surface membrane like so many blades of grass. Each of these projecting molecules has a specific job: to serve as a landing and attachment point for whatever substance they are constructed to hook onto. Collectively called receptors, they are very specific. If substance A meets up with receptor A, a chemical change occurs in one or both, and a series of chemical events follows. It may be the incorporation of substance A into the cell, or it may be an alteration in the structure of receptor A which then triggers a series of chemical events in substances already in the cell. Receptors are very specific, but sometimes mistakes occur. For instance, a receptor on the cell surface routinely attaches to a particular protein of the body, but a protein on a virus or a bacterium may assume the proper shape so that it, too, can bind to the receptor.

Cytokine. The cells of our body communicate with each other chiefly using chemical signals. When one cell experiences something, it often emits a chemical, usually a peptide or a protein, that wanders around the body until it comes to a receptor on another cell's surface that will bind it. This binding changes the receptor, either incorporating the bound substance into the cell or chemically or physically changing itself. Both reactions alter the receptor's cell, initiating one or several chemical responses.

One type of such substance prominent in the immune system is known as cytokines, "cyto" for cell and "kine" for activity or action. During infection, cytokines play a vital role in alerting and activating critical parts of the immune system into action.

A related word is chemokine. Chemokines function like cytokines but act specifically to attract a type of white blood cell. The term cytokine is often interchanged with chemokine.

Vacuole. Our cells all contain small internal membrane-bound areas known as vacuoles. There are several types of vacuoles, often containing food or waste products. The membrane surrounding the vacuole isolates the substance it holds from the rest of the cell and serves to concentrate it.

Each cell, whether part of the immune system or not, contains vacuoles that aid immunity. When a microbe enters the cell after attaching to a receptor on the membrane, part of the cell membrane surrounds it and forms a vacuole as it enters the cell's interior. The vacuole formed is called a phagosome. Also present in each cell are vacuoles that contain enzymes and other substances that can destroy microbes. These are called lysosomes. When an invading microbe such as a virus or bacterium enters a cell, it is routinely encased in a phagosome, which combines with the engaged lysosome, and the killing enzymes are activated.

Actin. A protein of immense importance in all cells is actin. It is a structural substance that gives form and structure to the cell. Without it, the cell would round up and lose its shape and ability to form tight junctions with its neighbor. Actin is vital for the formation of the cell's cytoskeleton.

Actin is important in infectious diseases because some organisms use it to move about. They can use it to move around inside the cell, or to transport themselves from one cell to another. The microbe attaches to actin and slowly moves like a train rolling on a track. In some cases, organisms or their toxins destroy the actin cytoskeleton, thereby initiating the cell's death.

Biofilm. Quite a few bacteria and yeast can establish a tough, complex layer known as a biofilm that forms a rigid attachment to parts of our body. Dental plaque is a good example. They can also develop on gallstones, kidney stones, and surgically implanted medical devices. Biofilms can also form on soft tissues.

To create a biofilm, the microbe's cells attach to a cellular or inanimate surface. Once attached, the microbial colony transforms itself. The secured layer sends out specialized appendages to achieve a firm grip on the substrate and also reproduces to form microbial cells on top of them. This adjacent layer also transforms to become a conduit between the top and bottom layers. The top, or third, layer is comprised of vegetative cells, albeit with molecular communication with the bottom two layers. So, the bottom layer attaches to the substrate, the middle layer connects the bottom cells to the top, and the top layer resembles a typical vegetative cell. Biofilms grow more slowly than typical bacteria or yeast, and since many of the bacteria are dormant, they are much more challenging to treat with antimicrobial substances.

CD. The initials CD have wide use, from a type of bank deposit to a computer storage disk. In biology, the term refers to "cluster of differentiation." Briefly, it refers to the presence of a specific protein on the surface of a cell that distinguishes it from other cells. The CD is always followed by a number, such as CD4 or CD8. Proteins in structure, they are a handy way of classifying types of cells, sort of like license plates that tell us which state a car is from.

MHC. Our cells have an elaborate, complicated system of communicating with the components of the immune system. It goes by two names. Originally called "major histocompatibility complex," or MHC, it is also called HLA, or "Human Leukocytic Antigen." Put very simply, the MHCs are large molecules located within the entrails of a human cell. When the cell digests and processes a substance, such as an invading microbe or toxin, the digested parts are mounted onto MHCs, which serve as vehicles to carry the substance to the cell's surface. It then exposes the carried substance on the cell's exterior so that cells of the immune system can encounter it and, if necessary, begin an immune response.

SECTION ONE

"You have to know the past to understand the present."
– Carl Sagan

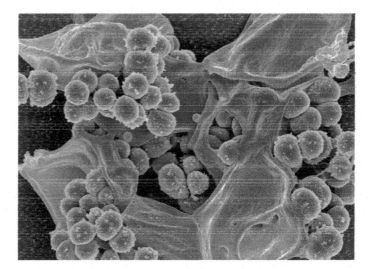

Chapter 1
Sanitation Transformation

Born to affluence,
Life committed to the poor.
Dear Filomena

Florence Nightingale was one of the most influential people of the 19th century. She was also one of the most enigmatic. Her very name conjures up an image, the context of which depends on the version of history one has read about her.

Her name is unusual, and how she came about it was even more remarkable. The original family name was Shore. William Shore's father had a wealthy uncle they called "Crazy Uncle Peter." Uncle Peter told William he would bequeath his fortune if he changed his surname from Shore to Nightingale. Nobody seemed to know why, but William complied. Shortly after that, William married Fanny, seven years his senior, and they and their fortune traveled to Italy. In Naples, in 1819, they had their first daughter Parthenope. A year later, their second daughter, named after the city of her birth, was born in Florence. They were the couple's only two children, but they were indeed a handful.

Right from the beginning, Florence was a bit unusual. She was exceptionally bright, as was her father, who didn't have to work. He spent much of his time educating his two daughters, who came to know several languages and were very familiar with classic literature and philosophy. Florence was one of the few girls of the era allowed to study mathematics, and she excelled in geometry and the newly formed discipline of statistics. She also developed a fondness for the natural sciences and religion.

The Nightingales were not among the super-rich, but they did live comfortably with two country estates. They frequently hosted lavish parties with very well-renowned guests. Florence had to perform her duties as hostess, but she took great delight in picking the brains of some of the intellectuals and politically well-connected. By a relatively young age, she became brilliantly educated and politically astute.

In those days, a young lady of the upper middle class had two choices about her life, no matter how well educated. She was either to marry or stay home and help care for her family. That was about it. Florence, though, sought another direction.

Tall and willowy, Florence was quite an attractive woman. She had several suitors, one interested her, and she came close to tying the knot. But a profound event in her early life played on her mind, and she was overwhelmed by it. She had had a "vision" and was "told by God to pursue her passion." We, of course, will never know the nature of this vision, but to her, it was intimate, personal, and profound. She truly felt God Himself called her to follow a career. She was especially attracted to nursing and assumed that was her destiny. There was just one problem, but it was a beaut: In those days, nurses were often the dregs of society. Women who couldn't make it in service took to "nursing" instead. Many women in the profession were coarse, alcoholic, and of low moral standards. One could imagine the reaction of Florence's family when she declared her desire to enter nursing as a profession.

Her mother was particularly incensed and perplexed. It wasn't that she was unkind. She and Florence often visited their less fortunate workers and neighbors, giving them gifts of food and other provisions. Florence was not only allowed but also encouraged to visit and care for their sick neighbors and tenants. But nursing as a profession and calling? Absolutely not.

Florence had a lot of skills and attributes, but her most robust feature was her tenacity. She just wouldn't let up. Finally, her mother allowed her to train as a nurse in Germany, where the profession had a higher standing, and to work part-time at a nearby medical clinic. Fanny probably was tired of the incessant supplications and threw her a bone, hoping the scene's reality would eventually dissuade her.

Then fate intervened.

Florence applied for and was given the chief administrator position of a clinic for indigent women. Before her arrival, the "clinic" was pretty much a place to go to die. Many workers were underpaid, untrustworthy, wretched women given to drink and debauchery. The clinic was poorly managed as to provisions and productivity. It was the type of place that would achieve prominence in a Charles Dickens novel.

Florence's influence was profound. She called upon all her skills in organization and administration to quickly clean up how the place was run, firing the poor workers and motivating the promising ones. She arranged the supplies and materials so the workers would be more productive and wouldn't waste as much time. She appealed to many of her contacts in the higher realms of society for extra funding. But most of all, she brought a sense of care and compassion to the workplace. She genuinely and deeply cared for the sick and dying; her example was a powerful motivation. Here was this attractive, wealthy woman of high intellect stooping down to make the lives of these unfortunate outcasts a little more bearable. The transformation of this one clinic in London in a few months set the tone for her entire career.

(It is interesting to note that the clinic at which she worked was the one closest to Broad Street in the Soho district, where Dr. John Snow made his famous discovery of the source of a cholera epidemic after removing the handle of a water pump, thereby halting the disease. Florence undoubtedly knew of this significant discovery).

In 1854, another set of circumstances formed Florence Nightingale's place in history. The Crimean War, in which Great Britain fought to curtail the advances of Russia in the Middle East, was underway. As in all wars, young men marched off to battle with visions of glory and adventure etched in their minds. Of course, the reality is much different. But the Crimean campaign was unique: The Times of London sent a reporter to the scene, William Howard Russell, who filed regular reports as an embedded journalist. With the invention of the telegraph and undersea cable laying, his words reached home in a few hours. People were appalled by what they read. The British military was poorly run, with corruption and incompetence evident. Most shocking was the deplorable state of the military hospitals. To say they were miserable, depraved, and indifferent to suffering was to understate the situation. With the public outcry that followed the reporting of the conditions under which injured and dying soldiers were treated, something had to be done. It was Florence Nightingale who intervened.

The Secretary of War, Sidney Herbert, and his wife were close personal friends of the Nightingales. They had met in Rome some years earlier. There was intense pressure on the government to do something about the deplorable conditions in the military hospitals, and Herbert turned to Florence. She gathered 38 of the best nurses she could find, and off they went.

Women in military settings in those days were unheard of. Military leaders and doctors regarded nurses as whores and derelicts, not exactly a welcoming environment. But Florence was persistent, and because of her upbringing and family status, she knew how the game was played. At first, the nurses were denied access to the hospital, but eventually, the conditions became so bad that out of desperation, she and her crew were permitted to work. And work they did. Florence was conscientious to see to it that the women under her direction strictly followed protocol. Anyone found to be of low moral character was quickly sent home. She and her nurses worked tirelessly under the most horrific of conditions. As in England, Florence used her administrative skills to see that things were run efficiently and productively. After some time, the conditions vastly improved.

In addition to raising the stature of the nursing profession, Ms. Nightingale was greatly responsible for introducing a concept and practice that we today find dogmatic but, in her time, was virtually unknown: sanitation. In the 1850s, the germ theory of disease was only a rumor and a very unpopular one at that. But Florence insisted on the essential practice of sanitary hospital care, such as clean linen, open windows to let air circulate more freely, changing bloody or soiled bandages, clean floors, and hand washing. Her reason for insisting on implementing these practices was flawed, as she felt disease was caused by "vapors" or "miasma." Still, her application of statistical analysis based on her observations showed that patient outcomes vastly improved when proper hygiene was enforced. It led to the wide adoption of efforts toward sanitation decades before the association between bacteria and disease was firmly established.

Florence profoundly felt that her devotion to her work should not gain notoriety. A person entered nursing not for personal notice and certainly not for money. Nursing was a way of carrying out God's love in a tangible way. So, it was incredibly ironic that things worked out the way they did. Russell's reporting, a poem by Henry Wadsworth Longfellow (*Santa Filomena*, also known as the *Lady With the Lamp*), and a painting depicting her on her nightly rounds made her the most famous woman not only in England but around the world. She could have been faced with the agonizing decision of whether to exploit her fame for the betterment of her profession or keep to a quiet, almost reclusive life. But she didn't have to make that decision. An infectious disease made it for her.

Today, we cannot be sure what disease Florence caught while serving in Crimea. She was exposed to several severe infectious diseases, including cholera, dysentery, tuberculosis, typhoid fever, typhus, and others. Post-traumatic stress disorder was undoubtedly possible. But the evidence of her symptoms points to one infectious disease: brucellosis, known at the time as Crimean Fever. Ironically, after dwelling and working under the most horrific conditions of filth, pestilence, and deprivation, she may have become seriously ill for the next twenty years by drinking a glass of fresh milk. That's possibly what happened.

Brucella, the bacterial agent of brucellosis, is passed to humans from animals such as goats and cattle by their milk. Pasteurization was unknown in the 1850s, so all milk and cheese were consumed untreated. She drank some during her time there; there is even one letter stating how grateful she was for some fresh goat milk she got from a general stationed nearby. The disease was to leave her a bedridden invalid for two decades.

Untreated brucellosis can be a severe disease, sometimes even fatal. The symptoms are often described as protean, a word derived from the Greek god Proteus, a sea god known for continual change. That pretty much captures the symptoms of brucellosis: all over the place. The incubation time can be quite variable; there is usually fever, either high or low grade, much or little joint pain, extreme fatigue, depression, and quite a few others. The symptoms of Florence Nightingale were severe.

She had intense joint pain, particularly in her back. Just getting out of bed and walking across the room was excruciating. Her fevers were constant. Every joint in her body was racked with pain. Her depressive states were deep and dark. And there was no resolution. In the 1860s, they didn't even know what caused the disease, let alone how to treat it. Despite this incredible hardship, her tremendous influence on the healthcare system is truly remarkable.

Knowing what we do about brucellosis, or "Crimean" or "Mediterranean" fever, as it was once called, gives us a greater appreciation for the tremendous accomplishments of Florence Nightingale, especially after her return to England from the Crimean War. Bedridden, in constant pain, and with a severe state of depression, she continued her excellent work, writing what amounted to "The Bible" for nurses and nursing schools across the globe, "Notes on Nursing." She was responsible for founding nursing colleges, which were imitated worldwide. Her use of statistics to establish proper procedures for care was the foundation of what we now take for granted in all medical fields. A prodigious writer, she influenced the nursing profession worldwide and was a tremendous force in establishing this indispensable and honorable profession.

From the perspective of us living over a hundred years following her death, one can make an excellent case that Florence Nightingale's most outstanding contribution to humanity was her forceful advocacy for the observance of good sanitary techniques when caring for the sick. For all of history up to Florence Nightingale's time, people didn't understand the importance of washing and cleanliness. Water is very heavy, and transporting and heating it was a tremendous burden, so most people went without regular bathing. Indeed, some felt that taking a bath was a vice, leading to illness. It was common for people to go several months without washing themselves, wearing the same clothes daily. Florence Nightingale was at the forefront of developing the doctrine that proper sanitation was necessary to prevent many infectious diseases.

"The amount of relief and comfort experienced by the sick after the skin has been carefully washed and dried, is one of

the commonest observations made at the sick bed." – Florence Nightingale

Thankfully, her symptoms suddenly dissipated about 20 years after her illness appeared. At around age 60, Florence could lead a relatively everyday life, and she spent much of her time traveling to encourage young members of her profession. Hers is a name that will last in history.

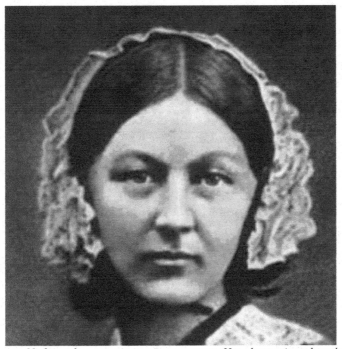

Florence Nightingale was a pioneer in many ways. Her observations, knowledge of statistics, and attention to protocol and detail changed the profession of nursing and the practice of medicine. They led to a deeper appreciation of the benefits of scrupulous sanitation. (Library of Congress, LOC)

Chapter 2
Louie Pasteur's Game Changer

A simple process,
But so profound its effects.
Pasteurization

Pasteurization, of course, is named for its inventor, the great Louis Pasteur. As simple as the process is, it revolutionized public health and the food industry on several levels. The procedure was one of a commercial enterprise's first scientific research and discovery applications. It also went a very long way in explaining some basic principles of biology. The ramifications of Pasteur's discovery and its application were of immense importance.

Today when we talk of pasteurization, most think of milk, but Pasteur was looking for a way to prevent wine from going bad. For a Frenchman, having your best wine turn into vinegar is about as bad as life can be. The task is monumental when a nation's livelihood is riding on saving the wine. A French gentleman named Monsieur Bigot, a wine manufacturer and the father of one of Pasteur's students, asked Pasteur to investigate the souring of wine after it was produced.

In 1856 Pasteur was up against two prevailing points of view. One was that life originated spontaneously, commonly called spontaneous generation. The other was that science was a philosophical enterprise, and scientists did science for science's sake. For a scientist to lower himself into the commercial realm was to demean the art.

Pasteur pretty much blew both of those notions out of the water. Though a chemist, he owned a microscope and brought his instrument to Monsieur Bigot's production facility. After making a few observations, he concluded that wine was produced because of the fermentation activity of the yeast present. The souring of the wine was created because of the presence of a bacterial species that contaminated the product. He didn't know it then, but the bacterium is called *Lactobacillus*, named for its strong production of lactic acid, which spoils just about anything. He noted that good wine just had the yeast; sour wine had the yeast and bacteria. (The spontaneous generation crew also noted the presence of yeast. They reasoned that the fermentation process produced the yeast).

To get rid of the contaminating bacteria, Pasteur showed that heating the wine briefly to about 160 degrees for a few minutes killed the microbes but left the wine unchanged. The process bears his name, pasteurization.

Some liquid foods you just cannot boil because it would ruin them. Beer, wine, and milk all come under the "do not boil" umbrella. But heating it for a few minutes to about 160°F (boiling is 212°F) can denature the enzymes the organism needs to survive while sparing the food product. A few enzymes in the food will be denatured too, but so be it.

Sterilizing raw milk from a cow or goat isn't just a matter of preventing the product from spoiling. Several serious infectious organisms are often found in milk, particularly *Brucella, Listeria, Salmonella,* and *Mycobacterium tuberculosis.* Of course, after Pasteurization, the product must be kept in a clean container and refrigerated. Dairy products left exposed at room temperature can still attract flies and other insects that can potentially transmit infectious organisms, most notably bacteria.

Pasteur's process revolutionized the dairy, beer, and wine industries, a major leap forward in preventing infectious diseases. With the necessary work and contribution of people like Florence Nightingale and the clear demonstration of the need for hygiene and sanitation, a new frontier was founded: the germ theory of disease. Biology itself was beginning to be revolutionized.

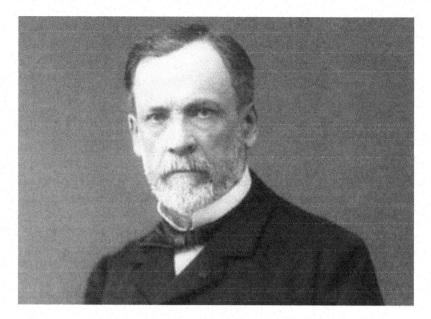

Louie Pasteur's many accomplishments added greatly to the advancement of medicine. Revolutionary in his day, they are considered commonplace today. (LOC)

Chapter 3
Nothing Small About It

The scourge, pestilence.
Extinct, but not forgotten.
Ineffable horror.

We humans like keeping score. Factoids such as the highest mountain, fiercest hurricane, longest river, oldest living human, fastest animal... The list is very long. Despite being macabre, some seek to ascertain the infectious disease causing the most deaths in human history. We have cholera, bubonic plague, typhus, tuberculosis, malaria, and others. All are formidable, but the one most often mentioned as causing the most deaths and human misery is variola.

The name variola was probably coined in the 6th century. It is formally attributed to Bishop Marius of Avenches, Switzerland, in the year 570. It comes from one of two Latin words, *"varius,"* meaning "stained," or *"varus,"* meaning mark on the skin. Common folk came to call it pocke, meaning sack. It was also called the "speckled monster."

In 1492 Columbus sailed the ocean blue. The introduction of European and African diseases into the New World is well documented, but such occurrences can go both ways. Shortly after Columbus and his crew's travels, a horrific disease appeared in Europe, beginning in Spain, and spreading eastward. It left its victims with huge red welts on their skin, which soon desquamated into foul-smelling, weeping sores. It became known as the "Great Pox." Most today would recognize it by its current name, syphilis.

To contrast it with the "other pox," variola became commonly known as the "small" pox. The name stuck.

The devastation that smallpox has wrought upon humanity cannot be overstated. Generations of people were killed and maimed, and their communities were ravaged. In some cases, entire civilizations were nearly wiped out. Those sickened but able to survive were often horribly disfigured by the pockmarks on their face and body, some left with life-altering medical conditions. Many went blind. Josef Stalin is said to have once remarked words to the effect that one person's misfortune is a tragedy; millions affected is a statistic. So it is with the history of smallpox. In the 18th century in Europe, over 400,000 people died each year from smallpox; but reading about the numbers afflicted and the areas of epidemics gives little insight into the horror of its victims. Smallpox has scarred the entire human race as indeed as it scarred its individual casualties.

For centuries, smallpox, or a disease of the pox virus family strongly resembling it, cursed humanity. One of the great pharaohs, Ramses V, is said to have a mark on his preserved skin resembling a pockmark. Theories abound, but it is possible that smallpox originated some 3,000 to 4,000 years ago in northeast Africa and was spread eastward to India by Egyptian merchants. Ancient texts in both China and India mention a strongly suggestive disease. It is likely that the virus first infected an animal, then jumped to humans, whence it became communicable, human to human, by the respiratory route. One theory holds that a pox virus that infected rodents in East Africa jumped to infect camels upon their introduction to that area as pack animals some three or four thousand years ago. The transformed virus in camels made it more likely to infect humans, who were just beginning to engage in travel for trade and commerce. That's the most likely scenario, but the scientific evidence to support it is deficient.

The disease probably entered Europe sometime between the fifth and seventh centuries AD. The only mobile people at the time were merchants and traders, and the virus likely traveled with them, either by land or by sea. The incubation period is around two weeks, so one could travel a considerable distance before becoming ill and transmitting the virus. Patients are infectious a couple of days before symptoms become severe, so there was no way to simply avoid an infected person. Outbreaks would come in waves, often with several years' quiescence. When it hit, it was ferocious. Most inhabitants of a town or village were affected. But two facts were obvious: it was transmissible from person to person, and it was a "one and done." Once you got the disease and recovered, you were immune for the rest of your life. Those known to have recovered from the illness were obliged to care for the sick.

12

Many remedies were attempted: application of cold cloths, herbal concoctions, not allowing fire in the room, leaving the windows opened, leaving the top of the patient's body uncovered, and "administering twelve bottles of small beer every twenty-four hours." Of course, nothing worked. For centuries humans were compelled to just suffer through the ailment and hope and pray for the best. Quarantine of sickened individuals helped but was not foolproof because of the possibility of transmission during the late prodromal stage, the few days before the time one becomes severely ill. Also, the virus is exceptionally hardy, able to survive for some time on environmental surfaces. It was a fairly common practice in Europe to steam open letters with a noxious agent in the hope of killing any virus that may have been applied during the sealing of the letter. Myths and folklore prevailed.

Medieval medical records don't document it, but somewhere in the history of the disease, a second, less virulent strain emerged. Known as variola minor (as opposed to the much more virulent variola major), this second strain had a much lower mortality rate. From an evolutionary perspective, this makes sense. A "good" parasite doesn't kill its host; if it does, it dies with it. Strains of the virus that were far less likely to kill would be more likely to be spread, therefore having a better chance of surviving. For evidence of this, we need to look no further than the "great pox," which invaded Europe around 1500. Syphilis is caused by a bacterial form known as a spirochete, an organism that is well-named because of its spiral shape. It slithers through our tissues like a corkscrew and can infect multiple organs after its transmission by sexual activity. The disease has three main stages: primary (a chancre on the genitalia), secondary (a rash), and tertiary (invasion of the deep tissues). It is the secondary stage of the disease that is of interest. When first introduced into Europe, the great pox was easy to spot. The infected patient in the secondary stage had many skin lesions, several of which became infected with other bacteria like Strep and Staph. The result was a patient who was very ill, had weeping sores, and obviously had a sexually transmitted disease. Such a person would be unlikely to engage in sexual activity any time soon, which is the chief means of transmission

13

of the spirochete. Strains that mutated to give a much-reduced skin rash activity would be more likely to be transmitted, so they out-competed their more aggressive cousins.

Could that scenario have been playing out with the variola viruses? One catastrophically severe, the other more benign? Could be. Unfortunately, historical records are too limited, and direct molecular evidence is not available to know just when the variola minor strain emerged, so it remains only a theory. But the minor strain did exist, and, with the help of human intervention, variola's days were numbered.

Mary Pierrepont was ahead of her time. Way ahead. Born in London in 1689, the daughter of the English Duke of Kingston, she grew up in the very highest reaches of British society. She had the best of everything and grew up knowing firsthand the finest life had to offer. At 23, she married Lord Edward Wortley Montagu, and her life and future seemed fixed. But in 1715, the "speckled monster" attacked, and her life and the disease's future were inexorably altered.

Lady Wortley Montagu was no ordinary aristocratic debutant. Incredibly brilliant and a gifted writer, she was limited only by her sex from becoming recognized as one of the best authors of her time. She also had a bulldog disposition. Females of her time were not allowed to learn Latin. She taught herself. Her father wanted her to marry a well-positioned aristocratic man she didn't like. She eloped with a man of her choosing. Feisty, fierce, and unwavering, she was not to be assailed.

But attacked and ravaged she was, by smallpox. Her beloved brother died of the disease, and she, while a survivor, was permanently disfigured. She was devastated.

In 1717 her husband, Edward Wortley Montagu, was appointed ambassador to the Ottoman Court. Contrary to custom, she and her children accompanied him to Constantinople (now Istanbul) and remained with him there for two years. Lady Mary was not one to sit around the embassy all day and engage only in the finer dignities of British society. She took delight in seeking out local customs and practices and writing about them in her own inimitable and prolific style. Being a woman, she had access to areas where English men

14

couldn't go – to the places where the local women congregated. There she was keen to observe and write about local activities and culture. Her *Letters From Turkey* became a classic and an inspiration for travelers for years to come.

During her preoccupation with local customs, one especially captivated her. Turkish folklore had it that if you took the scabs from smallpox patients, ground them up, and injected (or inoculated) them onto the upper arm of a healthy individual, it may make them ill for a while. But they invariably recovered and were immune to smallpox for the rest of their lives. She witnessed the procedure herself. In a dimly lit back room, a woman came in, ground up the pustules from a smallpox patient in a walnut shell, and used a knitting needle to scratch the material onto the arm of the person to be protected. The practice was said to have been handed down by word of mouth for centuries in several countries, like China, India, and some in Africa. Eventually, it made its way to the Middle East.

Rather than being frightened to death by such a strange procedure, Mary Montagu was enthralled. With her strong personality, writing skills, and nearly maniacal hatred of smallpox, she went on a mission to have the procedure introduced in her native England. To say she ran into some obstacles and roadblocks understates it immensely. One can almost hear an English physician say something to the effect, "You want to prevent someone from getting smallpox by giving them smallpox"? The very thought of it was preposterous, bordering on lunacy. To make it even worse, it was proposed by a woman in the early 18th century: an aggrieved woman, no less. To have the procedure used routinely, as it must, required winning over not just a handful of physicians but some of the most ardent critics. Her chances of pulling something like this off were slim and none, with a strong bias toward the "none" side. But she did.

She used all her tools and advantages. Her intelligence, daring, guile, passion, and tenacity played a role. So did her first-hand knowledge and insight into the procedure. But she had something else going for her: the acquaintance and friendship with Caroline, Princess of Wales.

Caroline was special. Born in Ansbach, Germany, she has been described by one historian as "the cleverest Queen consort ever to sit on the throne of England." King George I had, to say the least, a very troubled marriage. So he allowed his son George II to marry a woman of his choosing rather than an arranged marriage. Young George chose wisely. Caroline was intelligent, well acquainted with the arts, and, by all accounts, a good and loving wife. She and George II had eight children, seven of whom survived to adulthood. She was to become the Princess of Wales and Queen of England. Popular with the people and looked upon with respect by the ruling class, Caroline carried much influence.

Like Lady Mary Montagu, Caroline had contracted smallpox. It was shortly after her marriage in 1705. Her husband, George II, devoted to her and unwilling to leave her sick bed, also nearly died of it. But they both survived and, given their royal position, were very concerned about the disease affecting their family, not just for personal reasons but for royal succession. Caroline and Lady Mary were soul mates.

Lady Mary had done, at the time, the unthinkable. She had her son and daughter inoculated with the variola virus. One was done in Turkey, the other in England. Both children survived and weren't all that sick, just a few days of fever and muscle aches.

Having Caroline's ear was Lady Mary's strong suit. She was very persuasive, and Caroline listened intently. It was authorized to have six criminals under sentence of death inoculated. All survived with a limited illness and no severe side effects. Next, it was tried on several children at an orphanage. All survived and thrived. Seeing this, Caroline agreed to have her children inoculated. It went well. Here was the first successful attempt at vaccination in Western culture. The children of two prominent women, one a famous aristocratic writer and adventurer, the other the heir to the throne of England, had their precious children deliberately inoculated with the pus from a scab of a person with smallpox, and they became ill for only a couple of days. It was the birth of what was to become known as vaccination.

16

Indeed, though, there was heated controversy. The term genocide wasn't used back then, but depopulation was. Experimenting on criminals and orphans left the government open to widespread criticism. In some circles, that assessment continues to this day. Some maintain that the use of vaccines is an attempt by influential individuals to curtail or even eliminate the "undesirables" of society. Science is often neglected.

As crude and dangerous as it was, inoculation with the smallpox virus, or variolation as it came to be known, was the first formal attempt by humans to intervene in the natural course of an infectious disease. Using a less robust strain (we presume, but don't know for sure, they used variola minor) and an inoculation site different than the natural entry point, the disease was not eliminated but curtailed. It was the first documented effort in what has become one of the great marvels of human invention, vaccination.

As dramatic and lurid as the variolation work was in England, it was no less duplicated in the American colonies.

The infamous Salem witch trials occurred in 1692-93. Over 200 people were imprisoned. Twenty died; one was stoned to death, and 19 were hung by the neck until they were dead. The ugly event and its psychology are still topics of conversation today. (A reasonable explanation of the precipitating event, the delirium and seizures experienced by two teenage girls, may have been due to a fungus, *Claviceps purpurea*, which infects grains such as rye, leaving a residue of mind-altering toxins, one of which is known today as lysergic acid diethylamide, or LSD). One notable clergyman of the day who had a tangential part in the proceedings was a fascinating gentleman named Cotton Mather.

Mather wrote a letter to the court designed to alleviate the tension and paranoia of the time. He implored the court not to consider spectral evidence, that is, testimony about dreams and visions. The court ignored his advice, and the travesty continued. Some felt that his admonitions didn't go far enough; he should have been more forceful in denunciating the events. His reputation became tarnished. He needed to redeem it.

Cotton Mather was among the more interesting figures of the American colony days. He entered Harvard when he was only 12; he received his master's degree at 19. Early in life, he thought about pursuing a career in science but ended up in the ministry instead. But his interest in science and nature never waned. He was a frequent reader of the publications of the Royal Society of London and other scientific literature.

In 1721, His Majesty's Ship, the *Seahorse,* sailed into Boston Harbor. It had been chasing pirates in the Caribbean and had spent time in Barbados, a center of a smallpox outbreak. Thomas Durrell, an experienced seaman, commanded her. At the time, it was the duty of ships sailing into Boston harbor that were known to have frequented epidemic areas to make for a place called Spectacle Island, where it should remain in quarantine. (Such a place was known as a pest house). For some reason, Captain Durrell made for Castle Island, a military base. While docked there for repairs, several of the ship's crew were given shore leave. What in the world Captain Durrell was thinking is anyone's guess. They almost certainly were the source of the Boston smallpox outbreak which soon followed.

Cotton Mather had read of the occurrences in London using variolation. He also was familiar with the procedure from another account written in Turkey. Still another source was a family slave named Onesimus. Onesimus had informed Mather that while in Africa, he had "been given an operation, which had given him something of ye small-pox, and would forever preserve him from it." He showed Mather the scar. It made a believer out of him.

Just as Lady Mary Montagu and Princess Caroline met stern resistance to variolation in England, so did Cotton Mather in New England. He was convinced the procedure could prevent or mitigate a calamity, but proposing such a preposterous idea invited ridicule and contempt. He was not a medical doctor, and his contributions to the scientific community had been minimal. But Mather was convinced of his opinion, and he made a great pest of himself in seeking to convince the medical establishment of the worthiness of the procedure. He finally found a doctor intrigued by his idea just as the disease was beginning to progress out of control. His name was Zabdiel Boylston.

Physicians in New England in the early 1700s rarely had a formal college education. They learned their craft much like tradesmen through an apprenticeship. They lacked formal foundational education; the day-to-day application of medical practice was learned from a "master" physician. Given the level of medical technology of the time, they did all right. Boylston first learned from his father, a military physician who also practiced in rural Boston. After his father's death, he apprenticed to a leading surgeon in the Boston area. After beginning his practice, Boylston became one of the top physicians in Boston.

Boylston had two circumstances in his past that left him open to the idea of inoculation against smallpox. One was that his medical experience frequently exposed him to Native Americans and their remedies, which he found to be sometimes beneficial. The other was that he, like Lady Mary Montagu, had a horrific personal encounter with smallpox. He nearly died from it. Most people who were as sick from variola as he had been developed long-term sequelae, like organ failure or blindness. He miraculously had none. But the disease left mental scars, and he was open to anything that could prevent its ravages. His wife, Jerusha, had also been badly affected by the disease. At age nine, she lost both of her parents and three of her four brothers to the malady. After living with an uncle, two of her foster brothers also died of it. She also had come down with smallpox.

Boylston's description of the disease is one of the most poignant ever:

Purple spots, the bloody and parchment Pox, Hemorahages of Blood at the Mouth, Nose, Fundament, and Privities; Ravings and Deliriums; Convulsions and other Fits; violent inflammations and Swellings in the Eyes and Throat; so that they cannot see, or scarcely breathe, or swallow any thing, to keep them from starving. Some looking as black as the Stock, others as white as a Sheet; in some the Pock runs into Blisters, and the Skin stripping off, leaves the flesh raw....Some have a burning, others a smarting Pain, as if in the Fire, or scalded with boiling Water....Some have fill'd with loathsome Ulcers; others have had deep, and fistulous Ulcers in their Bodies, or in their Limbs or Joints, with Rottenness of the Ligaments and Bones: Some who live are Cripples, others Idiots, and many blind all their Days."

As in many dramas, Mather and Boylston had a formidable antagonist. William Douglass was a young, recently arrived physician from England. Born in Scotland, he was educated at some of Europe's top universities, and he let everyone know. Arrogant and outspoken, he disdained an equally arrogant and outspoken Cotton Mather and the minimally educated physicians of the area. Politically connected, he was a daunting foe.

The main character list of the time reads like something out of a dime novel: Cotton Mather, a fire and brimstone Puritan preacher best known for his involvement in the Salem witch trials; Zabdiel Boylston, a prominent local physician familiar with folk medicine who had a near-death experience with smallpox, and William Douglass, a brash, young, but knowledgeable physician. The drama that ensued did not disappoint.

In late June of 1721, Dr. Boylston took pus from several smallpox lesions of one of his patients and placed it into a vial. He then scratched the material onto the upper arms of three individuals: his slave Jack, Jack's two-year-old son Jackey, and his own son Thomas. We don't know if the strain was of the variola minor variety. Still, Boylston wrote that he used material from a discreet lesion, not malodorous (that is, not secondarily infected by bacteria). After about eight days, the two boys came down with a fever and several scars. The disease lasted two or three days, after which the boys resumed their everyday activities. Jack, the slave, had only a blister or two, indicating that he had probably had the disease previously.

The uproar was virulent. Boylston and Mather were accused of misconduct of a criminal nature. Dr. Douglass was most emphatic in seeing the procedure halted, suggesting that the act of giving smallpox in such a way was threatening patients' lives and spreading the disease. He enlisted the town's politicians, physicians, and newspapers to fight against Boylston

20

and Mather. (One of the journalists at the time was a 16-year-old apprentice, Benjamin Franklin).

The melodrama continued as Boylston continued to inoculate, and townsfolk presented themselves to receive the procedure, especially for their children. People were dying from naturally acquired smallpox much more than from the variolation procedure, and word of mouth was much in the procedure's favor. In the end, the conclusions were clear: variolation, while a crude, dangerous, and sometimes fatal technique, did, in fact, usually prevent most people from getting a much more virulent form of the disease. Even William Douglass, by 1730, had endorsed the method.

Zabdiel Boylston eventually was admitted to the Royal Society of London and traveled there to share his experience and statistics with variolation. His results, combined with those seen in England, allowed for the general acceptance of variolation, especially when an outbreak was not well contained and threatened mass devastation. It was humans' first bona fide attempt to alter the natural course of an infectious disease by using a strain of reduced virulence and altered route of administration. The characters, a British Lady of high breeding and strong personality, a Princess, a fire-breathing cleric, and a self-taught British colony physician, were certainly an odd lot. But they were on to something. For the next eighty years, variolation was used widely but selectively, primarily for protecting the military, the affluent, or the children of royal families.

Edward Jenner was born in England in May 1749, the son of a vicar. Orphaned at age five, he went to live with an older brother. At age eight, he was inoculated with smallpox in the county of his birth, Gloucestershire. He was one of the thousands of children variolated that year, as the procedure was considered the lesser of two evils.

Jenner was a very bright student, and at a young age, he developed an interest in science and nature. At thirteen, he began to serve as an apprentice to a country surgeon; then, at age 15, he apprenticed to a renowned physician named George Harwicke. At age 21, he went to London and studied under one of the eminent surgeons and biologists of the time, John Hunter. Jenner developed a strong bond with Hunter and was closely tied to him for the next two decades. He was well-connected.

Jenner's professional reputation came not so much from the practice of medicine but from his interest in nature. He came very close to accompanying Captain Cook on an exploratory mission. He worked in many areas, including comparative anatomy, species classification, geology, and ornithology. He even built a hot air balloon and sailed it some 13 miles. He also researched medical treatments and natural science, including studying human blood. He played the violin and wrote poetry. Edward Jenner was a true Renaissance man.

In 1773 Jenner returned to the area of his birth, Berkeley, to establish a medical practice. He was very professional, skillful, and quite popular with his patients, many of whom worked in agriculture. Berkeley was a leading dairy farming district of the time because of the favorable weather and verdant pastures, so many of his patients and acquaintances were involved with milk production. Of course, the cows had to be milked by hand, and many hands were required, both the farmers' families and professional milkmaids.

Being native to the area, Jenner had heard for some time that dairymaids who had contracted vesicular lesions on their hands after milking infected cows were rendered immune to smallpox. The locals were adamant in their belief in it. The naturally curious Jenner set about proving or disproving the theory. For years, he interviewed dozens of farmers and dairymaids to hear their tales of infection with cowpox and their experience when a smallpox epidemic came through the area. Jenner wrote about many of these case histories and submitted them to the Royal Society of London for consideration. Dairy cows are susceptible to diseases on their udders, including pyogenic organisms such as Staph and Strep. Dairy workers often referred to these diseases as "the pox," so care had to be taken to be sure the correct diagnosis was made. In what was referred to as "cowpox," a characteristic bluish-purple nodule appeared on the udder surrounded by a red, inflamed area. Cowpox today is a sporadic disease. It is not found on cows but instead on mice and voles. That may have been one way the disease spread from farm to farm.

Cowpox in a human is not a benign disease. The infected person has numerous painful pustules on their hands and forearms, which may spread to other body parts by touching. The infected person is quite ill for several days, with body aches, chills, and fever. But it's not nearly as bad as variola. Recovery is rapid, and the patient returns to good health in a few days.

When a smallpox outbreak occurred in May of 1796, Jenner decided to test the hypothesis that cowpox exposure prevents smallpox. A young dairymaid, Sarah Nelms, had draining cowpox lesions on her hands and forearms. He expressed some of the fluid from her lesions and collected it in a vial. Taking a needle, he scratched the material onto the skin of his gardener's eight-year-old son, James Phipps. He carefully observed the boy for two weeks, noting he became "indisposed" around the eighth day, with some pain in his armpit and a mild fever. In just a day or two, he was back to normal health.

Jenner was experienced with the variolation procedure, having administered it multiple times (he had been variolated at age eight). With an outbreak of smallpox in the community, he had no trouble finding a suitable variola lesion. About six weeks after the boy's cowpox inoculation, he applied the variola material to little James Phipps the same way the cowpox was administered. He was gratified that the boy did not react to the smallpox. He was completely immune. A new era of fighting disease had begun. (Because the infectious material came from a cow, Jenner called the procedure "vaccination," after the Latin word vacca, or "cow," and vaccinus, "from cows").

Using a pox virus from a cow to establish an immune state against smallpox was not unique to Edward Jenner. There is good evidence that a local Berkeley farmer, Benjamin Jesty, had performed the procedure on three of his family members some twenty years before Jenner. Seeing as they lived in the same area, it is reasonable to assume that Jenner had heard of it. Indeed, the act of contracting cowpox naturally and its rendering one immune to smallpox was common knowledge in the dairy community. But Jenner gets, and deserves, the credit. He wrote and published detailed descriptions of the cowpox lesions, the case histories of infected persons, and distinguished the pox lesions on cows from other cutaneous diseases. He also showed that the material from the cowpox vesicle on the arm could be used to inoculate other humans and that going back to a sick cow was unnecessary. He was doing good reproducible scientific research, writing about it, professionally sharing the knowledge, and giving an accurate description of obtaining the infectious material. This allowed for the wide dissemination of the procedure.

Of course, people don't get smallpox by having it scratched onto their skin; they breathe in the virus after being exposed to an ill individual. Jenner, and those who followed, had to wait and see that vaccinated people were immune to the natural disease. Their reckoning proved correct, and, though it took some time, variola was beginning its journey to extinction.

No medical procedure, including vaccination, is free of risks and side effects, particularly in early attempts. Vaccination is never 100% effective. Some vaccinated people will still get the disease, and a few individuals will react badly. But to those who knew smallpox firsthand, and the horror and devastation it brought, the risks were worth it.

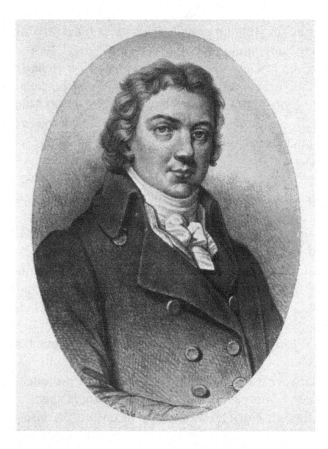

Despite an utter lack of knowledge of microbes or the immune system, Edward Jenner developed and reported on the successful inoculation of a mild virus to prevent the infection by a much more serious one, a procedure he called vaccination. (LOC)

Variola, the agent of smallpox, belongs to a family of viruses known as the Orthopoxviruses, or "true" pox viruses. In the virus world, they are enormous. While many viruses infecting humans have less than thirty genes, the pox viruses have nearly two hundred. Other viruses have single-stranded nucleic acid, either RNA or DNA. Variola is double-stranded DNA, the same as higher life forms. Other DNA viruses, such as Herpes and Varicella (the cause of chicken pox and shingles), replicate in the host cell's nucleus, but the pox viruses replicate in the cytoplasm. The RNA polymerase, which copies the DNA and forms messenger RNA, is very efficient and rarely makes an error in transcription, unlike RNA viruses. Therefore, the mutation rate for smallpox, while it exists, is relatively low. Pox viruses are not architecturally elegant; they look like a weathered old brick, somewhat rectangular with rounded ends. Because they are so large, the pox viruses can be seen with a well-made light microscope. They look like a little black dot inside a cell, but they are the only viruses that can be seen with a light microscope. All the others require an electron microscope.

Each pox virus, including variola, exists in two forms: the mature virion, or MV, and another known as the enveloped virion, or EV. The name is a bit misleading since the mature virion is encased in an envelope. It just so happens that the enveloped virion has two envelopes. The MV are pretty tough little creatures; their role is to exist outside the host animal and infect a new host. The EVs, on the other hand, are somewhat fragile, and their role is to infect other cells inside the same host. So, when we catch smallpox from another person, we get the virus's MV form. When the virus spreads within our body, we see the effects of the EV form.

Many viruses have but one attachment protein for host cell surfaces. Not so the pox viruses. Variola has at least a dozen. They all work harmoniously to ensure the virus enters the host cell. For some of the pox viruses, it also means that the virus has a wide range of host cells available to it, from mammals to insects. This doesn't apply to variola, however, as it has mutated to such a degree that it can, as far as we know, only enter human cells. This poses a problem that has long puzzled investigators of smallpox: where did the virus go between epidemics? The people it infects will all be either dead or immune. There is no carrier state. But the virus must reside somewhere between outbreaks. Now that the virus is extinct in nature, it is a riddle that will perhaps never be solved.

When the variola mature virion is packaged up and ready to leave the cell, it is excreted and moves freely away, as most viruses do. This usually happens when the host cell breaks down. On the other hand, the enveloped virion has a loose chemical bond with the surface of the cell that produced it. After it is made, it travels up a set of actin proteins to the cell surface, kind of like a train moving on a track. Once it reaches the surface, it forms a bond with the cell's membrane. Since the bond has a moderate avidity, some enveloped virions escape, and others remain attached. Those that escape spread throughout the body to infect other cells. Those that remain attached can adhere to neighboring cells, and the two host cells are made to combine. Such a cell combination is called a syncytium (from the Greek, *syn,* meaning "together," and "cyt" from the Greek *kyto*, meaning container or vessel, usually referred to as a cell). The syncytium is a large mass of cytoplasm with multiple nuclei because it comprises fused cells. They are characteristic of the skin lesions of smallpox. By staying attached to the membranes of cells and quickly being once again incorporated into the giant cell, the virus can avoid antibodies and some of the immune cells.

After a virus enters a cell, for it to be successful, it must accomplish several things:

It must take over the host cell's protein-making apparatus. In other words, assume control of the ribosomes, primarily in the rough endoplasmic reticulum. This usually means eliminating or significantly curtailing the host cell's ability to make its own proteins.

It must, at least for a short time, greatly diminish the host cell's ability to chemically stimulate the immune system, primarily the innate system. The production of cytokines, such as interferons and various members of the interleukin group, must be sharply reduced.

Finally, the virus must prevent the host cell from dying, either by the process of apoptosis (self-destruction) or by notifying members of the immune cell network to take it out.

The successful virus must be good at each of these tasks. Variola virus is among the best in the business.

Variola virus enters us mainly by way of saliva. Someone with the virus coughs on a susceptible person, and the virus enters and attaches itself to the receptors in the nose and throat cells. After entering the cell, the virus is very active, but the patient has no symptoms whatsoever. For about 12 days, the patient is in the incubation phase of the disease.

After completing its reproduction cycle in the respiratory cells, the virus starts to emerge. The encapsulated variety makes its way primarily into the circulation and is carried around the body to attach to different types of cells, mainly those of the liver and spleen. After reproducing there and creating a very large number of virions, the virus again enters the blood and many wind up in the cells of the skin. Why they gravitate to the skin is not known, but there must be a receptor that is amenable to it, and the virus prefers to grow at a temperature a little less than body temperature, obviously accommodated in the skin. Within the skin cells, it reproduces and spreads mainly from cell to cell, with the enveloped forms creating syncytia.

While the virus is very good at suppressing the body's immune response in the early stages, there is a limit to what it can do. With massive amounts of virus circulating around the body, the chemical alarm bells finally go off. And they go off in a grand way. It is not the mere presence of the virus that makes us sick. It is the immune response the body generates to combat the intruder that gives us our symptoms. With so much virus present, the release of cytokines is overwhelming.

After the incubation period, most patients have two to three days of prodromal illness. (The word prodromal comes from the Greek word *prodromas*, meaning "precursor"). The symptoms are non-specific, such as slight fever, headache, and muscle aches. Following that, all hell breaks loose. The virus has entered the skin tissues, and the immune system releases enormous quantities of cytokines, activating many white blood cells of various types.

Clinically, there are four general types of smallpox. About 90% of smallpox cases are called the "ordinary" variety. The patient has a high fever, prostration, and a severe skin rash. The extent of the rash in ordinary smallpox is quite variable: some have a discrete rash, that is, the individual pustules do not connect with one another, while others have a confluent rash. The mortality rate correlates with the extent of the rash. With an "ordinary discrete" rash, the mortality rate is less than 10%. If the rash is "ordinary confluent," the mortality rate exceeds 50%.

In about 5% of smallpox cases, the patient develops what is known as "flat" smallpox. It was more common in children. As the name suggests, the lesions are not raised but low and spreading, barely above the skin's surface. Patients with flat smallpox were extremely ill, and the death rate was well over 50%.

The rarest form of smallpox, seen in less than one percent of patients, was the most lethal. In hemorrhagic disease, patients bled profusely into the skin and mucus membranes and suffered terribly. Death was inevitable.

All four types of smallpox, ordinary discreet, ordinary confluent, flat, and hemorrhagic, were seen in single outbreaks, indicating the same viral strain infected each victim. The different disease presentation, therefore, is almost certainly due to differences in the innate immune reaction of each patient. Some of us might have a more robust means of inducing cell apoptosis. Others may have cells with a stronger signal to natural killer lymphocytes. Or something else. All our proteins are made at the direction of our DNA, which is subject to mutation, either in ourselves or in that which we received from our parents and ancestors. Just like we have unique physical characteristics, we have unique intracellular protein differences to a certain extent. Subtle as they may be, they can profoundly affect the reaction to a microbial intruder.

Smallpox is now extinct in nature, and a big reason for that was the use of the smallpox vaccine. It's a bit ironic, really, because the smallpox vaccine, a live preparation of the virus vaccinia, is, far and away, the worst vaccine that we have in our arsenal. Being a live unattenuated virus scratched into the upper arm, it causes an infection. It is usually mild but an infection, nonetheless. Most people who receive a smallpox vaccination develop a noticeable scar at the inoculation site. A benefit of placing the vaccine virus on the skin's surface is that it can be observed if the vaccine infection took place or "took." If not, the vaccination could be reapplied. With other vaccines, we cannot easily know if the vaccination was successful. Still, a live virus deliberately scratched into the skin is a bit risky.

The original viral agent used by Jenner and others in the Berkeley farmlands was called cowpox for the obvious reason that it was harvested from the udders of infected cows. But the virus itself does not exclusively infect cows; it is, in nature, a pathogen of rodents. Cowpox seems to get into cows by mistake, as it can infect a wide variety of animals. The pox viruses are endowed with many surface attachment proteins and can enter not just multiple cell types but multiple animals. Interestingly, the virus used currently to immunize against smallpox is not cowpox at all, but rather one we refer to as vaccinia.

Just where vaccinia originated is not known. It's not cowpox. So desperate was humanity for a better smallpox preventative measure than variolation, it didn't take long for the use of cowpox in the place of variola to take root. Jenner and others showed conclusively that the cowpox virus, once applied to the skin of a susceptible human, could induce a relatively minor disease. The material from that infection could be taken and injected into another person and achieve the same result, person to person; the material didn't have to come from another cow. An entire industry of inoculation sprang up in a relatively short time. In those days, of course, there was no pharmaceutical industry, no such thing as lyophilization (freeze-drying viruses whereby they could be reconstituted and remain viable), and no Food and Drug Administration to oversee the safety of the entire affair. It was very much an open market. Some practitioners were conscientious, trained professionals, while others were, well, less so. Accidents, and tragedies, ensued. The cowpox virus could not be stored and used whenever necessary. It had to be kept viable, and the only way to do that was to keep passing it from susceptible person to susceptible person.

One of the first recorded international issuances of the smallpox vaccine was by the Spanish in 1803. They commissioned a large-scale program of vaccination in South America. To get the virus there from Spain, they enlisted 22 pre-adolescent boys to voyage on a Spanish ship to the New World. The venture was called the Royal Expedition of the Vaccine, and it was ordered by King Carlos IV. Each week during the trip, two boys were inoculated with cowpox. The material from the vesicular lesions of at least one of the boys was used to inoculate another two. (Two were used because sometimes the vaccine doesn't "take," that is, the inoculated person doesn't develop the characteristic skin lesion and disease). That was the only way in those days to keep the virus alive during the trip to the Americas. After reaching the northern part of South America, teams of vaccinators split up, one group heading south and the other north into Central America and Mexico. After reaching the west coast of Mexico, the virus was transported in a similar way to Manila, the Philippines, and then into China. It was the world's first mass vaccination campaign. Jenner wrote, "I don't imagine the annals of history furnish an example of philanthropy so noble, so extensive as this."

Cowpox is not a benign disease. You get sick from it. Not as ill as from smallpox, but sick nonetheless. The skin lesion begins several days after inoculation, and about eight days into the infection, the inoculated person becomes quite ill with fever, chills, and significant muscle aches. Jenner described it as being "indisposed for two or three days." It's clearly not as severe as smallpox, but overt illness is induced. Over the years, as the practice spread, other pox viruses were apparently tried and found effective. Some speculate that horse pox, instead of cowpox, was used. Somehow, and we don't know just how, a pox virus was used in vaccination that made the patient less ill. One theory has it that a horse pox virus was used early in conjunction with cowpox, producing less illness in recipients. After repeated passages through humans and animals to keep it viable, it attenuated to the extent that it was even less invasive. People would naturally select the less invasive strain and continue to do so until the current vaccinia strain emerged. Perhaps it arose from the constant merging of two or more pox viruses during vaccination. Wherever it came from, that was the one selected for general use. The name **Vaccinia** was assigned to the virus used to administer smallpox vaccination.

Interestingly, there is not just one but several vaccinia viruses available. They reside in different jurisdictions, including the U.S.A., Europe, and Russia. Each has its own characteristics and history, but all are equally effective. They all cause a minor, localized skin infection, usually without the chills, fever, and muscle aches of cowpox. They all confer long-lasting immunity to smallpox. While vaccinia is less virulent than the original vaccine strain, it is not without risks. A healthy, immunocompetent individual, child or adult, can get the virus inoculated on their arm and expect nothing more than a mild skin infection with a slightly draining vesicle at the inoculation site. But it is a live virus, and occasional complications are inevitable. If given to a person with a defect in their immune system, the virus can cause severe complications. Therefore, it should not be given to people who are immunocompromised or pregnant, or live with someone who is. It should not be given to alcoholics, people with heart conditions, or other serious illnesses. It's interesting to speculate whether the American Food and Drug Administration would even approve such a vaccine today, given its potential side effects. When compared to the ravages of smallpox, of course, the potential side effects of vaccinia are slight. For the most part, the people of the early 19th century had no hesitation in adopting Jenner's replacement for variolation. Desperate times call for desperate measures. But, if, God forbid, smallpox vaccination is needed again, a better vaccine must be developed.

There may be one. Shortly before smallpox had gone extinct, a potentially better vaccine was developed. The modified vaccinia virus Ankara, or MVA, was made by passing a strain of vaccinia obtained from Turkey through tissue culture cells over 500 times. The result is a virus that can infect a host cell but cannot complete its replication cycle. It can, however, produce most of the proteins that the immune system will develop immune cells to combat, both T-cell and the B-cell lines. Because smallpox was extinct by the time it became available, there is no way to know if it does indeed confer immunity to the natural form of smallpox. But it does look promising.

Modern technology has given researchers the ability to manipulate the DNA sequences of viruses. Given the proper equipment, whole segments of viral genomes can be deleted, or foreign genes that code for specific proteins can be introduced. The technique is used to produce vaccines for infections such as

Ebola and Covid-19. Using material from frozen victims in the Arctic, the entire genome of the influenza virus that caused the 1918-19 epidemic has been produced, and the virus has been brought back to life.

While scientists' ability to mix, match, and recombine genes to create a preventative cure for a disease is laudable, there is a dark side. Variola is now extinct in nature, meaning nearly every living human being is susceptible to it. Many pox viruses still exist among a wide variety of animal species, and they are very much genomically related to variola. The typical pox virus has about 200 genes. The RNA polymerase that copies the viral DNA is very good; it rarely makes mistakes, so the genome is highly conserved. So, the genes of the pox viruses strongly resemble each other. The main differences are in the dozen or so genes at each end. It is now technically feasible to take a pox virus, for instance, camelpox, strip off a dozen genes at either end, and attach to the remaining core a series of nucleotide base pairs identical to the known sequence of variola. The newly created variola virus can be made in bulk by passing it through appropriate cells in tissue culture. This procedure would be quite easily accomplished, given the proper equipment and trained personnel. It would be less difficult than creating a miniaturized nuclear device to sit on the head of an intercontinental ballistic missile.

The consequences of releasing variola as a biological weapon would be enormous. Travel is now imminently more robust than it was when smallpox was in its heyday, and the spread of the virus would be virtually uncontrollable. Vaccine production could be ramped up, but many would become very ill and die before it could be effectively distributed. The currently available vaccine, vaccinia virus, applied in the viable form to the skin of the upper arm, is not without risks, and many people are vulnerable because of an underlying medical condition. They would become ill from the circulation of the live vaccine virus. The consequences resulting from the deliberate release of variola are incalculable.

Chapter 4
Chemical Warfare

Elusive Potion
For myriad maladies:
The quest for a cure

For thousands of years, mankind has sought substances that would cure diseases, including those that are infectious. Some were quite effective. The Egyptians left records of a poultice they used for treating wounds. It consisted of grease from animal fat, honey, and bits of linen. Honey has antimicrobial properties, and the fat helped keep bandages from adhering to the wound. Linen was a "sponge" to remove some of the dead tissue and pus from the area.

The sap of the balsam tree, which grows in the Middle East, was found to have anti-infectious properties. Applied to wounds, it can help prevent infection and promote wound healing. It is the root of the word "balm."

There were many others. By far, though, the most popular and enduring was a potion attributed to a Hellenistic king, Mithridates VI, who ruled the area of Pontus on the south Black Sea around the year 120 BCE. He was looking for something to help treat poisonous snake bites, and he created a potion containing lots of herbs and somewhat toxic plants, including opium, cinnamon, myrrh, and castor. It also included the flesh of venomous reptiles. Some ingredients, like hemlock, were dangerous, but they were used in diluted form, much in keeping with the Greek theory that "if it doesn't kill me, it makes me stronger." After experimentation on prisoners, he took what seemed to work and blended it into a concoction initially called *mithridatium*, named after its inventor. It later became known as theriac, from the Latin "theriaca," or antidote to poison. (From the Latin *therapia,* we get the word "therapy").

Amazingly, theriac sometimes seemed to work. Distinguishing actual therapeutic benefits from the placebo effect is difficult, especially several hundred years after the fact. Who knows which of its many ingredients was effective, as it took the "shotgun" approach: throw a bunch of stuff against the wall and hope that some of it will stick.

The Greeks, of course, were very influential. (It is often said that the success of Rome was founded on Greek philosophy). The reputation of theriac spread far and wide. And just like a story that goes around and changes slightly with each telling until it is altered substantially, so did the formulation of theriac change by location and time. Some recipes called for as many as 100 ingredients, some half that. Making it was a big deal, with whole communities involved in a festival atmosphere. Theriac was the absolute go-to drug for nearly 2,000 years. Today, very few people have ever heard of it.

Even theriac, though, was ineffective against the ravages of many infectious diseases that battered humanity over the ages: smallpox, bubonic plague, influenza, malaria, typhoid, typhus, dysentery, tuberculosis, and many others were unaffected by this complex concoction. Much more was needed.

The first bona fide drug used to treat a specific infectious disease has an amazing history. Its story is one of exploration, treachery, science, and exploitation. Drugs today can be developed, tested, and marketed in a few years. This one took centuries. But it was the first formulated pharmaceutical that was specific and effective for a severe infectious disease. Its name was quinine, and the disease was malaria.

The Quechua people were inhabitants of the highlands of the Andes in Peru, parts of Bolivia, and extending up into Ecuador. Theirs was an agrarian culture; they lived close to the land. An herbal remedy they were devoted to was the bark of a tree that populated the forested area where they lived, one they called Quina Quina. (The name comes to us from the Spanish, who probably put their mark on it. To the Quechua, it meant "holy bark"). For a long time, they used the tree bark to treat quite a few maladies, primarily the chills we experience when beginning a fever. It helped reduce the fever and shorten the time of illness.

The Spanish entered the area we now call Peru in the early 1530s and established settlements there. The disease we know as malaria did not exist in the Americas before the presence of the Europeans, but it became prevalent shortly after their arrival. Certainly, there were severe local infections, but the introduction of infectious organisms from Europe and Africa created a whole new array of maladies. The Quechua people used their tree bark remedy to help with the infections.

Most likely, some Spanish settlers were introduced to the holy bark tree, but it took the cure of a ruling-class woman to popularize it in Europe. The viceroy's wife in Peru was a Spanish countess named Anna del Cinchon. While in Peru, she came down with a case of what might have been malaria. The local Indians suggested she bathe in a pond near her home beneath a Quina Quina tree and drink some bitter water from the tree bark. Her fevers ended in a few days, and she was cured. Whether this story is true or merely apocryphal, it carried weight. The tree was named after her. The scientific name of the tree assigned by Carl Linnaeus is *Cinchona*.

It became apparent to the Spanish that this local tree bark effectively reduced malaria symptoms. Some of the bark was brought back to Europe and tried there. Jesuit missionaries did most of the first transport and application, so the colloquial term became "Jesuit bark." Later it came to be called quinine. It found some usefulness in southern Europe, Spain, and Italy in the early days, but there were problems. There are around two dozen species of cinchona trees, and they don't all produce the same amount of active ingredient. Different growth conditions, such as soil, rain levels, and elevation, can alter the tree's underlying chemistry. Fraud and deception were inevitable with how it was brought back by sailors and tradesmen seeking profit. Also, the active ingredient is an alkaloid, which doesn't dissolve very well in water. Mixing in a bit of alcohol in the right amounts helps. So, some batches worked quite satisfactorily with malaria patients, others not as well, and some not at all. Add to that the problem of accurately identifying a genuine malaria case without laboratory equipment and confusion reigned.

The big "breakthrough" for quinine, if that's the right word, came in England in the 1670s. King Charles II suffered tremendously from what was most likely malaria. Court physicians tried in vain to alleviate his symptoms. In near desperation, the king called upon a Mr. Robert Talbor, who was said to have a "miraculous cure for the ague," as malaria was called at that time. Talbor's secret recipe worked almost miraculously, and the king recovered his health. A little later, in 1679, the son of the king of France, Louis XIV, contracted the disease. Talbor cured him too. It was later revealed that Talbor's formula was rose leaves, lemon juice, ground-up cinchona, and wine. The alcohol in the wine helped dissolve the active ingredient. With the cure of these two high-ranking individuals, the cinchona bark gained respectability and was widely recognized.

The reputation of the bark grew. Here, for the first time in history, was a substance that, when taken orally, could cure or reduce the symptoms of a severe infectious disease. While valuable in treating individual cases, quinine assumed an immense role in world affairs. The Industrial Revolution demanded a supply of natural resources, many of which came from malaria-infested areas. Quinine helped ensure that the workers in these areas were more productive. Infected individuals and their employers were willing to pay large sums for the antidote. Scientists of the time were interested in studying the tree and its bark, and it was planted in different areas of the world. The cinchona bark became more valuable than gold, and it literally grew on trees.

Quinine is an alkaloid that works in several ways, but its activity against the *Plasmodium* species that cause malaria was fortuitous. Malaria didn't exist in the New World when the Quechua people started using their tree bark. They used the bark to control fever and the chills accompanying it. For them, it was non-specific, just like we might take an aspirin tablet to reduce a fever. (Aspirin is also derived from a chemical found in the bark of a tree. Salicin, from which aspirin is derived, is found in the bark of the white willow tree). But it just so happens that quinine interferes with the malarial parasite's ability to digest hemoglobin. Even though the bugs sit in the middle of a red blood cell filled with the stuff, they essentially starve to death. It works best on *Plasmodium falciparum,* the most virulent species of malaria. But it is not 100% effective, depending on the malarial species and stage of the disease. Still, its introduction to medicine was monumental: an oral medication that could effectively treat an infectious disease.

(Quinine is still helpful today. The World Health Organization lists it as the number one choice for treating severe malaria in adults, and all types of malaria in young children and pregnant women. Also, quinine water, the "tonic" in the British beverage gin and tonic, is still going strong).

The half-century from 1890 to 1940 had to be most frustrating for doctors and other healthcare workers. By the late 1880s, the nature of infectious diseases was emerging: microbial organisms acquired from various sources were the cause. By the turn of the century, it was often possible to accurately identify the microbe causing a disease, along with a logical prognosis. It was becoming more common to isolate the offending organism in the laboratory and study its characteristics. The little creatures were given names, classified, and discussed at length in scientific papers. Most were easily seen under the microscope, and many chemical agents could destroy them in the laboratory. But successful treatment for many serious infectious diseases was elusive. The drugs and poisons used to kill microbes also greatly damaged the patient. Many formulations were tried, but nothing gave a satisfactory result. It was a bitter pill to swallow.

Pharmaceutical companies are major industries today. They even have their own nickname, "big pharma." But it wasn't always that way. What we recognize as a pharmaceutical company existed only in an embryonic form less than a hundred years ago; they were fledgling chemical companies, mostly turning out inorganic substances, usually for a particular industry. The infrastructure for developing pharmaceuticals did not lie with huge companies. It was up to small, independent firms to develop new technology.

One potentially lucrative area of investigation and marketing was the dye industry. Dyes for textiles have been around for thousands of years. In the early 1800s, they were all derived from natural substances–indigo is a pigment of a deep blue color derived from a plant native to India, yellow is found in several flowering plants, and a deep purple dye is derived from an invertebrate called Murex, a mollusk found in the eastern Mediterranean Sea. (Thousands of the mollusks must be ground up to produce the dye; because of its expense, purple became the color of royalty).

Because of the relative rarity and need to transport natural dyes, several European workers sought to produce synthetic dyes. Sometimes, major breakthroughs come from the strangest places. An 18-year-old English student named William Henry Perkin learned in his chemistry class at school that quinine came only from trees. It would be revolutionary if someone could make quinine synthetically in a laboratory and then in a factory. The British military, diplomats, industrialists, and workers in malarial-infested areas of the world would be more easily protected, and great progress could be made. On his Easter vacation in 1856, the young Perkin set about finding a way to produce synthetic quinine in a crude laboratory he set up in his apartment. He didn't find it. But what he found instead began a whole new industry. He somehow produced an aniline compound that stained fabrics a bluish purple. Perkin called the color mauveine. Most today would call it mauve or violet. It stunned the world. For the first time, fabrics could be stained with a substance created entirely in a factory. Queen Victoria put her seal of approval on it by wearing several garments dyed with the stuff. Perkin went on to develop other dyes and became a wealthy man. The wheels had been set in motion: producing and applying aniline dyes became commonplace.

Aniline is a simple organic compound, a single benzene ring with one amino group. It is pretty reactive, as the formulation of so many dyes illustrates. The dye industry took off and became very important after Perkin's work. Importantly, it was subsequently discovered that aniline dyes had another beneficial application: the staining of living tissue.

Different materials can be stained with select aniline dyes; some can stain living materials. These discoveries were made mainly by German chemists working in the 1880s. We still use many of the same formulations discovered and applied back then. Every clinical laboratory in the world uses aniline dyes for diagnostic work: looking at blood cells in the hematology lab, tissue sections in pathology, and examining bacteria and other microbes in the microbiology lab. Two aniline stains discovered in the 1880s in Robert Koch's lab remain standard practice today, the Gram stain for bacteria and the acid-fast stain for tuberculosis.

The acid-fast stain was discovered by a brilliant and gifted researcher, German physician Paul Ehrlich. While Ziehl and Neelsen modified his original method, the principle he established was elegant. A physician by training, he became a knowledgeable chemist and combined his various talents to become one of the pioneers of modern medicine.

The growth of the dye industry meant enormous profits for some of the biggest chemical companies of the time. That meant funds became available for basic research, which was rare in the past.

A theory proposed by several researchers in the late 1800s made a lot of sense: If aniline dyes could enter and stain bacteria, perhaps one could attach a poison to the molecule that was harmful to the bacteria or parasite. Aniline could then serve as a "Trojan Horse" to bring the poison in concentrated form into the bacteria and kill it.

Of course, this would take a lot of money to pay researchers and buy lab equipment, and there was no guarantee of success. It was a "shotgun" approach: take as many noxious chemicals as possible, attach them to aniline, and see which, if any, worked. It would be long, laborious work without any real guide for making the right choices. But there was much to be gained if successful. Paul Ehrlich was at the center of the operations.

There were a lot of infectious diseases afflicting people at the time, but the one Ehrlich and his colleagues were concentrating on was syphilis. Historically, there had been some success in treating the disease, most notably using heavy metals like arsenic and mercury. This, of course, was dangerous, but if one could concentrate the poison onto a carrier molecule, then perhaps its full strength could be directed at the microbe and less of it toward the patient. At least theoretically.

Syphilis was a disease of immense devastation and significance for hundreds of years. The disease typically exhibits three clinical stages, primary, secondary, and tertiary.

The primary is a sore, called a chancre, on the genitalia. It is usually considered soft, unlike the hardened skin we associate with a callous. The secondary stage is a body rash that appears about six weeks after the chancre. The rash can vary from barely noticeable to obvious. The third stage is devastating. The organism invades the body's tissues and causes irreparable harm, with cardiovascular and neurologic sequelae that significantly impact the quality of life until a fatal outcome. Not all cases progress to the tertiary stage, but the disease is horrific when it does.

Not all patients with syphilis react the same way. The symptoms, particularly those in the late stages, are variable. The disease rightfully gained the monikers "The great imposter" and "The great imitator" because the symptoms can mimic those of other conditions. In 1906 bacteriologist August Paul von Wassermann developed a diagnostic test for syphilis. It had many false positives but was still very helpful in establishing a diagnosis. Tests at the time indicated that around 8% of the population of large cities had at some time contracted syphilis. Not all develop severe late-stage deterioration, but the quality of life for many can be significantly altered. It's interesting to note that the Wassermann test uses the fixation of complement in the reaction. Paul Ehrlich was one of the original scientists to describe the complement system.

Various therapies and palliative treatments have been tried over the centuries for treating patients with syphilis. Two that survived the test of time were using heavy metals like mercury, antimony, and arsenic, and heating the patient to very high temperatures. Sometimes both were used. So desperate were some to treat syphilis that doctors resorted to deliberately giving patients malaria, knowing that it raised the patient's body temperature enough to possibly rid the patient of syphilis.

One popular chemical remedy was a preparation that used a salt of arsenic. This was a dangerous deal. In the early 1860s, a French biologist and physician made a modified arsenic salt that he hooked onto aniline. He claimed it was about 50 times less toxic than unattached arsenic since it was an organic compound. Optimistically, he called it "atoxyl," the "a-"

meaning without or lessened, the "toxyl" part from the word toxic. It was used sporadically for the next 40 years.

As European countries entered the frontiers of Africa in the latter half of the 19th and early 20th centuries, tropical diseases presented a significant problem. Malaria could be treated with some success using quinine, but another terrible disease, African sleeping sickness, was a far more severe matter. The name "sleeping sickness" suggests a relatively mild, annoying disorder, but the disease is usually fatal. If not deadly, it is excessively debilitating. It is a parasitic disease caused by the blood parasite *Trypanosoma brucei,* and the bite of the tsetse fly spreads it. It was fortuitously discovered in the early 20th century that atoxyl, the arsenical compound, could successfully treat African sleeping sickness, at least when it is used in its early stages. Side effects, including blindness, were significant, but its success provoked interest in European research circles. At first, Ehrlich showed little interest, but as time passed, he became curious. His knowledge of chemistry helped him develop a vast number of formulations using a combination of aniline and arsenic compounds. He was determined to find one to treat African sleeping sickness safely, but he found the first chemical antibacterial agent instead. The stuff worked against syphilis, of all things.

The new compound was called arsphenamine, the "ars" from arsenic, the "phen" from the phenol ring it contained, and the "amine" from the chemical group attached to aniline. Arsphenamine is kind of hard to say, so the trade name Salvarsan came to be. The drug wasn't, by any stretch, perfect. The medicine was unstable when it contacted air, so it had to be kept in tightly sealed containers. The administration was cumbersome, and there were significant side effects. If the drug Salvarsan was invented today, it's doubtful the Food and Drug Administration would approve it. But in its day, it was something to behold. One year after its release, Salvarsan became the most prescribed drug in the world.

It's strange, if not downright bizarre that the first antimicrobial agent would be helpful against *Treponema pallidum,* the bacterium that causes syphilis. The organism cannot be grown in an artificial culture like most pathogens, and it's impossible to do any *in vitro* testing. Another strange fact is that, among bacteria, arsphenamine only works against this one organism. The word serendipity reportedly comes from the Persian fairy tale "The Three Princes of Serendip," in which the heroes keep finding things they weren't aware of. It certainly applies to the discovery of Salvarsan. Sometimes it's better to be lucky than good.

The discovery of a chemical agent effective against an infectious disease, as crude as it was, should have paved the way for similar findings. It might have moved faster, save for one obstacle: World War I. Most of the work in research was done by physicians, and the onset of war and the exigency of the situation demanded that all available devote their time to matters at hand, regardless of their specialty in civilian life. Also, the financial resources needed for research and research facilities dried up. All European countries were affected, and research on anti-microbial agents ground to a halt.

Surgical techniques had advanced significantly in the two decades preceding WWI. Anesthetics were widely available, and medical schools turned out many qualified surgeons. Very often, especially with war wounds, patients got post-operative infections. Wounds were cleaned, debrided, and properly bandaged, but infections are inevitable without antibiotics. War, especially trench warfare so common in WWI, is also a predisposing factor in communicable diseases. The horrible 1918-1919 influenza pandemic spread rapidly among troops confined to close quarters for long periods. Many other infectious diseases are readily spread because of living conditions during a war. Not having antibiotics when one knew the cause of the illness was exasperating.

Paul Ehrlich accomplished many things, and it's hard to state his greatest achievement. He was involved with formulating and applying aniline dyes that made diagnosis much more accurate. He headed the team that developed the first successful antimicrobial agent, Salvarsan. He produced numerous scientific research papers on chemistry and medicine.

But perhaps his most outstanding contribution to mankind was his work illuminating the immune system.

For centuries people have known that with some diseases, immunity is developed by nearly all members of the population after one has been infected. Smallpox was a good example, but there were others like measles, chicken pox, and bubonic plague. It was "one and done." Ehrlich appreciated that something in the body produced this immunity, and he sought answers. One factor he helped discover and wrote about was complement, an essential contributor to immunity. He was also very aware of antibodies and the acquired immune system. His, and of course, others, research into the immune system helped pave the way for the use of a form of antimicrobial therapy used for a quarter of a century. Some of the treatments are still used today. It's called passive immunity.

Many movies from the 1930s with a medical theme often referred to serum as if it were a magic potion. One of two scenarios played out: either the brilliant scientists were trying to perfect a "serum" to relieve mankind of some horrible affliction, or there was a heroic rush to get the precious "serum" to a sick patient to save their life. Drama always surrounded the attempts. It probably never occurred to many moviegoers to enquire as to what the "serum" was. They just believed it was good for you when things were looking grim.

The word serum is Latin. It means "watery fluid." It makes sense since serum is the fluid portion of blood obtained when blood clots. Many chemical substances are found in serum, but the ones that stirred much interest in the early 20th century were antibodies to organisms or toxins responsible for the symptoms of infectious diseases. Antibodies are the critical components of passive immunity. When born, antibodies from our mother cross the placenta and enter the baby's circulation, helping protect the vulnerable infant from infections and toxins for the first six to twelve months of life. Several workers in the early 1890s, including Emil Adolf von Behring, Ehrlich, and visiting Japanese scientist Kitasato Shibasaburo, collaborated on producing serum that contained antibodies to the toxin produced by *Corynebacterium diphtheriae*. Diphtheria at that time, and for centuries beforehand, was a scourge for all people.

Nicknamed "The Strangler," the toxin produced by the bacteria induces the production of a thick, mucus-fibrin mass called a pseudo-membrane that blocks the airway. Mortality can reach up to 20%. It had been noted for some time that if a person, usually a child, contracted but survived diphtheria, they remained immune. This prompted the theory that something in the blood protected the individual. Perhaps, it was thought, the serum of a person who recovered from the disease could be administered to another, thereby saving them. In many cases, it worked. von Behring became the first recipient of the Nobel Prize in medicine for the discovery.

Serum containing antibodies to diphtheria toxin does not, however, protect indefinitely. Also, the person afflicted who donates the serum must have recovered from the disease relatively recently, while the antibody level is still high. The serum must have been obtained more than three weeks following the onset of the illness so that a high enough level of the right antibody has been produced. All of this was discovered over time, mainly through trial and error. Passive immunity isn't perfect, but it is much better than nothing.

We still use passive immunity today. Virtually all antidotes to bites by poisonous reptiles use antibodies produced after venom is injected into animals, usually horses. In several infectious diseases, most notably hepatitis A and B, it is recommended to administer so-called hyper-immune gamma globulin, e.g., passive immunity, to mitigate the disease progression.

Because of the paucity of success in the search for anti-microbial agents versus the limited but better success resulting from the administration of immune serum, the use of the serum for treating recently infected patients became the trend in research and applied medicine in the first quarter of the 20th century. The treatment hit its high point in a well-publicized case in Alaska in 1925. It was the stuff of movies and dime adventure novels.

In the winter of 1925, there was a severe diphtheria outbreak in Nome, Alaska. Nome, once one of the most populated cities in the territory of Alaska, is located on the Bering Sea. Because of fierce winter storms in the area, sea travel to the city was out of the question. The only way to get the afflicted the life-saving serum containing high levels of diphtheria antibody was by dog sled through the harsh conditions. Alaska at the time had a system of dog sleds set up like the Pony Express, with a relay-type operation. Each musher would typically go about twenty miles, pass off the mail, or in this case serum, to the next individual at the appointed location. Conditions at the time were unimaginably harsh: Temperatures as low as -80°; snow drifts twenty feet high or more; winds up to 60 knots. But the intrepid mushers made it through, and in a short time, the epidemic abated. It was the stuff of legend. Hollywood noticed.

In the eyes of the media and Hollywood, the hero of the magnificent undertaking weren't the men who courageously risked their lives to get through. It was a dog. The lead sled dog on the last leg into Nome was a feisty pooch named Balto. Balto's name and image were plastered across every newspaper and newsreel in the country. A bronze statue of him was erected in Central Park, New York City. The message accompanying the news was that the "serum" was delivered, and it saved lives. It made a believer out of many people about the miraculous abilities of "serum." (It's interesting to note that the true dog hero, according to the owner of both dogs, wasn't Balto, but another dog named Togo. At age twelve, Togo led the most extended leg of the relay, over 200 miles. But when the media hype gets a full head of steam, it's hard to set it right).

The two broad approaches for treating infectious diseases, one using chemicals to poison the invading microbe directly, the other using the body's natural defense systems to accomplish the job, were much discussed and tried during the first thirty years of the 20th century. Both had some limited success, but progress for both was painfully slow. Salvarsan's updated version of Neosalvarsan used arsenic and was helpful against only a single infection, syphilis. Side effects were often severe. No other formulations seemed promising. The use of passive immunity had more success. Still, by its nature, it could only be used against a specific disease, and the shelf-life of the donated serum was limited, especially when refrigeration was unavailable. The use of passive immunity and perhaps other ways of enlisting the immune system was the path that most researchers considered the most promising. Using chemicals seemed to most a dead end.

One corporation that hadn't abandoned the idea of a chemical attack against bacteria was the giant German chemical company I. G. Farben. It was one of the largest corporations in the world, with a broad range of interests, including medicine. There was a theory in the late 1920s that the way to find a chemical that would kill bacteria and not harm the patient was to investigate them in the way Ehrlich had done to discover Salvarsan: keep chemically modifying promising ones until something worked. Farben's scope of operations and financial resources could fund and provide for an investigation of the matter. Research started in the late 1920s using aniline dyes as the basis of the attack.

Following animal experiments, it was discovered that azo dyes, as opposed to aniline, were less toxic. Researchers started the laborious task of chemically substituting side chains to the azo dyes. They would add chlorine, iodine, arsenic, and others, methodically making sure each new compound was unique. After four years, over 3,000 compounds were produced and presented for testing.

Most of the testing was done by a physician-turned-researcher named Gerhard Domagk (pronounced Doe-mock). He had interrupted his studies in medical school to serve as a medic in the German army during the first world war. He saw it all. Stationed in the eastern front of Ukraine, Domagk helped treat not only war wounds but a wide array of infectious diseases, including cholera, typhoid, pneumonia, meningitis, and a host of others. After the war, he finished his medical school studies and became a physician. He preferred research and obtained a post at the University of Munster. Like others at the time, he was convinced that the key to treating infectious diseases was using the immune system's power, and much of his early research centered on that. But the research done by Farben provided a steady income, and Domagk became instrumental in the search for a chemical anti-microbial.

Dr. Domagk's role in the research was to inject about two dozen mice with an especially virulent strain of the pathogenic organism *Streptococcus pyogenes*. The strain used showed a nearly 100% death rate for the mice. Half of the mice tested got the modified azo dye being investigated, and the other half got nothing but the pathogenic microbe. They were looking for a chemical agent to prevent the mice from dying. The research went on for over four years, and all they had to show was a lot of dead mice.

History gives us a lot of facts and figures, not so much emotion. Just what Dr. Domagk and his associates felt on the day they walked into the lab and saw one cage full of dead mice, the other full of rambunctious playful ones, we don't know. Awe? Joy? Skepticism? Whatever it was, it was justified. The lively mice should have been dead. They were given the same lethal injection of deadly *Streptococcus* as the ones in the next cage that died. But the live ones were also given a chemical treatment known to the researchers only as KL-695. It was an azo dye that was linked to a compound called sulfanilamide. Repeated testing bore out the results: this stuff worked. In 1931, for the first time in history, humans produced a substance in a laboratory that killed bacteria but did not significantly injure the infected animal. It seemed like a miracle, and, indeed, the term "miracle drug" was coined.

Science is, by its very nature, empirical. Charts, graphs, numbers, statistics, and other forms of enumeration are part and parcel of the scientific method. But sometimes, it is the personal, emotional aspects of applying science that make a difference. In the case of sulfanilamide, or Prontosil as it came to be called commercially, it was Dr. Domagk's 6-year-old daughter Hildegard who made a remarkable difference.

Little Hildegard was running around the house holding her doll and carrying a knitting needle when she slipped and fell, the needle piercing deeply into her hand. She was taken immediately to the hospital, where the needle was removed and her hand stitched up. But it was apparent in a couple of days that she was not well. Her hand had become swollen and red and very painful, the result of an infection that had set in. Bright red marks streaked up her forearm, signaling the presence of a

48

severe streptococcal infection. Her status deteriorated rapidly. The attending physician recommended amputation of her arm, but even that was a long shot: she was near death. Such was the case at the time: a seemingly minor event could become life-threatening. Out of desperation, her father, Dr. Domagk, administered the new drug he had been working on. In a couple of days, young Hildegard's fever broke, and she regained her usual state of health. In the 1930s, it was the stuff of miracles.

Still, testing had to be done, and questions answered. The biggest question, unanswered for some time, was why the substance worked when injected into live animals but failed to kill bacteria grown in culture in the laboratory. Domagk subscribed to the widespread opinion that the immune system cured diseases and that any chemical agent would work by augmenting the body's defenses. Just how the azo-sulfanilamide combination worked against the bacterial invader was a mystery to the research team. It turns out they made a major error in their assumptions.

By being so devoted to the idea of using a dye compound as a carrier to get material into a bacterial cell Dr. Domagk and co-workers failed to do what seems now to be an obvious experiment: test sulfanilamide by itself. This was done by French researchers at the Pasteur Institute in Paris. They showed that the sulfanilamide by itself produced the result; the azo dye had nothing to do with it. This discovery sent shockwaves through the boardroom of the Farben Corporation. They were all set to make a fortune on this newly discovered, revolutionary, and patentable medicine. Today we would call such a medication a "blockbuster," ensuring the good fortune of all involved. Again, the emotion of the time is not recorded. Still, one can imagine the sense of shock that went through the company's directors when it was revealed that it was sulfanilamide, a substance discovered some twenty-five years previously and not subject to patent, that was the "miracle drug." No patent, no profits. Anybody could make the medicine and make it they did. After the results of Domagk and colleagues' work were published in 1935, numerous modifications to the new "miracle drug" emerged. But it was another individual case that really got things rolling.

The benefit of sulfa drugs is dramatically illustrated by the fate of the sons of two U. S. presidents. In June of 1924, Calvin Coolidge assumed the presidency of the United States upon the death of Warren G. Harding. The Coolidges had two teenage sons, John, 18, and Calvin Jr., 16. They were both robust, healthy boys from their days working on the family farm in Massachusetts. Shortly after the family settled into the White House, the boys played tennis on the garden courts. For some reason, young Calvin neglected to wear his socks. He wore just his tennis shoes, probably just being a teenager. The next day Calvin developed a blister on his toe. Nobody thought much of it, but a couple of days later, the blister became infected, and the red streaks, typical of a pyogenic infection, were seen on the boy's ankle. The best doctors from Bethesda and Walter Reed were called in to attend, but they could only give palliative relief. In five days, young Calvin Coolidge Jr., the son of a sitting president, died, despite being attended by the best physicians in the country. His death was greatly dispiriting to the nation.

About a decade later, another president's son, Franklin Roosevelt Jr., age 22, got a sinus infection. Seemingly not too serious an ailment, it quickly got out of control. Today we use the term "flesh-eating" bacteria, describing strains of *Streptococcus* that manufacture a virulent toxin that dissolves flesh. That is probably what young Franklin had. The infection was progressing rapidly, and the best physicians were at a loss for ways to stop it. But one of his doctors, George Loring Tobey, was field testing a new drug from Germany, Prontosil (sulfanilamide). To Dr. Tobey, the drug was still experimental, but he was up against the blades: let the young man die or try the new drug. After a thorough discussion with young Franklin's parents, he proceeded with the treatment. Franklin developed a red skin pigment, typical at the time of Prontosil's side effects, but he recovered completely in a few days. Naturally, this made the headlines nationwide, and the "miracle drug" Prontosil was the nation's talk.

Sulfa drugs changed the course of human history on three major fronts. For one, people could now be successfully treated for otherwise serious or fatal bacterial infections. Cases of pneumonia, meningitis, skin and soft tissue infections, gonorrhea, and many others were now often amenable to therapeutic intervention. Sulfa had its drawbacks, notably some potentially serious side effects and the ability of bacteria to develop resistance quickly, but afflicted patients now had at least a fighting chance.

Another "benefit" of the discovery of sulfa as a chemotherapeutic agent was the creation of the government agency we now call the Food and Drug Administration or FDA. With the actively regulated pharmaceutical and healthcare industries today, it may be hard to envision what things were like in the early 1900s. For one thing, there was nothing that closely resembled the drug manufacturers we have now. Back then, it was perfectly fine for any company to make any drug and just go ahead and market it without testing either for efficacy or side effects. The marketplace was the arbiter of the value of the product. Corporations could obtain patents on substances they discovered, but there were often ways around that. Commercial products often contained additives that had medicinal use. Many products had enhanced advertising campaigns. Some interesting examples of products we know well today are soft drinks: The "coca" in Coca-Cola referred to the cocaine that was in the original recipe; the "7" in 7Up comes from the molecular weight of lithium, initially put in the beverage as a mood enhancer; Dr Pepper was marketed with the slogan 10, 2, and 4, implying that drinking it at those times gave the person a pick-up at the time of day when blood sugar was naturally low. The only laws at the time required the label to state the content of the product accurately. Claims about effectiveness or safety were left to the consumer to decide.

When sulfa became available, and the claims about its power reached a high level, hundreds of companies produced their own version and marketing strategies. The demand from people was robust, despite the general lack of knowledge about the new drug, even among physicians. To find a niche in the market, one company, the S. E. Massengill Company of Bristol, Tennessee, sought a way to make a sulfa drug available in a syrup. Cough syrups were very popular then and would appeal to a significant market segment since the sulfa drugs were only available in pill or injectable form. One problem, though, is that sulfa drugs, as a group, are not very soluble in water or alcohol. The company set about to find a liquid solvent for sulfanilamide. Unfortunately, the one that worked best was diethylene glycol, an organic liquid commonly used at the time as a solvent for personal care products like deodorants and skin creams. It has a slightly sweet taste and is practically odorless. Sounds good, but it also has a sinister side. It is the main component of brake fluid, and it is poisonous. It doesn't injure or kill you as fast as something like cyanide; its symptoms develop over several days. Most patients initially feel nausea, vomiting, diarrhea, and abdominal pain, then develop neurologic symptoms.

All of this was most likely unknown to the chemists at Massengill. They were happy to develop this new "elixir" of sulfanilamide, and it was marketed throughout the country. But soon, the reports of tragedies became widely known. The product was quickly taken off the market, but much damage was done. Scores of people were dead, and many more had become very ill. Something had to be done.

For several years, there were proposals made in the U.S. Congress to pass legislation intending to safeguard medical products and demand truth in advertising. None met with definitive action, but the "Massengill affair" could not be ignored. It provided the perfect reason to enact such legislation, and the national and public health outcry was overwhelming. In June of 1938, Congress passed, and President Roosevelt signed, the Federal Food, Drug, and Cosmetic Act, the forerunner of today's FDA.

(In the present day, a new drug or medical device must pass through three Phases to be approved for sale. The Food and Drug Administration must approve all three. In Phase I, the medication is administered to volunteers to evaluate its safety in humans. Drug efficacy is not the goal; ensure it is safe enough to continue testing. In Phase II, a relatively small number of patients diagnosed with the investigated malady are administered the drug, with drug efficacy and safety carefully monitored. If indicated, Phase III testing is undertaken, with a much larger number of patients tested. Following Phase III, the results are presented to an FDA Advisory Committee, made up of experts in the medical field in which the drug is proposed to be used. They then recommend adopting or denying the manufacturer's medication or device. Final approval is up to the full FDA panel).

Although not quantifiable, perhaps the most significant effect of the sulfa drug discovery was the paradigm shift among medical researchers in infectious diseases. So much work had been done to discover a substance that would kill invading microbes without damage to the patient, and so little progress had been made, that many believed such a thing was not possible, or only to a limited extent. Enhancing the body's immune system seemed the logical way to go. The discovery and application of sulfa drugs compelled many workers to renew their search for additional anti-microbial drugs. The result of their investigations was beyond their wildest dreams.

Ernst Chain was a voluble fellow. While a brilliant biochemist passionately devoted to his work, no one who worked with him would have ever recommended him for a "nice guy of the year" award. The son of a Jewish father, he had emigrated to England from Germany in the early 1930s, first working at Cambridge University, then at Oxford. His intelligence and memory were awe-inspiring. It was not uncommon for him to quote accurately from scientific journal articles published several years before, giving direct quotes and relevant sections. Not only was he a prodigious scientist, but he was also a gifted concert pianist. For a time, he struggled to decide between the careers of scientist and musician.

Like Ernst Chain, Howard Florey was an emigrant to England, coming there in 1922 from Australia as the recipient of a Rhodes scholarship. Extremely intelligent in his own right, Florey had an essential quality that Chain lacked: the ability to mix and mingle with the right people. He also was blessed with the skills of an administrator, bringing together the highest quality researchers and presenting cogent arguments to philanthropic organizations about raising funds.

Norman Heatley was a mild-mannered, modest English gentleman who began his career at Oxford in the late 1930s. Courteous to a fault, he assumed the roles he was given eagerly and with as much dedication as anyone. His unique ability was developing, modifying, and jury-rigging equipment to maximum use. Today we might call him a "techno-nerd."

This Oxford triad of Chain, Florey, and Heatley may not have comprehended the enormity of their work when they set about it. Still, their accomplishment represents one of the outstanding achievements in human history. Working under austere conditions in a cramped laboratory known as the Dunn building at Oxford University in England, they were the first to isolate and purify a substance produced by a living organism and direct it against bacteria causing an infection in humans. The substance, of course, was penicillin.

On paper, penicillin doesn't look like a highly complex chemical; just two amino acids, L-cysteine and D-valine. However, a few characteristics of the fungus that produce it make its isolation a challenging problem. L-cysteine-D-valine doesn't exist in nature as a free molecule; as it emerges from the mold, it is attached to a short protein called a peptide. The mold doesn't produce it all the time, just when under stress and when growing in the proper environmental conditions. And it doesn't make very much of it, only minute quantities. The mold that produces it is within the genus *Penicillium*. (The genus name *Penicillium* comes from the Latin word for paintbrush, "*penicillus*," a description of the mold's spore structure under the microscope).

The Oxford team at the Dunn Pathology Institute had worked in the late 1930s on the enzyme lysozyme, discovered by Alexander Fleming some fifteen years before. Chain had determined that lysozyme was an enzyme that attacked certain carbohydrates in a bacterial cell wall, disrupting them and causing their lysis. There is controversy as to who suggested investigating another of Fleming's discoveries, what he had called penicillin after the mold he obtained it from, *Penicillium notatum*. Still, it was extremely fortunate that someone, either Chain or Florey, did.

The first breakthrough in the investigation was made by Heatley, who succeeded in inducing the mold to produce maximum amounts of penicillin and constructed the laboratory equipment necessary for its harvest in quantities that could be

54

used in research work. Chain determined that penicillin was not an enzyme like lysozyme but a much smaller molecule. And it was Florey who convinced philanthropic donors that this substance, penicillin, was crucial and got the money to keep operations going.

After several years of complex and intricate research, Ernst Chain could harvest minute quantities of purified penicillin. The first trials of penicillin were like those Domagk used to test sulfadiazine: several mice were injected with a deadly form of streptococcus, some getting penicillin, others nothing. The penicillin group survived and showed no ill effects from the penicillin injected. It was like a miracle.

The development of penicillin brought on a whole new dimension to the practice of medicine. Going from a laboratory curiosity to an academic challenge to one of the great discoveries of all time was unprecedented. The Oxford workers knew they had something unique. But it was also hard to produce; only minute quantities were available. Enter again Norman Heatley, the so-called "forgotten man" of the penicillin saga, who fiddled with the equipment and the culture broths to enhance the yield of the substance manyfold. Still, a war raged, and Britain was directly in the firing line. The decision was made to transfer operations to the United States, where it was much safer. Just as important, adequate funding was available. When one thinks of the world's great centers of academic development, the name Peoria, Illinois, doesn't usually leap to mind. But that was where the main early work on penicillin was done.

A seemingly incidental but nonetheless essential step in the process was finding a different strain of the mold *Penicillium*. The one found in England did not have a high substance yield. In the U.S., an attempt was made to find a more vigorous strain, and sure enough, one was found. The find is attributed to a Peoria bacteriologist named Mary Hunt. It may have been because she was a woman, but she was assigned the task of visiting markets in Peoria to look for moldy fruit and vegetables. One of the world's great discoveries came from this unlikely source: a species of *Penicillium*, isolated from a rotten cantaloupe, that was the "mother of all penicillins." Ms. Hunt's find has become the ancestor of all modern penicillins, *Penicillium chryseogenum.*

Profits and fame account for a lot. As the clinical successes of penicillin grew, it became apparent to many influential people that a historical event was unfolding. Penicillin showed itself to be much better than sulfonamides, with a better spectrum of activity and fewer side effects. All strains of *Streptococcus* were susceptible, as well as other species. The floodgates in antibiotic research were opened.

Over the two decades following the work on penicillin, new antibiotics were discovered, tested, and released regularly. One could call the 1950s and 60s the "golden age" of antibiotic discovery. Not only were molds found to produce them, but soil bacteria also. Drugs were assigned to a "class" based on their mode of action and chemical composition. Pharmaceutical firms chemically modified them to gain a broader spectrum or more convenient administration means. The supply of new classes of antibiotics seemed limitless.

Until it wasn't. By the early 1970s, the discovery of new antibiotics produced by molds or soil bacteria came to a screeching halt. New antibiotics were tested and released, but they were modifications of existing drugs. Several new classes of drugs were introduced in the 1990s, such as fluoroquinolones and linezolid, but they were not produced by microbes but by chemists in a lab. The dried-up pipeline for new antibiotics wasn't for lack of trying. Thousands of soil samples and fungi from around the world were sent to pharmaceutical companies by their employees and other connections. They were meticulously screened for any hint of an antibiotic producer. Alas, nothing significant was uncovered.

Pharmaceutical firms today still release new antibiotics, but they are invariably a "variation on a theme:" taking a known antibiotic and modifying its chemical structure to create a drug that microbes haven't encountered before, so resistance has not yet developed. Either that, or the new drug has what appears to be superior pharmaceutical properties like fewer doses needed, oral versus intravenous, or fewer side effects. The challenge to antimicrobial research today is finding one to which bacteria are still susceptible. Resistance to antibiotics has reached a critical point.

When Ernst Chain worked on penicillin in the early 1940s, he noticed that some bacteria, mostly Gram-negative rods, were naturally resistant to it. But he also noticed that a few strains of *Staphylococcus,* which were on initial investigation susceptible, had become resistant to the drug. The antibiotic resistance mechanisms bacteria had developed in the natural setting eons before were fully operational when antibiotics were introduced. It didn't take long before the phenomenon of antibiotic resistance was well-known.

The genes that code for the resistance proteins can be passed between microbes by several means, giving rise to clones of resistant bacteria. Because of the widespread use of antibiotics in healthcare, these genetic resistance exchanges play out on a dynamic scale. The more antibiotics are used, the more resistance mechanisms are pushed. When exposed to an antibiotic, resistant bacteria survive, passing on their resistance genes—simple survival of the fittest.

Not all bacteria behave the same way. Some are prone to acquiring and passing on antibiotic-resistance genes, others hardly. The best examples are two genera of pyogenic Gram-positive cocci, *Staphylococcus aureus* and *Streptococcus pyogenes.* Both can cause severe infections in humans. It wasn't long after the introduction of penicillin that strains of *S. aureus* began to emerge that were resistant to penicillin at a very high level. They were found to produce an enzyme called penicillinase (now more appropriately called beta-lactamase) that destroyed the central part of the penicillin molecule, rendering it useless. This resistance mechanism spread like wildfire so that by the 1960s, just around half of all *S. aureus* isolates were resistant to penicillin and the related compound ampicillin. Today, over 90% of *S. aureus* is penicillin resistant.

Contrast this with the other serious Gram-positive coccus, *Streptococcus pyogenes.* It has never developed resistance to penicillin. The drug works against it as well today as it did in 1945. That's not to say resistance of this organism can never happen; *S. pyogenes* has developed resistance to other drugs. Antibiotic resistance is a very complex field, and clinical laboratories must be vigilant in keeping track of the problem so that some appropriate measures can be taken to contain it when it does occur.

Some researchers have hinted that humans may be beginning to enter the "post-antibiotic era," as the antibiotics available to us are no longer effective against a wide range of microbes. We're not there yet; it's still very rare that a bacterium causing an infection is resistant to all available antibiotics, a condition called pan-resistance. Most bacteria are susceptible to a few antibiotics. The main problem with antibiotic resistance is that most infections are initially treated empirically; the physician uses the best "guesstimate" of the most likely successful drug-bug combination. Lab studies take at least a day, more likely up to two days, to come back, and if the guesstimate is wrong and the patient has a resistant microbe, that means the patient has gone a couple of days without appropriate therapy. In less severe infections, that may not matter too much. But it is life and death in acute infections involving sepsis and other serious symptoms—the more resistant the microbe, the more likely treatment failure in those initial "guesstimate" situations. Hospitals are encountering this phenomenon more and more each year.

An unfortunate term that has come into vogue in recent years is "superbug." The name conjures an image of this plague-like beast of a microbe that infects and destroys with impunity. That's not it at all. The term superbug refers to microbes that have acquired resistance to a set of antimicrobial agents and therefore are difficult to treat in the initial stages of infection. They generally don't possess any characteristics of virulence and infectivity that distinguish them from any other opportunistic pathogen. If a species of *Klebsiella*, a common Gram-negative rod, develops resistance to imipenem, ceftriaxone, levofloxacin, gentamicin, and piperacillin, all usually effective broad-spectrum antibiotics, that's bad. Really bad. But a few antibiotics may still work, perhaps amikacin and/or colistin. The issue is that those antibiotics that are effective are not first-line drugs and are administered after appropriate laboratory testing results are available. The organism has a leg-up, a couple of days to make its mischief before a proper drug is given. If the patient is badly compromised, that may be too late. Sepsis can progress rapidly, and time is precious.

With antibiotic resistance becoming a larger and larger problem, some researchers have reverted to the once-popular philosophy of using the body's defense mechanisms to thwart infections. So far, not much clinical success has met the effort. But research today is light years ahead of where it was just 50 years ago. Perhaps some viable alternative to antibiotics may one day be developed. We'll just have to wait and see.

Chapter 5
The Sad Saga of Mary Mallon
Serving wholesome meals.
Oh, Mary! So contrary!
Guilty innocence.

History has given us nicknames that have become more famous than the name of the person they represent. Many will recognize the name "Billy the Kid," but few would be familiar with his real name, Henry McCarty, or even his alias, William Bonney. He apparently had a very youthful face and a goatee that made him look something like a billy-goat, a kid goat at that. "Tokyo Rose" was a familiar radio personality during the Second World War. She was an American of Japanese descent who graduated from the University of California at Los Angeles. Late in 1941, she traveled to Japan to attend to a sick relative but was stranded there when the war broke out. Her real name was Iva Toguri D'Aquino. "Wild Bill Hickok" reportedly got his nickname because of his large nose, which reminded some of a duck's bill. His real name wasn't William, but James Butler Hickok. He changed the first part of his nickname from "duck" Bill to "wild" because it sounded better. "Blackbeard the Pirate" was the name given to a British sailor who developed a reputation for being a ruthless cutthroat. In real life, he relied more on his tactical skills and the art of negotiation. His real name was Edward Teach.

The discipline of infectious diseases has its own famous nicknamed person whose real name is obscure to most people. She was a hard-working woman of Irish ancestry who simply wanted to make a good living and enjoy a few creature comforts now and then. An intelligent woman with meager formal education, she became embroiled in some of history's most important medical and legal questions. Her Christian name was Mary Mallon, but she is mostly referred to by her assigned nickname, "Typhoid Mary."

Mr. and Mrs. George Thompson were wealthy. They owned several lavish properties in the northeastern United States, their primary residence being in the upscale neighborhood of Oyster Bay on Long Island, New York. It was a beautiful home in the middle of a very exclusive, high-class setting. Not far away was the summer residence of Theodore Roosevelt, and there were equally impressive residents nearby.

Most years, the Thompsons' custom was to rent their Oyster Bay home for several months and spend the summer in the Catskills. In the summer of 1906, they rented it to the family of Mr. and Mrs. Charles Warren of New York. Mr. Warren was a banker to some of the industrial giants of the time, and he and his wife enjoyed the relaxed setting of the Oyster Bay community with their four young children. Theirs was something of an idyllic summer.

For some reason, the Warrens lost their cook in early August. Perhaps she was fired or had some personal issues, but the household needed a cook quickly. Mrs. Warren did what was commonplace then: she paid a visit to Mrs. Stricker's Employment Service in New York. They recommended a cook with impeccable references, one who had worked for some of the most prominent families in New York. Her name was Mary Mallon.

Family cooks of that time worked extremely hard and were very talented. They were the first of the household to arise each morning, and they worked close to 14-hour days. They were responsible for the entire kitchen, from buying groceries, cleaning ovens and sinks, washing dishes, and cooking. It was rough, hard work, and the meals had to be varied, engaging, and delicious. The cook typically prepared meals for the family first, then for the help. The Warrens had four children, and there were four servants besides Mary. After breakfast and the kitchen cleaned, it was time to prepare lunch. A day that began around 6 AM for a cook might end around 8 PM unless there was a party. Then it might be even longer. Challenging work, but Mary Mallon was up to it. She was a trained professional at age 37.

The trouble began in late August 1906. One of the Warren's children, Margaret, age 9, became ill. She had a fever and some diarrhea and felt listless. "Summer diarrhea" was a common malady of the time and still is today. Likely, Mrs. Warren didn't worry too much when her daughter first became ill. A little castor oil would fix her right up. But the disease persisted. Her fever spiked to 105 degrees, and she became delirious. Her stools became bloody, foul-smelling, and frequent. The child had become acutely, seriously ill. Then the tell-tale sign: a rash, or "rose spots," on her abdomen. A doctor was promptly summoned, and he confirmed the diagnosis: typhoid fever.

In 1906, there was no specific treatment for typhoid; care was merely palliative. Just do the best you can, pray, and wait it out. Shortly thereafter, four others became ill with the same disease: Margaret's older sister, two servants, and the gardener.

It was well known at the time that the primary source of typhoid fever was contaminated water. Whether you drank the water or it was used to wash fresh produce, most cases could be traced back to the water supply. How this house, at this time, had contaminated water was anybody's guess. Theirs was the only home in the neighborhood affected. Once the crisis was over, the Warrens did what any typical, thinking family would do. They high-tailed it back to their residence on the Upper East Side in New York, thanking their lucky stars that their daughters and employees had survived the disease. Mary, for her own reasons, did not accompany them.

When the Thompsons returned to their Oyster Bay home in mid-September, they expected to find the Warrens gone and their house in good order. What they found instead was the scene of a calamity. Typhoid was something you just didn't see in an affluent community like Oyster Bay. It was associated with filth and deprived living conditions. The Thompsons were now residing in what the locals and others were calling the "typhoid house." It was presumed that the disease arose from the water supply in their home, and any who entered there were at risk. This would not do. Mrs. Thompson, above all, was incredulous. She immediately notified the local public health authorities, who thoroughly inspected the entire home and its plumbing. Nothing. They interviewed the fruit and vegetable vendors and checked to see if any other cases in the community were noted. Nothing. They even considered a nice older woman who sold clams she dug herself in Oyster Bay. Nothing. The health workers finally just gave up, assuming the event was idiosyncratic. Case closed.

Mrs. Thompson was having none of it. Their standing in the community, let alone their ability to rent the property (who would want to live in the "typhoid house"), set her on a mission to find the best disease investigator available. Her inquiries led her to a rather unusual little man, Dr. George Soper, the "epidemic fighter." The "Dr." part of his name was somewhat misleading; he was not a medical doctor. His Ph.D. degree was in mining. But he liked to read medical literature, especially those articles dealing with disease outbreaks and their causes. The 36-year-old was officially classified as a "sanitary engineer," as "epidemiologist" had not yet been coined.

People had long known that contaminated water could cause infectious diseases. The seminal work on the matter was that of an obstetrician named John Snow, who elegantly demonstrated that a common source of contamination caused a cholera epidemic in the Soho district of London in the 1850s. It took a while for the concept to take hold, but by the early 1900s, it was accepted as fact. It was also well known that a person ill with an infectious disease could spread it to others. What wasn't appreciated, though, was that a perfectly healthy person could also be the source of a communicable disease.

In the early 1900s, most investigations into infectious disease outbreaks and epidemics involved looking at physical facilities and things like fresh water supplies becoming contaminated by sewage. In that regard, someone like George Soper, with his expertise in mining, would be a good fit for the job. Soper went further than most, though, as he kept abreast of the latest scientific literature in the field of medicine, especially articles related to the spread of infectious diseases. One article intrigued him. It was written by the eminent German microbiologist Robert Koch. In it, Koch described a person who was entirely well but could pass viable microbes which could infect other people and make them sick. It was just a single example that occurred in Europe, but it was nonetheless provocative.

Dr. Soper did the same inspection of the Oyster Bay house that the local officials did and also came up empty-handed. But he took it a step further. He traveled to New York City to interview members of the Warren family. During the conversation, he learned that the only real change that had taken place between the time the family moved into the home and the outbreak of the disease was the firing of the old cook and the hiring of her replacement. Using his investigative instincts, he contacted Mrs. Stricker's Employment Service (which was actually owned and run by a man). The owner was very cooperative and freely gave Dr. Soper a list of all the families to which his firm had connected Mary Mallon, the Warren family's cook. From there, it was plain old gumshoe detective work, paying a visit to each household to see if any incidents had happened when Ms. Mallon was employed.

What he found astounded him. Six of the seven families on his list for whom Mary Mallon worked as a cook had had a typhoid outbreak while she worked there. In one family, there were nine people afflicted. The only ones not sickened were the male head of the house, who had contracted the disease as a young man, and Mary, the cook. All told, Dr. Soper uncovered twenty-two victims. The only family not affected was an elderly couple, who probably had caught the disease in their youth and were naturally immune.

Continuing his search, Dr. Soper tracked Mary to a house on Park Avenue. Unfortunately, he was too late. At the home of Mr. Walter Browne and his family, he encountered their 25-year-old daughter, Effie, horribly sickened with typhoid. She soon died. Also ill was a household servant. There were now twenty-four known victims associated with Mary Mallon, which was only from the list he had obtained at the single employment office. No doubt there were others from jobs Mary had found on her own. Firm action was indicated.

Dr. Soper confronted Ms. Mallon in the kitchen of the Browne home in a surprise visit. In such a situation, tact is essential. A little charm doesn't hurt, either. Dr. Soper displayed neither. He later wrote that he "bungled the interview." Mary became indignant and defensive. It was the most absurd thing imaginable that she could be making people sick with typhoid when she was perfectly well and didn't recall ever having the disease. Dr. Soper explained that he just needed to get a few specimens of her blood and feces. That would prove it once and for all. But the more he spoke, the more upset she became. Finally, she picked up a carving fork and lunged at him, sending him racing out the back door in fear for his life. The tangled legal case of Mary Mallon had begun.

Several attempts to get Mary to cooperate were unsuccessful, to say the least. The more she was implored, the more belligerent she became. After doing their darndest to get Mary to comply, Dr. Soper and Hermann Biggs, the head of the New York Department of Health, enlisted the services of a female doctor, Dr. Josephine Baker. The diminutive "Dr. Joe," as she was called, was one of the few women practicing medicine in the New York area. She worked for the Public Health Department and was used to attending to poor, working-class people, especially women. If anyone could turn Mary Mallon, it had to be Dr. Joe.

She got a more hostile reception than the men did. On March 19th, 1907, Dr. Baker, several police officers, and an ambulance showed up at the front door of the house where Mary was working. Mary saw them coming and bolted out the back door. After a two-hour search of the neighborhood, they found her hiding behind some trash cans. The policemen pulled her out and "escorted" her to the ambulance. Dr. Baker's description of the episode of Mary's detention is quite descriptive:

"She came out fighting and swearing, both of which she could do with appalling efficiency and vigor. I made another effort to talk to her sensibly and asked her again to let me have the specimens, but it was of no use. By that time, she was convinced that the law was wantonly persecuting her, when she had done nothing wrong. She knew she had never had typhoid fever; she was maniacal in her integrity. There was nothing I could do but take her with us. The policemen lifted her into the ambulance, and I literally sat on her all the way to the hospital; it was like being in a cage with an angry lion."

After basically holding her as a captive at the Willard Parker Hospital in New York, a facility used to treat patients with infectious diseases exclusively, the precious stool specimen was obtained, sent to a microbiology laboratory, and, sure enough, tested positive for the typhoid bacillus.

The word "quarantine" in the early 1900s was invoked quite frequently. It comes from the Italian word "*quarantena*," referring to 40 days, as in the forty days of Lent. Centuries ago, it was the custom for ships coming into Italy to be isolated for 40 days so that cases of plague and smallpox could not spread from the crew to the community. Many areas of the world adopted this approach.

New York had a 13-acre island in the middle of the East River, North Brother Island. The facilities there were referred to as Riverside Hospital. It was mainly a series of small cottages where residents were given medical attention while they bided their time. Most patients were quarantined there voluntarily, but not Mary Mallon. She was effectively a prisoner.

This raised a serious legal question: she had committed no crime and was given no trial or legal representation, but here she was being held prisoner by state agents. One of the founding legal principles of the United States is that of *Habeas corpus,* which is *"A legal term meaning that an accused person must be presented physically before the court with a statement demonstrating sufficient cause for arrest. Thus, no accuser may imprison someone indefinitely without bringing that person and the charges against them into a courtroom. In Latin, habeas corpus means "you shall have the body." '* But the reality of the situation was apparent: a woman who was a carrier of a deadly disease who worked in a profession that practically guaranteed the transmission of that disease to unsuspecting people. Her unrepentant and uncooperative nature clearly demanded intervention by those protecting the populace. It was a genuine conundrum.

After some legal battles, the health authorities prevailed. Mary Mallon was held in a small bungalow on the island's edge. Her residence was pretty decent, with a living room, a kitchen, and a bathroom. She even had a small fox terrier for company, and she reportedly made a few friends and was permitted to have visitors. But she wasn't allowed to leave, and she certainly wasn't allowed to prepare meals for the other island residents.

Today in the United States and many countries, we have laws to protect the identity of patients and their personal information. In the U.S., we often refer to these rights as the HIPAA regulation, which stands for "Health Insurance Portability and Accountability Act." Everyone in the healthcare industry is familiar with the letter and the spirit of the HIPAA regulations: you never breathe a word about any patient to anybody outside of their immediate family. These regulations didn't exist in the early 1900s. Even though one would think patient privacy is a moral and ethical imperative, private information of a sensational nature was often leaked to the press. Adding to the maelstrom was the pervasiveness of what was known as "yellow journalism," a contest between publications to see who could come up with the most electrifying story (and sell the most newspapers). In June of 1909, Mary opened a copy of *New York American*, a newspaper owned by William Randolph Hearst. She saw banner headlines giving her name and calling her "the most dangerous woman in America." It went on to list details of her predicament and suggested she could remain "a prisoner for life."

Controversy and legal battles ensued. Somehow, Mary got an attorney, who argued a perfect legal case, but the court sided with the health department. While acknowledging they couldn't lock up every typhoid carrier, this case was unique. Everyone seemed to sympathize with her, but Mary Mallon was condemned.

Finally, in February 1910, Mary relented. She signed a paper promising to report to the health department for monthly testing and never work as a cook again. She was free from her island confinement, but more problems were just beginning. Her image, name, and story were plastered in the mainstream press. Who would hire the "typhoid carrier," even if it was a laundress or a maid? In 1910, there was no unemployment compensation, government assistance, or social security disability. Find a job or become a charity case. She was unmarried, and at age 40, her prospects were minimal.

Mary faithfully reported to the health department for testing for the first year. Then she just faded away.

During this time, one might be justified in feeling somewhat sorry for Mary Mallon, perhaps even taking a devil's advocate position for her. She wasn't sick, did not intend to hurt anyone, and was the victim of a miserable biological situation. Her life was in turmoil through no fault of her own. But any humane feelings for her evaporated in early 1915. A typhoid epidemic occurred at the prestigious Sloan Hospital for Women in Manhattan. Twenty-five cases of typhoid fever had broken out, with 24 victims being doctors, nurses, or other hospital staff and one patient. Two died. This was unheard of at a hospital like Sloan, well known for its impeccable attention to hygiene. Hospital officials were distraught and perplexed, so they called in "the epidemic fighter," Dr. George Soper.

Three months before the outbreak, the hospital had hired a new cook, Miss Mary Brown. She was very good at her work, well-liked by the staff, and dependable. Take three guesses about the true identity of "Miss Mary Brown." She must have known something was up because she disappeared right before being summoned for an interview by Dr. Soper. Some good police work found her hiding in a bathroom at a friend's house, and several policemen once again took her into custody. At age 46, she had cooked her last meal and infected her last person.

Mary Mallon lived out her days on North Brother Island. She liked to read, had a few friends, and eventually got a job preparing specimens in the laboratory at Riverside Hospital. On December 4th, 1932, Mary didn't show up for work. She had suffered a stroke in her cottage, completely paralyzed on her right side. For the last six years of her life, she remained bedridden in Riverside Hospital, and on November 11, 1938, she died of pneumonia.

One might say that Mary Mallon gives testament to the oft-quoted phrase of historian Laurel Thatcher Ulrich that "well-behaved women seldom make history." If she had been more interested, concerned, and willing to assist during that first encounter with Dr. Soper, we would have never heard of her or her famous nickname. (The name "Typhoid Mary" originated during a medical conference concerning typhoid carriers. During the discussion period after a lecture on the subject, one of the physicians attending the conference referred to the woman discussed by that moniker. The name stuck). However, she chose a different path; as they say, the rest is history.

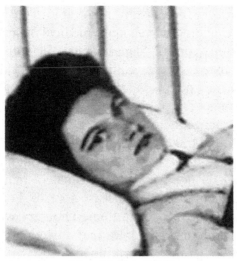

Mary Mallon (LOC)

The cases of Mary Mallon and others bring up many interesting questions in medicine and law. It also highlights the critical field of epidemiology. The term comes from two Greek words, *epi*, meaning "among or upon," and *demos*, meaning "people." The term epidemic, an outbreak of disease not usually seen in an area or group of individuals, is contrasted with endemic, indicating the condition exclusively belongs to a particular region or place. The description and study of disease outbreaks, some of them of monumental proportions like the bubonic plague, have captivated humans for millennia. But only in the last 150 years or so has the discipline of epidemiology become the straightforward practice it now is.

The epidemiologist must be a natural multi-tasker. As seen in the case of Mary Mallon, things to consider include the science of the organism(s) involved, physical facilities, geography, statistics, and pharmacology. Beyond the science and engineering components, it is often necessary to consider history, sociology, criminology, and psychology. Finding out why an epidemic occurred is one thing. Getting people to cooperate to eliminate it can be something else entirely.

Today, epidemiologists work in two main areas: governmental public health departments and healthcare facilities. The two very often overlap in their work.

Many diseases are, by law, reportable to the public health department. Attending physicians, medical laboratories, and hospital infection control departments file reports of the occurrence of listed severe, communicable diseases. These reports include the patients' names, addresses, diagnoses, and laboratory findings. The public health epidemiologist then takes the information and, much like a detective, follows up on two major themes: determine where the patient got the illness, and keep it from spreading. Most often, the information about the disease outbreak is not widely disseminated, mainly because there is no imminent danger of disease spread. For instance, if someone returns from a trip to a foreign country with a case of shigellosis, a communicable intestinal infection, there is not much to be done other than informing the patient of the threat of possible spread and going over good hygiene practices.

Sometimes, however, the appearance of a disease, especially when multiple persons are involved, is concerning enough that public notification is necessary. Sometimes this means press releases and product recalls. Listeriosis is a relatively rare disease in the U.S., but it can be dire to some people, especially the elderly, immunocompromised, and pregnant. So, a complete health department offensive is required when it turns up in cantaloupes all over the country. Press releases, news conferences, product recalls, on-sight investigations, and statistics gathering are in full swing. The information about individual patients is scrupulously guarded, but the public must be given as much accurate information as possible. Lives are at stake.

Public health epidemiologists get most of their initial information from medical laboratories, usually those based in hospitals. Identifying the organism causing an infectious disease is very helpful to the physician treating the patient, but it can also benefit the public health department. The finding of a couple of patients with *Salmonella* may not seem much out of the ordinary to the individual lab worker. Still, the plot thickens when several other medical labs in the same geographic area report similar findings. That is especially true if all the isolates are of the same serotype, the same strain. That would indicate a common source, and it's a clue to the public health epidemiologists that something is afoot.

Clinical laboratories are known as sentinel labs in the public health context. The formal name given to the system is Laboratory Response Network or LRN. Prompt isolation and reporting of critical infectious organisms and good communication channels are essential for public health.

(It is speculated that the outbreak traced to Mary Mallon on Long Island was caused by some homemade ice cream she prepared. She sliced fresh peaches by hand and left them in the cream mix for several hours while preparing the ice machine. In the warm August afternoon, that would have been an ideal way to cultivate *S. typhi,* which likely would have gotten onto the peaches from her hands).

The practice of good sanitation, the discovery of anti-microbial agents like antibiotics, the development of vaccines, and the employment of tools to make us aware of the presence and extent of infectious diseases have combined to provide a phenomenal decrease in the suffering of people around the world. Gifted pioneering workers like Florence Nightingale, Louis Pasteur, Paul Ehrlich, Gerhard Domagk, Edward Jenner, and so many more have laid the foundation for a field of science that not long ago was not known to exist. The road to success was not straightforward, with trials, tribulations, heartache, and exultation paving the way. We will never eliminate infectious diseases, but the knowledge and wisdom gained from experience aid greatly.

SECTION TWO

"Symptoms of a sickness are not necessarily signs of weakness, rather they imply that your body is actively fighting the sickness. And when all the resources of the body fall short to fight the sickness, that's when the real trouble begins."

– Abhijit Naskar

Chapter 6
What's Bugging Us

Overt and covert,
Looking for an opening.
Tiny predators

Bacteria. Viruses. Mold. Microbes. Bugs. Yeast. Microbial agents. Parasites. Fungus. Organisms. Germs. Pathogens. Microorganisms. Cooties.

There sure are a lot of names for the tiny creatures that can make us sick. For the uninitiated, they all kind of run together and are perhaps even interchangeable. But there are tremendous biological differences between the various groups, and the therapies and prognoses of the diseases they cause greatly depend on which one we're talking about.

For most of human history, people had no idea these microscopic beasts existed. Their effects, such as infectious disease, fermentation, and putrefaction, had to be explained, and what sounds to us as some pretty weird interpretations were thought to be reasonable. Spontaneous generation was held as absolute truth. Divine intervention was the default reasoning. There were innumerable folk medicine theories and remedies. The more erudite descriptions of disease came from philosophers, men like Plato, Aristotle, and Galen. Accepted medical theory for over a millennium maintained that health was held in the balance of "humours:" the body's reflection of the natural elements of air, water, earth, and fire, that is, blood, phlegm, black bile, and yellow bile. When one of these got out of balance, illness, including infectious diseases, resulted. In this context, bloodletting was a perfectly reasonable remedy.

The first glimpse of what was actually behind it all was provided by the work of a Dutch cloth merchant in the late 1600s. Antonie van Leeuwenhoek was born in Delft, Netherlands, in 1632. His Christian name was Thonis, but it somehow morphed into Antonie. The name van Leeuwenhoek, which means "Lion's Corner," referred to the shop his father ran in Delft.

Antonie's private life was troubled. His father was a shop owner, and his mother was from a wealthy family. His father died when he was five years old, and his mother remarried. His stepfather died when he was sixteen. Antonie married, and he and his wife had five children, but only one, a daughter, lived to adulthood. Other than those simple facts, not much else is known, but reportedly as a youngster, he spent time with an uncle, who provided him with his primary education. He never attended a university. At the age of sixteen, he was sent off to apprentice in a linen drapery establishment where he learned the trade of the cloth merchant.

It is often said that one picture is worth a thousand words. In the case of Antonie van Leeuwenhoek, though, one picture, or portrait, is worth considerably less. Images of him mostly portray a rather pompous, supercilious-looking fellow without much substance. He looks grandiose, self-absorbed, and perhaps pretentious. But such was not the case. Despite his lack of formal education, he was highly intelligent, industrious, and had a passion for knowledge. He used his skills to set up his own business and became quite prosperous. He also secured positions with the city government, working as a sheriff's assistant, chief surveyor, and census taker. He was apparently rather highly regarded in his community.

One of the tools of the trade of the better cloth merchants of the 17th century was the magnifying glass. The quality of a garment or drapery was in the details of the stitching, and a simple magnifying glass allowed the observer to quickly make an evaluation. Certainly, van Leeuwenhoek used one in his work.

Microscopes existed in the 1600s, but they were crude, and their magnification was very blurred. The preferred type was the compound microscope, which has two lenses. One lens is located near the observer's eye, so it has the name ocular lens. The other rests near the object being observed, so it's the objective lens. It's the type of microscope commonly used today. The quality of the instrument depends mainly on the quality of the lenses. If there is an aberration in one of the lenses, it is magnified in the other. If both lenses are flawed, that makes it that much worse. There were severe limits on what could be observed because of lens quality issues.

The top microscopist of the day was the esteemed British scientist, Robert Hooke. He had published papers detailing his observations, the most important of which was the visualization of red blood cells. But because of the poor resolution of his microscope, that was the limit of his observation. It's not recorded in history, but it is reasonable to believe that van Leeuwenhoek was familiar with Hooke's work, having visited London in the early 1660s.

Armed with his working knowledge of the magnifying glass in his work and his awareness of the work of Robert Hooke, Antonie set about constructing a better lens. With his great diligence and attention to detail, he succeeded beyond his expectations. We don't know what technique he used, but it probably involved taking two glass rods, heating them in a flame, touching them together, then slowly pulling them apart to form a thread of hot glass. The product of this he then ground down methodically to form a very tiny but very flaw-free lens. Rather than use them in a compound scope, he used them individually, like a very refined magnifying glass. The results were nothing short of astounding.

Imagine that only one single human being could visualize what no other person in the history of the human race could see. That guy was Antonie van Leeuwenhoek in the 1660s. His little lenses could magnify objects over a hundred times and, in some cases, 300 times. He could see simple and single-cell animals, like rotifers and paramecium. He even saw bacteria. van Leeuwenhoek described what is thought to be the microscopic parasite *Giardia* in his own stool specimen, the first description of an infectious disease agent. He literally discovered, by himself, a whole new world.

Such breakthroughs do not come without issues. Antonie had some of what we today would describe as character flaws, the chief of which was his extreme reluctance to share his lens-making techniques with anyone else. He apparently assumed, and probably correctly, that if others had his instrument, they would make all kinds of important discoveries and write scientific papers, thereby overwhelming his personal accomplishments. He made a couple of dozen of his lenses, but his secret of how he did it died with him. One of the great virtues of science is the sharing of knowledge. van Leeuwenhoek, in this regard, failed miserably. After he died, no one had a clue how to construct his precious lenses, and his secret remained just that.

Old dogmas are not often put to easy rest. When van Leeuwenhoek's discoveries hit the scientific establishment, they were met with derision and outright ridicule. The very idea was preposterous, especially since it came from this uneducated Dutch cloth merchant. His most repulsed idea was his description of single-cell animals, or "animalcules," or little animals, as he called them. It took some decades and hundreds of scientific papers submitted to London's Royal Society before the powers that be began to change their mind and reluctantly accept the Dutchman's reports. Still, there wasn't universal acceptance. van Leeuwenhoek spoke only Dutch and never authored a book on his findings. All that he notably recorded were letters written to the Royal Society in London, and since no one could verify his findings, the idea of a microbial world was very slow to catch on. But Antonie van Leeuwenhoek unquestionably was the first person to make detailed descriptions of the tiny creatures that inhabit our world. For that, he is sometimes referred to as the "Father of Microbiology."

In the world of the agents causing infectious diseases, there are four groups: bacteria, viruses, fungi, and parasites. We may refer to them collectively as "germs" or "bugs," but they are biologically distinct. Within each group are certain species capable of making us very sick, or worse.

Bacteria. Bacteria are small, single-cell creatures that are found everywhere. They aren't very big, much smaller than a red blood cell, but they can replicate at a tremendous rate yielding millions of cells in a very short time. Inside, bacteria have a lot of the things we have in our cells. They have DNA, RNA, ribosomes, lots of enzymes and protein structures, and a cellular membrane. It's the level of organization and complexity that really distinguishes bacterial cells from ours. The most obvious difference is the structure of the nuclear material. Our DNA is arranged in highly specialized chromosomes encased inside a nuclear membrane, segregating it from the rest of the cell. In bacteria, the DNA is just one long, tightly coiled string intimately associated with the cell's cytoplasm. This different type of nuclear material arrangement is named prokaryote for bacteria, and eukaryote for human and other developed animal cells. The terms are from the Greek, *pro* meaning "before," and *karyon,* meaning "nut" or 'kernel." The *eu* for our more advanced form refers to the "true" nucleus.

Another major difference between bacterial and human cells is the presence of a cell wall in the former. We don't have rigid cell walls, but bacteria must have them in addition to their outer membrane if they are to survive in the environment. Their small size gives them high internal pressure.

Cell walls differ markedly between various groups of bacteria. Most bacteria have a common backbone to their walls, the stuff called peptidoglycan, which helps hold the whole thing together. In some, the layer of the peptidoglycan layer is thick; in others, it is thin. We call those with thick cell walls Gram-positive; those with thinner peptidoglycan layers we call Gram-negative. The thicker walls of the Gram-positives don't easily allow the penetration of organic solvents like acetone and alcohol. The thinner-walled Gram-negative bacteria do. There are considerable differences in what other materials each type of bacteria allows inside the cell, including antibiotics. Several antibiotics can wreak havoc with the bacterial cell wall, causing it to leak and pretty much come apart at the seams. Little pieces of the aborted cell wall then go flying off into the environment. Other antibiotics must enter the internal part of the bacterial cell to damage the organism. The cell wall type is important in allowing or preventing these antibiotics' entrance.

Bacteria translate their DNA into proteins and peptides in the same general manner as more advanced cells. The DNA unwinds, enzymes known as polymerases copy it into messenger RNA, and the mRNA migrates to ribosomes for transcription. Ribosomes have two parts, each of a different size. When the reading of messenger RNA is initiated, the two ribosome sections come together and work to transcribe the genetic code. The general system is the same in bacterial and human cells.

There is a big difference, though, in the structure of the ribosomes. The arrangement of components within the bacterial ribosomes is very different from ours. This provides another potential target for antibiotics, which can zero in on the bacterial protein-making apparatus while sparing ours.

The reason antibiotics are effective against bacteria but don't work against viruses is that viruses have neither cell walls nor ribosomes. The target of antibiotics is not present in viruses.

Bacteria can be divided into many groups, but those that infect humans can be easily placed into just six. Four depend on the organism's shape, either round or rod-like, and the way they take up certain stains. Another group is the spirochetes, the corkscrew-like organisms. Finally, some bacteria must reside inside the host cell to grow and infect.

Bacteria that exist outside of animal cells need a rigid cell wall to keep them from exploding or at least severely leaking. They are so small that the internal pressure of their cell, about 5x atmospheric pressure, would quickly result in the rupture of the cellular membrane, and they would die very quickly. One of the most common ways we have to kill bacteria is to disrupt their cell wall, using antibiotics like penicillin.

There are two types of bacterial cell walls, those that easily allow the entrance of organic solvents like alcohol or acetone and those that don't. This difference was discovered in the 1880s by a worker in Robert Koch's lab in Germany, Hans Christian Gram. He developed a staining procedure to help easily discern the difference, and the technique he perfected forever bears his name, the Gram stain. We call bacteria resistant to organic solvents "Gram-positive," and those much less resistant "Gram-negative." The difference has much to do with the thickness of the cell wall stabilizer, peptidoglycan. Gram-positive organisms have a lot of it, Gram-negative not so much. There are other differences as well. The distinction between the two is usually clear-cut.

We use the term coccus for the round bacteria, which comes from the Greek word for berry. The longer straight or cylindrical ones are given the technical name bacillus, which comes from the Latin *baculum,* or "staff." Most microbiologists just use the term rods.

So, four of the groups of bacteria infecting humans are Gram-positive rods, Gram-positive cocci, Gram-negative rods, and Gram-negative cocci. (The latter are mostly of one genus of bacteria called Neisseria, and they only exist as pairs or diplococci. So, in infectious diseases, we don't ever say Gram-negative cocci but Gram-negative diplococci). These are, of course, further subdivided into numerous genera and species.

Another group of bacteria is the spirochetes. Technically, they are Gram-negative, but they stain very poorly and are so distinctive that they are always referred to separately. They look like corkscrews and make their way through the environment by that type of motion. The best-known members of the group cause the diseases syphilis and Lyme disease.

The sixth and final group of bacteria is the obligate intracellular species. Like the spirochetes, they are technically usually Gram-negative, but in fact, they can only cause infections while dwelling inside a mammalian cell. They don't stain well, and special procedures are often needed to visualize them. More well-known examples of this group are *Chlamydia* and the organisms that cause typhus.

Another distinction we observe among the bacteria is their requirement for oxygen. Some can't live without it, some die if exposed to it, and a lot can go either way. Another word for oxygen-tolerant bacteria is aerobe. Anaerobic bacteria grow only when air is absent. Obligate means just what it says. So, an obligate aerobe needs air to grow, and obligate anaerobes die in the presence of air. Facultative means the organism can grow whether oxygen is present or not.

Each of these designations helps us identify and characterize a bacterial pathogen. The identification of the organism and the diagnosis and prognosis of the disease is made much easier when we know the fundamental characterization of the bacterial pathogen.

Bacteria	Description	Examples
Gram-positive cocci	Round; stain purple on Gram stain	*Staphylococcus; Streptococcus*
Gram-negative bacilli	Rod-shaped; stain red on Gram stain	*E.coli; Salmonella*
Gram-positive bacilli	Rod-shaped; stain purple on Gram stain	*Listeria; Clostridium*
Gram-negative diplococci	Round; stain red on Gram stain	*Neisseria gonorrhoeae*
Spirochetes	Corkscrew-shaped	*Treponema pallidum*
Intracellular	Small rod-shaped	Rickettsia

(The Gram stain was developed by Hans Christian Gram, a Danish physician working at a hospital in Berlin in the mid-1880s. The stain is easily done. First, the material to be stained, usually either material from a bacterial culture or a specimen obtained from a patient, is allowed to dry on a glass slide. It is then "fixed" to the slide by gently heating; the slide should be "mildly uncomfortable to the back of the hand." Chemical fixatives may also be used. The slide is then flooded with crystal violet, an aniline dye, for about a minute. That stain is then washed off with water, and a solution of iodine (elemental iodine plus potassium iodide) is applied. After about a minute, that solution is washed off with water. The iodine is a "mordant," forming large chemical complexes with the crystal violet, allowing the dye to adhere firmly to the bacterial cell membranes. The next step is the crux of the stain. An organic solvent, either ethyl alcohol or acetone, is added to the slide for a few seconds and then washed off with water. Cells that allow easy penetration of the solvent are known as Gram-negative; the crystal violet-iodine complex is dissolved and washes out of the cell. Organisms known as Gram-positive are resistant to the penetration of the organic solvent and retain the crystal violet. They appear purple under the microscope. The Gram-negative cells at this point are colorless. To visualize them, a counterstain, usually the red-colored safranin, is applied. Gram-negative bacteria thus appear red under the microscope).

Gram-positive cocci.
The primary human pathogens are *Staphylococcus* and *Streptococcus*.
The organisms frequently initiate the formation of pus and are often called pyogenic. Numerous non-pathogenic species colonize humans.

Gram-negative rods.
Myriad Gram-negative rods colonize and infect humans. They range in size, appearance, and motility. All share a toxic cell wall component, Lipid A.

Gram-positive rods.
Four genera predominate in human infections, *Listeria*, *Corynebacterium*, Bacillus, and the anaerobic genus *Clostridium*. The latter two produce spores.

Gram-negative diplococci.
A single genus causes human infections, Neisseria, which has two pathogenic species, *N. gonorrhoeae* and *N. meningitides*.

Spirochetes.
The spirochetes do not stain by Gram stain and cannot be grown in traditional bacterial culture. Several human diseases are known to be caused by them, most notably syphilis and Lyme disease.

Intracellular pathogens.
Several bacteria must reproduce inside a living cell. They cannot be cultivated in artificial culture. Examples are *Chlamydia*, and the agents of typhus and Rocky Mountain spotted fever.

Bacteria are a part of us. We cannot live without them any more than we could live without our kidneys. They help defend us from pathogens, aid with our nutrition, and help our immune system develop and stay acutely active. We have trillions of bacterial cells colonizing us always.

Still, there are quite a few folks who feel that the only good bacterium is a dead one. One claim of a commercial anti-bacterial detergent was that it instantly killed 99.999% of bacteria!! At the first sign of a cold or other infection, many people head straight to the doctor and all but demand an antibiotic to "cure the infectious disease." They don't realize that antibiotics are non-specific poisons, killing any and all bacteria we have that are susceptible to it, whether it needs killing or not. Antibiotics can act like neutron bombs, taking out not only the infection-causing critters but everything else.

Bacteria have what can be described as a broad-spectrum association with us. Many of the bacteria we have are usually very passive, not giving us any trouble and often doing us some good. But sometimes, our circumstances change. That benign, harmless microbe can suddenly turn on us, causing grave illness. The name applied to these usually benign but occasionally virulent organisms is "opportunistic." It is a very apt term.

A very good example of this type of pathogen, and there are many, is the organism *Streptococcus agalactiae*, commonly known as Group B Strep. It is a common colonizer of our intestinal tract and of the vagina. Billions of people are walking around right now with Group B Strep somewhere on their body, and they don't even know it. But if given the right opportunity, the organism can turn on us in an instant. Newborn infants are at particular risk of developing life-threatening meningitis and sepsis when they encounter the organism during vaginal birth. Many people with diabetes develop skin ulcers caused by Group B Strep, and the infection can sometimes lead to a life-threatening situation.

Many other bacterial species are like that: a benign lifelong companion that can go over to the dark side in a very short amount of time. Without the opportunity, they just colonize. Given the correct set of circumstances, though, they can ravage us without mercy.

Bacteria contain a group of genes that produce proteins known as universal stress proteins. These aren't unique to bacteria and are found in many different life forms like plants and fungi. As the name implies, these proteins become active when the organism is subjected to some form of stress, be it an altered pH, lack of nutrients, the presence of a noxious chemical or physical agent, and many others. They either directly or indirectly influence the release of gene products the organism may use to address the stress factor, often resulting in a quite different organism. These universal stress proteins can become activated when the organism is inside us. They are an extremely complex and somewhat enigmatic system, and they allow bacteria to greatly alter their activity.

Many bacteria possess an important faculty: the ability to form a layer of themselves over a surface, a structure known as a biofilm. The example most of us are familiar with is dental plaque. The biofilm is comprised of three layers and is remarkable in its complexity and effectiveness. By forming this film, the host's innate defenses are mitigated, and the organism can grow rapidly.

A typical biofilm has three layers. The bottom layer attaches to the underlying structure, whether it be a sheet of epithelial cells or the surface of a plastic device like a catheter. Adherence is from tiny hairs called fimbriae and the stickiness of the carbohydrates on the outside of the bacterial cell. On top of the adherent layer is a film of vegetative cells that provide a bridge between the lower and upper cells. They exist in a state of reduced metabolism, existing in a near-starvation form. The top layer is composed of cells that behave much like typical bacteria, metabolizing and reproducing actively. A biofilm has what amounts to a primitive circulatory system, with nutrients from the top shunted down to the cells below. The tight junction of the bottom layer leaves them very resistant to the effects of neutrophils, which have difficulty engaging and dislodging them. Hence, the entire structure is very resistant to the effects of the innate immune system. In the example of the biofilm of dental plaque, which must be scraped off with a sharp instrument, we can see the resiliency of a biofilm in full engagement. Depending on where a biofilm forms, such as an implanted medical device, it can make life miserable.

Some bacteria are just flat-out bad. If you have them, you are sick. *Yersinia pestis* and the bubonic plague. *Bacillus anthracis* and anthrax. *Treponema pallidum* and syphilis. Many organisms cause significant disease but can be harmlessly carried by some individuals, such as *Salmonella typhi*, the cause of typhoid fever, or *Neisseria meningitides*, a cause of a deadly form of meningitis.

Many bacteria that are associated with us, though, are not only innocuous but beneficial. The dictum that all bacteria are "all bad all the time" is unfounded. Our bacterial flora is very much a part of us, and the killing of the pathogenic varieties must be undertaken judiciously.

Diagnosing a bacterial infection is usually, but not always, straightforward and routine. Most bacteria multiply rapidly and can grow on nutrients outside the human body. Bacterial growth on this artificial nutrient media is called a culture, as millions of the same strain of bacteria grow together. If the hardening ingredient agar is added to a liquid media, the organisms form discreet round entities called colonies. The colonies of each species of bacteria are often unique and can be identified by a lab worker. Sometimes tests are applied for specific identification.

The specific identification of infecting bacteria can often be enough to guide therapy, but antibiotic resistance is such a problem that laboratories usually conduct further tests to determine which antibiotics would most likely be successful in treatment. The test is called an antibiotic susceptibility. When a specimen is taken and submitted to a laboratory to determine the infectious agent, culture and susceptibility (C&S) is most often requested. (Sometimes, the term "sensitivity" is mistakenly used in place of susceptibility).

While culture and susceptibility is the routine procedure for bacterial identification, some infectious agents defy easy diagnosis, and alternative methods must be pursued. The culture is very useful when several species may cause the same symptoms, such as a urinary tract infection or pneumonia. Some tests are specific for unique bacterial pathogens. Organisms that cause syphilis, tuberculosis, Lyme disease, and others must be diagnosed using specific techniques, not routine culture. For some infections caused by bacteria, a "shortcut" technique is sometimes available, such as a screen for Group A *Streptococcus*, the agent that causes Strep throat.

The diagnosis of any disease is no better than the specimen being submitted. It must reflect the active infective site, either tissue or fluid.

The word **parasite** can have several meanings, depending on the context of the discussion. We may describe a particularly obnoxious freeloader as being a parasite. Bacteria can parasitize us. The derivation of the word comes from the Greek, *para*, or "beside," and *sitos*, meaning "food." A parasite is a creature that takes nutrition from another, offering no benefit in return.

In infectious diseases, the term parasite is reserved for small, or maybe not so small, animal species that infest us. Some can be easily seen, like roundworms or tapeworms. Some are microscopic organisms, such as those that cause malaria or giardiasis. The word "infest" is used here advisedly, as they often do not elicit a vigorous immune response but merely live on us as something of a nuisance. A "good" parasite does not want to kill or damage its host.

Parasites run the gamut in both size and severity of illness. They range from the single-cell amoeba to the enormous tapeworm, and from benign organisms we don't even know we have to those that cause severe diseases like malaria and African sleeping sickness. They can enter our bodies in all sorts of ways, like ingestion, inhalation, blood-borne by insect vectors, or sexual transmission. They can even enter our bodies if we step on them with bare feet, the typical entry means of hookworm. Some, like lice and leeches, don't even bother to enter the body.

One of the most unheralded accomplishments of Western medicine has been the near-complete elimination of parasites from developed populations. We don't take our children to the pediatrician to have them "de-wormed." In developed countries, malaria is only seen in people who have traveled to or emigrated from an endemic area. Our public water supplies only rarely are the source of microscopic parasites, and when that happens, the remedy is readily available. One could probably take thousands of Americans, do a routine search for parasites on all of them, and not find a single one. We still see the occasional case of giardiasis or toxoplasmosis, but infrequently.

It wasn't always this way. For nearly all of human history, people have been infested by parasites. Almost every person in every part of the world, from the mightiest king or pharaoh down to the lowliest serf or peasant, had something. In many cases, individuals had multiple parasites at the same time. Parasitic organisms were as much a part of humans as our intestinal bacterial flora is with us today.

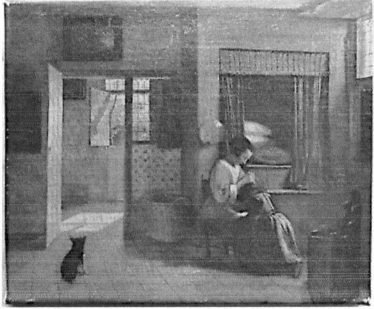

A painting by Dutch artist Pieter de Hooch from the late 1650s entitled "A Mother's Duty." It shows a mother carefully pulling lice and nits from her daughter's hair. The Dutch at the time were notorious for their clean habits, as depicted in the rest of the painting, yet, like everywhere else in the world, parasites were an everyday fact of life. (LoC)

There are no vaccines for parasites used in the developed world for the simple reason that we just don't need them. The reason for the near eradication of almost all parasites in the developed world has been sanitation. Measures taken to rid us of bacterial pathogens like typhoid and cholera have also prevented the spread of parasites. While they are certainly not extinct, parasites play only a minor role in the practice of infectious diseases in the developed world.

Parasites begin the infestation of our body in a very small way. Small size that is. Even those that will eventually become good-sized worms start out in an embryonic form. The immune system cells can usually surround and either engulf or latch onto them and inject toxins, bringing about their end.

From the parasite's perspective, this won't do. It wants to set up housekeeping and not be bothered by these pesky immune cells. Over the eons, parasites have developed many unique ways to deflect and evade the cells and chemicals designed to take them out. Some try to hide inside host cells, like malaria inside a liver or red blood cell, or *Trypanosoma cruzi* inside a muscle cell. Others have developed the ability to rapidly alter their protein coats, cranking out a new surface protein every few days, making antibodies produced against the old form obsolete before they even get produced. *Trypanosoma brucei*, the agent of African sleeping sickness, and *Giardia lamblia* are particularly good at this.

Some parasites have developed the ability to produce a substance that can mitigate an important factor in host defenses. There are a lot of them.

A few examples: *Schistosoma mansoni*, a worm known as a trematode, or fluke, lives in the blood vessels surrounding the intestinal tract. It makes a product that prevents the maturation of dendritic macrophages, an essential type of defensive cell.

Strongyloides stercoralis is a small worm that usually enters the body through the skin and lives in the small intestine. A protein given off by *Strongyloides* binds to macrophages, partially inactivating them and inducing the production of interleukin-10, a strong anti-inflammatory cytokine, thereby reducing the general immune response.

Necator americanus, the hookworm, produces a protein that inactivates eotaxin, the chemical attractant for eosinophils, thus significantly reducing the recruitment of those vital anti-parasitic cells.

And on and on it goes. Every successful parasite produces something to reduce the effectiveness of the immune system. Otherwise, they would not be a successful parasite.

All of this raises a rather interesting question. We in the developed world have a powerful, sophisticated immune system that evolved to thwart and contain parasites. It may have evolved with the "understanding" that parasites would always be around to temper its activity. But most of us in the developed world no longer have any parasites. Could our immune system, in some cases, be more than enough, perhaps too powerful? The question is more than rhetorical, as millions suffer from allergic and autoimmune diseases. Much of the immune machinery that protects us from parasites is the same that is involved in autoimmune diseases and allergies. There is a theory, and it is still just a theory, that the human immune system evolved over the millennia to accommodate itself to the reductive power of parasites. Now that parasites are not a problem in the developed world, we may have too much of an immune system for the lifestyle many enjoy. In addition to a lack of parasites, we have reduced our exposure to bacteria due to sanitation, cleansing agents, and antibiotics. The problem of an excessive immune system burden, if it exists, worsens. Over a century ago, the population suffered from some horrific infectious diseases. But the number of autoimmune disorders was reportedly minor. Today we no longer have the same staggering numbers of severe infectious diseases, but allergies and other autoimmune disorders have significantly escalated. Coincidence is not evidence of cause, but one must still ponder the possibilities and what to do about it. Some have suggested putting a few worms *back in* rather than doing everything possible to eliminate them. It will be very interesting to see where this whole matter goes.

The laboratory diagnosis of intestinal parasitic diseases is often routine. A stool specimen is obtained, processed, and examined under the microscope for the tell-tale eggs of the culprit. Special stains are applied to a blood film examined under the microscope for blood parasites such as malaria or trypanosomiasis. In some cases, special tests must be used.

Just about all of us get a **fungal** infection. Sometimes it starts early in life with a diaper rash. It might be athlete's foot, jock itch, "ringworm," toe or fingernail onychomycosis, or mouth or vaginal yeast infection. It is usually a relatively benign, nuisance type of infection. Treatment, even if needed, is generally readily available and usually effective. But some people get serious, even fatal, fungal infections with nothing benign about them. The fungi are the ultimate opportunistic pathogen.

Two types of fungi can infect humans, molds and yeasts. Some, especially the most serious ones, are mold and yeast together, depending on their environment. Our immune system is very good at preventing these more serious fungal infections. Still, a severe fungal infection can be among the most challenging infectious diseases to treat when our guard is let down, whether because of an underlying serious illness or an immune defect.

The most common molds that cause infections are known as dermatophytes, those fungi that infect our skin. They like moisture and are most commonly found between the toes or other moist places on the body. Any person can be susceptible to a dermatophyte infection, even if their immune system is fully intact. The most common infections caused by molds are athlete's foot, jock itch, nail infection, and ringworm. "Ringworm," of course, has nothing to do with worms. It is a skin infection caused by a dermatophyte fungus. The predominant genera among the dermatophytes are *Tinea, Trichophyton, Microsporum,* and *Epidermophyton.* They all require keratin in the skin to grow, so their infections are limited to the skin.

People with an underlying illness requiring serious immune-damaging therapy are susceptible to mold infections deep within their bodies. Usually, benign molds are kept at bay by an intact immune system. But when our defenses are low, some of them can pounce. Once they do, they can be tough to eradicate. The common fungus *Aspergillus* is a good example of such an opportunistic fungal pathogen. There are several others.

Then there are the deep mycoses caused by what is known as dimorphic fungi. ("Di" means two, and "morphic" means forms). These organisms exist as molds in the environment but as yeast or yeast-like organisms once they enter the body. They are serious pathogens, like *Coccidioides immitis, Blastomyces dermatididis,* and *Histoplasma capsulatum.* Most people who encounter these organisms don't get seriously ill, but a few, perhaps owing to their immune status or genetic makeup, do. Treatment can be harrowing and sometimes more toxic than the disease itself. The dimorphic fungi are deep, severe pathogens for some people.

The yeasts are interesting biological entities. We often associate them with commercial food products like wine, beer, and baked goods. But a couple of yeasts, *Candida* and *Cryptococcus*, can cause infections in humans, some of which are very serious. Most yeast infections don't occur spontaneously; some underlying problem must allow them to take hold. Like all fungi, yeasts are not susceptible to anti-bacterial antibiotics. When an antibiotic is used, it knocks out a good bit of the endemic bacterial flora in an area, allowing the resistant yeast to take hold and cause an infection. This often occurs in the vagina or mouth, where we always have a solid bacteriologic flora. These infections tend to be self-limited and relatively harmless, but some deeper yeast infections can be severe and even life-threatening. These deeper yeast infections, usually with members of the genus *Candida*, occur much more commonly in the healthcare setting, where antibiotic use and invasive procedures are often used. *Cryptococcus*, when it infects, is always serious once it sets up an infection. It is an environmental organism, but for people with a damaged immune system, such as those with HIV or undergoing cancer chemotherapy, it can cause meningitis. Once it develops an infection, it's not easy to eradicate.

The fungi are eukaryotic organisms. They have a nucleus and lack the peptidoglycan cell wall that bacteria contain, and their ribosomes differ from those of bacteria. Therefore, antibiotics used against bacteria don't touch the fungi. However, we have anti-fungal agents, some of which are very effective.

Fungi have a cell wall that differs from that of bacteria. It consists of several chemical compounds. The most common part is polysaccharides (sugars). Various substances such as chitin, β-Glucan, and a few proteins are interspersed with these. The whole thing is a gel-like substance. Most anti-fungal agents we use target parts of the fungal cell wall or the cell membrane underneath it, which human cells don't have. The effectiveness of the agents varies depending on the drug and the fungus. Some, like terbinafine, are so safe that you don't need a prescription. It's used to treat athlete's foot and other skin infections. Others, like amphotericin B (the first antifungal agent), are toxic and reserved to treat only severe deep-seated infections. Unlike antibiotics for bacterial infections, antifungal agents kill a substantially lesser number of infecting fungi. Treatment failure often occurs, prompting a second course of therapy or a trial of a second agent.

The term **virus** derives from the Latin root "vir," meaning husband. Women can make of that what they want, but it also gives us the words virtue, virile and virulent, quite a mix. The viruses were the last discovered infectious agents, even though they are the most abundant. There has always been a great debate over whether they are living creatures or merely chemical agents. A good case can be made on both sides. But it's indisputable that they are formidable infectious disease agents, covering a broad range of illnesses.

The viruses are not visible under a light microscope, nor can they be cultured in routine laboratory culture media. They are strands of nucleic acid, either DNA or RNA, and they cannot do anything outside a living cell. Without a cell to infect, they just sit there and eventually "die" and become non-infectious. Pretty much every living creature is susceptible to some virus, including bacteria.

For decades, scientists suspected the existence of something like a virus. Bacteria, fungi, and parasites were well-known after the 1880s, but there were many infectious diseases for which the causative agent was unknown. Influenza was a classic case. Despite the explicit infectious nature of the illness and the enormous social ramifications, scientists could not isolate the cause. One bacterial species, given the name *Haemophilus influenzae*, was thought to cause it but was later shown to be a secondary invader of respiratory tissue. It was highly frustrating for early researchers because they had very fine micro-filters which could trap bacteria, yet the agent of some diseases could pass right on through and not be sifted out. After years of study, this so-called "filterable agent" was identified by electron microscopy and tissue culture techniques. The term virus applies to these tiny infectious agents that every person encounters at some time.

There are many different viruses infecting many different types of cells, anything from mammals to plants to insects to bacteria. Yes, some viruses can infect bacteria. We call them phages. All viruses operate on the same principle. A virus consists of a strand of nucleic acid made of either DNA or RNA. Some are single-stranded, and some are double. It gets itself into a cell, uses the cell's metabolic mechanisms to make copies of itself, reorganizes into a mature virus, then escapes to infect another cell. Sometimes the presence of the virus is relatively mild, and life goes on as if it was never there. However, the host cells often mount a vigorous immune response, and damage to the entire host ensues. The severity of a viral infection very much depends on the virus involved, the type of host cell infected, the immune response to it, and the ability of the virus to mitigate the immune response.

In humans, there is an extensive range of consequences accompanying the infection by a virus, from you don't even know you have it to death. Most times, our immune system can handle them, but others, such as rabies and Ebola, run unchecked with dire consequences. As with any infectious agent, the immune status of the person infected is also vitally important. Herpes simplex in one individual may result in a cold sore, while a much more severe infection in an immunocompromised individual may ensue.

Viruses are classified according to the type of nucleic acid they possess, either RNA or DNA. Also important is the number of strands of each, single or double-stranded. When a virus infects, it goes about the job of forcing the host cell to manufacture many more viral copies. Some of the most virulent types code for proteins that result in shutting down part of the immune system. Some can interfere with the host cell's ability to discontinue operations and destroy itself through apoptosis, enabling the manufacture of more virions. (A virion is a single, intact, virus particle able to infect). Most viruses have just one long strand of nucleic acid. A few, such as influenza, divide their nucleic acid into segments, allowing for greater mixing and biological diversity.

Viruses are much smaller than bacteria, and they lack the essential features that are the targets of antibiotics, like cell walls and ribosomes. So, when we want to kill a virus, we are limited in our choice of drugs. Using an antibiotic to fight the virus causing a common cold is just a waste. It may even be counterproductive as it may help lead to the emergence of antibiotic-resistant bacteria. There are anti-viral drugs, but their use is limited, and treatment failures are not uncommon. Like bacteria, virus genetic material can mutate, rendering it resistant to anti-viral therapy. This is especially true of RNA viruses.

Diagnosing viral diseases can be easy, or it can be tricky. Some viral infections are diagnosed simply by examining the patient: chicken pox, warts, genital Herpes, and others are usually obvious from their presentation. In many other cases, however, laboratory tests are required to establish the causative viral agent. There are significant differences in diagnosing viral infections in the laboratory as opposed to those caused by bacteria.

Most, but certainly not all, of the bacteria that cause human infectious diseases can be cultured on artificial media. You take a sample of the infected body part or fluid and inoculate it into a well-defined amalgamation of ingredients on which the organisms grow well. Originally this medium was a soup or broth. Later a hardening agent, agar, was added so that the growing bacteria would form discreet colonies on Petri dishes. The hardened broth is often supplemented with blood products to support the growth of a wide array of bacteria, from *Acinetobacter* to *Yersinia*. Lab workers can then identify with a high level of certainty the organism causing the disease.

Not so with the viruses. They don't grow on routine laboratory culture media. They can only grow on living cells, and while living cell lines are widely available, they are expensive and require well-trained lab workers to maintain them. Viral cultures on living cellular material take several days to grow out. Viruses are usually very trophic, or specific as to what types of cells on which they can develop. Select the wrong cell type, and the infecting virus doesn't grow. Many viral infections are of limited duration and do not require specific therapy, so there is often the question of "why bother" when the test is expensive and may or may not grow anything relevant. The patient is recovered by the time the results are back. In severe infections, of course, viral cultures can be very important.

Three other tests besides viral culture are used to detect viral infections: serology, EIA tests for viral antigens, and polymerase chain reaction. Each has its uses but also its drawbacks.

In the field of serology, a sample of the patient's serum or other body fluid is examined for antibodies to the suspected virus. When positive, it indicates that the patient has been exposed to the virus or something that chemically resembles it, but it is not definitive proof that the infection is current. Sometimes multiple samples must be analyzed over several weeks. Sometimes the type of antibody detected, IgM or IgG, is a valuable clue. Serology gives a "most likely" kind of diagnosis.

EIA, or enzyme-linked immunosorbent assay, is a fancy name for merely taking a sample of infected material from a patient, either a fluid like serum or spinal fluid or a swab from an infected site and exposing it to a known antibody to the infecting organism. It's the opposite of the serology test. The drawback to the test is that it takes a relatively large number of viral particles (virions) to give a positive test. So, an EIA that is positive is usually diagnostic. A negative test does not rule out the suspected infection. EIA tests are routinely used for all types of infecting organisms, not just viruses.

Polymerase chain reaction, nearly always called PCR, is a very useful laboratory test for diagnosing a viral infectious disease. The test determines the presence of the virus' RNA or

DNA, not the entire virus or its proteins. In short, the sample to be tested is exposed to a known part of the suspected organism's known nucleic acid, called a primer. After a series of test procedures, the target organism's nucleic acid, if present, will multiply, and the result may be measured. The test is very specific but usually done for a particular infectious agent. If that virus is absent, one doesn't know what the infecting organism is. The test is excellent for ruling out some diseases or confirming a suspected diagnosis, but its scope is narrow.

Identifying the virus causing an infection is more complicated and often less conclusive than other types of organisms. Quite often, the diagnosis just goes down as "viral infection."

All the organisms that infect us can be classified into four groups: bacteria, parasites, fungi, and viruses. Each of those can be classified into various groups and subgroups. Some organisms cause infections that are relatively easy to recognize and treat. Some are enigmatic, some deadly. One thing is sure: the healthier our immune system, the better our chance against them.

Chapter 7
Little Sacs of Poison

Multi-lobed blood cells,
Always ready for action.
Granulated bombs.

Our immune system is one of immense, mind-boggling complexity. Various nouns have been used to give an overview: system, network, matrix. None of them give it justice. Layer upon layer of sophisticated cells and chemical signals work to ensure our protection from invading microorganisms. The invaders are constantly on the threshold of doing us harm, and a robust, properly functioning immune system is essential to keep the attackers at bay. Immunity to infectious organisms has been an inherent part of living creatures for eons, and because of the nature of the biological process, it is never done evolving.

At the heart of immunity is the signal. Chemicals of several classes have evolved to sound the alert about the presence of an invader. The emitted chemical signals mobilize different types of immune system cells and proteins and direct them to the infected site, alter some physiologic processes to allow for more efficient cell and protein migration, direct armaments against the pathogen, and, when the threat has abated, order the downregulation of the inflammatory response and the repair of damaged tissue.

Central to the immune response to many infectious organisms is a cell technically known as the polymorphonuclear neutrophil, quite a mouthful. Common appellations include white blood cell, leukocyte, WBC, poly, PMN, granulocyte, and neutrophil. Whatever you call them, we wouldn't last very long without these little guys. The bone marrow churns out about 100,000,000,000, or a hundred billion, daily. Most of them stay put in the bone marrow, but many enter the bloodstream, ready to receive a chemical signal directing it to an invader. Others get into the body's tissues and roam around like sentinels looking for microbial intruders. Without any action, they last just a day or two. They stick around for several days if they encounter a bacterium or a virus. They are the SWAT team of the immune system.

Neutrophils begin in the bone marrow as stem cells, then become part of the myeloid line of cells. Myeloid comes from the Greek word *myelos*, meaning marrow. The myeloid line contains several cells, including neutrophils, the cells that will become blood platelets (responsible for the clotting process), eosinophils, basophils, and the real workhorses of the immune system, monocytes. Neutrophils are the "shock troops" of the network, the shoot-now-ask-questions-later guys who are the first to arrive on the scene. They are endowed with unique components to help them do their job.

As they mature in the bone marrow from stem cells, neutrophils undergo a development pattern that takes about 14 days. They go through several stages, each characterized by their change in appearance and the addition of components that allow them to do their job when released into circulation. During bone marrow maturation, they gain the ability to directly detect the presence of an invading microbe (or to pick up the signal from another cell type alerting of an invader's presence), the ability to signal other cells as to an invader's presence, and the power to engulf the invader and destroy it. They can also damage human tissue.

Central to the neutrophil's killing power are destructive enzymes in vacuoles attached to their cell membranes. The vacuoles (from the Latin, *vacuus*, or empty) are spaces surrounded by a membrane within the neutrophil. They contain molecules that can quickly be converted into substances highly poisonous to microorganisms. The vacuoles are attached to the cell's surface membrane to facilitate quick release. As they mature in the bone marrow, three types of vacuoles form. The first is the primary or azurophilic type, and the second is the specific or secondary type. The third type is known as tertiary granules. When examined under the microscope, the vacuoles are very small and referred to as granules, hence the common term granulocyte as a synonym for neutrophil. (The term neutro-phil refers to the non-acid, non-alkaline appearance of the cells when stained with aniline dyes; they appear neutral).

The azurophilic granules are called that because they stain blue when exposed to the dye azure or similar aniline dyes.

They contain proteins that can kill microorganisms by themselves or in combination with other chemicals. Most of their contents, but not all, stay within the neutrophil during the encounter with the microbial invader.

The specific (secondary) granules also contain anti-microbial substances but have proteins that serve as receptors for signaling compounds from other cells and tissues. Most of their material is transported to the neutrophil's surface during activation, either to aid in killing invaders or to receive chemical signals to instruct the neutrophil on which way to travel.

In the mature neutrophils, there is a difference between those in the blood vessels (vascular system) and those in the extravascular tissues. Those in the blood vessels don't need to move around much since they just go with the flow of the circulatory system. And they don't need to produce much energy since they are in a relatively passive state. Neutrophils outside the blood vessels need to trigger two systems to function: activate internal structural proteins called actins to aid their motility, and switch on their glycogen system to provide energy as they migrate and entrap microbes. When a blood vessel neutrophil leaves the circulatory system, it starts to genetically transform into a tissue neutrophil.

One of the more intriguing characteristics of neutrophils is their ability to stick to the interior lining of blood vessels. The cells forming the inner lining of blood vessels form a wall. It is a smooth, watertight layer known as the endothelium. Neutrophils circulate in the blood vessels, but when an organism invades, they must get to the infected site as soon as possible. They do this in a fascinating way. As they travel along in the bloodstream, they have an attachment protein that forms a very loose bond with the endothelial cells. It makes for a touch-and-go landing, just slowing down to see if anything is happening in the area. Proteins on both the neutrophil and the endothelial cells, called selectins, interact to allow the neutrophil to come to a very brief slowing along the endothelial lining.

When something big is happening nearby, the endothelial cells lining the blood vessels receive chemical signals from the infected site. They then release a chemical signal of their own, an extended protein, letting passing neutrophils know there is trouble afoot. When the extended protein is displayed, the neutrophil makes a firm attachment to this endothelial protein, one strong enough to halt its movement in the blood circulation. Then it migrates out of the bloodstream and into the neighboring tissue. Like a bloodhound following a scent, it follows a chemical trail until it reaches the infected site within the body.

The chief chemical attractant for neutrophils is interleukin-8 (IL-8). Many cells, including macrophages and epithelial cells, can send out IL-8 after encountering a microbial invader. Because IL-8 attracts a cell, it is technically called a chemokine rather than a cytokine, but very often the term cytokine is used. Genetic differences exist in the construction of IL-8 in different individuals and populations. Some people have a more vigorous engagement of neutrophils than others, resulting in more or fewer neutrophils arriving at a site. This can influence the outcome of the disease condition. (Another abbreviation for IL-8 is CXCL-8). Another important chemical attractant is interleukin-17 (IL-17), which is produced by a type of lymphocyte.

Once they arrive at the infected site, they do what they were born to do: kill. Neutrophils are endowed with an incredible array of toxin-containing granules to carry out their mission. First, the bacterial prey is surrounded by a neutrophil, phagocytized (from the Greek, *phagein*, to eat, devour), and placed in a vacuole called a phagosome. The bacteria-containing phagosome is then brought into contact with those toxin-containing granules of the primary or azurophilic type. These then merge with the phagosome, and the killing power of the neutrophil is unleashed.

Some bacteria have derived the means to evade neutrophils. Some have motility that helps them scoot away, or they have a gooey capsule surrounding them that can repel the neutrophil's advances. To assist the neutrophil in its quest to surround the invader and engulf it, other members of the immune system pitch in. The complement system is most notable in the endeavor. It can act alone or in concert with antibodies. The invading organism is anchored to the neutrophil's surface, allowing phagocytosis. This assistance given to the neutrophil enabling it to capture its prey is known as opsonization.

After the killing is complete, the neutrophil dies. The cell death is usually self-induced, a process called apoptosis (from the Greek, *apo*, off, and *ptosis*, falling, or falling off. It is pronounced two ways, either pronouncing or omitting the second p). Generally, the process is relatively orderly, with the dead neutrophils and their contents consumed and carried off by friendly cells called macrophages. But when the infectious process is heavy, the dead white blood cells accumulate, and pus is formed.

Pus is technically called "liquor puris," but everybody just calls it pus. It is usually some shade of whitish yellow, but sometimes it has a greenish hue because it contains the enzyme myeloperoxidase from the neutrophil's azurophilic granules. When pus becomes locked in a compartment, it is referred to as an abscess, a sure sign of an infectious process. Quite a few medical words begin with the prefix Pyo..., which refers to the presence of pus. The term pyogenic refers to a pus-generating type of infection. The presence of significant numbers of neutrophils and various chemical activators in a body site is known as inflammation.

In the book, *The Healing Hand,* an insightful review of the practice of medicine in the ancient world, Guido Majno wrote a colorful summary of the significance of pus:

"Pus is therefore a noble substance: it is made of brave cells that never sneak back into the blood vessels to escape; they all die in the line of duty. Note also the double meaning of suppuration: it indicates that there is an infection, but also that the body is fighting it well. The outcome of the battle can be predicted, to some extent, from the aspect of the pus, as was observed even in ancient times. The whitish, creamy kind (and therefore rich in polys) is "prefer-able," because it indicates that an infection is being fought effectively. Hence its ancient Latin name of pus bonum et laudable, 'good and laudable pus.' Thin or malodorous pus suggests a poor defense of especially vicious bacteria."

100

When everything works well, the process of infection protection by neutrophils is orderly. Billions of neutrophils are produced in the bone marrow. Some enter the bloodstream and circulate; others roam around the body's tissues seeking invaders. When an invader is detected, chemical signals are sent from the site to the cells lining the inside of the nearest blood vessel. Proteins are projected to halt the circulating neutrophils, which usually slow down momentarily as they float in the blood. After it is speared, the circulating neutrophil begins to change into a roaming type and wiggles its way out of the bloodstream, following a series of chemical "breadcrumbs" to the infected site. Once there, it starts gobbling up invading microbes, kills them, then dies a peaceful death.

The details of how this all transpires are, of course, extremely complicated. By their very nature, neutrophils are a hazardous material. The enzymes and substances contained in their granules harm not only their microbial prey but also human tissue. Like a hand grenade with a safety pin, the immune system is endowed with checks and balances to prevent an unfortunate release of harmful chemicals.

The materials released from the primary granules are an impressive array of substances poisonous to bacteria. Perhaps the most important is one known as **myeloperoxidase** or **MPO**. After a complicated set of reactions, MPO activation results in the microbe's exposure to what amounts to bleach.

Defensins are tiny proteins widely found in nature. They are an integral part of the primary granules. Their job is to become stuck in the invading microbe's membranes to allow the leakage of cytoplasmic components. Defensins are active against a broad range of bacteria, fungi, and even some viruses.

Lactoferrin is a protein found widely in bodily fluids, including breast milk, tears, saliva, and nasal secretions. It is also one of the essential components of the secondary granules of neutrophils. It plays several different roles, but a major one is to act as an iron sponge, thus depriving bacteria of an essential growth requirement. It can also directly damage bacterial membranes, causing leakage and cell death. In addition to directly damaging invading microbes, lactoferrin has several effects on the immune system. It is stored in the secondary granules and is thus secreted out of the neutrophil and not thrust into the phagosome. It reduces the surface charge of the cells, thus promoting the cell-to-cell "stickiness" and adherence of neutrophils to local tissues and other neutrophils, concentrating the cells in the affected area. It also reduces the release of specific signaling molecules, thus helping to control the level of the immune response.

Lysozyme is an active protein found in both the secondary and primary granules. Like lactoferrin, it is also found in tears and other bodily secretions. Lysozyme disrupts the structure of bacterial cell walls, causing leakage and death. (The first scientist to describe the effect of lysozyme was Scottish microbiologist Alexander Fleming, who noticed in 1922 that drops of sweat from his nose killed colonies of bacteria on his culture plate. Six years later, Fleming noticed that a mold growing on his culture plate similarly inhibited bacterial growth. The mold was *Penicillium*).

In addition to myeloperoxidase, defensins, lactoferrin, and lysozyme, neutrophil primary granules contain many other antimicrobial substances. These include about a dozen different types of enzymes that assist in the killing and degradation of invading organisms.

The secondary granules, also known as specific granules, release their contents mainly to the cell's exterior. Before doing that, however, they have a significant role in initiating the killing process. They contain what is known as the NADPH oxidase system, which is responsible for creating an "oxygen burst" that begins the degranulation process. The result of this oxygen burst is a significant lowering of the pH of the phagosome with resultant activation of the contents of the primary granules.

The secondary granules also play an important role in producing substances that aid in recognizing immune signaling and adhesion to surrounding tissues and assisting in opsonization.

There is a third type of granule, less abundant than the primary and secondary but nonetheless important. They are the tertiary granules containing substances necessary for the neutrophil's migration through tissue.

With their many weapons, neutrophils are very effective at actively killing intruders. Perhaps even more remarkable is that they very often kill invading microbes even after they have completed their job and are dead. When the cell's mission is complete and it begins to degrade, its DNA and some RNA are released, taking with it some of the cell proteins and material from the granules. This soup of chromatin, granule proteins, and some assorted proteins forms a web that can entrap microbes. The bugs can either be killed directly by the natural antibiotics present or held in place to be attacked by other cells. This phenomenon is known by one of the best acronyms ever, NET, for neutrophil extracellular traps.

Endowed with such an array of weapons, neutrophils are incredible killing machines. But with all that firepower, they must be directed appropriately. Indiscriminate activation and release of all that poison would be catastrophic to our health. The superoxide radical produced during the oxygen burst is highly destructive to human tissue, as are the following products of hydrogen peroxide and hypochlorite (bleach). Collagen is a substance that is the "glue" holding normal tissue together, but the neutrophil produces collagenase, essentially dissolving the organic cement to allow for the migration of immune cells through the tissue. All these substances must be tightly controlled and shut down when the danger of the invading microbe is passed. One very influential component of this control apparatus is the macrophage.

When a neutrophil and a macrophage randomly bump into one another, usually in the bone marrow, the two hook up, and the cells lock together. If the neutrophil is OK, that is, undamaged and just going about its business; it emits certain chemical messengers that notify the attendant macrophage that all is well. If, on the other hand, it is not OK, either it is too old or has been eating and destroying too many microbial invaders, the macrophage is equipped to take it out, liquidate it, basically, to eat it. Without this orderly process of spent neutrophil removal, all hell would break loose, and we would suffer grievous consequences.

Once the threat of infection is over, chemical signals are sent to various body areas. These signals essentially end the profusion of neutrophil migration and infiltration into infected tissues and begin the process of tissue repair. Much of this signaling comes from the macrophages.

One of the primary chemical signals designed to end the inflammatory condition is interleukin-10 (IL-10). It is secreted by several cell types, including macrophages, and has the very important effect of reversing the emission of pro-inflammatory chemical signals. It and several similar chemicals put a brake on neutrophil infiltration into tissues. Without this anti-inflammatory measure, life would not be at all pleasant.

The neutrophils and their entourage of cells and chemicals are a formidable force in protecting our bodies. Without our knowing about it, they guard us against harmful microbial invasions around the clock for our entire lives. Their level of performance is truly amazing. But bacteria and other little critters are resourceful; some have developed the means to overcome the neutrophil's best efforts. Some examples:

The organism *Staphylococcus aureus*, usually called just Staph, is equipped with several means to defeat neutrophils. They form an enzyme called catalase that destroys the hydrogen peroxide produced during the oxygen burst. As its name aureus implies (*aureus* is Latin for gold), colonies of the organism are golden in color owing to the production of a gold pigment. This pigment is an antioxidant that allows the organism to escape the effect of superoxide in the phagosome. Staph can clot plasma and tissue fluid, surrounding itself with a gooey mass that inhibits its being engulfed by neutrophils, the process of phagocytosis. A similar substance clots the tissues surrounding the infected site inhibiting neutrophil migration. (These clotting substances are called coagulase. One is bound to the bacterial cell; the other is freed to clot surrounding tissues). A staphylococcal protein known as Protein A binds the Fc portion of an antibody, effectively reducing its ability to engage with complement and hence inhibit opsonization. Staph also makes a rather vile substance called the Panton-Valentine Leucocidin (PVL), which can destroy neutrophils and other tissues.

Other organisms have their own set of similar or unique anti-phagocytic faculties. Some of these can be transferred to other organisms genetically. The body's defenses are constantly evolving because the threats upon it are never at rest. It's a truly fascinating game.

Indicators of infection. Since neutrophils are called upon when an infectious process is underway, they can be a good indicator of such. In the laboratory, we can measure the number of neutrophils and other white blood cells in a blood sample and observe their presence in other bodily specimens. An increase in their numbers can tell us that an inflammatory condition exists. After that, further investigation is needed to determine the nature and cause of the infection or other malady.

Blood samples from normal individuals show a range of neutrophils, other white and red blood cells, and platelets. A standard laboratory test is called the complete blood count, or CBC. When the proper equipment is available, it is a quick and easy-to-perform test that measures the numbers and condition of the red blood cells, white blood cells, and platelets. Each of these measurements has normal ranges. If the normal is exceeded, further testing and examination are usually needed to determine the cause of the ailment and possible treatment.

Humans normally have around 4 to 10 billion white blood cells in every liter of blood, clearly too many to count, so a small amount of blood is taken, and the result of the count is expressed as the number of cells in a microliter, or 1/1000, of a liter. The abbreviation for microliter is mcl. A normal range for all white blood cells (WBC) is 4,000-10,000 WBC/mcl. Neutrophils also have a normal range among the total white blood cells. An observation is made of the percentage of each type of white blood cell present. This is called the differential. The normal range for neutrophils is usually 1,500 to 8,000 cells/mcl.

High white blood cell numbers in the blood is known as leukocytosis (*leuko* referring to the white, *cyto* referring to cells, and *osis* referring to a condition). Conversely, a reduced white blood cell count in the blood is known as leukopenia (*penia*, from the Greek, meaning poverty or lack). The words high or elevated are relative, and there is no magic number above which one can conclude an infectious process is going on. Markedly elevated WBC, say over 20,000, raises a red flag in clinical settings. Mildly elevated, for instance, 11,000, might increase one's suspicions, especially if other clinical signs are observed. Of course, a high white count doesn't say what type of infection it is or where it is. It is an indication that one should diligently seek out a cause.

The neutrophils' level of maturity in the blood can also indicate a recent or current infection. While in the bone marrow, maturing neutrophils have a round nucleus. When they are ready to leave the bone marrow and enter circulation, their nucleus becomes multi-lobed. But if the body needs a sudden burst of neutrophils to fight an ongoing infection, the cells are released from the bone marrow a bit early, before the nucleus has had time to divide into its usual 3-5 segments. While not round, the nuclei of these immature cells have a "C" shape or an indented oval. Such cells are traditionally called "bands." On charts picturing the entire neutrophil maturation from nascent blast cell to mature form, the cells are typically illustrated with the least mature forms on the left of the diagram. So, an increase in the number of band neutrophils, from a normal of 1 or 2 percent to considerably more, is often noted as a "shift to the left," meaning the bone marrow has diligently pumped out neutrophils at a high rate to meet a current need. A significantly elevated WBC with a neutrophil shift to the left indicates a probable infection occurring somewhere in the body. Usually, but not always, an infection with this type of white cell response is caused by bacteria.

We can also observe neutrophils in specimens other than blood. Many types of body fluids and tissue samples can be examined under a microscope in a laboratory. Neutrophils are a good indicator of an inflammatory condition, quite often infectious. A good example would be urine. Normal urine has very few white blood cells in it. When we put a sample of several milliliters of urine in a tube, centrifuge it, and examine the sediment under a microscope, we see very few white cells. Perhaps an occasional one, after reviewing several fields under a magnification of 400 times. But if there is an infection in the bladder or the kidneys, there will be many WBC in the urine

106

sediment. Of course, it doesn't tell us what organism is causing the infection and its exact location. Still, it indicates that further testing and examination are needed, especially if the patient displays symptoms of urinary tract infection.

The neutrophils are a genuinely great segment of our immune system. Produced at a rate of over one hundred billion a day, present in our blood and tissues, and ready to attack an invader in a relatively short time, they represent the core of the innate immune system. The acquired immune system is more specific and fine-tuned but takes several days to get up to speed. The neutrophils hold infections at bay until the immune system is entirely on board.

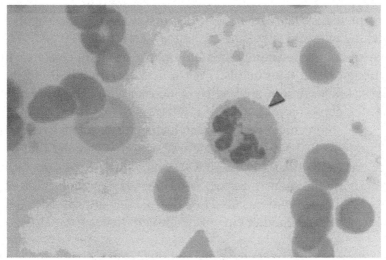

Neutrophils have a multi-lobed nucleus and are interspersed with numerous granules (PHIL).

Chapter 8
First Responder

Works well with others.
Complicated complement
Can still work alone.

An essential immune system constituent at the center of several operations is an array of proteins collectively known as complement. It's a rather odd label. The original name assigned to it in the latter 19th century was alexine (from the Greek *aleksis*, or "defender," "to ward off"). It was later changed to complement for its role in "complementing" the immune system. An antibody would bind to an antigen on the invading organism. Then the antibody would also bind to complement. Complement then acts as a bridge, assisting the neutrophil in latching onto and engulfing the antigen-carrying pathogen. This system envisioned complement as only working in concert with antibodies and neutrophils. We now know it acts in several ways, often without antibodies or neutrophils. Maybe alexine was the correct term after all.

Complement is not one molecule but a system of around 30 proteins that act in a cascade-like action. Once the first one becomes activated, it turns on a second, which turns on a third, and so on, through number 9. Some of the molecules are proenzymes or zymogens. They don't enter the cascade; their role is to signal another enzyme or protein to become active.

In what is known as the classical pathway, an antibody combined with its specific antigen meets up with the complement protein known as C1q. Two other molecules, C1r and C1s, attach, creating the C1 complex. Since this system was discovered first, it has been known as the classical pathway.

Now that the first component of the complement system, the C1 complex, is formed, a cascade of chemical activation events occurs. Components C2 and C4 are rapidly engaged. The whole group, C1 complex-C2-C4, is called C3 convertase. C3 convertase activates a very potent destroyer of microbes, C3. In a way, that's an unfortunate name. C3 is not just another complement factor. It has a history. A long history, say a few hundred million years. C3 is not just found in people or other vertebrates; it or its close chemical relative is present in almost every invertebrate. It is the original antimicrobial force.

C3 contains a magic bullet of microbe destruction, the *thioester bond*. Combining a sulfur atom and a carboxyl group confers on the protein the ability to attach to and disrupt just about any fatty acid, including those of membranes. The thioester is so powerful that it must be hidden inside the folded protein. Once the C3 contacts the C3 convertase (the combination of C1, C2, and C4), it opens, exposing the thioester.

The microbe is now getting it from two directions: While complement factor 3 unleashes its destructive forces on the microbial membranes, the whole complex becomes firmly attached to the neutrophil's surface. Phagocytic cells such as neutrophils and macrophages have on their surface several proteins that adhere to activated C3. The most prominent of these is complement receptor 1, or CR1, but there are others. So one part of C3 is attached to the invading microbe, the other to the phagocytic cell that aims to engulf and destroy it. After docking, the process of phagocytosis begins.

C3 is a potent force. It has the inherent ability to destroy an invading microbe directly, and it aids in the attachment of the microbe and its bound antibody to the neutrophil surface, setting it up for entrapment and destruction. But there's more. C3 splits into two parts, one known as C3b, the destructive and attachment part, and into C3a, a smaller part that drifts away. But it doesn't just drift away and disappear. When little C3a contacts an epithelial surface, mast cell, or macrophage, it signals to the immune system that an invader is present. The result is an influx of more complement molecules and a large part of the innate immune system. Even the liver is activated, producing more defense-type proteins of all classes. It's teamwork at its finest.

Another accomplishment of complement factor 3 is its ability to signal the activation of other members of the complement cascade, notably C5. Like C3, activated C5 divides into two parts, C5a and C5b. The C5a is smaller and behaves much like C3a in activating the rest of the immune system. With the C5b now active, the other members of the complement cascade, C6, C7, C8, and C9, are all turned on and attached, giving this great big aggregate known as the MAC, or membrane attack complex.

The MAC is powerful stuff; once active, it can take out just about anything with a membrane, including us. We can envision it as a tube, with the final product, the hammer-like C9, oriented at a 90° angle to the surface. The whole thing can insert itself into the pathogen's membrane, with the C9 part extending down the deepest. The C9 molecules form a channel, allowing for the two-way flow of water and solutes. The microbe is then subjected to a sudden imbalance in pH and nutrient content, disrupting the integrity of the cell. Death to the microbe is the usual result.

All this activated complement is powerful, and it can take out membranes at a very rapid rate. Viruses do not have traditional cellular membranes, so they are spared the complement attack. But bacteria, fungi, and parasites all have cell membranes and are vulnerable.

Of course, all our cells have membranes and are just as vulnerable to a complement attack as an invading microbe. All the complement factors are constantly in the bloodstream, and it is not unusual for them to activate spontaneously. The system must be very tightly controlled.

The primary safeguard against a complement attack against self is that C3b is rapidly degraded if it doesn't attach immediately to a membrane surface. Water molecules will inactivate the thioester linkage that is so important. Since the C3b is usually activated and deposited on the pathogen surface, it doesn't have time to float around and attach to a host cell membrane. But it can happen. The same is true for the MAC.

All our cells are equipped to rebuff an inadvertent complement attack. Proteins are present in our cell membranes that can dissociate the activated complement. Several are normally present, and they usually act by inactivating C3b, inactivating the C3 convertase so that C3b is never formed, or inactivating the membrane attack complex. A protein called CD59, or protectin, is particularly effective in this latter task. With the C9 component, the MAC is effective. Removing C9 from the complex significantly inactivates it. CD59 is very good at doing this, and our cells are usually not at risk. If a person's CD59 is defective, much trouble can ensue.

To sum up, complement assists the neutrophil in microbe destruction by linking to an antibody attached to a microbe's surface, unwinding itself to become active, and directly destroying the microbe's membranes while attaching the whole complex to the surface of the neutrophil to facilitate phagocytosis.

The attachment of the antibody complex plus the appropriate complement components to the neutrophil surface is known as opsonization (from the Greek *opsonein*, "to prepare for eating"). The complement-antibody complex is known as the opsonin. All cells naturally have a net negative charge, so without the opsonin to bind the neutrophil with its prey, much energy would be lost with the cell chasing it down. Opsonization is a well-coordinated system that has evolved into a very effective killing machine.

But what if there is no antibody? Complement can still be activated by not just one but two other pathways. Many microbes have on their surface a carbohydrate known as mannose. When encountered, the presence of mannose activates the C2 and C4 components of complement, resulting in the activation of C3, just as in the classic pathway. Because mannose is a carbohydrate and is bound by a protein, it is in the general chemical class known as a lectin. The mannan-binding pathway is called the lectin pathway.

The other pathway is remarkable. It's been given the name alternative pathway because the "classic pathway" was discovered and described by scientists first, but it was the original way complement factor 3 functioned. C3, the ancient defense molecule, sometimes spontaneously opens to pick up a water molecule, becoming $C3_{H2O}$. When it does, it is very destructive, capable of destroying cellular membranes, whether they belong to an invading microbe or the body's tissue. Fortunately, the survival time of $C3_{H2O}$ is extremely limited, just a few milliseconds. Without the proper additives, it disintegrates.

Those needed "additives" are three proteins found in the serum and tissues. The liver produces them, and their amounts increase in times of inflammation, so we have a lot more of them when we become infected by a microbe. They are all rather complex proteins but go by the simple names of Factor B, Factor D, and Properdin (sometimes called Factor P).

When C3 adds the water molecule, its shape changes. Usually, it self-destructs, but if there happens to be a molecule of Factor B floating close by, along with a molecule of Factor D, the picture changes. Factor B is cleaved by Factor D as it binds to C3. This complex isn't very stable, but if a molecule of properdin is readily available, it also bonds and stabilizes the mixture of C3 and a big part of Factor B. This big thing, C3-Factor B-Properdin, can then bind to and disrupt the membrane of an invading microbe and act as a catalyst to initiate the rest of the complement cascade. It's pretty incredible.

Our bodies are equipped with a guardian against the reckless release of the alternative complement cascade. It is Factor H, a protein that can be found free in the serum or as part of the surface molecules of our cells. Factor H binds and inactivates the reactive complement. If the invading microbe is attacked first, so be it. If no microbe is present, Factor H takes care of our cells.

When all goes well, our complement system is highly efficient. Every day it is there for us, either assisting other immune system components or removing a potential invader on its own. Once it is initiated either by contact with an engaged antibody (classic pathway), directly attaching to an invading microbe's mannose component (lectin pathway), or spontaneously hooking up with Factors B, D, and P to initiate the cascade on its own (alternative pathway), complement provides us with a strong and dependable defense against invaders.

Many molecular parts are involved in complement's activities, and all are subject to genetic alterations, either large or small. A fundamental defect in a component of our complement system sometimes results in a defect in our immunity to infectious diseases. Perhaps one of the best-known involves the pathogenic bacterium *Neisseria meningitides,* a cause of a potentially lethal type of bacterial meningitis. The organism invades by first colonizing the epithelial cells lining our respiratory tract, then directly enters the cell and travels right on through, reaching the tissues underneath. It is up to our innate immune system, including complement and neutrophils, to arrest the infection right at that point. But some people, estimated to be around one in every 20,000 to 40,000, have a defect in a complement component between numbers 5 and 9, preventing the complete elimination of the pathogen, allowing it to spread into the bloodstream and settle in the meninges, often with a fatal outcome. This one fact illustrates the vital role of the complement system in helping preserve our health.

Chapter 9
Safety Net

Roaming our bodies,
Defending us, aiding us.
True multi-tasker

If we think of the neutrophils as the ground troops in the war against infectious diseases, then the macrophages are the special operations guys. They're like the Navy SEALS, Delta Force, Force Reconnaissance, and the British SAS. They can do the work of the neutrophil, detecting and annihilating microbial invaders, but they take the warfare to another level.

Macrophages come in all shapes, sizes, and functions. An important group are mobile macrophages roaming around the body, always looking for action. Like neutrophils, some are produced in the bone marrow each day in large numbers and make their way into the bloodstream. When a macrophage enters the bloodstream from the bone marrow, it is called a **monocyte**. When common stains are applied to a blood film in the lab and the slide is examined under the microscope, the monocyte is easy to recognize. They are quite a bit bigger than neutrophils, and their nucleus ranges from round to a "C" shape. The outer edge of the cell is very even, with a well-formed border. In the healthy state, about 5-10% of the white blood cells in our bloodstream are monocytes.

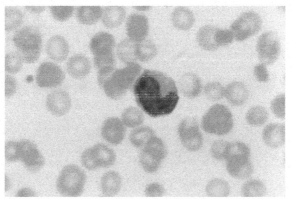

Monocytes are larger than neutrophils, have a smooth outer edge, and a large nucleus. (PHIL

114

The monocytes circulate and bump along the blood vessels just like the neutrophils do. Like neutrophils, when they are needed in the tissues, they are stopped in their tracks by chemical structures displayed on the endothelial cells lining the blood vessels. They leave the bloodstream and enter tissues like their neutrophil cousins. But when they leave the bloodstream, monocytes are transformed. They are now known as **macrophages**. Chemically, they undergo several changes enabling them to better recognize and destroy microbial invaders and alert the immune system's other components of the impending danger. They also change physically, with their formerly smooth outer membrane appearing fuzzy and ruffled.

Wandering macrophages are divided into two main types. Some resemble an amoeba, more or less round, with a prominent nucleus. And some look like trees. These odd-looking things are called the dendritic cells, from the Greek *dendrites*, meaning "tree." Like trees, they are characterized by having many branches. All the better to detect and latch onto an invading microbe.

Mobile macrophages are much bigger than neutrophils. The blood monocyte is about twice as large, and after they leave the blood and mature into macrophages, they get even bigger. Compared to neutrophils, they are also a lot slower. If we think of the neutrophils as jeeps and half-tracks, the macrophages are tanks. They are the last to arrive on the scene but hang around the longest. One great advantage the macrophage has over the neutrophil is that the former can handily synthesize proteins, whereas the latter is, with a few exceptions, dormant in that regard. That makes the macrophage much more adaptable to varied conditions and circumstances.

Macrophages and neutrophils share some important qualities. They both are built to respond to chemical signals leading them to the infection site and engulf and destroy microbes. The molecular direction-givers, or chemical attractants, are known as chemokines. Given off by cells at the affected area, chemokines are strewn out along the path the phagocytes travel to their destination. They also send a powerful signal to the endothelial cells lining the local blood vessels to begin to trap the circulating white blood cell and allow it to leave the capillary and start on its extravascular way. They signal the monocytes to exit the blood vessel and head off to the infected site. They also get the monocyte to "grow up," mobilizing its antimicrobial armamentarium. Without the chemokines, the neutrophils and macrophages would waste valuable time searching for a target. They can't just stop and ask for directions.

Once the mature macrophage reaches the infected site, it performs several duties. First on its list is to eat up, or phagocytize, the microbial invader. It is also designed to send chemical messengers to other immune cells, enabling them to mobilize and join the battle. These two tasks are part of the innate immune system, the "put out the fire" first response mechanism. But the macrophages, as opposed to the neutrophils, have another important job. They must process the little parts of the invading microbe and present them for recognition by the cells of the adaptive immune system, the lymphocytes.

Macrophages are equipped with several chemical "sensors" that can detect various microbial invaders. Just as we can readily distinguish between a mammal, a bird, and a reptile, the macrophage can distinguish a virus, a bacterium, a fungus, and a parasite, by detecting unique chemical groups associated with each type of organism. When it does so, it sends out chemical messengers called cytokines that travel to the sections of the body where they are active. In doing this, the macrophage initiates a cascade of events designed to eliminate the current threat of the invading microbe and ensure that it doesn't happen again. They also are involved in the repair of the damaged site.

Macrophages are not a single, homogenous population. They can be divided into two main groups. Those that are aggressive microbe fighters are known as the M1 population. They are pro-inflammatory. The other main category of macrophages is known as M2. They are the damage control group, involved in tissue repair; they are anti-inflammatory. Chemical signals from the affected site tell monocytes which way to go: Interferon-gamma and other cytokines stimulate them to become the M1 type, while interleukin-4, among others, leads them toward the M2 type.

116

Phagocytosis by macrophages is essentially the same as phagocytosis by neutrophils. When available, an opsonin, such as complement bound to the microbe, binds to the receptor on the macrophage, and the microbe is then surrounded and engulfed. The internalized macrophage membrane containing the microbe, known as the phagosome, is then joined inside the cell by a lysosome, which contains a variety of anti-microbial substances. Here the macrophage differs from the neutrophil, which has three different types of lysosomic granules. The macrophage has just one type, but it is very powerful. Filled with digestive enzymes, the macrophage lysosome is efficiently walled off from the cell's cytosol. But when the macrophage engulfs a microbe, the bug-containing phagosome and the poison-containing lysosome merge. The merged lysosome releases its powerful anti-microbial contents, killing and digesting the microbe. This action is like the neutrophil. But the macrophage takes it to another level. The digested material is broken down into peptides of about a dozen or so amino acids in length. This little piece of the microbe is then displayed on the surface of the macrophage so that other members of the immune system may detect it and develop an immune response explicitly directed toward the microbe that bore it. This is the beginning of the process we call acquired immunity.

Our bodies are equipped with numerous mechanical means of repelling microbial invaders. Our skin, mucus, urine flow, sweat, tears, hairs, cilia, saliva, gastric juice, vaginal secretions, and nasal secretions all help us ward off the tiny creatures that would penetrate us. But, of course, they do get through. It's crucial that we have a backup. And we do. We have a "safety net." Spread adroitly throughout our organs, the cells making up the Mononuclear Phagocyte System are a marvelous scheme of well-positioned cells designed to monitor for and attack invaders. While many monocytes and macrophages are usually on the move, either rolling along in blood vessels (monocytes) or meandering through tissues looking for microbial prey (macrophages and dendritic cells), the cells of the Mononuclear Phagocyte System are relatively stationary, embedded in the tissues they protect. They, too, are indispensable to our health.

Members of the Mononuclear Phagocyte System associate themselves early in life with the tissue in which they'll spend their career. They are assigned jobs besides simple pathogen recognition and removal, such as red blood cell removal and recycling, bone sculpture and remodeling, and removal of extraneous material in sensitive areas such as the brain.

For a long time, this system was called the reticuloendothelial system, or RES. "reticulo" comes from the Latin word for net, *reticulum*. Endothelial refers to the position the cells would assume, the single cell layers bordering blood flow. Historically, they were given names according to where they were found, the name of the person who first described them, or what they looked like. They assume roles unique to their location and situation.

A partial list:

Kupffer cells, liver. These cells line the liver sinusoids and are thus exposed to large amounts of blood surging through their area, being intimately connected with the endothelial cell lining. They have a very irregular surface that extends into the space where the blood flows, giving them a lot of surface area. They look something like the teats on the udder of a cow. Their job is to constantly monitor for and remove microbial and other bloodstream debris. Since they are near the intestinal tract, they have a lot to do. Being macrophages, albeit fixed in place, they are well equipped to send various chemical signals alerting the rest of the immune system of potential dangers. Kupffer cells are especially good at hooking onto bacteria coated by complement, removing it from the blood, and processing it to initiate antibody or cellular immunity. They also play a major role in removing and breaking down old, worn-out red blood cells. They comprise about 80-90% of the body's Mononuclear Phagocyte System.

Alveolar macrophages, lungs. Another set of resident macrophages with a lot to do are those located in the lungs, the alveolar macrophages. As the name suggests, they are located deep in the lungs, at the terminal bronchi, and adjacent to the alveoli, where air exchange occurs. Unfortunately, the air we breathe is likely to contain lots of stuff besides air: bacteria, mold spores, viruses, dust, pollen, and who knows what else comes into us, along with oxygen and other gases. The body is very good at filtering out a lot of this stuff with the lining of the upper airway, with things like mucus, hairs, and cilia. But, alas, something will manage to get through.

The alveolar macrophages are good at gobbling up and digesting microorganisms, but they also clean up much of the non-microbial gunk that gets in. So important is their work that they have a helper, the alveolar type II epithelial cells, also known as type II pneumocytes. These helper cells have several important roles in lung function. A critical one is to make two proteins, Surfactant Proteins A and D, which can attach to microbes that enter the deep part of the lung. These recognize and bind to specific markers on microbes, then act as opsonins, presenting the attached microbe to the alveolar macrophage for phagocytosis and digestion. When functioning correctly, the system is very good at preventing infection.

Langerhans cells, skin. The macrophages take on three very different shapes, depending on where you find them. In the blood, they are known as monocytes, large white blood cells looking somewhat like a big neutrophil, with a nucleus the shape of a letter C. The outer part of the cell is well-defined. The macrophages wandering in our tissues have a much more scattered and rough outer membrane, and the nucleus is round. Then there is a third type of macrophage, the dendritic cell. It looks like a starfish, with appendages appearing as tentacles. The first one discovered was in the skin, described in 1868 by a rather remarkable medical student named Paul Langerhans. Remarkable in the fact that at age 21 he discovered not just one but two cell types later named after him, the islets of Langerhans in the pancreas and the Langerhans cells in the skin. Because of their appearance, he thought those cells found in the skin were nervous tissue, but they were a type of macrophage with " tentacles " resembling the dendrites of nerves. The Langerhans cells of our skin are firmly embedded within the living skin tissue to encounter any invaders that come in that way. Like any good macrophage, they can ingest, digest, and present any microbe they encounter. Most importantly, they send out numerous chemical signals alerting several types of immune cells to the presence of an invader in the area. Dendritic cells form a vital part of the immune system, and the Langerhans cells of the skin were the first described.

Bone Marrow and spleen macrophages. Red blood cells and white blood cells have entirely different appearances and functions in the body. We naturally think of them as distinct, sharing only their site of origin in the bone marrow and their circulation in the bloodstream. But red blood cells, those noble, tireless oxygen carriers, owe their very existence to the activity of macrophages. So too, they owe their death. And lots of close supervision in between.

Red blood cells (called corpuscles, from the Latin *corpusculum*, or "small body") arise in the bone marrow from erythroblasts, similar to the means that give rise to leukocytes. As they mature in the bone marrow, erythroblasts attach themselves to a central macrophage through a chemical bridge known as a ligand. As many as a dozen erythroblasts can connect to a single macrophage in an erythroblast island. While attached, two vital things happen. Iron is transferred from the macrophage to the growing red blood cell for incorporation into hemoglobin. When the developing red blood cell matures, it aborts its nucleus, which the macrophage picks up and metabolizes. When mature and ready to circulate, the macrophage escorts the newly formed red blood cell (often called a reticulocyte since it is a little bit larger than a typical RBC and still retains fragments of nuclear material) to an area of the bone marrow where it can gain easy access to the bloodstream. This is quite an operation. We make about ten billion RBCs per day.

Typical red blood cells remain in circulation for about 120 days. They have a rough time of it, squeezing through capillaries, rolling around and bumping into things, and never getting a rest. At the end of their 120 days, they are worn out.

120

They signal this senescence by displaying several chemical markers on their cell membrane. When detected by a resident macrophage, either in the spleen or liver, they are gobbled up and removed from circulation. A very detailed process recycles their hemoglobin; some parts are used again, and some are excreted through the bile duct as bilirubin. The iron they contain is precious, and potentially dangerous. If iron circulated freely in large amounts it would be toxic. Also, invading pathogenic bacteria need iron to survive. Sequestering it onto carrier proteins makes it much less available to the microbe and less toxic for us. The macrophages scoop up the iron and attach it to a carrier protein, transferrin. The transferrin makes its way to the liver, where the iron is transferred to a storage molecule, ferritin. When needed for the formation of new RBCs, the iron is transferred back onto transferrin and carried back to the bone marrow, where it is incorporated into the bone marrow macrophages and then into the erythroblasts. A pretty complicated system, but it works.

Iron management is a vital function. Not only is it required for red blood cell function, but it is also an essential element in many other metabolic systems. That applies not only to humans and mammals but to all life forms, including microbes. For bacteria to infect us, they must have iron. Since all our iron is tied up either attached to hemoglobin inside an RBC or on a protein of either transferrin or ferritin, no free iron is available for the bacteria. So, just like people who take what they want at gunpoint, the bacteria have devised a method to get what they need. They produce a protein known as a siderophore (from the Greek, "iron carrier"). When environmental iron is low, a molecule inside the bacterial cell, called *Fur* (ferric uptake regulation), is activated, producing a siderophore. Once created, that molecule goes out and steals iron from the human carrier protein, either transferrin or ferritin. The outer surface of the bacterial cell has a receptor for the iron-loaded siderophore. When it binds, carrying its precious iron molecule, it is quickly incorporated into the bacterial cell. Clever.

But not clever enough. Human cells can also bind iron-bound bacterial siderophores, and they bind it more emphatically than the bacterial cell can. So, we just take the iron back. This cat-and-mouse game in the fight for iron has been going on for many years. Sometimes we win; sometimes, it's the bacteria.

Successfully hiding or stealing iron from bacteria is an essential defense against infectious diseases. People with conditions that result in excess iron release and circulation are at risk of certain infections or have a worse prognosis than those with normal iron levels. Alcoholics with liver disease are the most obvious example. Infections with some bacteria, especially Gram-negative rods, can be more virulent when the bug gets an ample supply of iron.

Spleen. The resident macrophages of the spleen are divided into two main sectors. Those which evaluate and tear down red blood cells and redistribute their remains are located in the area known as the red pulp. Another vitally important group of tissue macrophages is situated in what is known as the white pulp. As blood flows through the white pulp area, it contacts the resident macrophages, which are constantly vigilant for any sign of trouble. Trouble can be a pathogen that has invaded the blood and is floating freely or attached to, or invaded, the red blood cell. Even little bits of non-self-protein and other extraneous materials are scrutinized and removed.

The spleen is an organ with several jobs. It serves as a reservoir for blood, about 300-400 milliliters, so that when we suffer a hemorrhage, blood can be quickly released to replace that which was lost. It serves as a "recycle center" for senescent red blood cells. And it serves as a "matchmaker" for antigen-presenting macrophages with a compatible lymphocyte. The macrophages play a critical role in the latter two tasks.

Microglial cells. Nature has gone to great lengths to guard our brain and spinal cord. It is encased in the skull and vertebrae, surrounded by the thick meninges, and secured by the blood-brain barrier. Our nervous tissue, the body's control center, is protected in many ways from outside injury and encroachment. We also have a highly developed protective mechanism inside the brain tissue, the network of resident macrophages known as microglial cells. The central nervous system is an incredibly busy place. Innumerable reactions occur every day, both inside the nervous tissue and between cells. This creates waste products. Since access to the brain by the bloodstream is restricted by the blood-brain barrier, less cleansing of the tissues is available as in other organs. The microglial cells act to compensate for this divergence by being the self-appointed garbage collectors of the entire area.

The suffix *glia* is a Greek word meaning "glue." Microglial cells exist in several stages, depending on what's going on in their environment. The initial form is the ramified stage, from the Latin word *ramus*, or branch. They look like tiny octopuses, with a small central body and tentacles swirling about. The central body just sits there, but tentacles wave around, searching for anything that's not okay. Once they encounter something, such as a microorganism or a strange protein, they react, rounding up and becoming phagocytic and sometimes moving around (amoeboid). Like any macrophage, they then play an essential role in removing pathogens (as well as brain waste products), sending out chemical signals about the current danger of infection, and helping repair the damaged area.

Osteoclasts, bone. Of the resident macrophages, the osteoclasts are the most unusual. They are derived from the same source as other macrophages, but when they get to where they do their work, they fuse, making one giant cell with numerous nuclei. They sit right in bone, in little grooves. Macrophages are designed to destroy microbes with their enzymes and acids. As osteoclasts, they use these properties differently. Their job is to tear down and reabsorb bone to keep it from overgrowing. An adjacent cell type, the osteoblast, makes bone. The osteoclasts and osteoblasts communicate with each other, resulting in harmonious bone formation and bone resorption. The osteoclasts recycle the calcium that is produced and help preserve it.

Two things can make this bone creation/bone resorption contract go awry. The osteoclasts are macrophages, and if the bone is infected, a condition known as osteomyelitis, other macrophages are induced to enter the area. They can turn into osteoclasts, upsetting the balance of bone-constructing cells.

Another problem with osteoclasts is that they receive chemical signals from the hormone estrogen. Estrogen reduces the activity of osteoclasts. When estrogen activity terminates, as in menopause, osteoclasts tend to overdo things and pull too much calcium out of the bone. Ingesting more calcium in the diet doesn't reverse the effect; what's done is done. The result is the disease osteoporosis.

The cells comprising the Mononuclear Phagocyte System, our network of resident macrophages, arise mainly from fetal mesenchymal tissue, if not exclusively. The cells are in place when we draw our first breath. They don't last forever, but it's hard to say if they are replaced by their reproduction in place or monocytes from the bone marrow that may transform into the resident macrophage when they get there. Whatever the method, the resident macrophages are an indispensable part of our immune system. Having macrophages firmly in place, strategically located to detect and respond to invading microorganisms, is a tremendous advantage.

Macrophages are a vital part of the innate immune system. They are non-specific. Any invading microbe, whether a bacterium, virus, fungus, or parasite, gets the same general action. Even a foreign body or damaged tissue receives a similar response. But macrophages have a much wider range of activity than only the innate immune system, as important as that is. They also begin the essential process of acquired immunity, working with the lymphatic system's cells to ensure this doesn't happen again.

Chapter 10
Our Own Worst Enemy

Monocyte power –
Failure to communicate.
They've gone off the rails

In all their forms, macrophages play an enormous role in keeping us healthy. Besides their prominent role in fighting off microbial predators, they are also involved in the proper function of every organ and tissue in the body. While we usually associate white blood cells with immunity, the macrophages do much more. Unfortunately, they are not sentient; they respond strictly to chemical reactions. Suppose the chemical stimulus comes from an invading microbe. In that case, engaged macrophages do an excellent job initiating an inflammatory response, enabling a wide array of immune cells and chemicals to respond appropriately. But if the stimulus is from a malfunctioning tissue or organ, the macrophages often react as directed by the chemical signals they receive. Unfortunate consequences may arise. Many diseases afflicting humans today originate not from invading microbes but from an off-kilter immune system directed at ourselves, with macrophages playing an important role. Here is a brief, partial list of examples:

Alzheimer's disease. In 1887, a brilliant young student received his medical degree from the German University of Wurzburg. At that time, it was difficult for a young doctor to become established in medical practice. Despite his desire to continue his studies in research after graduation, he needed to earn a living and was compelled to accept a job with a wealthy family. It was common for the rich to travel a great deal at the time. If a family member were afflicted with a medical problem, a medical doctor would be hired to accompany them. The young doctor had never been interested in the embryonic field of psychiatry, but his assignment was to care for a young woman with a mental illness, and his interest in psychiatry was piqued. When his commission was over, he applied for and was given a position at one of the most prestigious research facilities in the world. The young doctor's name was Alois Alzheimer.

Dr. Alzheimer was always interested in anatomy, even at the microscopic level. He knew how to use a microscope. As fate would have it, one of his colleagues and friends was the eminent researcher Franz Nissl, one of the great neurologists of the time. Dr. Nissl developed a very useful stain visualizing neural tissue microscopically. The Nissl stain is still used today. Dr. Alzheimer was well acquainted with his methods.

A patient of Dr. Alzheimer's intrigued him. She was a 51-year-old woman named Auguste Deter who had developed severe memory loss and other psychiatric symptoms. He followed her for five years until her death, after which Dr. Alzheimer requested and received the woman's brain removed at autopsy. While working with a group of physicians like Dr. Nissl, he felt the basis for some psychiatric disorders might be organic. He was interested to see if any changes had occurred in Ms. Deter's brain to explain her dementia. When he looked at her brain tissue under the microscope, he made a remarkable discovery: many of the cells in her cerebral cortex contained a stringy material that he described as "tangles," which was not observed in healthy brain tissue. He made the same discovery in similar cases.

Dr. Alzheimer reported his discovery at a medical meeting in Germany. Not much interest was aroused, as it seemed to be some rather unique, seldom seen condition. However, one of Dr. Alzheimer's colleagues, Dr. Kaepelin, was publishing a book listing psychiatric disorders. He included the condition his colleague described. Since it had no name, he named it after its discoverer, Alzheimer's disease.

From this inauspicious debut arose awareness of one of the most devastating diseases of our age. Any serious medical condition is, of course, terrible. But the thought of losing one's mind, becoming utterly dependent on others to take care of us, and having that drag on for years, is for many one of the worst ends possible.

Those little "tangles" that Dr. Alzheimer described in the brain cells of his patients arise because of the accumulation of a waste product, **β-amyloid**. The term "amyloid," as used here, is a poor one, as it derives from the Latin *amylum*, which roughly means starch. The tangle material is a protein, but when it was first discovered in the 19th century, it was thought to be a starch-like, or carbohydrate, substance. Also, the designation "beta" often is written before the word amyloid. Technically, the designation should always follow the primary substance, as in "Interferon-α." But beta-amyloid it is, through conventional use.

The role of beta-amyloid in the cause of Alzheimer's disease is not fully understood. The substance is not unique to neurons and is associated with many different types of cells. Also, studies have shown that people with normal mental function had some accumulation of beta-amyloid around their neurons at the time of their death. There is certainly no linear cause and effect associated with the accumulation of beta-amyloid in the brain, but it seems to be one determining factor.

Beta-amyloid comes from a protein called Amyloid Precursor Protein, or APP. Just what APP does has yet to be fully understood, but it is known to be a protein that originates in the inner part of the neuron and extends through the cell membrane into the environment. It must be some sort of signaling receptor. Once it has been activated by contacting the appropriate molecule, it is cut in half by a protein called BACE. The severed part that floats away is the beta-amyloid. This is all a natural process, and it occurs in all of us. For some reason, those who develop Alzheimer's disease either make more beta-amyloid than is normal or have difficulty disposing of it adequately. It tends to accumulate around the neuron's surface, giving rise to "tangles."

Another protein of neurons that may play a role in Alzheimer's disease is found inside each nerve cell. **Tau** proteins are not just one type but several of similar construction, essential in maintaining the microtubules responsible for transporting materials inside the cell. For some unknown reason, in some people, the tau proteins, like beta-amyloid, can become malformed and involved in the formation of the notorious tangles symptomatic of the disease.

The resident macrophages of the brain, the microglial cells, have the job of helping to remove various types of debris and waste products. That would include beta-amyloid and mangled tau. The microglials are assisted in this mission by monocytes that arrive on the scene from time to time. There are some people who, because of a genetic predisposition, develop Alzheimer's disease in middle age. Frau Deter was 51 when she began displaying symptoms. But usually, it is one of old age, and the macrophages in some individuals may change as time marches on. One theory is that the accumulated sheets of beta-amyloid and some tau protein resemble the biofilms of bacteria. Indeed, some theories implicate incorporating products of several different microbes in forming such a biofilm. As we age, the lining of our gums and intestinal tract may become more porous, allowing the permeation of either bacteria or their by-products into our circulation. Some of it may make its way into the brain and become attached to the developing beta-amyloid tangles.

Macrophages have a receptor on their surface, Toll-like receptor-2, that recognizes bacterial biofilms and subsequently mounts an inflammatory reaction. The reaction of Alzheimer's may be a case of mistaken identity: the beta-amyloid complex looks to TLR-2 like bacterial biofilm and the resulting inflammatory response damages the neuronal synapses and harms brain function. Whether that theory is accurate, the action of macrophages may play a significant role in the onset and course of Alzheimer's disease.

Parkinson's Disease. Doctors in the early 1800s weren't called doctors or physicians. They were known as apothecaries. One whose name is now associated with a severe disease was James Parkinson, an English gentleman whose life's work included medicine, politics, geology, and paleontology. In 1817, he wrote an "Essay On The Shaking Palsy," the first known English description of the disease that would eventually bear his name. In it, he described a half dozen patients with the symptoms of the illness he called *Paralysis Agitans:*

"involuntary tremulous motion, with lessened muscular power, in parts (limbs) not in action and even when supported; with a propensity to bend the trunk forward, and to pass from a walking to a running pace: the senses and intellects being uninjured." Of course, in 1817, he could only describe the

apparent symptoms, not the cause or explanation for the illness. Some 60 years after his death, the disease was named after him by one of the top early scientists in the field of neurology, Jean-Martin Charcot.

In typical Parkinson's Disease, the onset of symptoms develops over time. These include shaking, rigidity, and slow movements, including difficulty walking. Patients are often afflicted by mental and emotional disturbances, including depression, anxiety, and, late in the disease process, dementia. The disease typically begins after age 40, with peak onset between the age of 58-62.

Normal motor function originates in an unusually named part of the brain, the substantia nigra, Latin for "black substance." It's not really black, but it is much darker in appearance than neighboring brain tissue due to the high concentrations of neuromelanin in the area. Two chemicals are essential in the smooth conduction of nervous impulses to the muscles: acetylcholine and dopamine. Acetylcholine is the "gas pedal" responsible for transmitting the nervous impulse. Dopamine is the "brake," or a "clutch," responsible for slowing down and smoothing the impulse. When it all works as planned, the nerve impulse is sent out in a controlled, regular fashion. The problem with Parkinson's Disease is the imbalance created by a shortage of dopamine. The neurons responsible for its manufacture are impaired or dead, so the "gas pedal" substance, acetylcholine, controls the impulse. The result is the symptoms of Parkinson's, muscle tremors and rigidity.

Just as beta-amyloid is associated with Alzheimer's Disease, a neural protein is associated with Parkinson's Disease. Alpha-synuclein (α-Syn) is a protein found in several different types of cells, but it is especially prominent in the neuronal cells of the substantia nigra. It seems to form an essential part of the channel through which dopamine is released into the synapse.

There is a great deal of evidence that Parkinson's Disease involves considerable inflammation around the cells of the substantia nigra that are responsible for the release of dopamine. This inflammation is directly related to the activity of the resident macrophages of the area, the microglia, that may be responding to increased levels of α-Syn. The microglial cells go from having a rather unassuming, business-like approach to being aggressive immune cells determined to wipe out an invading predator. The result is the ultimate destruction of the dopamine-releasing cell, with the resulting symptoms of Parkinson's Disease. Just what makes this all happen, the overexpression of α-Syn and the ramping up of the activity of the microglial cells, is unknown, as is the best way to make it stop.

Atherosclerosis. The disease atherosclerosis is one of the most pervasive in the world. It is impossible to say how many people have it because the disorder begins and progresses insidiously. Also, its development may halt and never be detected. When it progresses to its highest form, it is life-threatening, and heroic medical procedures are often needed to save a patient's life. The cost of human lives and the expense of treatment is tremendous.

The name atherosclerosis is an odd one. The term "sclerosis" means hardening. The term "athero" is the odd part. It comes from the Greek *athere*, which means "gruel," a soft, mushy substance. When the lesion first begins deep in the wall of an artery, it is relatively soft and pliable. As it progresses, it becomes hardened, even calcified. So the name makes sense when looking at the entire progression of the condition.

Macrophages are intimately involved in atherosclerosis. When most people think of the disease, commonly known as "hardening of the arteries," they naturally consider cholesterol the culprit. But cholesterol is not the entire story. The reaction to cholesterol in the lining of the arteries, chiefly by macrophages, is a major part of the condition.

Cholesterol is necessary for life. Every cell in our body can make it, but the liver has taken on the job of mass production. The synthesis of cholesterol is, to say the least, complicated, with over 35 chemical reactions involved. We can utilize the cholesterol in our food, especially in the first few hours after eating it, but most is made in-house.

The word cholesterol comes from the Greek words *khole*, meaning bile, and *steros*, meaning stiff or hard. That's because it was first found in gallstones over a hundred years ago.

Cholesterol is located in the membranes of all our cells, providing strength while allowing for pliability. It also allows for communicating the cells' interior with the surrounding fluids and tissues, enabling the smooth integration of nutrients and other chemicals into the cell. It serves as a building block for essential chemicals, like steroid hormones (such as testosterone and estrogen), bile acids, and vitamin D. Clearly, cholesterol has a lot to do. The body expends considerable energy seeing to it that it is well managed.

Cholesterol is a lipid, or fat, some 25 carbon atoms long. Of course, lipids (also called oil) and water don't mix, so cholesterol cannot be dissolved in serum. It needs a transporter to carry it around the body, just as transferrin and ferritin harbor iron. The "cholesterol ferry" is a lipoprotein, the "lipo" for lipid, the protein for, well, protein. The lipoproteins designed to carry cholesterol are complex, much more than a simple modified protein. They have compartments with an array of several thousand molecules attached. One can think of lipoprotein as more of a particle than a simple molecule; its size approximates that of a virus.

There are four types of lipoproteins, but the two that come into play as major cholesterol transporters are low-density lipoprotein and high-density. The density part of the terms refers to the ratio of lipids to protein in the particle. The low-density lipoprotein has a higher amount of lipid; the high-density lipoprotein has a higher amount of protein. For the most part, the low-density lipoprotein (LDL) carries cholesterol from the liver out to the cells of the body that need it; the high-density lipoprotein (HDL) carries cholesterol back to the liver for denaturation and removal. In a nutshell, LDL cholesterol inserts cholesterol into cells, while HDL removes it.

Somehow, we have created the terms "bad cholesterol" and "good cholesterol." The "bad" isn't really bad; we couldn't live without it. But sometimes things go awry, and the LDL cholesterol ends up where it shouldn't, in the wall of an artery.

Arteries have several layers, the thickness of which depends on where the artery is and the blood pressure and flow amount it receives. The cells lining the artery lumen are endothelial cells. Just below that is the intima, a thin layer of connective tissue. Under a layer of elastic fibers resides a layer of smooth muscle known as the media. Then another layer of fibers, to the adventitia. The LDL cholesterol must go through all of this to get where it needs to go. Unfortunately, sometimes it gets "stuck." Just why that happens in some people is mysterious. Having a high level of LDL cholesterol increases the likelihood. Still, there may be other reasons. Perhaps a microbe first attacked the area, like a virus or a bacterium. Maybe it is related to the level of sheer force and pressure from the blood coursing through. Whatever the cause, in some people, LDL cholesterol builds up in the tissue just below the surface of an artery.

Because LDL is a particle, its removal is assigned to macrophages, which respond dutifully. After engulfing the LDL, a couple of things happen. One is that the macrophages send out chemical signals, like TNFα and IL-1β, that initiate an inflammatory response. Also, when something goes wrong in the intimal layer of the artery, the cells called upon to help repair the damage are the local smooth muscle cells, which migrate to the area. They, too, can engulf LDL. The result is the presence of what are known as "foam" cells, or phagocytic cells laden with LDL and cholesterol. They are given their name because they have so much fat that they look foamy.

The inflammatory response doesn't stop there. The more active the macrophages and other involved cells become, the more chemical signals are sent to expand the operation. One is a signal sent to the nearby endothelial cells of the artery to put out a chemical "hook" to attract more monocytes that swarm into the area. Also, platelets are attracted to the site, stimulating fibrin production. With these cascading events, the more LDL cholesterol in the blood, the more it adds to the growing plaque.

It doesn't happen overnight, but after a while, the plaque in the artery starts to grow. There are layers of dead cells, fibrin, and lipids. At some point, calcium starts to become deposited. Given enough time, the plaque can grow so much that it begins to occlude the lumen of the artery. Two catastrophic events are now possible: the artery becomes blocked, or pieces of the plaque disengage and travel to another part of the body. A heart attack or stroke may ensue.

Septic shock. With macrophages and dendritic cells playing a major role, the immune system is very good at restricting bacterial invaders to isolated, sometimes remote locations. Bacteria have specific molecular structures on their surfaces that macrophages recognize through a surface receptor. The microbial molecule is referred to as a **PAMP** for pathogen-associated molecular pattern. The macrophage molecule is called the **PRR**, for pathogen recognition receptor. Once the bacterium enters the body, the PAMP hooks up with the PRR. The macrophage is then activated. This leads to a series of chemical reactions inside the macrophage or dendritic cell that ultimately release potent cytokines like TNFα and IL-1β. These, and others, initiate an inflammatory response with the characteristic increased porosity of the arterial lining and attraction of more phagocytic cells in the area. White blood cells and various anti-microbial chemicals pour into the site.

Also activated is the blood coagulation cascade, resulting in the formation of blood clots. These mini clots serve to contain the bacteria in one area, sort of like a spider web trapping an insect. This keeps the bacteria from spreading through the body, making them more of a stationary target for phagocytic cells. It's very effective when the organisms are confined to a small space.

But sometimes, organisms break out of the local tissues and enter the bloodstream. When that happens, monocytes in the blood are activated much like tissue macrophages for local infections. The same chemical and cellular control tools are employed, but on a much larger scale. Suppose many organisms are present in the blood. In that case, massive amounts of cytokines like TNFα and IL-1β are released, wreaking havoc on the permeability of blood vessels, not just the local ones but throughout the body. Adding to the problem is the activation of the blood's coagulation cascade, not just in the local tissues but all through the bloodstream.

The word disseminated comes from the Latin words *dis*, meaning apart or away, and *seminare*, meaning to "sow;" it refers to widespread effect. The word intravascular refers to the area inside blood vessels. Of course, coagulation refers to the clotting of blood. The complete term for a perilous consequence of large numbers of bacteria in the blood is disseminated intravascular coagulation, usually called DIC. This is a life-threatening situation for two reasons. One is that blood clotting in critical areas can lead to the malfunctioning of an organ downstream from the clot, which doesn't receive enough blood to function. Also, there are just so many clotting chemicals normally present in the blood, and if they are all used up, there isn't enough to form a clot where it is needed. The patient can become a relative hemophiliac. With DIC and hypotension secondary to blood vessel dilation, bacteria in the blood present a critical condition. And it all starts with monocytes engaging the bacteria and sending out their usual stream of chemical signals.

Septic shock secondary to bacteria in the blood occurs commonly with Gram-negative bacteria. That's because they have a toxic substance in their cell walls that is easily recognizable to monocytes, a substance known as endotoxin. The PAMP of endotoxin is the lipid A portion of lipo-polysaccharide, and all monocytes and macrophages are very good at recognizing it. Some more common causes of Gram-negative septic shock are urinary tract infections, infections with *Neisseria meningitides,* hospital-acquired pneumonia, and infections in the peritoneum. There are many other potential causes.

Gram-positive bacteria can also cause septic shock, but the most common way they do it differs. They lack lipid A endotoxin, but they sometimes produce **exo**toxins that react with blood monocytes. Exotoxins are relatively small proteins given off by the organism when they grow to high numbers. Certain strains of a few bacteria, like *Streptococcus* and *Staphylococcus,* make exotoxins known as "superantigens," which are impressive in their power. Superantigen activity results in the activation of millions of lymphocytes, and they release massive amounts of the cytokines that lead to the symptoms of septic shock. As in the case of the reaction to endotoxin, the result is often critical illness. If left untreated, it often results in death.

Osteoporosis. The disease osteoporosis is not new. Female Egyptian mummies were observed to have had what is commonly called the "dowager's hump," often a characteristic of the ailment. In 1830 a French doctor with the unwieldy name of Jean Georges Chretien Frederic Martin Lobstein noticed that the bones of some patients at autopsy had more holes, or pores, than normal bone and suggested the name osteo (bone) porosis (holes).

Quite a few factors may cause the degradation of bone. An important one is the overactivity of the osteoclasts, a giant amalgam of resident macrophages in bone. For some individuals, bone degradation and calcium resorption are overdone, resulting in greater bone porosity and susceptibility to bone fracture. It has been estimated that in the United States, yearly, around a million fractures occur due to bone fragility, at the cost of perhaps $14 billion, with, of course, loss of mobility and reduced quality of life. Sometimes bone fractures result in complications such as pulmonary embolism and pneumonia, possibly leading to death.

Peak bone density is achieved during our early adult years. As we age, starting around the fourth decade of life, bone mass begins to recede, like the graying of hair. On average, we lose around 0.7% of our bone mass every year. An eighty-year-old will naturally have less bone density than a thirty-year-old, regardless of sex. But sometimes, this slow process is accelerated. This can be due to several reasons, but a significant cause in women is reduced estrogen, usually following the onset of menopause or the surgical removal of the ovaries.

Osteoclasts are specialized resident macrophages of bone. Their job is to tear the bone down. They work in harmony with the osteoblasts, which build more bone. Normally, the two cell types strike a balance resulting in strong bone formation.

To help maintain this balance, the hormone estrogen affects the activity of the bone-destructive osteoclasts. It does this in two ways, one indirect, the other direct. Cytokines, such as TNF-α and interleukin-1β, promote the enhanced activity of macrophages, including osteoclasts. With more osteoclasts, there is potentially more bone destruction. Estrogen keeps the level of the cytokines under control, indirectly limiting the number and activity of osteoclasts. When the estrogen level is markedly reduced, these cytokines are produced in increased amounts, producing more osteoclasts. This can lead to more bone resorption. The osteoblasts (the bone makers) try to keep up, but in some women, they are unable to, perhaps because of genetic reasons.

Estrogen also seems to affect the osteoclasts directly, initiating the process of apoptosis, or programmed cell death. By systematically reducing the number of operating osteoclasts, estrogen helps strike a balance between bone-forming and bone-destroying cells. When this balance is upset by the absence of estrogen, osteoporosis results.

Simple X-rays are not sensitive enough to visualize the early stages of osteoporosis. They don't reveal anything until late in the disease progression. But there are imaging studies that measure bone density that are very good, and it is wise for older people to be screened occasionally.

Estrogen replacement therapy is an often-recommended treatment, despite its possible complications. A proven preventative measure is a regular exercise regimen, especially working with weights. Bone remodeling is a continual process, and the more we stress our bones into activity, the healthier they become.

Inflammatory bowel disease. Names assigned to diseases arise in numerous ways. Some come from traditional parlance, a term that was used centuries ago persists. Latin and Greek figure prominently in many conditions. Some diseases have two names, one popular and one scientific, like smallpox is variola, and chicken pox is varicella. There are quite a few whose name briefly defines the condition. Often the phrase is shortened to an acronym or set of initials, like gastric esophageal reflux disease becomes GERD. Some diseases are named after an individual, usually the person who published a scientific paper first describing it, like Parkinson's Disease.

Inflammatory bowel disease (IBD) includes the conditions ulcerative colitis and Crohn's disease. Both disorders have no doubt existed for millennia, but distinguishing them from other ailments and each other was not possible until modern means of diagnosis became available.

"Ulcerative colitis" (UC) gives a physical description. It was first proposed by Samuel Wilkes in 1859 and reinforced by William Hale White in 1888. A major advance in understanding UC came in 1909 at a symposium in London, where a thorough description of the condition was presented. Also in 1909 sigmoidoscopy was introduced as a routine diagnostic tool. After that, ulcerative colitis became a commonly used term.

Crohn's Disease is named after Dr. Burrill Crohn, one of the authors listed in a seminal paper on the subject in 1932. In an oddity of history, Dr. Crohn, an eminent gastroenterologist, was not the primary researcher for the publication. Drs. Ginzburg and Oppenheimer did most of the work. The authors suggested the term "regional ileitis." At the time, authors of scientific literature were listed alphabetically. Hence, Dr. Crohn's name appeared first, and for some reason, other researchers referring to this descriptive work used the name of the first author listed. The disease now bears the name Crohn's Disease.

The submucosal tissues of the intestines, both large and small, are replete with macrophages. Because they are exposed to so much material that comes into the bowel, their inflammatory tendencies are mollified by chemical messengers from the adjacent intestinal cells. They are very good at phagocytizing microbes and other materials, but their cytokine production is naturally much reduced to prevent overreaction and the symptoms that go with it. In inflammatory bowel diseases, the macrophage population, for some reason, does not receive these mitigating signals, and they function more like macrophages in other parts of the body, sending out extensive cytokines and chemokines. The result is a hyperactive immune response instead of a routine one.

Rheumatoid arthritis. Like inflammatory bowel disease, it is difficult to trace the history of rheumatoid arthritis because some of its symptoms overlap with other disorders, such as gout and osteoarthritis. The word rheumatic was first used in the early 1800s. It derives from the Greek word *rheuma,* which means roughly a "liquid discharge from the body." It was felt at the time that the ailment was caused by excess drainage from the upper part of the body to the lower, throwing the entire system out of balance. (Another condition attributed to excess water retention was called dropsy, from the Greek word for water, *hydrops*. Today it is called edema. "Rheumatism" and dropsy were two of the diseases that formed the rationale for a commonly used therapeutic measure to reduce bodily fluid, bloodletting).

Rheumatoid arthritis (RA) is characterized by joint inflammation, swelling, cartilage and bone destruction, and auto-antibody formation. There are usually systemic features involving the heart and lungs. Some patients also exhibit psychological disturbances as well. The exact cause of RA is unknown, but there seem to be three predisposing factors: genetics, environment, and luck. As in other autoimmune diseases, the inflammatory process is initiated by an antibody or activated T-cell that directs its attention to the synovium. One hallmark of RA is a marked increase in the integrins and selectins that protrude from the endothelial lining of the small blood vessels, the chemicals that "hook" neutrophils and macrophages from the circulation. Once the many phagocytic cells enter the synovial space, it is difficult for them to get out, leading to an enclosed area that becomes a maelstrom of immunologic activity. An enormous array of macrophage and other immune cell signaling occurs, with the resultant production and release of toxic and proteolytic enzymes and acids. Osteoclasts notably increase in number, with consequent bone destruction.

Lupus. The derivation of the word lupus is rather odd. It comes from the Latin word *lupus*, meaning wolf, intimating that the condition "devours" the patient. A striking fact about the condition is that it affects women about six times more frequently than men, primarily women between the ages of 20 and 40. There are two general types of lupus. One is confined to the skin, most commonly the face, with a characteristic "butterfly" rash. It is called discoid lupus. The other type, systemic lupus erythematosus or SLE, involves the entire body and is the more serious. These two types of lupus, discoid and systemic, should not be confused with the disease lupus vulgaris, a cutaneous infection by *Mycobacterium tuberculosis.*

Lupus is characterized by antibodies directed against the patient's molecules and tissues, including nucleic acids, erythrocytes, coagulation proteins, phospholipids, lymphocytes, platelets, and many others. Which autoantibody is produced and its quantity varies with each patient. The most characteristic autoantibodies are directed against nuclear material: single and double-stranded DNA, histones, ribonucleoproteins, and others. Our bodies constantly have nucleic acids and associated molecules in the blood from the normal metabolism of our cells. The level goes up during times of trauma or infection. These nuclear products are typically removed effectively in the liver, but when attached to an antibody, their removal is less effective. The immune complexes tend to get deposited in tissues, inducing an inflammatory response. SLE is the most common and potentially one of the most severe autoimmune disorders.

Macrophages and dendritic cells play a vital role in the progression of SLE. There is an overexpression of "monocyte hooking" molecules, those that extend out from the endothelial cells of blood vessels to slow down and trap circulating phagocytic cells. This is most likely caused by the inflammatory nature of the deposited immune complexes in the tissues, resulting in even more chaos in the affected tissues. Also noteworthy is the increased production of type I interferons (both α and β), which adds to the accumulation of macrophages and dendritic cells in tissues. Several abnormalities in molecules found in the cell membranes of macrophages are present in the disease. As a result, the production of various cytokines is potentially abnormal. Which ones and to what extent vary with each case. SLE can be difficult to diagnose, as the symptoms are not unique and are often transitory.

The collection of cells we refer to as macrophages are remarkable in all their forms. Monocytes, macrophages, dendritic cells, or resident macrophages are on the front lines of combating invading microorganisms by killing them and engaging other parts of the immune system and bodily tissues to join the fight. They are also vital to the "mop up" operation, helping to direct the calming down of the inflammatory response and assisting in the reconstruction phase. They are engaged in many normal bodily functions, from molding our bones' shape to managing our red blood cells. Unfortunately, they can also become involved in acute and chronic diseases when the chemical signals they receive and respond to are aberrant. Much research is now devoted to minimizing the potential harm done by macrophage over-involvement without jeopardizing their critical role in our fight against invading pathogens. That battle is just beginning.

Chapter 11
The Attack of the Killer Lymphocytes
Cellular Hit Men
By way of the thymus gland.
Defends by self-destruction.

We each have about 600 lymph nodes scattered strategically throughout our bodies. They aren't very big, usually around a half to one centimeter in diameter. They tend to cluster in areas where they may be most needed, bearing the names of their general location. The most prominent are the cervical (back of neck), axillary (armpits), supraclavicular (along the collarbone), mediastinal (sternum and lung area), mesentery (abdominal), inguinal (groin), and femoral (upper inner thigh). Also, inside the lining of our intestinal and respiratory tracts are clusters of cells known as lymphoid tissue, going by the names of tonsils, adenoids, and Peyer's Patches. And our spleen is replete with lymphoid tissue called the white pulp. All of this is connected by pipelines coursing through our body, constructing a complex known as the lymph system. This elaborate setup aims to create unique places within our bodies to clear debris, microorganisms, and waste. One of its primary functions is matchmaking, bringing certain types of cells into direct contact to acquire long-lasting immunity.

The word lymph comes from the Latin word for water, *lympha*, but it is far from ordinary H_2O. Lymph originates from blood plasma as it leaks through the capillaries into the tissues, accumulating in the equally thin-walled lymph vessels. It contains salts, proteins, some fat, and, importantly, the cells of the lymph system, the lymphocytes. Macrophages and dendritic cells also flow along the lymph channels. Because it doesn't have any red blood cells, lymph is nearly colorless, with just a hint of opacity because of the cells it contains.

The lymph vessels don't have a pump like the heart. The fluid movement through them is mainly due to the action of the surrounding skeletal muscles contracting and putting pressure on the neighboring tissues. Like blood vessels, lymph vessels vary in size: very small at the point of the beginning (lymph capillaries), progressing to larger (lymph vessels), then much larger before they empty into a vein (lymph ducts). Like veins, lymph vessels contain valves to prevent backflow. After circulating through the channels, lymph re-enters the bloodstream through the superior vena cava, and the fluid becomes part of the bloodstream again.

Like neutrophils, lymphocytes originate in the bone marrow but are a very different type of cell. Neutrophils are quintessential members of the innate immune system. They arrive on the scene of an infection or injury shortly after it has begun and get right to work. If complement, antibody, or serum proteins are engaged, fine, but neutrophils are active in attacking and engulfing invading microbes or damaged tissue on their own. On the other hand, most lymphocytes are intimately involved in the acquired immune system. Some form a bridge between the acquired and the innate systems.

Neutrophils are of one type. When they leave the bloodstream and enter the surrounding tissues, they become more active, but all neutrophils have the same inherent characteristics and jobs. Lymphocytes are much different. They start in the bone marrow, all looking alike, but they are far from a monolithic group. There are several groups and subgroups of lymphocytes, and their roles are decidedly different.

One of the more captivating names in human cellular biology is "natural killer." Sounds ominous. But it's an excellent description of one type of lymphocyte whose job is to kill human cells that have gone awry. To the uninitiated, it may come as quite a surprise that we normally have millions of cells in our body that are there to destroy some of our very own cells. But that is very much the case. All our cells die and are turned over at some point, but sometimes that process must be speeded up.

Natural killer lymphocytes have the unique job of detecting cells that have become abnormal and getting rid of them before they get out of control. Commonly abbreviated NK cells, these lymphocytes are better described as being in the innate immune system than the acquired because they act independently of the typical factors of the latter. Most lymphocytes are created to do battle with one, and only one, protein. If it was formed to attack a cell infected by, say, measles virus, that's all it can handle. And it's just one little piece of a protein on the measles virus that it keys into.

On the other hand, the NK cells carry on their work against an extensive array of microbes, primarily viruses. But, unlike neutrophils, they don't go after the microbe directly. They attack the cell that harbors it, inducing the host cell to kill itself, thereby destroying the enclosed organism.

The natural killer lymphocytes are the body's armed patrolling hit squad. They roam around all body parts, randomly bumping into myriad cells, most of which are perfectly normal and going about their routine business. Their activity can be likened to an old movie scene where the policeman commands a citizen to "show me your papers!" If the proper documents are immediately produced, the policeman walks away. But if not, stern measures are taken. So it is with the natural killer lymphocytes and their activity. They are armed with two types of surface proteins. One is an activator that commands the delivery of a lethal dose of granules into the host cell it encounters; the other is an inhibitor, which calls off the mission and allows the encountered host cell to live. A lot depends on which of the two is dominant in an encounter situation.

MHC is an essential protein. It's easy to see that from the first word of its name: "M" stands for Major. The "H" stands for Histocompatibility, with the "histo" part coming from the Greek word *histos*, or "web of a loom." In medicine, it refers to tissues. The word compatibility is used because the discovery of the substance in the 1930s dealt with rejecting transplanted tissue from one individual to another. The "C" stands for Complex, a very apt term. MHC is not a simple protein. It is made up of several sections, and it is the product of several genes. Because of that, individuals vary in the chemical makeup of their individual MHC, creating problems when tissues and organs are transplanted. MHC often goes by another name, and another set of initials, HLA. "H" stands for human, simple enough. The "L" stands for leukocyte, a somewhat unfortunate designation because all our cells (except red blood cells) have it. The "A," for antigen, is used in the context of transplants because one person's tissue is foreign, and therefore antigenic, to another.

Whether you call it MHC or HLA, this set of proteins serves a vital function. We can think of them as "ferry boats," carrying pieces of the cell's busted-up proteins and carbohydrates to the surface. Our cells constantly create waste products, whether peptides or carbohydrates, and enzymes break down these wastes. The cell may also be infected with an infectious organism, and those are inactivated and digested. The MHC particles' job is to pick up pieces of the degraded protein or carbohydrate, whatever its source, and ferry them to the cell's surface. There the MHC molecule sits, the passenger molecule prominently attached and displayed. Three types of lymphocytes can then encounter the MHC. They are either the natural killer cell, or one of the two antigen-reading types of lymphocytes, CD4 or CD8. The NK cells don't care what the antigen presented is. They are reading for the presence of MHC molecules. The CD4 and CD8 lymphocytes have a great interest in the presented antigen. They will only react if the molecule displayed on the MHC molecule perfectly matches the receptor they are carrying.

Natural killer lymphocytes are equipped with two "triggers." One is designed to release chemicals that can destroy the human host cell. The other is designed to stop the destructive process.

The substance the NK cell activator is searching for is produced by cells during times of stress. Viral infection and cancer indeed come under that heading. Small amounts of these stress proteins are routinely released, but the amount goes up when something inside the cell is off-kilter. The "killer" trigger protein, when activated upon contact with the stress proteins displayed on the host cell, initiates the release of several substances. One of them perforates the membrane of the cell being attacked. Others, known as granulozymes, flow through the perforated cell opening. The contents of the granules then start a process of the cell's self-destruction, apoptosis. This destructive process requires the attachment of phosphate ions.

144

Unless stopped by the inhibitor proteins, the killing process proceeds.

The substance on the host cell surface that activates the inhibitory protein is MHC. We normally have plenty of it as the routine by-products of cell metabolism and the subsequent transport of digested pieces of it to the cell surface. When activated by MHC, the inhibitory protein starts to wiggle and squirm, thus binding the phosphate molecules necessary for the killer proteins to complete their activation. When the inhibitor molecules are functioning at a high level, that is, there is plenty of MHC present to activate them, they bind much of the phosphate ions needed by the activator molecule, thus preventing the activation of those enzymes required by the killer protein, and the process is halted. It's something like taking the bullets away from a potential assassin.

But when the MHC isn't present or is present only in substantially reduced numbers, the inhibitory signal is not activated. Then the killer protein cascade receives its phosphate, the activator system dominates, and the host cell is killed. There are several circumstances when normal levels of MHC are lacking, but two important ones result from infection by some microbes or when a cell has developed cancer. Some microbes produce proteins that shut down MHC activity directly. Others disable the host cell's ability to create it. In either case, MHC isn't made in the usual quantities, and the NK cell is not inhibited from releasing its cell-killing package. Some cancerous cells also result in the under-production of MHC.

The NK activator won't be triggered if we have a normal amount of MHC. When we have a lot of stress proteins and reduced MHC, the killing process runs its course.

The killing of cells by apoptosis is an orderly one. The dead cell doesn't just explode and splatter its contents all over the surrounding tissue. Apoptosis is a step-by-step system. Macrophages are enlisted to contain the dead cell, and its contents are catabolized, just as when a senescent cell needs to be removed. If the cell contains a virus, pieces of the virus are displayed on the macrophage's MHC molecules, and acquired immunity, employing other types of lymphocytes (CD4, CD8, and B cells), begins.

Lymphocytes comprise about a third of our circulating white blood cells during normal conditions. The natural killer lymphocytes are about one-sixth of that or around 3-5% of our usual circulating WBC. They are produced and mature in the bone marrow. When a virus infects the body, chemical signals, mainly interferon, are sent to the bone marrow, instructing it to crank out many more natural killer lymphocytes. Within a day or two, NK cells can increase by 20 to 100-fold. NK cells constitute a vital first line of defense.

Like the natural killer lymphocytes, CD8 cells contain granulozymes that promote cell death by initiating apoptosis. But the CD8s belong to an entirely different class of lymphocytes called T-cells. The "T" stands for thymus, the organ in which the CD8 cell (as well as the CD4 cell) develops. Like the NK cells, the CD8s are formed in the bone marrow, but for maturation, they migrate through the bloodstream to the thymus, a small organ in our upper chest.

Situated behind our sternum and between our lungs, right in front of our heart, the thymus is an odd organ. It's been known for millennia, having been first described by the Roman philosopher Galen, who noted an unusual feature: it is of its largest size when we are born and shrivels to a small size as we age. By the time puberty is over and we enter our adult years, the thymus starts to recede so that when we reach old age, the thymus is very small, with primarily fat tissue. Its work isn't done but much lessened. But such important work it is! Without our little thymus gland, our lives would be much different, if not prematurely terminated. It is an integral part of our immune system, giving nourishment and a controlled environment to our CD8 and CD4 lymphocytes, allowing them to mature and be ready for action with whatever challenges are thrown their way. A healthy thymus is essential for a good life. None of this was known to people centuries ago, and the function of the thymus could only be guessed. The term "thymus" comes from the Greek word for "soul," *thumos*, because of its juxtaposition to the heart.

The function of the thymus is to screen lymphocytes sent to it from the bone marrow, allowing the good ones to mature and proliferate while eliminating the bad ones. It's kind of like a person serving as quality control on a conveyor line of fruit, inspecting product as it passes, picking off the bad ones, and allowing the good ones to progress.

We might think of the thymus gland as a cave with many compartments. Immature lymphocytes (usually called naïve lymphocytes) enter from the bloodstream and settle in one of these "caves." Hanging from the top of the cave are "stalactites," or projections from the wall of the compartment. These projections are actually fingers of the epithelial cells that line the thymus, and their role is to assist in the maturation of lymphocytes. When they enter the thymus, lymphocytes come into direct contact with the epithelial projections and form an intimate relationship. The epithelial cell is a guide for the lymphocyte's maturation, and it is very demanding. Only about 2% of lymphocytes entering the thymus live long enough to emerge; 98% are commanded to kill themselves through apoptosis.

The first order of business is to determine if the lymphocyte (inside the thymus, it is more appropriately called a "thymocyte") can determine the difference between self and non-self. In a highly complicated fashion, lymphocytes each receive a different gene coding for the antigen to bind and ultimately inhibit. The process is random. During this creative development, it is inevitable that some lymphocytes will receive a molecule that readily binds an antigen that is inherent in the body's own construction. Clearly, the lymphocytes with these self-binding molecules must be eliminated: a chemical signal is transmitted to the cell to self-destruct through apoptosis. If it is convincingly demonstrated that the cell binds only to a non-self, or foreign, antigen, it is spared and can progress. The MHC molecule produced by the thymus epithelial cell is key to this sorting-out system, which can bear both self and foreign antigens. This is a critical action, as having lymphocytes that attack our own cells is never good. Unfortunately, the system isn't fool-proof, and auto-immunity may result from the occasional cell that slips through.

The second important function of the thymus is to aid in determining what type of T-lymphocyte the candidates will become, a CD8 cell or a CD4. The former is cytotoxic and can kill aberrant cells, similar to the natural killer lymphocytes' mission. The CD4 cells are known as T-helper cells, and, as their name suggests, they don't directly kill the host cell gone bad but rather help other cells of the immune system to become engaged.

MHC also directs this differentiation between CD8 and CD4 cells. There are two types of MHC. (Actually, there are three, but one and two are the most important). Cells destined to become CD8 types bind strongly to MHC I and are chemically encouraged to produce more of their surface marker, CD8. Those that will become CD4 will bind strongly to MHC II and create more of their surface marker, CD4.

The initial screening process occurs in the thymus's cortex, the outer compartments. Typically, dense numbers of these "baby" lymphocytes are clustered around the projected appendages of the thymus epithelial cells, each undergoing scrutiny as to their "worthiness" to enter the circulation. Those that emerge as useful and not potentially harmful migrate to the thymus medulla, where they end their maturation process. They are then ready to enter the circulation, destined for a lymph node, lymphoid tissue, or general circulation.

During the early part of our lives, the thymus is at its most active. As life goes on, it becomes much less active. After puberty, it begins to atrophy until in old age it becomes a tiny organ of just a few grams. It never ceases to function; its main job is to ensure a full complement of active, functional lymphocytes throughout life. The lymphocytes emanating from the thymus are collectively called T-lymphocytes, whether they be of the CD8 or CD4 type. Of course, the "T" stands for thymus, a vital, under-appreciated organ.

Like the natural killer lymphocytes, the CD8 T-cells have the power to destroy their fellow human cells. When they encounter a cell that has had the misfortune of being invaded by a virus or another microorganism, and the proper safeguard signals are exchanged, the CD8 lymphocyte releases granules that contain enzymes that initiate the cell's self-destruction. They also make an enzyme, a permease, that allows the entry of the destructive enzymes into the cell. The natural killer lymphocytes act similarly. But there is a big difference between the CD8s and the NKs: The former are very specific in the individual cells they work on, while the latter are much more general. The NK cells detect an imbalance between the number of normal MHC molecules on a cell's surface and molecules indicating underlying trouble. When there is an imbalance, they spring into action. The CD8 lymphocytes don't detect an imbalance of different molecules. They search for one, and only one, small piece of protein or carbohydrate displayed within the MHC I molecules on a cell's surface. The CD8 cells have a protein shaped like an antibody on their surface. Unlike antibodies, it doesn't float away but is firmly attached. This anchored antibody must hook up with the antigen molecule being carried in a groove on the MHC that will excite it into action. The CD8 molecule will lock onto the scanned host cell. The solid docking of its anchored antibody molecule with the displayed antigen releases the lymphocyte's deadly cargo— failure to detect the tell-tale surface antigen lodged on an MHC 1 molecule results in no activity.

Once a CD8 cell encounters the antigen that reacts with it, it begins to replicate, making clones of itself. These new cells are duplicates of the mother CD8 cell, including the attached antibody. Instead of just one CD8 cell that can bind to a specific antigen, there will soon be millions. Moreover, the cells continue to replicate over many years, helping to give us immune memory. It is one big reason we get some infections only once, on initial exposure.

While the CD8 cells are called cytotoxic, their fellow T-cells, the CD4 lymphocytes, are known as "T-helper" cells. They don't kill the embattled cell but help empower other cells, notably macrophages, to attack the invader.

The CD4 lymphocytes are not a monolithic group. By their actions, they are categorized into several different types; the main ones are given the abbreviations TH1, TH2, TH17, and Treg. They are not only responsible for activating an inflammatory response but for moderating it as well. When a member of the immune system, usually a wandering dendritic cell, encounters a pathogen, a chemical signal is sent to the thymus epithelial cells. They then direct which type of CD4 cells are required. Generally, The Th1 cells combat intracellular pathogens; the Th2 cells are marshaled against extracellular parasites.

Monocytes are, of course, the real workhorses of the immune system, being responsible for the engulfment of invading pathogens and the signaling to the rest of the troops about what is needed. Monocytes don't have a simple on-off switch. They operate at different levels. Their contents are so toxic to human tissue they must be carefully controlled to prevent the inappropriate release of these destructive enzymes.

When a pathogen is recognized and engulfed, it is encased in a tiny bit of the monocyte's surface membrane, called a phagosome. The phagosome containing the microbe is isolated inside the cell, and the killer granule, known as the lysosome, is engaged to combine with the organism-containing phagosome, and the encased microbe is destroyed. This is what happens most of the time. But some bacteria have developed the means to prevent the combination of the destructive lysosome with the phagosome, preventing its killing. This is where the Th1 CD4 lymphocytes come in. They detect a piece of the microbe on the surface of the monocyte, not by MHC 1, but by a related MHC 2. If it is a match, a potent chemical signal is given to the monocyte to "ramp up" its destructive power and release destructive enzymes and other toxic material not contained in the lysosome. This hyper-reaction can destroy the monocyte but often the invading microbe as well. In addition, the monocyte is chemically instructed to release inflammatory cytokines, such as TNFα, which also brings in many more monocytes and CD4 lymphocytes.

The most often used example of this activity is the organism that causes tuberculosis, *Mycobacterium tuberculosis*. When the bug invades tissues, usually the lung, it is immediately encountered and engulfed by local macrophages. Still, the bacterium can prevent its immediate destruction by forming an enzyme that controls the combination of the monocyte's lysosome with the bacteria-encasing membrane. T helper cells, in this case, Th1, will carry out the function of signaling the monocyte to take its deadly game to a higher level, and the process of cellular immunity is in full swing.

Of course, this process takes some time, often a few weeks. CD4 cells of the right type must be activated and arrive where the monocyte engages with the pathogen. If we have encountered the microbe before, the T cells active against it are already circulating. All they need to do is replicate to present a higher number of cells, and the containment effort is speeded up.

Because of the delay in our initial encounter, the organism can sometimes gain a foothold in its monocyte hosts. As Th1 lymphocytes become active in the area, a stalemate sometimes occurs with a vigorous cellular immune response but not total killing. *Mycobacterium tuberculosis* is a very slow-growing microbe, and its cell wall is especially tough, containing a significant amount of wax. The result is a stand-off, with a few microbes remaining encased in some monocytes and a vigorous cellular response of monocytes and CD4 lymphocytes accumulating around it. The term "granuloma" is used to describe the histologic structure resulting. Granulomas are not unique to TB and may be formed following infection by other microbes. When seen on biopsy material by a pathologist, they are a helpful clue that an intracellular infection is occurring in the organ of the tissue being examined.

The Th1 CD4 lymphocytes send out several chemicals to signal cells to alter their metabolism and genes to challenge the invader. The most prominent and probably important one is interferon-gamma. There are three types of interferons, 1, 2, and 3. Type 1 includes alpha and beta and their subtypes. Type 3 is called lambda, consisting of four subtypes. Type 1 and 3 interferons are most useful against viral infections. Type 2 interferon consists solely of the gamma type. Our cells are equipped with receptors for IFN-gamma, especially the macrophages. When a CD4 Th1 cell encounters its target antigen presented in an MHC 2 molecule on the surface of a macrophage, it immediately releases interferon-gamma, most of which binds to the adjacent macrophage. A progression of chemical reactions is then initiated within the macrophage, activating or suppressing at least 200 genes. This activity boosts the macrophage's ability to contain and destroy the pathogen it contains.

Most times, organisms that invade cells are handled very efficiently by the combination of macrophages and helper T-cells. Infections such as those caused by the microorganisms *Cryptococcus neoformans*, *Cryptosporidium parvum*, *Toxoplasma gondii*, and others usually occur unnoticed by the infected person. There are only very mild or no symptoms, and the infection is cleared without our knowledge of its presence. But when there is a problem with the helper CD4 cells, this changes dramatically. In the early 1980s, a virus that had been rare in the developed world burst onto the scene. Initially, the virus was unknown, but infectious diseases usually controlled by CD4 lymphocytes started appearing in significant numbers. While these diseases were known, their sheer numbers and mortality rates were astounding. People were dying from diseases previously seen only in patients with severely compromised immune systems, often secondary to the chemotherapeutic therapies used to treat cancer. The new condition was assigned the moniker *acquired immune deficiency syndrome* or AIDS. It was later shown to be caused by a virus that invades the lymphocytes, with a predilection for CD4 cells. The virus was named *human immunodeficiency virus*, or HIV. The severity of usually benign infections like cryptococcosis, toxoplasmosis, and cryptosporidium illustrates the enormous importance of our T-lymphocytes in fighting infections.

Another important T-helper cell is the Th2 variety. Like the Th1 cells, they are of the CD4 type, but their mission is decidedly different. The Th2 cells are outfitted to help combat large invaders, primarily parasites, that exist outside cells, not within them. Suppose a person walks barefoot through an area contaminated with human fecal waste. If present, the larvae of hookworms can attach to the skin and work their way into the bloodstream, which carries them to their destination, the lining of the small intestine. An important weapon the body uses to combat such infestations is a specific antibody, known as IgE, that works against the parasite. It essentially pokes holes in it.

152

We have several different types of antibodies, the most common of which are IgG and IgA, both produced by our B-lymphocytes. When a Th2 CD4 lymphocyte becomes activated, it performs as the Th1 CD4 cells do: it reproduces to make many copies of itself, then these daughter cells go into action. But instead of engaging a monocyte that has encased the microbe, the Th2 cell contacts the B-lymphocytes making the antibody and chemically signaling them to make the IgE type instead of its usual IgG or IgA. In addition to directly attacking the parasite, engaged IgE attaches to the potent mast cells, enabling their release of active chemicals. Th2 lymphocytes are also very good at releasing chemical signals for the creation and specific migration of eosinophils, the type of granulocytes that are very active against parasites.

One of the main molecules sent out by the Th2 lymphocytes is interleukin 4 (IL-4). It stimulates the active B lymphocytes to produce IgE instead of the more common IgG or IgA. Another cytokine produced by the Th2 cells is interleukin 5 (IL-5), which stimulates the bone marrow to create more eosinophils. These white blood cells are effective against an invading parasite. Also produced is interleukin 13 (IL-13), which has several functions, including augmenting the activity of IL-4. Still another cytokine is amphiregulin, which stimulates epithelial tissue growth, aiding in the expulsion of a parasite.

With two CD4 lymphocytes termed Th1 and Th2, it would seem most likely that a third commonly encountered one would be designated Th3, but instead, it's called Th17. This CD4 lymphocyte derives its name not by being the 17th member of a sequence but because it helps the immune system by secreting an important cytokine, interleukin-17 or IL-17. The Th1 cells assist in combating intracellular organisms, and the Th2 cells help defend against extracellular parasites. The Th17 variety's primary foes are extracellular bacteria, creatures such as Staph and Strep, which are very common invaders. When the Th17 cell encounters these types of bacteria, it secretes interleukin-17, which acts on the local tissues, instructing them to secrete other cytokines such as interleukin-8, a powerful attractant for neutrophils. Since neutrophils are firmly entrenched in the innate immune system, the Th17 variety of CD4 lymphocytes bridges the innate and adaptive immune systems. It's a T-cell originating in the thymus but working to stimulate the first attack against invading extracellular bacteria. Their role is vital, as these species of bacteria are a common, everyday occurrence. Failure to mount an aggressive initial response to their presence can result in an overwhelming infection in a short time.

All the responses initiated by the various T-helper cells must be carefully controlled. They instruct powerful cells to release their killing machinery at a breakneck pace. Sooner or later, the response must be shut down or mitigated. That job is given to another type of CD4 lymphocyte, commonly designated Treg, short for regulator T-cell. Like its CD4 cousins, the regulatory T-cells are developed in the thymus but receive very different instructions. The T-helper cells work by dispensing chemical signals, usually cytokines, into or around the cells they are trying to help. The regulatory T-cells also produce cytokines, but their actions are much different. They instruct the target cell to shut down what it is doing. A major Treg cytokine is interleukin 10 (IL-10), which has a depressing effect on other cytokines responsible for cellular inflammation. Normally, about 10-15% of our circulating CD4 cells are of the regulatory type, but their numbers increase when it is necessary to reduce the activity of other CD4 cells. What drives this increase of Treg cells is not clearly known, but as their numbers increase, the activity of other T-helper cells decreases, and the healing process begins. A critical factor in the severity of autoimmune diseases is the failure of the body to produce an adequate number of regulatory T-cells. The hyper-immune response is not controlled, and the condition expands accordingly.

T-cells can go in several directions when they enter the thymus following their creation in the bone marrow. Their fate is not pre-determined. On encountering the epithelial cells of the thymus, they are given "instructions" on how to develop. These instructions come from a chemical signal directed from the thymus cells. If the body needs more CD8 cells to fight a viral infection, the T-cell will rev up the genes to display the

CD8 molecule on its surface and suppress the genes that code for CD4. Just the opposite happens if CD4 cells are needed. The type of CD4 cell needed (Th1, Th2, Th17, Treg, or another less common type) is also taken care of by chemical instructions received from the thymus, which receives its chemical instructions from the affected body part. Genes within the chromosome of the T-cell are either triggered or suppressed, depending on the chemical signal received.

Through a very complex process of gene manipulation, T-cells have a particular protein on their surface. Each T-cell has one that is unique; there are millions of different T cells, each displaying a special protein. They are designed to bind with a unique protein or carbohydrate on an invading organism, like an antibody binding to an antigen. The usual process calls for a monocyte, macrophage, or dendritic cell to encounter a pathogen, process its parts, then expose a tiny bit of each of it on an MHC 1 or MHC 2 molecule. The particle-carrying MHC is then displayed on the cell's surface. That phagocytic cell then makes its way to some lymphoid tissue, either a lymph node or another type. It keeps bumping into lymphocytes until it encounters one containing the protein that matches up with the displayed little part of the microbe (called an epitope). Once that happens, the engaged T-cell is stimulated to divide and make many more copies of itself, which enter the bloodstream and enter tissues searching for the same epitope. The protein receptor never leaves the T-cell; it is firmly attached to its surface and can only go where the lymphocyte carries it as it searches for the key protein or carbohydrate.

Before the complex nature of lymphocytes was worked out, one of their major products, antibodies, was well known. The immune system has been conveniently divided into two parts, cellular and humoral, the latter word coming from the Latin *umor*, meaning "body fluid." Antibodies, complex proteins that bind with little pieces of microbes, are transported in the serum to all the fluids and tissues of our body so that they can attach to the bug and work with other parts of the immune system to eliminate it. The work of antibodies was known by the late 1800s.   In 1906, a German bacteriologist used his knowledge of antibodies to develop a test for syphilis, the Wassermann test. By today's standards, it was very crude, but after this work, using antibodies to aid in diagnosing infectious diseases became routine.   For over half a century, the big, unanswered question was, "Where do antibodies come from?". They are specific to infectious agents and abundant in sick individuals and not others, but how are they produced?

The answer was initially proposed by a budding British ornithologist, Bruce Glick, in 1956. He was doing his doctoral thesis on bird anatomy and was especially interested in a hitherto mysterious little structure, the bursa of Fabricius.   Sitting adjacent to the cloaca, it is a structure common to all birds. First discovered by a man with a challenging name, Hieronymus Fabricius, back in the early 1600s, the birds' bursa was not given much attention. (The term "bursa" refers to a small pouch; the root of the word is the same as for the word "purse"). Glick was doing some surgical work on birds and had taken the bursa of Fabricius out of several of them. Coincidentally, one of his colleagues asked him if he could inject a few of his birds with some antigenic material from a species of *Salmonella* to collect antibodies for his experiments. Much to their surprise, the birds in Glick's collection with their bursas removed produced no antibody. It turns out that the bursa of Fabricius in birds was the organ responsible for making antibody-producing cells, somewhat analogous to the thymus of mammals. The cells were given the nickname "B" cells, obviously from the bird organ from whence they came.

After Glick's discovery, much work was done on lymphocytes and their ability to produce antibodies. Different types of antibodies are known (IgG, IgA, IgM, IgD, and IgE, distinguished by their chemical structure and function). Some amazing work has been done to illustrate the elaborate genetic machinations needed to produce such a wide array of antibodies. After injecting a human with a protein or a carbohydrate, we'll make an antibody to it, whether it comes from a common microbe or some obscure substance from the bottom of the ocean or the top of the highest mountain in the Himalayas. Just as remarkable, we don't (in most cases) make antibodies against

156

our own tissues. Lymphocytes that do are effectively eliminated from the process. It's a stupendous operation, and we still don't know all the secrets of the process.

We humans don't have a little pouch next to our intestinal tract for the maturation of lymphocytes into the B cell type. In mammals, that job has been turned over to the bone marrow, at least for the most part. That's rather convenient since both bursa and bone marrow start with B, so there is no need to change the designation.

Just as there are several kinds of antibodies, there are several kinds of B-lymphocytes. The follicular, or FO, is the most prominent B-cell responsible for the classic antibody response. Produced in the bone marrow, the FO B-cells migrate to the lymph nodes or the spleen. Each cell is equipped with a unique receptor on its surface, one that will only react with a single molecule. There are millions of different receptors, so there are millions of different B cells. Their job is to mix and mingle with other cells in the lymphoid tissue until just the suitable dendritic cell or macrophage comes along, bearing an exact match for the B-cell's receptor on the macrophage's MHC molecule. When the two get together, the B-cell is triggered to multiply and begin cranking out more of its unique receptor, not as an isolated molecule but as one attached to a molecular stem. This complex of stem and receptor is known as an antibody. The type of stem molecule to be produced depends on the job to be done. A T-helper cell usually gives the chemical signal to the B-cell, directing the proper anchor molecule. So, if IgE is needed to combat a parasite, then the chemical signal is provided to make that happen. The appropriate signal is transmitted if IgG, IgA, or IgM are required. The resulting large molecule, consisting of the specific receptor attached to a unique stem, is known as an antibody.

Unlike the T-cells, which hold on to their receptors, the B-cells let theirs get away to circulate. Antibodies penetrate all human tissue and are extremely valuable in combating microbial invaders. They are ultra-specific, designed to combat a unique structure, whether it is still attached to a microbe or floating free. They act in several ways, depending on the situation. Some are called neutralizing, as they hook onto a microbial protein and interfere with its activity. Some bring the microbe to a neutrophil, helping the phagocyte engulf the invader. Others link the microbial protein or carbohydrate with complement, which can attack the microbe or enable a neutrophil to phagocytize it, known as opsonization, or "assist with eating." Still others, the IgE class, link parasite antigens to mast cells and basophils, initiating a cascade of chemical reactions designed to rid the body of the invader.

The IgA class of antibodies is different than the others. They are commonly called secretory antibodies because they don't circulate around the body in the bloodstream or in the tissues. They are designed to be released into the respiratory and gastrointestinal tracts, and then are then eliminated from the body. The job of IgA is to attach to and neutralize a microbe before it enters the body. The structure of IgA antibodies differs from the others. They lack the molecular stem called the Fc portion because they work alone and don't need to dock to a human cell.

Immature or "naïve" B cells can go in any direction once released from the bone marrow. Which path they follow is dictated by the circumstances they find themselves in and at the behest of T-helper cells.

When a B cell and a T cell collaborate on the formation of antibodies, the results are what we call the acquired immune system. The B cell multiplies into many clones of itself, each able to produce the same antibody. Not only that, but some of the B cells also continue to reproduce indefinitely, giving rise to immunologic memory. The appropriate T cell does the same. Ordinarily, producing a specific antibody can take up to two weeks to reach full operation. With memory cells, the process is much shortened to a day or two. That's why some diseases affect us only once; the second time, the needed antibody response is much quicker.

Some B-cells have the ability to enter a quiescent state, staying alive but not metabolizing or producing antibody. Most of these are sequestered in the bone marrow. They are ready to spring into action when the need arises. These quiet, previously activated B-lymphocytes are an essential part of immune memory.

When B cells are activated and begin to make copies of themselves, they are usually no longer referred to as B cells. They are now called plasma cells. The terms plasmacytes and activated B cells are also sometimes used. The new moniker is used because they appear somewhat different under the microscope than their inactivated kin. Their nucleus appears "clock-faced." They contain abundant endoplasmic reticulum and Golgi apparatus, all the better for manufacturing copious amounts of antibodies.

Like the T cells, there are different kinds of B cells. The FO is by far the most common, but two other types exist. One is known as the B1 lymphocyte. Unlike typical B cells, they are not formed in the bone marrow but are initiated by the liver. They reside in the chest and abdomen, and for the most part they produce a not-very-specific IgM antibody. These antibodies usually form against bacteria and viruses' surface molecules but often cross-react with other substances. They also create some members of the IgA class, those that are secreted in our body fluids. Some circulate all the time freely and form a valuable part of the innate immune system, combining with complement to repel a potential invader more rapidly.

The third type of B cell is the marginal zone, or MZ, lymphocyte, which is similar in activity to the B1 cells. While they can hook up to protein and be stimulated by T cells, the MZ B cells' main job is to react to carbohydrate antigens, the best example of which is the capsule of invading bacteria. They make IgM antibodies primarily and are among our first lines of defense in attacking encapsulated bacteria, such as pneumococcus, which often causes pneumonia.

Lymphocytes, in all their iterations, form an immensely complicated yet vital component of our immune system. They bridge the gap between the innate and acquired systems and protect us from every type of microbial invader. Failure of these cells to act properly, as seen in diseases such as AIDS and lymphoma, clearly results in ill health, sometimes death.

Working in concert with the other cells and molecules of the immune system, they are vigilant in protecting us.

Chapter 12
The Auxiliary

Acute-phase proteins;
Invaluable assets,
Often overlooked

Streptococcus pneumoniae is well-named. It causes pneumonia, often the most severe kind. Of the dozens of microorganisms that can be the etiologic agent of pneumonia, *S. pneumoniae*, usually called pneumococcus, is the most common cause of cases acquired in the community. It can attack directly and without warning or invade secondarily following another infection, such as influenza. It is one serious pathogen.

The most obvious virulence factor on pneumococcus is the slimy carbohydrate capsule surrounding the cell wall. It repels the neutrophil attack, allowing the organism to bounce off the predatory white blood cell like a bar of soap. Complement and antibodies to the capsule are beneficial in hooking the bug to the neutrophil, allowing phagocytosis. But it can take almost a week for antibodies to form, with the infection proceeding to a sometimes dangerous level. In the age before antibiotics, rapidly progressing pneumonia was often fatal. It still can be today.

In the early 1930s, one of the body's backup systems to thwart the invader was discovered at the Rockefeller Institute in New York. William Tillet and Thomas Francis Jr. worked with pneumococcus and the body's antibody response to it, measuring serum antibody levels and trying to find a treatment for the disease. At that time, before the age of antibiotics, it was common to take the serum from a previously sickened and recovering patient and administer it to a patient in the early stages of the same illness. In their work, they discovered something very interesting: a substance in the serum of sick patients seemed to attack the organism, but it wasn't an antibody. Rather than attack one single strain of pneumococcus, as an antibody does, it attacked all members of the genus. Its target wasn't the capsule but a carbohydrate attached to the organism's core lining. This material of pneumococcus, called the C-substance, is common to all strains of the organism and plays a role in its pathogenesis. The serum substance they found seemed to act like a routine antibody, but unlike antibody, it didn't last long in the serum of sick patients. As soon as the patient was over the crisis and recovering, this C-reactive substance quickly disappeared from the patient's blood. They named it **C-reactive protein**, which has come to be known as CRP.

The early researchers who first identified CRP associated it with pneumococcus, but CRP has a much wider range of action than one species of bacteria, as significant as that is. Instead, it is designed to hook onto substances that have exposed choline, a chemical common to humans and bacteria alike. Produced in the liver, CRP is only released when something in the body has gone awry, and choline is expressed: a bacterial infection, tissue destruction, atherosclerotic plaques in the arteries, and many other conditions. Whatever brings about an inflammatory response, the liver, primarily through the stimulation of interleukin-6, starts manufacturing large amounts of C-reactive protein, an extremely useful substance.

Choline, a relatively simple chemical, plays an enormous role in our bodies. It is an integral component of every cell membrane. The vital neurotransmitter acetylcholine allows our muscles to receive signals from our nervous system and allows muscle contraction. There are many other molecules, primarily lipids, in which choline is found, and life would quickly cease to be in its absence. It is strange, then, that CRP directly attaches to choline and removes it. Fortunately, a couple of safeguards regulate CRP: it only acts to scarf up released choline produced from decaying cells, and it can attach to choline present on microorganisms, such as pneumococcus, rendering the organism inactive. CRP can bind the substance or microorganism to complement, enhancing the neutrophils' ability to phagocytize it. Compared to antibodies, CRP's action is rather crude, but it nonetheless is a very good thing to have to work for us before antibodies can be produced. CRP has a half-life of about nineteen hours, so it diminishes quickly once the crisis is over.

C-reactive protein is one of many chemicals the body produces that generally behave in our defense, either to thwart the advance of microorganisms or to aid in the mopping up and recovery of damaged areas. Collectively known as *Acute-Phase Proteins*, they are always present in the circulation, but their numbers are increased when the body is stressed. The liver or some other organ receives a chemical signal from the challenged area, intensifying their production.

When a crisis develops, interleukin-6 and a few other signaling proteins contact liver cells, bind to them, and start the process by which the genes coding for acute-phase proteins are activated in larger numbers than usual. The initiating signal comes not only from infectious diseases but also from tissue injuries, burns, cancer, and other physiologic disturbances. Even severe psychological disorders like schizophrenia have been shown to stimulate the release of some acute-phase proteins. Just which acute-phase proteins are mustered and in what numbers depends on the nature of the condition and its severity.

Serum amyloid A proteins, like C-reactive protein, increase dramatically in the serum following an acute inflammatory condition. There are at least four different serum amyloid A proteins in humans, usually abbreviated SAA, followed by their number (e.g., SAA1). When certain infections hit, the liver is signaled by cytokines to increase the production of the serum amyloid A proteins. After production, they attach themselves to high-density lipoprotein (HDL), which carries cholesterol from the body's cells to the liver.

Serum amyloid A proteins have many functions. For one, they act as an attractant for white blood cells, signaling them to slow down when they enter the infected zone. They also signal cells in the infected area to secrete enzymes to degrade the matrix substance around them, allowing the easier penetration of immune cells and molecules. They assist HDL in carrying cholesterol away from the area to eliminate it in the bile.

Like CRP, the blood level of serum amyloid A proteins can be used as an indicator of the presence of an acute infectious disease or inflammatory condition. Also, like CRP, its elevated numbers don't give a definitive diagnosis but can strongly indicate that an infection or other inflammatory event is occurring.

The proteins of complement are decidedly increased when the body is under assault. This would include mannose-binding lectin (MBL), which can bind to surface receptors of many pathogenic organisms and initiate the complement pathway. Also, like CRP, complement proteins can bind to damaged tissue and facilitate its removal by macrophages.

Several proteins of coagulation are significantly increased during an inflammatory event. Certainly, they are essential when hemorrhaging is involved, but they are also increased during quite a few infectious diseases. Fibrin clots can help wall off a budding infection and prevent its spread to other parts of the body.

White blood cells, especially neutrophils, carry a powerful armamentarium of destructive enzymes. We need these to help destroy invading pathogens, but alas, the proteins released by neutrophils can cause harm to our own tissues as well. Counteracting these WBC-associated proteases are a series of molecules known collectively as anti-proteases. There are several. One of the most studied is the one known as **alpha-1 antitrypsin**. It goes by several names, but whatever you call it, it has an important function: bind and help inactivate destructive enzymes released during combat with an invading microbe. Despite its name, trypsin isn't the only enzyme it can inactivate; it can act against a variety of them. Not only that, but it binds the deactivated enzyme to regional cells and, in so doing, serves as a beacon to circulating lymphocytes to slow down and remain in the area. The anti-proteases protect us from the collateral damage generated during the battle against invading microbes.

The collateral damage of injured tissue needs to be cleaned up. Just as immediate action needs to be taken following a sewage spill, the toxic materials released from wounded cells may cause harm and need to be quickly ameliorated. Several

164

proteins normally present in the circulation are rapidly manufactured in greater numbers following tissue injury, whether infectious or traumatic. **Ceruloplasmin** is a complex protein with several tasks. Chiefly, it transports copper ions throughout the body. But it also functions in iron metabolism. When tissues are damaged, iron may be released, an undesirable occurrence for several reasons. One is that free iron is potentially toxic to the body. Also, bacteria with access to iron ions grow much faster than those without it. Ceruloplasmin assists with the metabolism and removal of iron by enabling it to be associated with transferrin and safely transported away. During stress, ceruloplasmin levels increase, reducing the immediate danger of iron overload.

Similarly, two other proteins, haptoglobin and hemopexin, increase following tissue damage. Their role is to ensure the proper metabolism of hemoglobin. Hemoglobin is safe enough when contained within an intact red blood cell. But if the red cells are damaged, hemoglobin can be released with toxic effects on various tissues, especially the kidneys. Haptoglobin and hemopexin are very useful in metabolizing free hemoglobin to mitigate the damage it may cause.

Other molecules come under the heading of acute-phase proteins. Our bodies are adept at quickly activating the genes responsible for their manufacture and release. Mainly produced in the liver, they are quickly released into the bloodstream and find their way to wherever they are needed. While not the primary workhorses of the immune system, they are invaluable in assisting both cellular and molecular responses. Mainly, the acute-phase proteins serve as enablers for the immune system in the fight against an invader. Some attach to receptors on the invading microbe to help damage it. They also help prepare the site of confrontation by allowing for the greater inflow of immune cells and proteins, assist with the clean-up of potentially toxic debris, and assist with the chemical signaling that is so important to a well-coordinated effort.

Besides quickly manufacturing an array of proteins to confront an invading enemy, we have another means of altering the playing field to put the battle a little more in our favor. By raising the temperature, either locally at the site of the infection or for the entire body, many microbes are put at a disadvantage, and the immune response to them is given the upper hand. Technically this elevated temperature is called pyrexia, from the Greek *pyrex*, meaning "hot" or "fire." Of course, very few use that term; fever is far more common. The word "fever" comes from *febris*, the Latin word for it. The adjective febrile is frequently used to describe a patient's condition, as "the patient was febrile (feverish) for most of the night." Normal body temperature is referred to as afebrile.

Many think that fever is all bad all the time, and the sooner we are done with it, the better. But nature has given us this means of aiding our fight against foreign invaders, and while we usually don't feel very well while feverish, it has its place in our anti-microbial arsenal. All mammals become febrile. It is a complicated scheme involving the nervous system and many bodily organs. We shouldn't be too quick to dismiss fever as an evil rather than a potential good. It has its place.

There are two general types of pyrexia. In one, often called heat stroke, the body's ability to control its normal temperature is compromised. The amount of heat built up by the environment and exercise is overwhelming, and the core temperature rises despite the usual physiologic functions to control it. Immediate measures are needed to reduce the body's temperature, namely hydration and placing the patient in a cool environment. In this case, the usual drugs used to reduce fever, such as aspirin or Tylenol, are useless.

The other, much more common type of fever, is intentionally produced by the body's nervous and immune systems to help thwart microbial invaders. It is a very complex system involving the stimulation of specific neurons in the pre-optic portion of the brain by chemical stimulators. These chemical stimulators may be either interleukin-1, tumor necrosis factor-α, interferon-gamma, interleukin-6 (the so-called pyrogenic cytokines), or prostaglandins produced by the activity of the cytokines. Prostaglandin E_2 is well known to induce fever.

The brain contains at least four different types of neurons that are involved in temperature regulation. One is stimulated

166

by warm temperatures, a second by heat loss, a third is temperature insensitive, and the fourth is responsible for heat production. Normally, they are in balance, so what we call the body's thermostat is normally set at 37°C. But when an appropriate chemical stimulator crosses the blood-brain barrier and lands on receptors on the neurons responsible for heat production, it takes the lead over the others. The body thermostat is set to a higher level, and various actions are taken to raise the temperature to that level. Shivering, narrowing of the blood vessels (vasoconstriction), increased metabolism, and increased heart rate result in increased body temperature. The core temperature will stay elevated as long as the neurons directing heat production predominate. Ironically, even though the temperature is rising, the patient feels chilled mainly because of the activity of shivering, which induces heat production. Once the immediate crisis is resolved, another group of neurons receives chemical signals and becomes active, overriding the effects of the fever-inducing neurons. It is a highly complex system, but it is designed to assist the immune system in addressing the presence of an invader.

Many microbes do not do well at temperatures significantly above 37°C (98.6F). Their enzymes don't function as efficiently, and they grow at a slower rate. With an elevated temperature, the heart rate and blood flow increase, allowing for the more rapid transport of microbe-fighting white blood cells and molecules. Interferons and several cytokines are more active at elevated temperatures. So is the activity of macrophages. Elevated temperatures also enhance tissue repair.

Most of us are aware of medications that reduce fever. Collectively called antipyretics, they can interfere with the production of prostaglandins, thus limiting the stimulation of heat-producing neurons. The body's core thermostat is set at a lower level, reducing fever. Aspirin, acetaminophen (Tylenol), and ibuprofen (Advil, Motrin) are effective antipyretics. Clearly, the temperature cannot rise too high. Still, one may legitimately question the wisdom of taking action to reduce fever, given its proven ability to help us control the spread of infectious diseases. Fever is not a disease but rather a symptom of invaders and a means of combating them. It has its place.

The increased production of the so-called acute-phase proteins and fever are vital, ancient means of addressing the acquisition of an infectious disease. While not confined to infectious conditions, they are an integral part of our immune system, enabling the fight or assisting with clean-up and repair.

SECTION THREE

"If you know the enemy and know yourself, you need not fear the result of a hundred battles. If you know yourself but not the enemy, for every victory gained you will suffer a defeat. If you know neither the enemy nor yourself, you will succumb in every battle."

– Sun Tzu, The Art of War

Chapter 13
The Big E

Constant companion.
Inauspicious force for good.
Also, pernicious.

Two popular metaphors for expressing vast numbers are "stars in the sky" and "grains of sand on the beach." Infectious disease investigators could add one of their own, "numerous as the bacteria in the human gut." Somehow, this one has never caught on, but it is just as apt. There are over a trillion (that's with a T) of them in each person. The gut microflora has its own ecosystem, with over a thousand species of bacteria co-habiting the length of each person's colon.

The first identification of one of the prominent members of this bacterial flora came from a remarkable man, Theodor Escherich. Born in November of 1857, he was the son of a medical doctor, public health administrator, and statistician, Dr. Ferdinand Escherich. His mother died when he was five years old, and the family moved to Wurzburg, Germany. Apparently, young Theodor was quite a prankster, and he was sent off to a Jesuit boarding school in Austria, presumably to help him mend his ways. After graduation and some military service, he entered medical school and became qualified to practice medicine in 1881. He must have gotten his priorities straightened out as he graduated with high honors and was selected to work with the esteemed pediatrician Karl Gerhardt. There, Dr. Escherich developed an interest in pediatric infectious diseases. Working with Dr. Gerhardt gave him access to some of the best of the newly established microbiology laboratories of the time.

Dr. Escherich was very interested in the bowel flora of babies. When developing in the uterus, our intestinal tracts are sterile, but shortly after birth we rapidly become colonized by many different species of bacteria. Dr. Escherich was interested in this colonization and the bacteria that were involved. He investigated the role they played in the health of developing children. He also studied breast milk and was among the first to give scientific evidence of its advantages.

During these very early investigations, Dr. Escherich discovered the bacterium that would one day bear his name, the organism about which today more is known than any other living creature. When he isolated and identified it, he called it *Bacterium coli commune*, but the name was later changed to honor its discoverer, *Escherichia coli*.

Dr. Escherich did much more in his illustrious career. He was a top administrator as well as a physician and researcher. He was responsible for creating and designing many top-rated pediatric medical centers, which were lacking in his day. He died at age 52. His contribution to medicine is stated most eloquently in this obituary in the Boston Medical and Surgical Journal:

"He was a contributor to numerous medical periodicals, a member of many learned societies, and was known as a pediatric consultant throughout Europe. His professional reputation was international. His energy for work was tremendous, and his disposition strenuous and masterful. He is described as impulsive, uncommonly strict, strong-willed, faithful, severe with himself but kindly towards others. That the children, his patients, loved him, is evidence that he loved them and, therefore, had a good heart. His career is an admirable example of the life of the German university physician, scientist, and professor."

People with names that are hard to pronounce often have them shortened. The guy who invented the radio is always referred to as simply "Marconi," probably because his first name is a little tricky to say (Guglielmo). So it is with the organism that is the most studied and researched in all creation. Very few say *"Escherichia"* coli; it almost always just comes out "E." But the man behind its discovery was nonetheless a remarkable individual.

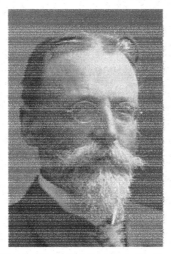

*Theodor Escherich first described a ubiquitous and important bacterium. He called it **Bacterium coli commune**, but in 1919 its name was changed to **Escherichia coli**.*

E. coli is a member of a vast family of bacteria known as *Enterobacteriaceae*. The rules of naming an organism, known as binomial nomenclature, are followed in bacteriology as in other areas of biology. So, bacteria have genus and species names, even though the distinction of some may seem arbitrary. A collection of genera having some common characteristics is known as a family. *Enterobacteriaceae* is a family of Gram-negative bacteria, the genera of which resemble each other in many ways. Some of the more common genera in the family that live on and sometimes infect humans include *Escherichia coli, Shigella, Klebsiella, Enterobacter, Citrobacter, Salmonella, Proteus, Providencia,* and *Morganella.* They all have unique characteristics that define the genus but also share many components and attributes that tie them together. The family is, in fact, enormous, with hundreds of different genera found in many natural habitats. The ones mentioned here constitute most of the genera involved with humans, both as commensal flora and as a cause of disease.

A term used in scientific nomenclature often confusing is the designation "strain." *Escherichia* is the genus; *coli* is the species. A strain is a subset of the species that can be singled out because of some unique characteristic(s). For instance, *E.*

coli that has become resistant to an antibiotic because they have acquired a collection of antibiotic resistance genes can be referred to as a "strain" of *E. coli*. The word strain usually indicates a common ancestor. A helpful way to envision the concept of strains of bacteria is to think of breeds of dogs. There are cocker spaniels, border collies, pit bulls, and many more. They are distinct from one another but are all members of the species *Canis familiaris*.

Enterobacteriaceae, usually called enterics, have been a part of us for as long as we have existed as a species. Most live in our bowel as commensals, living out their existence in the most benign fashion. But others have gone over to the dark side. They have become pathogens, organisms that can make an otherwise healthy person quite ill, sometimes worse. Most of them can and do make us sick when the opportunity is presented, such as injury or medical condition. Because of our intimate relationship with them, we will always have infections by *Enterobacteriaceae*.

E. coli is the most studied organism. More is known about its genetics, enzymes, structure, and other attributes than any other biological entity. But, to the public, it is also greatly misunderstood. Very commonly, one can read a news article about health matters and notice a concern or warning about that terrible "*E. coli*" that may infect us as if it were a distinct pathogen like *Yersinia pestis,* the organism that causes bubonic plague. A statement like that is misguided. Every human being, every single one of us, has *E. coli* in our bowel. If you get a stool sample from any human and give it to a clinical lab to grow out the organisms it contains, the first and most apparent organism recovered is *E. coli.* Obviously, then, not all *E. coli* strains are created equal. There is a great deal of difference between the normal, commensal strains and the pathogenic ones. Knowing which *E. coli* strain is present is just as important as knowing it is an *E. coli.*

The differences between *E. coli* strains start with its genome, the long strand of DNA that encodes most of the organism's genes. It's often referred to as a "chromosome" because its function is the same as that for higher animals, the coding of genetic information, but it isn't a true chromosome like ours. Instead, bacterial DNA is a long strand of the classic double helix, tightly coiled and rambling throughout the bacterial cell. Bacteria don't have nuclear membranes to contain it.

The bacterial DNA is transcribed into messenger RNA (mRNA). That mRNA goes to a ribosome to be translated, the same process as ours. Bacterial ribosomes are different from ours, but they belong to the organism. That differs from viruses, which don't have their own ribosomes and need to use those of the host cell. The mRNA is translated into protein, the building blocks of life. *E. coli* is very good at this process of making protein. When they get going strong, the entire cell can divide in 20-30 minutes, an amazingly efficient system. Dividing unobstructed, a single cell, with the reproduction of its progeny, can produce up to a billion organisms in a little over a day.

In addition to the long, coiled strand of DNA we call a chromosome, bacteria often have additional, much shorter, independent strands of DNA called plasmids. Bacterial cells may contain one or several. Although they are not nearly as big as the main chromosome, they code for proteins just the same, and they usually divide in harmony with the rest of the cell.

Much of what we know about molecular genetics comes from studying *E. coli.* Its entire genome is known. A major part of the chromosome comprises what is known as "housekeeping genes," or genes that create products needed for routine physiologic functioning like structure, energy production, motility, etc. In pathogenic organisms, though, a set of genes clustered close to each other and away from the housekeeping genes gives the organism its virulence capabilities. These gene clusters are commonly known as "pathogenicity islands." The genes which code for products needed for host cell adhesion, invasion, toxin production, and immune cell avoidance or disruption are concentrated in these genetic areas. Sometimes, they appear not to be derived from other *E. coli* but imported from entirely different organisms. The pathogenicity islands contain the genetic material that can make an innocent, tame commensal into an aggressive pathogen.

The plasmids harbor information that allows the organism to adapt better to its environment. They are best known for containing genes whose products enable the microorganisms to produce enzymes that combat antibiotics, either destroying the antibiotic or altering its binding site, rendering it ineffective. Plasmids do other things, of course, such as enabling the organism to take advantage of an environmental change, such as acquiring a nutrient.

As with any creature subject to the biological laws of natural selection, the bacteria which can rapidly adapt to changes in their environment will be the most likely to survive and pass on their advantageous genetic information to their progeny. *E. coli,* and the other members of the *Enterobacteriaceae,* are very good at this. They reproduce by binary fission, so mixing genes, as in vertebrates, is impossible, but they have several methods of exchanging genetic information.

One means of gene transfer is bacterial "sex," or **conjugation**. On the periphery of each *E. coli* cell are appendages called pili (or fimbriae), tiny hair-like structures commonly used by the organism to adhere to a cellular surface. Some of these become specialized to serve as a tube through which genetic material, mainly a plasmid, can travel from one organism to another. One organism "docks" with another, the specialized pilus is hooked up to the adjacent cell, and the plasmid transfer occurs with the genetic material flowing right through the pilus tunnel.

Many people don't realize it, but a virus can infect a bacterium. It's very common. The virus that infects a bacterium is called a phage, and there are lots of them. Quite a few phages integrate themselves onto the bacterial chromosome. When they leave, they can take with them small bits of bacterial DNA and transfer them to the bacterium they next infect. It's a way in which chromosomal DNA is transferred between organisms. It's called **transduction**.

As we all know, James Watson and Francis Crick reported that DNA strands contain the genetic code. That was in 1951. But Watson and Crick didn't operate in a vacuum. Some twenty-three years before them, in 1928, British bacteriologist Frederick Griffith made a discovery that "transformed" the biological world. Griffith's experiment was to take two strains of the bacteria known as pneumococcus, a species of *Streptococcus* that is sometimes highly pathogenic due to a slimy capsule surrounding the cell, aiding it in evading white blood cells. Of Griffith's two strains, one contained a polysaccharide capsule enabling it to cause disease leading to the death of mice when injected. The other was a non-virulent strain that lacked a capsule. When injected into mice, the encapsulated strain rapidly killed the mice. The non-capsulated strain does nothing; the mouse immune system gobbles it up.

Griffith took some encapsulated deadly bacteria and killed them, rendering them, of course, non-infective. He injected them into mice along with some live non-virulent bugs. One would think that nothing would happen to the mice since the only living strain injected was the non-capsulated, nonvirulent type. But one would be wrong. What Griffith found eventually changed the course of biology, although it went virtually unnoticed at the time. The non-virulent strain became virulent by acquiring a capsule from the dead organisms, killing the mice. It was transformed. It took some dozen or more years for anyone to figure out why, but Oswald Avery and his co-workers at the Rockefeller Institute in New York figured out that the transforming factor was DNA. The non-capsulated pneumococci picked up some DNA from the dead bacteria and incorporated it into their genome. Knowing that DNA was the molecule responsible eventually led Watson and Crick to do their work explaining the DNA double helix.

Frederick Griffith was killed in a bombing raid in London in 1941, and his discovery received little notice during his lifetime. Still, his research laid the groundwork for some of the most important discoveries in biology.

E. coli, and many other bacteria, can retrieve DNA strands deposited in their environment on the death and lysis of other organisms, and integrate them into their own genome. The term used for it harkens back to the one used by Griffith, **transformation**. Not only can *E. coli* capture DNA from other *E. coli,* but it can also get it from other genera, such as *Klebsiella, Enterobacter*, and *Proteus.* DNA transformation is a potent tool bacteria use to pass on genetic information.

176

Another genetic discovery of great importance in the pre-Watson and Crick era was made by a botanist who specialized in genetic studies, Barbara McClintock. She was unique in two ways: one of the few elite women scientists of her era, and one of the few scientists interested in and working on genetics. Her discovery came using the corn plant *Zea mays,* commonly called maize. This variety of corn plants has multicolored kernels and lends itself well to the application of Mendelian genetics. Dr. McClintock described what is commonly called "jumping genes," or genes that are movable from one part of the chromosome to another. Like Griffith's discovery, her work received very little notice at the time of her discovery in 1941, but as time went on, the profound nature of the discovery was more appreciated. She received the Nobel Prize in physiology in 1983, over 40 years after her work was published.

Jumping genes are technically called transposable elements, or TEs. "Jumping genes" is much more fun to say, but they are now usually referred to as **transposons**. They exist not only in plants but are very common in bacteria like *E. coli.* By having its genes move around and not be held in a fixed location, the encoded information has much more of a chance to be displayed, copied, and actualized. Transposons give the organism much more flexibility in adapting to environmental changes.

One of the most significant early discoveries of molecular genetics was made by a French biologist and doctor who was nearly not around to uncover it. Francois Jacob was born in Nancy, France, in 1920. A devoted scientist, he trained to be a doctor and wanted to become a surgeon, but he faced a formidable obstacle: World War II. After joining the army, he fled France for England when the Germans overwhelmed his country. He served in the Allied military as a doctor and saw considerable action. Severely wounded at Dunkirk, he nearly lost his life. Dr. Jacob was hospitalized for seven months and survived but could never become a surgeon because of his extensive wounds. Still, he was determined to carry on work, in his words, "into the nature of things," and ended up as a bacteriologist at the Pasteur Institute. There, he teamed up with

Jacques Monod to make one of the most critical molecular genetic discoveries of all time: the lac-operon.

Until the work of Jacob and Monod, it was assumed that organisms cranked out the proteins and enzymes encoded in their genes all the time, whether they needed them or not. If there is a gene on the chromosome for something, it gets transcribed into messenger RNA like all the others, and that's that. But Jacob had noticed that *E. coli* didn't always make the enzymes necessary to ferment lactose, the sugar found in milk. If much glucose is present or lactose is missing, the enzyme that breaks down lactose, known as galactopyranosidase, is not made, nor are any other enzymes needed to bring lactose into the cell. This puzzled him greatly until he had an "Aha!" moment while sitting in a movie theatre with his wife. He reasoned that the genes coding for lactose fermentation were covered up and not copied until lactose was present in the environment and glucose was missing. The covering-up molecules were called **operons**, and since the first one described was for lactose fermentation, it was abbreviated to "lac-operon." Jacob and Monod were awarded the Nobel Prize in Physiology or Medicine in 1965 for their discovery.

We now know that this shielding of specific genes on the DNA strand doesn't apply just to bacteria. The phenomenon is widespread and plays a major role in the expression and repression of the cells of our immune system. Not expressing and copying genes whose products would have no immediate role is a very efficient way to conserve precious energy. It gives those organisms that employ it a great ecologic advantage.

A spontaneous **mutation** is still another way bacteria can adapt to environmental changes. With the nucleotides of DNA being transcribed by RNA polymerase billions of times a day, there are sure to be a few errors that occur. Most of the mistakes result in minimal alteration in the protein produced. A few can be detrimental to the organism. But now and then, changing just one amino acid of a protein can make a profound difference in the way the protein operates, giving the altered organism an ecological advantage.

In summary, *E. coli* and other bacteria have multiple ways they can alter and manipulate their genetic foundation to survive better and take advantage of changes in their environment. A single gene may become slightly altered, giving rise to a modified protein. Bacteria can absorb and incorporate into their own genome the genetic material from another bacterium (transformation). Genetic material can be passed from one organism to another through a specialized pilus (conjugation). Genetic material can be carried from one strain of bacteria to another by a virus (transduction). Genes can move around on the chromosome and plasmids to be more accessible (transposons). Plasmids are little DNA fragments that code for proteins independent of the main bacterial chromosome. They similarly can be transferred from one organism to another. And, of course, much of the genetic material is covered and controlled by operons, enabling the organism to display "just in time" efficiency.

From an infectious disease perspective, we think of two important outcomes that result from this genetic adaptability. One is the ability to acquire and employ virulence factors making the organism a more potent pathogen. The other is the capacity to become resistant to antibiotics and other antimicrobial agents. *E. coli* is very good at doing both.

We all have an intimate relationship with *E. coli*. It lives inside us from the time we're about two days old until we die. Just as human relationships can be nurturing and fulfilling, then suddenly turn dark and ugly, so can our association with our little bacterial companion. The pathogenesis of *E. coli* takes on several forms, ranging from somewhat of a nuisance to deadly. The difference depends on what genes have been acquired by the organism, and our own immune status.

The most common infectious disease in which *E. coli* is involved is in the urinary tract, which is conveniently divided into two parts, lower and upper. The lower urinary tract consists of the urinary bladder and the urethra, which carries the urine out of the body. The upper urinary tract involves the kidneys and ureters. The ureters carry urine from the kidneys to the bladder. Lower urinary tract infections tend to be mild, usually easily treatable with common antibiotics. Upper urinary tract infection is also usually easily treated in uncomplicated cases, but it has the potential to become a severe infection. Many different organisms can infect the urinary tract, but by far, the most common is *E. coli.* Urinary tract infection, whether upper or lower, is commonly abbreviated as UTI.

If you're a bacterium, the urinary tract is not a very hospitable place. Urine is normally sterile, and there are good reasons for that.

Obstacle number one is the regular flow of urine, which by its nature, flushes out anything that isn't firmly attached. (The technical term for urination is micturition, from the Latin word for it, *micturitum*). The urinary tract lacks the cilia and mucus of the respiratory tract, but the regular gush of urine is a powerful force against any would-be invaders.

Some strains of *E. coli* contain a unique means of attachment to the lining of the urinary tract, tiny hair-like structures emanating from the bacterial surface called fimbriae. They tightly attach the organism to epithelial cells so it doesn't get easily washed away. For this, the kidneys have an answer: the Tamm-Horsfall Protein, or THP. Discovered in 1952 by the individuals it is named for, many years went by without a clear understanding of its purpose. It is the most abundant protein in the urine, and it is produced not by the liver or other organs, but by cells in the kidney, presumably for excretion in urine. We now know that THP can latch onto an attachment appendage of *E. coli* known as type 1 fimbriae, thus binding it up and preventing the organism from attaching firmly to the urethral cell surface. (It has long been claimed by some that cranberry juice is a good remedy for a UTI. While it is not a good cure, there may be some validity to its preventing UTIs because of the presence of high levels of quercetin, a flavonoid. It has been shown in experiments that quercetin prevents the adherence of *E. coli* to epithelial surfaces as the Tamm-Horsfall Protein does).

When *E. coli* is in the bowel, nutrients are easy to come by. We eat the food for them, digest it, and all they need do is grab onto it. Not so in the urinary tract. Urine has some nutrient value for bacteria, and some strains can use it as a culture media and grow quite readily. But it doesn't supply all the nutrients needed by *E. coli.* The bacteria need to be able to synthesize two amino acids, arginine and glutamine, as well as the

180

nucleoside guanine. When in the bowel, organisms can get a little "lazy" and shut down the synthesis of these compounds since they are provided for them. In the urinary tract, however, they need to ramp up the genetic and protein synthesis machinery required to create these substances.

The epithelial lining of the urinary tract doesn't have a resident macrophage population like some other organs. Instead, the only white blood cells patrolling and protecting the tissues are neutrophils. Since complement and antibodies don't survive very well in urine, neutrophils are on their own in encountering and killing invading bacteria. The epithelial cells lining the urinary tract are very good at recognizing and responding to bacteria that adhere to them. Chemical signals attracting neutrophils (commonly called interleukin 8 or IL-8, but now technically named CXCL8) are sent out, and the WBC are well-positioned to migrate onto the scene quickly. Their job, of course, is to kill the invading bacteria.

Bacteria need iron to reproduce and develop. They don't need much, just trace amounts, but a complete lack of iron shuts them right down. One component of the neutrophil granules that is very effective in thwarting an invasion is lactoferrin, a member of the transferrin family. Lactoferrin attaches to and sequesters iron, making it unavailable to the bacteria. It can also directly damage the cell membrane of bacteria, leading to their death. In addition to lactoferrin, the granules of neutrophils contain defensins, which are small peptides designed to disrupt bacterial cell membranes. The epithelial cells lining the urinary tract also secrete lactoferrin and defensins.

The epithelial cells lining the urinary tract have a "buffer zone" on top of them designed to thwart the attachment of invading bacteria. Part of this surface lining is mucus; another is a complex substance known as glucoaminoglycan, a highly polar molecule that attracts water. It serves as a natural lubricant for the cell surface and is very helpful in repelling the attachment of bacteria.

We don't often think of our resident bacterial flora to be a part of our innate immune system, but they are in fact a very powerful factor. Bacteria are engaged in a little battle of their own with each other to gain a foothold on some part of our body where they can enjoy a carefree existence. When more than one species attempt to access the same area, the winner will be the one that can eliminate its competitors while not incurring the wrath of the host immune system, a delicate balance. One of the best bacteria at doing this are members of the genus *Lactobacillus,* which is prominent in our gut, the vagina, and, to a lesser extent, the mouth. Some species of *Lactobacillus* produce surfactant compounds that can destroy some species of bacteria, like *E. coli,* and prevent their bacterial rivals from adhering to various surfaces, including epithelial cells and catheters. Rather remarkably, they also make a protein that down-regulates our immune system, therefore reducing the amounts of cytokines released while at the same time up-regulating interleukin 10, the cytokine that slows down the immune response. This latter endeavor no doubt allows them to get along with the host immune system in a symbiotic relationship: the lactobacilli keep away the harmful bacteria, and the human host enables them to live in their chosen place peaceably.

Males have an advantage over females in resistance to UTIs on two obvious fronts: Their urethra is longer, about 20 centimeters (8 inches) versus 4 cm (1.5 inches) in the female, and men have a prostate gland that secretes fluid that contains antibacterial ions and molecules. The prostatic antibacterial factor, or PAF, uses zinc ions to damage bacteria.

It's no wonder that urine is sterile when it leaves the bladder. *E. coli* and other would-be invaders have many seemingly insurmountable entrenched obstacles blocking their path.

Urinary tract infections are endogenous or "generated from within." We don't "catch" a UTI like we do Strep throat, influenza, or *Salmonella.* The bacteria that cause UTIs are part of our normal bowel flora, living peacefully within us for a long time. It is only when a series of events come together which allow the organism to successfully invade the urinary tract that the trouble begins.

Potential urinary tract pathogens must overcome a hostile resident bacterial population in the form of

182

Lactobacillus, develop a way to obtain iron from an area where it is rare, dodge the assault coming their way from neutrophils and their products such as lactoferrin and defensins, attach themselves to the urinary tract epithelial cells despite the repellent mucus and glucoaminoglycan layer and the competitive attachment of Tamm-Horsfall Protein, and, in males, evade the killing effect of prostatic fluid. In the face of all these impediments, there is also the overwhelming force of urine flow, washing them away every few hours.

But obviously, they do get through. Each year in the United States, about seven million women go to the doctor and receive a diagnosis of urinary tract infection. And that's only the outpatients. Millions more patients in healthcare facilities develop UTIs, especially those who are catheterized. There's credible evidence that about half of all girls and women will get at least one UTI in their lifetime. Males also develop urinary tract infections, especially those over 60 years of age, but the incidence in males in the United States is much less, about $1/30^{th}$ of that of females. Urinary tract infections are one more affirmation that life isn't fair: some people never get a single one, while others are plagued by them constantly. Mostly they aren't serious, but sometimes, in the case of urosepsis, it can be a matter of life and death.

The lactobacilli in the vaginal introitus are not wholly successful in limiting colonization by enteric bacilli. If a swab of the vagina, or a urine sample, is cultured, a few Gram-negative rods from the colon invariably appear. Not all of them can invade the urinary tract, however, as those capable of ascending the urethra to reach the bladder must have the proper virulence factors.

Escherichia coli is listed as a single species, but, in fact, there are many varieties. About 10 of the recognized 700 serotypes of *E. coli* can cause a urinary tract infection. They possess key factors that allow them to invade more readily than the other strains.

One important factor is fimbriae, the little hairs on the bacterial surface that allow them to attach to the cells lining the urinary tract. (Oddly, the same structures have two names, the

183

other being pili. Singular is fimbria and pilus). There are many types of fimbriae, but two greatly help *E. coli* attach to the cells of the urinary tract: type 1 and P. The former is most beneficial to the organism in attaching to the cells of the bladder, and the latter to the cells of the kidney.

Fimbriae have two main sections, a firm stalk that anchors it to the bacterial cell and provides a rigid pole to support the "business end" of the whole thing, the small "hook" at the end of it that flops around looking for a compatible attachment site. We can think of a flagpole with a flag waving at the top.

E. coli strains that possess the P fimbriae are the most likely to cause the most serious type of urinary tract infection, pyelonephritis. That could lead to sepsis, or bloodstream invasion, a potentially fatal condition. The P fimbriae allow the organism to adhere more strongly to the lining of the intestinal tract, migrate from the perineum into the urethra, and ascend the urinary tract. While red blood cells and the urinary tract epithelial cells are embedded with the P antigen receptor, neutrophils are not, so the bacteria don't adhere readily to their surface. If a gooey polysaccharide capsule is added to the bacterial surface, neutrophils have difficulty surrounding and engulfing the P fimbriae-laden bacteria.

Type 1 fimbriae attach to a cellular receptor different from that used by the P fimbriae. They bind to proteins that contain the simple carbohydrate mannose, which, like glucose, has six carbons. The mannose-containing proteins of the body function mainly as a shuttle between the cell's interior and the surface, and when exposed, the type 1 fimbriae form a secure attachment to the mannose portion of the anchored protein. *E. coli* possessing type 1 fimbriae are much more likely to cause bladder infection alone and not kidney infection.

Like all Gram-negative bacteria, *E. coli* contains lipopolysaccharide (LPS) in its cell wall. Lipopolysaccharide is a force. It doesn't directly damage our tissues, but our immune system is well programmed to recognize it and react since it is a unique part of the bacterial cell wall. The reaction includes the release of numerous cytokines that have the combined effect of making us feel sick. At the very least, we feel chills, fever, muscle aches, and fatigue. At the worst, we become septic and close to death. When *E. coli* or some other related organism grows to large numbers in our urinary tract, we have much lipid A present. Severe illness results if it gets into the blood and the general circulation.

Besides these outer structures, uropathogenic *E. coli* produces several chemicals which aid it in invading cells after they have attached. These are not connected to the organism but are extruded from them to influence human cells. Collectively known as exotoxins, or secreted virulence factors, they are just as important as the surface attachment and immune avoidance organelles.

While we don't "catch" a urinary tract infection like we might catch a cold, we do have to acquire the strain of organism capable of causing the infection. There is no certain way of knowing how this comes about since the organisms involved reside quite calmly in our intestinal tract until the opportunity arises for them to make their way up the urethra and into the bladder or kidneys. They can be with us for years or a very short time, say, following travel. It's possible that a newly acquired strain itself doesn't infect, but it possesses one or more of the necessary virulence genes on the pathogenicity islands of its genome and can pass these along to another potentially infectious strain.

Just having the more virulent strain of *E. coli* in our bowel doesn't automatically lead to infection. Many people are colonized by such strains with no untoward effects. Quite often, the initiating factor is unknown; you just wake up one day with the symptoms of a UTI. Other times there is a most likely precipitating event: recently taking an antibiotic that disrupts the protective vaginal flora of lactobacilli, vigorous sexual intercourse, insertion of a catheter (especially if it is left in for several days), a kidney stone that gets stuck in the urethra. Once we leave ourselves vulnerable, the organism able to infect us will take advantage. Very often, the condition is idiopathic, meaning an unknown cause (from the Greek, *idios*, meaning "private," and *pathos*, "suffering").

Since the urinary tract is sterile in most people, the defense mechanisms in place are clearly effective. The bacterial growth never gets a chance to become established. Beginning with urine flow, the avoidance of bacterial invasion lies chiefly with preventing bacterial adhesion to epithelial cells. The Tamm-Horsfall protein binding to type 1 fimbriae, the formation of a thin layer of mucin on the epithelial surface, and the formation of defensins to disrupt the surface of bacteria all help. When bacteria do attach, there is the "self-destruct" option: the epithelial cells are programmed to undergo apoptosis and die and slough off, taking the attached bacteria with them. The dying epithelial cells also send chemical signals, mainly interleukin 8, to get neutrophils to migrate to the scene and start killing bacteria. It's a very effective strategy.

The chemical signal sent out by infected epithelial cells is designed to attract neutrophils, which are bacteria-killing machines. Unfortunately, neutrophils come with some baggage. The granules which contain the enzymes so destructive to bacteria also can damage human tissue, in this case, the lining of the urinary tract. Collateral damage is inevitable and must be minimized. Such a destructive force must be rigidly controlled. The epithelial cells lining the urinary tract are endowed with several mechanisms to ensure rapid, effective signaling of neutrophils, but in a responsible way.

Bacteria have chemicals exposed on their surface that we don't have. Called pathogen-associated molecular patterns, or PAMPS, they are parts of large numbers of organisms, and our cells have evolved chemical receptors to bind to these microbial pieces, such as LPS and fimbriae. After recognizing the presence of the PAMP on the bacteria, the detecting cell is programmed to send chemical messengers to alert the immune system of an invader. They also signal the immediately surrounding tissues to accommodate the soon-to-arrive defensive cells. In the urinary tract, three important things happen following the attachment of the PAMP to the host cell:

Neutrophils are activated to prepare to be drawn into the infected area.

A chemical signal is sent to the endothelial cells lining nearby blood vessels to send out a chemical "hook" to snag neutrophils as they float by.

A chemical attractant trail is laid between the blood vessel and the bacterial attachment site, showing the way for the neutrophils to find the microbes.

Like the lac-operon of bacteria, our cells have genes on them that are chemically covered up and are not routinely expressed. If our genes were all copied all the time, it would lead to a chaotic situation. Rather, some genes are covered, and the proteins for which they code are manufactured only after a stimulating event around the cell occurs. In the case of *E. coli* invading the urinary tract, the stimulating event is the attachment of LPS to the receptors on the epithelial cell's surface. This sets up a chain reaction of molecules inside the epithelial cell.

Nuclear factor kappa B (NFκB) is the key compound for allowing the transcription of covered genes of the immune system cells. It is always present but kept in check by the molecule IκB, or inhibitor of kappa B. The detection of invading microorganisms starts the process of a complex cascade of reactions resulting in the removal of IκB from NFκB, which then allows the copying of previously sequestered genes of the cytokine system. Interleukin 8 is an important molecule in this group as it is the main chemical attractant for neutrophils. Others include tumor necrosis factor α (TNFα) and interleukin 1β (IL-1β), which aid the inflammatory response, but unfortunately, both stimulate the systemic symptoms of fever and muscle aches.

The reaction of the epithelial cells lining the urinary tract to invasion by *E. coli* and other bacteria is forthright and effective. Once the invading bacterial cell is attached, the epithelial cell sends out chemical signals to attract and accommodate neutrophils and anti-bacterial chemicals, and destroys itself by apoptosis. The latter task ensures that the affected cell will sluff off and be carried away by a urine stream, taking the attached bacteria with it. It's a very efficient system.

But some bacteria have developed ways to circumvent it, especially the uropathogenic strains of *E. coli*. Type 1 fimbria and the P fimbria can penetrate the small mucin layer and gain a foothold. Tamm-Horsfall protein doesn't attach to all bacteria present.

One means bacteria use to ascend the urinary tract and eventually localize is creating a sophisticated structure known as a biofilm. Biofilms are formed by a wide range of bacteria that can infect humans. The example most of us are familiar with is dental plaque, a hard, encrusted material. A typical biofilm has three layers. The bottom layer attaches to the underlying structure, whether it be a sheet of epithelial cells or the surface of a plastic device like a catheter. Adherence is from the fimbriae and the stickiness of the carbohydrates on the outside of the bacterial cell. On top of the adherent layer is a film of vegetative cells that bridge the lower and upper cells. They are in a state of reduced metabolism, existing in a near-starvation form. The top layer is composed of cells that behave much like typical bacteria, metabolizing and reproducing actively. A biofilm has what amounts to a primitive circulatory system, with nutrients from the top shunted down to the cells below. The tight junction of the bottom layer leaves them very resistant to the effects of neutrophils, which have a hard time engaging and dislodging them. Hence, the entire structure is very resistant to the effects of the innate immune system. From the model of the dental plaque biofilm that must be scraped off with a sharp instrument, we can see the resiliency of a biofilm in full engagement.

The biofilm serves in one respect as a scaffold. Bacteria ascend the urinary tract, but do it one step at a time. The top layer of cells on the biofilm reproduces, laying down more of the bottom layer, and eventually, despite regular micturition, climb all the way to the bladder. There they keep doing the same thing, making more biofilm.

Bladder infection goes by the name cystitis, which is a bit odd when you think about it. We don't think of the urinary bladder as a cyst, but in traditional medical terms, that's what it is: a sac filled with fluid. "Bladderitis" just doesn't sound right, so cystitis it is. If the infection stops there, it is self-limited in most cases. Antibiotics can speed recovery remarkably, but even without them, cystitis is usually cleared in a week's time

188

by the innate immune system. In many infections, the macrophages are the principal active cell, but in cystitis, the neutrophil is called upon. Interleukin 8 is excreted in large amounts by infected epithelial cells, and neutrophils follow the IL-8 trail and enter the bladder and urethra en masse. Because the macrophages and dendritic cells are minimally involved, there is no significant release of the cytokines TNFα or IL-1β, so the person afflicted usually doesn't display the systemic signs of chills, fever, and myalgia. Rather, three symptoms predominate, and they all come under the heading of dysuria, or "bad" or "disordered" urination.

One characteristic symptom of cystitis is frequent urination. When our body is infected, some physiologic functions go into hyper mode. If the respiratory tract is infected, larger quantities of mucus than normal are produced and forced out by increased smooth muscle action, taking some of the invading pathogen and cellular debris with it. Similar activity is seen in the intestinal tract, giving us diarrhea, or "increased stool." In the urinary tract, increased urine flow has the purpose of flushing out the offending organism. Along with increased urination is the symptom known as, for lack of a better term, "urgency." The infected patient often feels the need to relieve themselves, even though there is very little or no urine in the bladder.

Another symptom of dysuria is pain during urination. The bowel doesn't have any pain receptors, so we don't feel the typical sensation of tenderness when we have an intestinal infection. But the urinary tract does indeed contain pain receptors. Just ask anyone who has had to try to pass a kidney stone. The irritation caused by the attachment of bacteria and the resulting inflammatory response usually gives a patient the sensation of pain, most often referred to as "burning," especially during urination when the urethra expands.

Normal urine is clear, although it varies in color. When infected, urine contains millions of bacteria and white blood cells, so it appears cloudy and dark and may be foul-smelling. Sometimes, but not often, it may also contain blood.

The diagnosis of UTI is usually quite simple, especially when common clinical laboratory supplies and equipment are available. Sometimes a good medical history is all that is needed: the classic symptoms are noted, no other explanation presents itself, and the patient denies this has been recurrent. Treatment can often be initiated on that alone.

Of course, this applies to otherwise healthy adults. Diagnosis can be more perplexing in young children and people with complicated medical histories. Good medical evaluation and quality laboratory testing help get it right.

Laboratory diagnosis is usually easily obtained. Two objects are typically seen in the urine during UTI, bacteria and neutrophils. Increased amounts of both are consistent with a UTI, but having one without the other is not. Examining a sample of urine under the microscope is all it takes to visualize both white cells and bacteria, but it does take a good microscope and trained personnel to do it. Alas, there is an even easier way to screen for UTIs.

A urine sample can be tested with a plastic strip, commonly called a dipstick, containing numerous chemicals designed to qualitatively detect the presence of substances in the urine. Among those indicative of UTI that may show up in a urine sample are nitrites and leukocyte esterase (LE).

Nitrites are produced by *E. coli* and other members of the *Enterobacteriaceae* from nitrate, a waste product normally present in urine. Nitrites are vigorously produced by all members of the enteric Gram-negative rods, which cause most UTIs. Unfortunately, other organisms sometimes causing it, like *Pseudomonas aeruginosa* or *Staphylococcus saprophyticus,* will give a negative test. Also, it takes the bacteria a few hours to reduce the nitrate, so if the test is done on urine that hasn't been in the bladder very long, it may test negative. So, while a very useful screen, the nitrite test is not 100%.

Leukocyte esterase (LE) is a screening test used to establish the presence of neutrophils. Of course, the best way to confirm neutrophil presence is to just look at a urine sample under the microscope, but sometimes that isn't available. LE is an enzyme found in the azurophilic, or primary, granules of neutrophils. When lots of neutrophils are present in the urine, there will be a correspondingly high level of LE, which is detected by the reaction of the esterase enzyme on an ester in the strip, forming an aromatic compound that then combines with a dye in the strip turning it purple. The whole reaction takes just about a minute. The LE test is not perfect. Some antibiotics can give rise to either false negative or false positive results. Also, vaginal infections such as those caused by the parasite *Trichomonas* can yield false positive results. Still, the LE test is very useful as a screening test and is a little more sensitive than the nitrite test.

While not always necessary, the urine culture, or cultivation of the invading organism on laboratory media, can be very helpful in both establishing a diagnosis and in guiding treatment. The urine culture is more expensive than the dipstick and urinalysis, and it takes a couple of days, but it can show the specific organism causing the disease, as well as the most appropriate antibiotic to use.

Once the diagnosis of cystitis is established, treatment is usually very effective. Several antibiotics are excreted in the urine in their active form, so their concentrations are relatively high at the site of infection. Often just a single dose of the proper antibiotic, such as amoxicillin or cephalexin, results in marked improvement.

A potentially much more serious urinary tract infection than cystitis involves infection of a portion of the kidney itself, a condition known as pyelonephritis (*pyelo* referring to pus, "nephro" from the Greek word for kidney, *nephros*). Like cystitis, most cases of pyelonephritis occur by ascending infection: an organism, most often *E. coli,* colonizes the distal urethra, then "climbs" its way up. It would seem logical to conclude that the organism first infects the bladder, then keeps on going up the ureters to reach the kidney. But such is not always the case. The strains of *E. coli* which cause pyelonephritis are often different than those that cause cystitis. While the strains containing the F1 or P fimbriae can cause either malady, the F1 type is more likely in the bladder, and the P-type is more common in the kidney. The prevalence of receptors on the cells lining the respective surfaces influences which strain will prevail.

The infection in the kidney most commonly involves the nephron, the filtering unit of the outer part of the kidney, known as the renal cortex. The end of the P fimbria has an affinity for a receptor on the cells lining the nephron. Once they attach, they begin an infectious process that can be difficult for the immune system to thwart. The formation of a biofilm within the nephron is key to the advancement of the infection.

Pyelonephritis can be either acute or chronic. One of the classic symptoms of both forms is flank pain, marked discomfort just above the hip bone on the back. The main danger of pyelonephritis is the possibility that the organism can enter the bloodstream. The kidney is endowed with abundant blood vessels, and it is not unusual for infecting bacteria to make their way into the circulation. Because of the presence of toxin on Gram-negative rods (lipid A, also known as endotoxin), sepsis may result. Known as urosepsis, prompt medical intervention is essential.

When an organism breaches the confines of tissue, it must be vigorously controlled to prevent its spread. One of the key ways this is accomplished is for the circulatory system, from the signals given by the immune system, to lay down a small clot around the organism and the infected tissue. The coagulation cascade is triggered by several reactions, resulting in a tiny clot at the local level. This works very well in controlling the infection, but when the bug can break through this and enter the circulatory system, especially when it does so in large numbers, the result is the formation of blood clots in the blood vessels throughout the body. Called disseminated intravascular coagulation, or DIC, the consequences are profound. Shock is the classic symptom, accompanied by multi-organ failure. Untreated, death is the usual outcome. Gram-negative bacteria are especially good at inducing this reaction because they contain lipid A in their cell walls. Lipid A is a very good stimulator of the cascade that forms blood clots and the accompanying cytokine storm, perpetuating the dramatic symptoms.

Modern hospitals are well equipped to handle the onset of septic shock caused by Gram-negative organisms. Prompt control of the infecting organism and stabilizing the conditions of shock, such as blood pressure maintenance and blood clotting, is essential and almost a routine procedure. What complicates the matter has been the emergence of Gram-negative organisms that are resistant to multiple antibiotics.

Initially, the administration of antibiotics is empirical, that is, giving several different antibiotic classes with the hope that one or more will be effective. When the lab results show the offending organism and the antibiotics it is susceptible and resistant to, the regimen can be tailored to suit the offending organism directly. An example of initial antibiotic therapy for Gram-negative urosepsis might be a third-generation cephalosporin like ceftriaxone, an aminoglycoside such as tobramycin, and perhaps a third drug such as the fluoroquinolone levofloxacin. Unfortunately, it is not unusual to encounter an *E. coli* or another Gram-negative rod resistant to all of those. By the time the lab results are available, it may be too late. As time passes and bacteria become more resistant to antibiotics, the problem will likely worsen. Such multiple antibiotic-resistant bacteria have given the moniker "superbugs" in the secular press, a bit of an exaggeration. The organisms don't possess any special means to create a more frequent or serious infection. They are merely more difficult to treat with the most common and safe antibiotics. But the trend is perilous: the bacteria resistant to an antibiotic will persist at the expense of the susceptible ones, and their many genetic transfer abilities can pass the antibiotic resistance genes to neighboring bacteria.

While *E. coli* with type 1 and P fimbriae are the most encountered uro-pathogens, they are not the only ones. Indeed, there are other attachment proteins within the species *E. coli*, some of which are located on fimbriae, and some are single proteins projecting from the bacterial surface. Organisms other than *E. coli*, such as *Proteus mirabilis, Klebsiella pneumoniae, Enterobacter cloacae* and *aerogenes, Pseudomonas aeruginosa*, and others, can also cause urinary tract infections. They can also cause urosepsis. And they can all develop resistance to antibiotics.

The words diarrhea and dysentery have different meanings. Diarrhea, from the Greek *dia*, meaning "through," and *rhein*, to "flow," means watery feces, and plenty of it, often occurring frequently. Dysentery, on the other hand, is far more serious. The name also derives from the Greek, *dys* meaning "bad" or "abnormal," and *entera* meaning bowels. We all get diarrhea occasionally, whether from an infectious disease or something we ate. Dysentery, on the other hand, is a much more serious pathological condition that makes us very ill and, in some cases, can kill us. Historically, there is good evidence that more soldiers died in some wars from the effects of dysentery than combat. Diarrhea can be troubling, sometimes a bit debilitating, but usually of limited duration. Proper rehydration is usually the only treatment needed. Dysentery, on the other hand, is a wretched illness that lays one up for days, possibly weeks. It's usually accompanied by prostration, muscle aches, fever, and dehydration. While ill, the patient doesn't take on proper nutrition, resulting in profound weakness. It's a serious, unrelenting ailment.

There are quite a few microorganisms that can cause infectious diarrhea. Bacteria, viruses, and parasites all can be involved. The most serious form of diarrhea is cholera, caused by the bacterium *Vibrio cholera*. Cholera can be life-threatening if not treated adequately. In some people, infection with the anaerobic bacterium *Clostridium difficile* is of major consequence. But most infectious diarrhea is somewhat benign and lays us up for just a few days.

Dysentery usually makes us very ill. It is caused by two very different organisms, one a parasite and the other a bacterium. The parasite is an amoeba, *Entamoeba histolyticum*, which occurs sporadically in undeveloped countries, usually confined to a small circle of individuals. It can be a very serious infection, especially when it spreads to the liver. Diagnosis and treatment are often problematic.

The most common form of dysentery is that caused by a bacterium, a Gram-negative bacillus, so it is sometimes called bacillary dysentery. It is an ancient disease of humans; Hippocrates wrote a somewhat detailed description of it. The bacillary form of the disease can occur sporadically like the amoebic form, but it also manifests as a horrific epidemic, sickening thousands. Dysentery is especially worrisome when sanitation breaks down, such as in wars and natural disasters. When confronted as a sporadic case in a country with good medical facilities, it usually isn't fatal unless the patient was previously debilitated with another condition. But the illness is profound, with loss of activity for days, sometimes weeks.

The organism that causes bacillary dysentery is closely related to *E. coli*. One could make a very good case that the organism, known to clinicians as *Shigella*, should more appropriately be classified in the genus *Escherichia*. *Shigella* and *Escherichia* are identical in 99% of their genomes. But convention and practical sharing of information demand that the name *Shigella* be retained. Most likely, in ancient times, members of the species *E. coli* began to accumulate the genes for invasive proteins, and as time went on, the distinctive creature known as *Shigella* came to be. Over time it became even more specialized, and today it is observed to be a distinct group.

Shigella has several characteristics that make it a unique pathogen:

It is very resistant to the effects of stomach acid and bile salts. The infective dose necessary to initiate disease is less than 100 organisms, perhaps as little as twenty. Most enteric Gram-negative rods are destroyed at a high rate by their passage through the stomach and upper small intestine, but not *Shigella*.

It reproduces in the small intestine. Garden variety *E. coli* must enter the colon to begin growing, but *Shigella* grows to very high numbers in the small intestine. From there, it enters the bowel in equally high numbers.

As the organisms enter the colon, they encounter, to say the least, formidable competition. Even millions of them are overwhelmed by the presence of resident bowel flora that number in the billions. Shigella's target is the lining of the bowel, especially the mast cells that serve as the entryway for several pathogens. Even though *Shigella* is not motile, some organisms do make it to their target site. It doesn't attach by the end of a pilus like its *E. coli* relatives do, but rather by a surface protein that hooks up with a receptor on the host cell's outer membrane. Once firmly attached, the pathogenic process begins.

Shigella's entry into the host cell is insidious. Once bound to the host cell's surface, the organism forms a series of proteins that create a spike that projects into the membrane of the cell it is trying to enter. It is a process like that used by *Salmonella.* At the end of the spike is a plug of a small protein. Once the proper interior cellular environment is detected, the plug dissolves, and several proteins enter the host cell. A couple of them induce the host cell to surround the bacterial cell with a membrane, form a vacuole, and the bacterium gains entry. After entry, the bacterium is contained in the vacuole, but the proteins that induced the penetration of the outer membrane perform a similar function to the vacuole, and the bacterium is freed inside the host cell.

Once free inside the cell, the organisms do two important things: one is to propagate, using the nutrients found in their immediate environment, and the other is to commandeer the structural proteins of the host cell, known as actin, and use them to migrate to adjoining cells. Unlike its *E. coli* progenitors, *Shigella* does not form flagella. It has the genetic material to make them, but the genes are not expressed. Rather, it takes control of actin, the host cell's proteins that are designed for structural integrity and shape, alters their direction, and rides them like a train, with the destination being the membrane of an adjacent cell.

Our cells are designed to destroy invading bacteria. By a process known as autophagy, invading microbes are encapsulated and subjected to deadly proteins. Autophagy is the "garbage disposal" of each cell, providing orderly maintenance of the by-products inevitably created during metabolism. For bacteria, being caught up in an autophagic vacuole is like being sent to jail with a death sentence. *Shigella*, though, produces enzymes that disrupt the system, and they can carry on their invasion.

With all this intracellular activity, the destruction of the epithelial cells lining the colon is rampant. Once engaged, the organisms stay inside the host cells, migrating from one to another, staying out of the reach of complement and neutrophils. Eventually, released cytokines like TNFα, IL-1β, and IL-8 attract large numbers of white blood cells. They also make the patient feel very ill.

With such a small number of organisms necessary to initiate an infection, it is no wonder that bacillary dysentery spreads rapidly throughout an enclosed population, especially when personal hygiene is low due to environmental factors. *Shigella* only grows in humans, so we don't get it by contact with animals or eating foods associated with animal waste. It's the classic example of "fecal-oral" transmission.

One could make a very good case that *Shigella* should be classified as a type of *E. coli.* But by convention, we recognize four distinct groups of the genus labeled as species *dysenteriae, flexneri, boydii, and sonnei.* These are often referred to as types A, B, C, and D instead of their species epithet. *Shigella* was named for Kiyoshi Shiga, the Japanese researcher who discovered and described the organism in 1898 during a severe outbreak in Japan. (Reportedly, over 20,000 people died). He named the organism *Bacillus dysenterie*, but in 1930 it was renamed.

In the early 20th century, as researchers worldwide studied the organism, one strain became notorious for causing an even more potent disease: *Shigella dysenteriae*, type 1. When epidemics were caused by this bug, bloody stools and other serious complications increased dramatically. The research discovered that these strains of *Shigella* had a means of virulence in addition to those of the invasive strains, namely, the formation of a toxin. Aptly, it was called Shiga toxin, abbreviated *Stx*.

Shigella is invasive because it contains a set of genes that code for about two dozen unique proteins. Most of these genes are not on the central bacterial chromosome but rather on a separate strand of DNA known as a plasmid. Because the proteins produced from this plasmid are necessary for invasion and virulence, it is known as the virulence plasmid or VP. Without that virulence plasmid, *Shigella* is just another type of *E. coli.*

The toxin, however, is not produced from the virulence plasmid. Instead, it comes from a very unexpected source: a virus. We often think of viruses attacking humans and other animals and plants, but viruses often infect bacteria. They are called bacteriophages, or usually just phages. Ordinarily, they are inconsequential, but rarely they take on a major role. The best example is the disease diphtheria. The organism causing diphtheria, *Corynebacterium diphtheriae,* is by itself innocuous. It does nothing. But *C. diphtheriae* infected with a particular virus becomes a virulent pathogen, producing an extremely serious disease. So it is with Shiga toxin. When *Shigella* is invaded by a phage known as a lambda type, it can potentially produce a toxin. And not just any toxin. Shiga toxin is the deadliest poison known to man. It has been reported that just one molecule of the stuff can kill a cell.

Several lambdoid phages can invade *Shigella.* The virus can insert itself into the bacteria's chromosome, where it then lies dormant. This stage of its existence is called the lysogenic phase. Encoded on the virus is the genetic formula for the Shiga toxin, so it's the virus that carries around the genes for the toxin, not the bacterium. As the bacterial chromosome is copied and transcribed, so are the virus and the toxin gene. Often the viral expression is suppressed, so toxin is not always produced. But, especially under stress, the Shiga toxin gene is transcribed, and the toxin flows from the organism. It is more likely to occur in times of stress, such as when the bacterium is exposed to an antibiotic.

Humans use several antibiotics that disrupt bacteria's ability to make proteins. Drugs like tetracycline, erythromycin, and streptomycin attach to a portion of the organism's ribosome blocking its ability to process messenger RNA. Shiga toxin acts the same way, only it acts against humans. The toxin attaches to the human 28S ribosome half of the 60S ribosome, removing a single adenine molecule. That doesn't sound like much, but it is enough to completely halt protein synthesis in the human host cell, leading to its death. We can think of it as a "reverse antibiotic," in which the bacteria use a drug (toxin) to disrupt human protein synthesis the same way we use antibiotics to disrupt theirs.

Shiga toxin is a complex structure. At its core is a large protein called the 'A' molecule. Surrounding the A portion are five 'B' molecules. After it is released from the bacterial cell, the toxin rolls around until one of the B molecules finds and attaches to a receptor on a human cell. The receptor has a long chemical name but is usually abbreviated Gb3. Once Gb3 on the human cell locks on to the B molecule, the whole toxin is incorporated into the host cell. Once inside, the B molecules act to free the entire molecule from the encapsulating endosome, releasing the deadly 'A' molecule. From there, it is just a matter of time until a portion of the A molecule hooks up with the 28S ribosome, putting the kibosh on protein manufacture and killing the cell.

Shigella and *E. coli* are very closely related, so it is no surprise that a virus that can infect the former can just as easily infect the latter. Several strains of E. coli are accommodative to lambda phages, but the most important for us is the one with the antigenic type of O157:h7 (it has the outer carbohydrate antigen designated 157 and the type 7 flagella). There is a slight difference in the Shiga toxins: the one on *E. coli* has a single amino acid difference from the one found in *Shigella dysenteriae*, but it acts in the same way, shutting down protein synthesis in animal cells. Since it is slightly different, the *E. coli* Shiga toxin is abbreviated *stx*1 instead of the *stx* found in *Shigella*.

E. coli O157 does not invade our cells like *Shigella*, moving about inside cells using actin molecules to propel itself. But it does have some characteristics which make it a formidable pathogen. Like *Shigella*, *E. coli* O157 can infect with a very small dose of organisms, most likely less than 100 bugs ingested. The organism attaches to a receptor outside of an intestinal epithelial cell. If it contains a lambda phage capable of producing Shiga toxin, serious disease may ensue.

A big difference between *E. coli* and *Shigella* is that the latter does not colonize animals other than primates. *E. coli* does. It is part of the normal intestinal flora of ruminants, including cows. Since such animals are an important part of our food chain, it is no surprise that an organism colonizing a cow could make its way into human food, whether it be the animal flesh itself or vegetables and fruits exposed to bovine waste matter. This situation is exasperating because adult cows are not sickened by the organism. They lack the Gb3 receptor on their cells necessary for the toxin to attach before invading. That's not true of calves, who have an *stx* receptor and can get sick and perhaps die if exposed. The receptor disappears as the cow matures.

As if the *E. coli* variant of the Shiga toxin (*stx*1) wasn't enough, a second Shiga toxin was found in *E. coli*, designated *stx*2. This second toxin is not found in *Shigella*, only in *E. coli*. It is chemically and antigenically distinct from *stx* and *stx*1, sharing only about half of the amino acid structure. But it functions the same way, with the B segments attaching and the A segment causing cellular damage. There are several subtypes of *stx*2, designated by subscript letters, for example, $stx2_a$, $stx2_b$, etc. If the culprit is of the *stx*2 variety, this information can come in handy in tracing the source of an outbreak.

The events in an infection caused by Shiga toxin-containing *E. coli* are usually straightforward. The patient eats some food contaminated with the organism. Like *Shigella*, the number of organisms required to set up an infection is extremely low, probably less than a hundred bugs. Organisms then attach to the cells lining the colon by a bacterial surface protein known as intimin. *E. coli* O157 is rich in this substance. Sometimes the organism just sits there, not doing much. After all, the virus within it bears the genetic code for the toxin, and the virus' genes are sometimes suppressed. But once activated, toxins pour forth from the bacteria, attaching themselves to the intestinal epithelium and entering the bloodstream. The illness thus shows considerable variability in infected patients: the higher the dose of infecting bacteria, the more accommodative the patient's bowel is to the bacteria's multiplication, and the more active the virus within the bacteria, the higher the toxin release and the more severe the illness.

The toxin acts on two fronts. In the intestine, it attaches to the bowel lining, leading to its erosion and hemorrhagic diarrhea. The toxin also enters the bloodstream, and as it circulates through the body, it randomly attaches to the Gb3 receptors of the cells lining blood vessels, the endothelium. It

200

concentrates most in the kidneys, where some cells have a high level of Gb3. It is most aggressive in the cortex of the kidney, in the renal tubules. As these cells are poisoned by the toxin and slough off, collagen exposure results. This activates platelets, which leads to the activation of thrombin and the laying down of clots. If enough renal tubules are damaged, kidney damage is profound, leading to incomplete filtering of the blood and the build-up of the waste product urea in the bloodstream, a condition known as uremia.

The toxin causes similar damage to other parts of the body with the attendant build-up of platelets and mini clots. As red blood cells flow through the blood vessel, they can bump into these irregular surfaces and become damaged. The damaged red blood cell is known as a schistocyte (from the Greek, *schistos*, or divided). Such cells are highly susceptible to breaking apart and releasing their hemoglobin, which damages the kidneys when free.

This cascade of events is known as the "hemolytic-uremic syndrome," or HUS. It can be deadly. When medical intervention is available, including fluid replacement and dialysis, the patient usually survives, but sometimes severe kidney damage results. As in most cases, when the afflicted patient is very young or very old or encumbered by a pre-existing medical condition, the outcome becomes potentially more critical.

(All scientific disciplines rely on abbreviations. There are some very long chemical words or phrases that would be simply too difficult to use even once, let alone numerous times. The proper form to use an abbreviation is to write out the scientific name or phrase completely, followed by the abbreviation in parenthesis afterward. Unfortunately, for Shiga toxin-producing *E. coli*, several abbreviations have been used through the years. Shiga toxin-producing *E. coli* is STEC; enterohemorrhagic *E. coli* is EHEC; an older reference to the toxin's effect on Vero cells, derived from Green Monkey Kidneys, is VTEC. They all refer to the same thing, with the EC for *E. coli*. It depends on the author's preference).

Tracing the source of a toxigenic *E. coli* outbreak can be difficult, if not impossible. If it occurs in a restaurant, and meat is the common source of infection, it is usually not too hard to discover the source of the offending food. But if the organism is contaminating fresh produce, like lettuce, it becomes very challenging to find where it came from and if it can occur again. The cows responsible are not sick. Investigators can't simply go to local veterinarians and ask them how many sick cows they've treated. Epidemiologists and lab workers require intense work to discover the strain of the organism involved and its common source.

Shigella and *E. coli* are bacteria; in the lab, it is very easy to kill them with an appropriate antibiotic. Unfortunately, for diseases in humans, it doesn't work that way. *Shigella* is an intracellular pathogen, so the antibiotic must penetrate tissues to reach the organism. Experience has shown that antibiotic treatment, even when the bug is highly susceptible to the drug, does not hasten the course of the disease. With toxigenic *E. coli,* using an antibiotic stresses the virus responsible for toxin production, inducing it to produce more of it, ironically worsening the situation. Palliative treatment is all that can usually be done.

Shiga toxin is known as an exotoxin. It is made inside the bacterial cell, then released to do its damage in areas remote from the bug that made it. It differs from endotoxin, the lipid A component of Gram-negative bacteria cell walls that all strains of *E. coli* possess. Endotoxin does not come into play for stx-positive strains. While sitting in the bowel cranking out the toxin, they are no different from any other strain of *E. coli*. The exotoxin does its dirty work remotely from the organism that produced it.

Travelers to foreign countries often experience symptoms of diarrhea when they return to their native land. This is especially true for tourists from developed countries to areas with less-developed public hygiene. One famous epithet of an affliction for American travelers who travel to Mexico and return with symptoms of diarrhea is "Montezuma's Revenge." The ailment can be anything from a day or two of runny, liquid stools to full-blown shigellosis (dysentery). Even people who

202

are diligent about their eating and drinking habits ("don't drink the water!") can be affected.

Pathogenic *E. coli* and its close relative *Shigella* cause damage by three different methods: production of toxins, invasion of cells, and, in infections such as those in the urinary tract, forming a biofilm. Strains of *E. coli* associated with traveler's diarrhea have been shown to do all three in unique ways.

Some strains of *E. coli* are known to invade cells lining the colon. Like *Shigella*, they hook on to the outside of the target cell, then promote their entry by injecting chemical agents which force the host cell to bring the bug inside. Then they hijack the actin molecules within the cell to promote their migration to the adjoining cells. These strains are referred to, appropriately, as **enteroinvasive** *E. coli*, abbreviated EIEC.

Other strains manufacture a toxin, but unlike the Shiga toxin, this toxin enters the cell that the *E. coli* has attached to. The toxin differs from the Shiga toxin, being much more like the one produced by *Vibrio cholera*, the bacterium that causes cholera. The resulting infection, therefore, involves only diarrhea, not systemic symptoms like kidney failure and anemia. These strains are known as **enterotoxigenic** *E. coli*, abbreviated ETEC.

Another strain of *E. coli* responsible for diarrheal disease endemic in areas of poor sanitation and sometimes seen in travelers forms a biofilm on the surface of the bowel lining. These organisms have surface attachment organelles that allow them to easily stick to one another, even before they firmly attach to the host cell surface. Once attached, they begin making a dense aggregation of bacteria, resembling a layer of bricks. They also produce a toxin that is injected into the cells they are colonizing. Diarrhea is the result of this invasion. They are known as **enteroaggregative** *E. coli*, abbreviated EAEC.

The strains of *E. coli* that cause travelers' diarrhea might be thought of as hybrids. They are usually not as virulent as the invasive *Shigella* or Shiga toxin-producing *E. coli but* possess virulence factors that distinguish them from common commensal strains. In contrast to the more virulent pathogens, they require a much higher infective dose to create an infection.

Shigella and STEC can colonize and initiate an infection when fewer than 100 organisms are ingested. But EIEC, ETEC, and EAEC require much higher doses, approaching ten million organisms. People residing in an area of the world colonized by these strains develop immune tolerance to them with significant levels of antibodies, mostly IgA, so after a single bout of diarrhea, they are no longer sickened by the bug. But they can carry it in their intestinal tract, and improper hygiene and poor sewage treatment may lead to the infection of an immunologically naïve traveler. Also, children living in the endemic area are at risk, and sometimes these organisms can wreak havoc on the local population. The need for adequate water treatment and sanitation cannot be over-emphasized.

E. coli is our constant companion. There are over 700 serotypes, most benign and probably helpful. A few others, though, are malevolent pathogens. The organism has well-developed systems for sharing genetic information within its own species and with other organisms. It passes along genes for both virulence and antibiotic resistance with impunity. We will never rid ourselves of its potential threat. The best we can do is contain its propensity for opportunism with good sanitation and hygiene, along with the judicious stewardship of antibiotics.

Chapter 14
GI Incursion

Dire affliction from
A simple drink of water.
Relentless typhoid.

One of the more sinister members of the bacterial family *Enterobacteriaceae* is the genus *Salmonella*. It looks like the name may have been inspired by a fish, but in fact, it is named after a veterinarian named Daniel Salmon, a pioneer in diagnosing and treating diseases of cattle and hogs. It was in Dr. Salmon's lab that Dr. Theobald Smith first isolated the organism now called *Salmonella*. It's appropriate that the organism is named after a veterinarian since most *Salmonella* infections originate in animals, such as cattle, hogs, and poultry. It can even colonize and infect reptiles and amphibians. But the worst of all the salmonellae only infects humans: *Salmonella typhi*, the agent of typhoid fever. (The name *Salmonella typhi* is technically incorrect. The rules of nomenclature have given us a rather complex way of identifying salmonellae. But it's easier to refer to the organism as its own genus and species. Most workers do).

Being a member of *Enterobacteriaceae*, *Salmonella* is structured in the same fashion as the other genera. It is a Gram-negative bacillus (rod), about two or three microns long and about half a micron wide. A complex part of the cell of all members of the *Enterobacteriaceae* is the outer membrane and cell wall. We can think of the cell wall of enteric rods like *Salmonella* as if they were a three-lane track in an oblong shape encircling the cell.

The lipopolysaccharide (LPS) component of the cell wall is a toxin. It is the same in *Salmonella* as in *E. coli* and other Gram-negative rods. The toxic component is lipid A, which is unique to bacteria. Our cells do not contain it. Lipid A is exceptionally reactive in activating the innate immune system. Small quantities are usually not troublesome, but when present in moderate to large amounts the immune reaction against it is so robust that the result is significant illness, sometimes sepsis and death. This is not due to the direct effect of lipid A on tissues but the immune system's overwhelming reaction to it and all the side effects incurred. Since lipid A is an integral part of the bacterial cell wall and is not easily released into the environment, it is referred to as **endo**toxin instead of the routinely released **exo**toxins.

The number of *Salmonella* it takes to make us sick is tough to figure out. If you give a volunteer a "Salmonella cocktail" and know the approximate number of organisms present, it takes about 100,000 bugs to make most people sick. But anecdotal evidence shows it probably takes far fewer, perhaps less than one thousand organisms in real life. When measured amounts are given to volunteers, the organism is grown in artificial culture media, which may attenuate some of its invasive properties. When we get a dose of the naturally occurring variety, it may be a much better invader and have a lower infective dose.

There are two types of *Salmonella*: non-typhoid and typhoid. Most infections come from the non-typhoid types, of which over 2500 known varieties have been described. These organisms are nearly always associated with animals, and we get sick by consuming the bugs in our food. There is a great range of animals infected. Cattle (beef and dairy), hogs, chickens, and turkeys can all have their unique infective strains of *Salmonella*, many of which can infect humans. The organism often lives in the animal without killing it or even making it ill. Like all the enteric Gram-negative rods, the salmonellae are pooped out with the animal's excrement. On a busy farm, that material can end up in many places, sometimes on food products not associated with animals, like lettuce or peanuts. Steer manure can contain viable *Salmonella*. In the case of poultry, the organism can infect the ovaries and become viable in the albumin and yolk of the eggs. Proper cooking kills the organism. Leaving uncooked contaminated food, utensils, or chopping blocks sitting around for hours heightens the threat. Of course, we can also contract a *Salmonella* infection when exposed to food, water, or other material contaminated by humans, much like we contract *Shigella*. There are about 1.2 to 1.5 million cases of *Salmonella* food poisoning every year in the United States.

To infect us, *Salmonella* must run the gamut of host defenses. It starts with stomach acid, then bile, then competing organisms in the bowel, then the layer of mucin covering the intestinal epithelial cells. Successful salmonellae have proteins and appendages to overcome each of these obstacles. Their destination is the cell layer lining the bowel, the enterocytes. They use their fimbriae and surface carbohydrates to form an attachment to a suitable receptor on the host cell's surface. With so many fimbriae and carbohydrates on their surface, that's not hard to do. *Salmonella* contains a collection of proteins that serve as a kind of syringe, able to inject enzymes into the host cell after the organism has attached itself. The pathogen *Shigella* and some strains of *E. coli* use a similar mechanism. This action by *Salmonella* directs the host cell to internalize the organism. After the bug enters the cell, actin molecules, which comprise the host cell's cytoskeleton, are overtaken and redirected. The cell's structural actin proteins are rearranged to encase the organism. This actin vacuole is called a "*Salmonella*-containing vacuole," or SCV. Once entrenched inside this vacuole, the organism uses it as mission control, directing activities to dictate its commands. Bacteria-killing lysosomes do not combine with the actin-lined vacuole containing the organism, so the organism is safe in its own cellular sanctuary.

As predators, salmonellae are endowed with many genes that code for molecules used in the invasion process. They are concentrated on a particular section of the bacterial chromosome called the "pathogenicity island." Close to one thousand genes are located here, most suppressed until the organism needs them. Also encoded are two secretion systems. They are of what's known as the T3 type, and since *Salmonella* makes them, they are called T3SS for *Salmonella* secretion. The first secretion system kicks in when the organism enters the cell, helping form the "syringe" by which invasive proteins are injected. The second set is created after it has overtaken the cellular machinery and taken up residence. The secretion systems enable the organism's gene products to be deployed wherever their function carries them.

The infected cell contains a poison-containing vacuole called a lysosome. Its job is to combine with the vacuole that contains the infecting organism, then release its toxin to kill the invader. Salmonellae possess gene products that help reduce the effectiveness of the activity of the host cell's lysosome. Some alter the membrane of the SCV so the lysosome doesn't bind strongly. Other *Salmonella* proteins inactivate or mitigate the action of lysosome's anti-bacterial molecules. They even have several molecules that travel to the cell's Golgi apparatus, where proteins and enzymes are packaged, and inhibit the delivery of antibacterial molecules to the vacuole. With all this, the bacteria can reproduce inside the host cell with little interference from the cell's anti-bacterial forces.

In summary, when *Salmonella* enters our intestinal tract, it binds to the cells lining the bowel. A spike protein then penetrates the intestinal cell, and its pathogenic molecules are injected. Once these molecules enter the cell, they round up some of the host cell's actin molecules, which are redirected to form a vacuole. The organism then enters this contrived vacuole, not the typical endosome made up exclusively of cell membrane material. This vacuole, termed a Salmonella-containing vacuole, protects the organism from the injurious effects of the cell's lysosomes, which bind poorly or not at all. The organism produces various chemicals within the vacuole, which helps shut down the cell's attack against it. It's like a burglar breaking into a building and disabling the alarms.

All this activity does not go unnoticed by the innate immune system. Chemical messengers are activated, and nuclear factor kappa B is eventually sent to the cell's nucleus to unleash the cytokines responsible for antibacterial action. One of the most important of these is interleukin-1-β, the inflammatory cytokine. Interleukin-1-β (IL-1β) is a powerful agent. The gene responsible for its production codes for a pre-molecule, which a specific enzyme must activate. Once made active, it is released by a complicated system that is not yet fully understood. Each cell possesses several failsafe mechanisms to help ensure against the overproduction of this cytokine because its influence is very great.

Originally called the "pyrogenic factor," interleukin-1 is responsible at least in part for the occurrence of fever. It activates other cells to produce several different cytokines, resulting in a profound inflammatory event. When we get a non-typhoid *Salmonella* infection, we often get that "just-got-hit-by-a-cement-truck" feeling. Our body aches all over; we have fever, profuse diarrhea, nausea, and vomiting. It will often lay us up for several days. It's hard to keep anything down, so we often become dehydrated and weak from lack of nutrients, which only makes us feel worse. Much of this reaction can be traced back to the release of IL-1β and other inflammatory cytokines. Their chief purpose is to rally the innate immune system to rid the body of the bacterial invader, but all we feel is terribly sick.

Salmonella typhi takes it to another level. Unlike garden-variety Salmonellae, it enters through the cells of the distal ileum of the small intestine, not the large intestine. It's hard to say if it enters through the intestinal epithelial cells or the microfold (M cells), but it could be both. Once inside, the organism aims for its target cell, the macrophage. Ironically, this is the cell designed to kill it. It's kind of like a bandit breaking into jail. But macrophages are mobile and can take the bacterium to greener pastures throughout the body.

S. typhi is equipped with a secret weapon, a tough carbohydrate capsule known as the Vi (short for virulent) antigen that surrounds the cell. This capsule makes it harder for the immune cells to get a bead on the outer structures of the bacterial cell, lessening the immune response. The typhoid bacillus enters cells like other Salmonellae by injecting invasion-enabling molecules, but the host cell's recognition of the invader is not as robust. *S. typhi* is something of a stealth invader. Some patients get some diarrhea and fever, but most patients have mild gastroenteritis or no initial response at all.

After entering the macrophage, usually in the lymphoid tissue known as a Peyer's Patch underlying the intestinal mucosa, *S. typhi* sets up its operation much like other Salmonellae. The vacuole in which it resides is joined by the cell's lysosome, replete with its antibacterial arsenal. Like other Salmonellae, *S. typhi* has a large pathogenicity island that becomes activated when the organism is safely nestled inside the phagosome. A bacterial protein known as Pho/G is switched on, probably by the acidic environment. It then migrates to the organism's DNA. Pho/G unwraps the molecular covering suppressing this gene array, and the proteins needed for intracellular durability come pouring out. The second secretion system is similarly activated, and the organism effectively controls much of the activity of its macrophage host. The vacuole membrane is modified, allowing the egress and entrance of molecules the organism needs.

Typically, antibacterial substances are numerous in the macrophage lysosome. When it combines with the phagosome containing the invading bacterium, it is just a short time until the bug is killed, drawn, and quartered, and its entrails are prominently displayed on the macrophage surface. There it is recognized by passing lymphocytes, and the process of acquired immunity begins.

S. typhi short circuits this whole orderly process. Many of the bacterial proteins unearthed by Pho/G inactivate or mitigate the effectiveness of the lysosomal antibacterial factors. The encased bacterium controls the activity of the Salmonella-containing vacuole to the extent that it is like its own preferred habitat. It begins to replicate, and many bacteria are present in a single cell in a short time. All this activity does not notably damage the macrophage itself, and it does what it always does–gets into the bloodstream and lymphatic channels and goes on about its business, unwittingly carrying this load of endotoxin-laden bacteria with it. Eventually, the macrophage ruptures, releasing its bacterial payload, and the organisms stream into the environment. From there, they can infect other macrophages, even the specialized ones in various tissues. The presence of the Vi capsule reduces its vulnerability to complement and neutrophils, but it doesn't eliminate it. Vi is antigenic, so antibodies can eventually reduce its effectiveness. During its stay in the macrophage, the endotoxin is modified to make it more difficult for toll-like receptor 4 to recognize it, but once outside the macrophage, it is exposed to numerous cells that can, and do, find it. The unmitigated reproduction of the organisms inside macrophages, and their destruction outside the cells, results in a great deal of endotoxin release into the bloodstream and tissues.

This presence of large amounts of endotoxin in the bloodstream and tissues results in a profound release of cytokines, accompanied by the symptoms typical of typhoid fever:

An *incubation period* of around 10-14 days. The organism is entering cells, enabling its invasive genes, and making itself at home in the macrophage. The typical sequence:

Active invasion. Infected macrophages migrate around the body, carrying their bacterial payload with them. Macrophages naturally like to go to organs of the reticuloendothelial system, so the liver, spleen, and bone marrow are priorities. The escaping *S. typhi* quickly encounters other macrophages in these areas. During this invasive phase, the patient experiences fever, usually low grade, and some muscle aches. Active invasion lasts about a week. Storm clouds are building.

Fastigium. The word fastigium comes from the Latin, meaning "ridge." It represents the peak of the disease—the pouring out of endotoxin results in a massive cytokine release with its attendant symptoms. Fever often reaches 105°F and can last up to a week. For some reason, fever spikes usually occur in the afternoon. Patients often experience delirium, hallucinations, and profound prostration. The name typhoid comes from the Greek word for "smoky" or "hazy," a general description of patients' mental states. (Typhoid should not be confused with typhus, an unrelated disease, but one with similar fastigial symptoms).

In its journey around the body, the organism is mainly active in the lymph system of the abdominal cavity. They often form macular lesions on the abdomen known as "rose spots." These little red dots contain viable organisms and are only seen on the abdomen and sometimes on the lower chest. About 50% of typhoid patients get them; they are a hallmark of the disease.

The lysis period. Following the violent fastigial period, there is a severe but less intense time in which the bacteria are mopped up and endotoxin removed. Antibodies have formed, and the humoral and cellular immune systems are highly active.

The patient is still quite ill, but the high fever spikes have stopped. There can be undulating low-grade fevers. The lytic period typically lasts a couple of weeks.

The convalescence period. After being sick for 3-4 weeks, patients are extremely weak and still need supportive care, but they are on the road to recovery. Unfortunately, around 20% of untreated patients relapse to some extent. Most patients recover without any long-term complications, but with all that endotoxin flowing through the body for so long, the complications of thrombotic lesions are not unusual. They are by their nature hard to predict, but sometimes damage to individual organs can trouble patients for the rest of their lives. A normal and valuable function of the immune system is to initiate the coagulation cascade, resulting in the formation of blood clots. When a bacterium enters the circulation through a capillary in a localized infection, the blood around it clots, preventing its spread and trapping the microbe so it can be better accessed by phagocytic cells. But the release of large amounts of Gram-negative bacilli into the circulation from around the body induces an overwhelming quantity of thrombotic activity, and the damage is potentially severe.

One of the organs most frequented by *S. typhi* in its bodily travels is the liver, an essential part of the mononuclear phagocyte system (sometimes called the reticuloendothelial system, RES). It is rich in tissue macrophages called Kupffer cells, a friendly environment for the organism. The resulting bacteria pouring out of the liver enter the common bile duct and end up in the gall bladder, another friendly environment. *Salmonella typhi* is notorious for colonizing the gall bladder and is exceptionally efficient if the patient has gallstones. Like most bacteria, it can form a biofilm around the stones. A biofilm is a specialized structure of bacteria that creates a hardened crust on the material surface, much like *E. coli* forms in the urinary tract. The gall stones are locked in place, and the organism is locked onto the stones, protected from the immune system. Organisms are then shed into the bile duct, ending up in the intestine, to re-infect the intestinal wall or be shed into the environment. It is the stuff of the carrier state. It is said that Mary Mallon (Typhoid Mary) was offered the choice of gall bladder removal, an operation known as a cholecystectomy, but she refused. In her time, the procedure was not the routine matter it is today. Post-operative infection was not uncommon, and there were no antibiotics. It's hard to fault her on that one.

In acute typhoid fever, many organisms are being shed into the bowel from the bile duct, so the patient is constantly re-infected in the intestinal tract. This leads to considerable irritation and symptoms that result from it. Fortunately, the cells lining the intestinal wall and the tissues immediately underneath them are constantly being replaced, so the inflammatory bowel condition is short-lived, usually resolving when the fevers subsist. But the diarrhea is dehydrating, just another thing to deal with when the disease is going full-bore.

In the developed world, there is very little typhoid fever. The few cases diagnosed in the U.S. are invariably imported from endemic areas. The three pillars of infectious disease prevention, sanitation, vaccination, and antibiotics have seen to that. Despite the existence of carriers, many of them asymptomatic, the disease has, for all practical purposes, been defeated in areas where good sanitation is practiced and quality medical care is available. But there remain vulnerabilities.

During natural disasters, especially flooding, the sanitation infrastructure can break down, at least temporarily. Fresh water supplies can become contaminated with sewage, and typhoid has a way of popping up. If not typhoid, then certainly non-typhoidal *Salmonella and* other illnesses. Rapid and effective control of water supplies is one of the priorities following natural disasters.

The first antibiotic shown to be effective against typhoid was chloramphenicol, discovered in the early 1950s. It is active against most Gram-negative bacilli and went a long way in controlling typhoid outbreaks. Unfortunately, chloramphenicol has a rare but potentially severe side effect: it can suppress and shut down the bone marrow, yielding a condition known as aplastic anemia. It is an irreversible, fatal condition. (Chloramphenicol-induced aplastic anemia affects about one in 25,000 to 40,000 people). But several drugs have been discovered that are effective, and modern antibiotics are very

213

good at knocking down the infection, even during the fastigial stage. The best antibiotic to treat typhoid is ceftriaxone, a member of the large family of antibiotics known as cephalosporins. Oddly, the cephalosporins are of no use in treating non-typhoidal *Salmonella* infections affecting the intestinal tract alone. But once the organism escapes that area and disseminates, the cephalosporins, especially the third-generation forms, are highly effective. Defervescence (the beginning of recovery) occurs within a day or two. One limiting fact about the third-generation cefs is that they must be administered intravenously over a regular schedule. In countries where typhoid is endemic, access to sophisticated medical care is only sometimes possible, so oral antibiotics must be used even though they are less effective. Members of the fluoroquinolone class of antibiotics, such as levofloxacin, have been effective. Trimethoprim/sulfa (Septra, Bactrim) has also been used effectively.

Antibiotic resistance is always a problem. When a patient's life depends on treatment outcome, it can be a huge problem. All members of the *Enterobacteriaceae* are very adept at acquiring genetic material rendering themselves resistant to various antibiotics. *S. typhi* is no exception. Some strains are resistant to multiple antibiotics. The over- and inappropriate use of antibiotics of all types contributes to the problem, as it encourages the survival of organisms equipped with resistance genes. Developing countries are no exception, and antibiotic resistance levels are often higher there than in developed countries.

Using antibiotics to treat a routine case of gastroenteritis due to non-typhoidal *Salmonella* does no good. The disease progression goes on the same, regardless of antibiotic use. Using an antibiotic to treat gastroenteritis may do more harm than good. Antibiotics are not specific: they are killers of a spectrum of bacteria, sometimes a very broad spectrum. Our bowel flora doesn't like the presence of *Salmonella* any more than we do. Various strains manufacture anti-bacterial substances to attack the invading organism. Using broad-spectrum antibiotics wipes the normal good flora out just as it takes out the invader. Also, *Salmonella* invades the individual cells lining the gut, meaning the antibiotic must be able to enter the host cell, so the access of the antibiotic to the organism may not be 100%. Using an antibiotic to treat *Salmonella* gastroenteritis doesn't help the patient get better faster, and it may help create antibiotic-resistant strains and prolong the infection or its complications.

Many people not in the medical profession do not realize this. Common "wisdom" says that if you have an infection caused by a bacterium and feel like death warmed over, you take an antibiotic. Some people are adamant about antibiotic use to the point of being obnoxious toward their physician. Others self-medicate; the antibiotic left over from a previous ailment that is sitting in the medicine cabinet seems like a logical choice. Neither of these mindsets is at all helpful.

After smallpox, anthrax, and rabies, one of the first vaccines developed was the one effective against typhoid fever. It wasn't that hard to do. Just grow the organism in culture, kill it with something like formaldehyde, and inject whole dead cells intramuscularly. It was effective, but not 100%. Also, it had one notable side-effect: injecting whole bacterial cells meant you were injecting endotoxin. It isn't that much, and since the organism is dead, the disease and its effects won't spread, but getting a typhoid vaccine most often resulted in being ill for a couple of days, mostly with muscle aches and chills. Also, the first typhoid vaccine involved only B-cell involvement, not T-cells, so the vaccine was relatively short-lived, only a few years.

Current vaccines avoid these problems. There are two of them, given together. One is a purified Vi capsule conjugated to a carrier. Putting the carbohydrate capsule onto a protein carrier gives a more robust and long-lasting immune response to the vaccine. The other vaccine uses live attenuated bacteria contained in a capsule taken orally. The live bacteria are immunogenic but do not produce disease.

In addition to *Salmonella typhi*, another sub-group of salmonellae cause a similar disease. Known as the paratyphoid group, the routes of infection and symptoms are the same. Typhoid and paratyphoid are easily distinguished in the laboratory.

Typhoid fever remains a serious problem in the developing world. It is most commonly found in the Indian subcontinent, parts of central Asia, and areas of Latin America. Without treatment with antibiotics, the mortality rate is 10-15%. It is higher in children. Of course, the death rate will be higher if a patient has a significant underlying medical condition. And there is always the threat of long-term sequelae due to tissue damage.

There are an estimated 9-10 million cases of typhoid fever in the world every year. That results from unsanitary living conditions, lack of access to clean water, and inadequate medical care. What a shame.

People in the developed world do not routinely get typhoid vaccinations. It is often given to individuals traveling to endemic areas but not anyone else, so most people are vulnerable to typhoid. That raises the possibility of the organism being used as an agent of bioterrorism. It is virulent, readily available in some areas of the world, and relatively easily transported and administered.

The greatest number of people in the United States involved in an attack using a biological weapon wasn't, as many think, the use of anthrax spores in 2001. It was the use of *Salmonella* in a rural area of Oregon in the 1980s. Hundreds of people were sickened, and some died. It wasn't an event commonly called bioterrorism because it wasn't done to create terror and panic but to achieve a purposeful end. Nonetheless, the means of the organism release and infection rate illustrate what could happen.

In the 1980s, an ashram in Oregon was reaching its capacity. It was a very popular establishment, with its spiritual leader, Baghwan Sre Rashneesh, the chief attraction. Hundreds of people lived in the compound. Such a facility needed quite a bit of administration and direction. The Baghwan took no part in such affairs. It was left to a chief administrator, a woman named Sheela, who took her job very seriously.

The ashram needed more land for expansion. But the area where it resided, Antelope County, had stringent zoning regulations preventing their plans. Their main hope was to put

216

a re-zoning regulation on the ballot and have the citizenry vote. But the county residents far outnumbered the ashram inhabitants, many of whom couldn't vote. The odds of electoral success seemed pretty grim to Sheela, but she developed an idea. What if many in the county couldn't vote because they were sick? And what could sicken many people in a short time, make them too ill to vote, but not kill anyone? It's unclear who proposed the idea, but *Salmonella* fills the bill. The incubation time for *Salmonella* gastroenteritis is about two days, it wipes you out so much you don't even want to get out of bed, and people usually get better in a few days. Perfect.

The ashram had an infirmary with a small laboratory. Lab workers often use a standardized strain of *Salmonella*, *S. typhimurium*, to perform quality control testing on their laboratory reagents. The organism was readily available in lyophilized form from commercial sources. You just drop it into some culture broth, and it starts growing. It's easy to grow as much as you want by transferring it to fresh culture material. The agent was easily procured in large amounts.

Salmonella usually infects by way of contaminated food. One planning an attack need only plant the culture material on some food and let nature do the rest. But what food, and how to inoculate it? If the culture material were put into food that was later cooked, the organisms would die, and nothing would happen. So, fresh food needed to be contaminated. The idea struck Sheela or one of her co-conspirators that a restaurant salad bar was just the place. Surreptitiously plant the culture material on the salad bar ingredients, including the salad dressings, and wait for the sickness to start.

It's one thing to think of such a despicable plot, another to implement it. Whatever her motivation, Sheela ordered her plan to be carried out. But they weren't sure it would work when the election came up. Best to do a trial run and see if they could pull it off. Several people were enlisted to visit restaurants in the community with salad bars, do their worst, and see what happens. What happened exceeded their estimates. Over 700 people in the area developed *Salmonella* gastroenteritis. Several dozen people, mostly older, were severely ill and needed hospitalization. A few died. The plan was an unmitigated success.

The local healthcare personnel and facilities were overwhelmed. The Public Health Department quickly responded and sought to track down the source of the infection. The diagnosis of gastroenteritis due to Group B *Salmonella* was easily made, but the source of the infection was not so easy. The first thought in such an outbreak is a common food product source. Countless hours and endless laboratory testing were done, but the offending food material was never identified. It was known that most of the infected people had eaten at certain restaurants, and others had attended or lived with sickened people. Still, the idea of the intentional release of the agent wasn't considered. No note was sent, and no claim for responsibility was made. The disease is common enough that contamination with an animal product is always the first, and usually only, consideration. The nefarious release of a biological agent was never suspected.

History doesn't tell us the thoughts going through the perpetrators' minds after the "trial" event. Their group's spiritual message was peace, love, and understanding. What they did was pure evil. Maybe they were jolted into some sensibility by the magnitude of the awful thing they had done. Still, the second release of *Salmonella* several days before the zoning election never happened. The vote went as planned, and the group's proposal for the ashram's expansion was turned down. Sometime later, the group disbanded.

That might have been the end of the story but for one public health microbiologist. About a year after the fact, he noticed that the offending organism was the same type commonly used by lab workers. He persuaded investigators to dig into possible sources, and they eventually got to the source of the infection: the lab at the infirmary at the ashram.

This case didn't involve the typhoid bacillus. But *S. typhi* can be propagated and spread in the same way. One cannot just order it from a commercial vendor, but with over 9 million cases occurring naturally around the world every year, getting ahold of viable organisms would not be a problem for determined individuals. The organism only infects humans, but it is easy to grow in artificial culture. Most of the residents of the developed world are susceptible to the disease. Antibiotic-resistant strains exist and are not hard to create by mixing wild-type *S. typhi* with drug-resistant members of the *Enterobacteriaceae*. The best treatment is given intravenously, so a large outbreak would quickly overwhelm hospitals. A well-orchestrated release of antibiotic-resistant typhoid would be an absolute nightmare. It would not kill too many people, but it assuredly emphasizes the "terror" of bioterrorism. Economic damage could also be profound.

Typhoid fever has left its mark on humanity. Once called "slow fever" because of the nature of the course of febrile episodes, it hobbled and transformed many communities throughout the world for centuries. It is now controlled in developed countries but still ravages the underdeveloped world. It is not extinct. Humans had best keep up their guard.

Chapter 15
A Most Difficult Infectious Disease
Disharmonious
Unintended consequence
Of healthcare systems

While working on the microbial flora found in the intestines of infants in 1935, workers Hall and O'Toole encountered a bacterium they had a hard time isolating in culture. They could see it with their microscopes, but cultivation proved elusive. Because of its size, shape, inability to grow in the presence of oxygen, and ability to form spores, it was surely a member of the common genus *Clostridium*. But, since it was mixed with many other organisms, isolation in pure culture was elusive. When they finally did get it to grow by itself on culture plates, the species name *difficile*, French for difficult, was assigned.

Today the organism is relatively easy to cultivate in the laboratory, but the name is nonetheless appropriate. Once thought to be a nondescript, mundane member of bowel flora, the organism has proven to cause an often incredibly difficult-to-manage infectious disease in hospitals and other healthcare settings.

The genus name *Clostridium* comes from the Greek word *kloster,* meaning "spindle," the cylinder gizmo on a spinning wheel that winds up the yarn or thread. The genus has over 200 species, and they live all over the place, primarily in soil and natural environments. Some are associated with humans, mainly in the large intestine. Three general facts about *Clostridium* are very important concerning their involvement in disease: (1) Most species are obligate anaerobes, so they do not grow when oxygen is around, such as the amount found in healthy human tissue. (2) They form spores, little seed-like, thick-walled structures within the bacterial cell. Spores persist even when the organism that produced them dies, and they can hang around in a dormant state for a very long time, often years. Spores are tolerant to oxygen. (3) Many Clostridial species form toxins that are released from the vegetative cell. Some of these toxins are very potent and often deadly—the diseases botulism, tetanus, and gas-gangrene result from toxins released by *Clostridium* species.

We are all colonized by thousands of species of bacteria, but only a few can cause disease. When an organism is found in patients suffering from an infection, it becomes suspect as the culprit. But association does not always indicate causation. The bug may just be well adapted to inhabit a diseased area caused by another organism. Also, an organism may induce disease in one person, but it can be a harmless commensal in another individual.

The classic means of assigning a causative role of a microorganism to a specific disease are known as "Koch's postulates." Developed by Dr. Robert Koch in the late 1880s, they make sense when the organism is a frank pathogen: (1) the organism must be isolated in pure culture from an individual ill with the disease; (2) when introduced into a healthy individual the disease in question must occur; (3) the organism must again be isolated in pure culture from the sickened individual. If we take typhoid fever as an example, typhoid bacillus (*Salmonella typhi*) can be isolated from the blood of sick individuals. Well persons inoculated with the typhoid bacillus develop typhoid, and the organism can be isolated from their blood sample. Simple. Unfortunately, with some diseases, it isn't so straightforward. Some organisms exist within us for some time without causing any sign of disease. Even when one person is ill and the organism is isolated in culture, it doesn't always cause disease when given to a healthy individual. Finding the cause of the disease is sometimes elusive and frustrating.

This was the case with the disease associated with *Clostridium difficile*. (Most health workers refer to it simply as C diff). In the late 1800s, a type of bowel inflammation that today sounds just like C diff infection was described, but no causative organism was found. After antibiotics were introduced in the 1940s, descriptions of this mysterious ailment kept cropping up, but, again, the infectious agent wasn't known. Because of the large number of white blood cells accompanying the disease, some speculated that a pyogenic organism such as *Staphylococcus aureus* might be involved. Still, too many patients with the disorder did not have that organism in their bowel flora.

The mystery persisted until the mid-1970s, when the causative agent was finally described. It was, in fact, a toxin, one that has a pernicious effect on the cells lining the colon. Once the toxin was described, it was just a matter of working backward to find the species of bacteria which made it. *Clostridium difficile* is the culprit.

In fact, C diff commonly makes two toxins, A and B, that produce the same result. Without the toxin, C diff is just another stool bacterium of no apparent consequence. But even when capable of making the toxins, C diff is usually not pathogenic. Millions of people are walking around today with toxigenic C diff in their bowel and don't even know it. They have no symptoms at all. Yet, others have their lives completely unsettled. Some even die from the infection. When we harbor the bug in our bowel, what happens to us is more a matter of the patient's circumstances than the organism.

Most bacteria that are pathogenic in the colon have special attachment proteins that allow them to adhere to the bowel lining. Once established, they can proceed with their virulence mechanisms, and the infection begins. *Salmonella, Shigella,* and *Vibrio cholera* all attach to the epithelial lining. Not so C diff. It grows in the middle, or lumen, of the large intestine, competing with hundreds of other species of bacteria for its nutrition. With good bowel motility, it gets pooped out regularly. The competition with other intestinal microbes for nutrients and frequent bowel emptying keeps its numbers relatively low.

Two things can upset this harmonious condition. One is antibiotics, which kill off many competing bacteria in the gut, leaving C diff unfettered to metabolize and multiply. Some antibiotics kill C diff like other bacteria, but C diff can produce spores that are oblivious to antibiotics. The second contributing factor is bowel stasis, commonly called constipation. Without regular bowel movements, C diff hanging out in the lumen can grow to much higher numbers than otherwise would be the case.

Both these factors, antibiotic use and bowel stasis, are prominently seen in one setting: hospitals. In the hospital, antibiotics are frequently used to treat and prevent infections. Opiates for pain management and anesthesia are also commonly used. These and other medications can slow down or stop bowel motility. Such conditions promote the advancement of C diff, sometimes to pathologic levels.

Sometimes we go to the hospital to receive treatment for one ailment, only to be forced to confront another. Two words describe these situations, nosocomial and iatrogenic (pronounced I-atro-genic).

Nosocomial comes from two Greek words, *nosos*, "the sick," and *komein*, "to tend." In the 17th century, nosocome was the word for hospital. Acquiring a nosocomial infection means one becomes infected during a hospital stay and treatment. Iatrogenic also comes from the Greek, *iatros* meaning "healer or physician." It refers to an ailment resulting from the actions or comments by a physician.

Acquiring a nosocomial infection is usually not a sign of negligence or poor-quality care. But it can be. Many procedures and techniques are used in hospital care, and some carry risks. For instance, the insertion of a bladder catheter is very often necessary, and it mostly goes off without incident. A small percentage of patients, however, acquire a urinary tract infection. That would be a nosocomial infection.

Iatrogenic refers more directly to the actions of a physician. If a patient enters the hospital for a knee replacement, and the wrong knee is replaced, iatrogenic is appropriate.

C diff infections are nosocomial because they result from a stay in a hospital and the medications and procedures accompanying it. Often the organism is acquired in the hospital, but not necessarily. Many of us harbor the bug in our intestinal tract without knowing it. When the right circumstances are present, the organism produces enough toxin to damage the cells lining the intestinal tract, and disease ensues.

Quite a few antibiotics give us a side effect of diarrhea. Termed antibiotic-associated diarrhea, or AAD, the mechanism is non-specific. Antibiotics don't just kill the organism they are used to target; they take out some of our normally colonizing bacteria. Around a thousand species of bacteria inhabit our colon, and a microbial balance is desired. Taking an antibiotic upsets this microbiome, and the disruption can lead to diarrhea. Sometimes an allergic reaction to the drug can produce that result. Usually the reason is elusive, but once the antibiotic is discontinued, the gut flora returns to normal, and diarrhea ceases.

Infection with C diff is different. It is due to the specific generation of a toxin that attacks the cells lining the bowel. The antibiotic allows the organism to flourish by removing competing bacteria; the proliferation of the vegetative cells of C diff and their production of toxins cause the malady.

C diff makes two toxins, conveniently called Toxin A and Toxin B. Some strains make only one of them; most make both. The two toxins work in much the same way. After being secreted from the bacterial cell, they hook onto a receptor of the cell they will attack, usually an enterocyte lining the large intestine. After being incorporated into the host cell, the toxins begin their dirty work.

Each of our cells has a series of proteins that give the cell its shape. Just like our bones give our body our configuration, the proteins making up the internal structure of the cell are known as the cytoskeleton. It is this internal cellular structure that the C diff toxins attack. Not directly, though. They go after the energy system that allows the structural proteins to be produced. They block the conversion of GTP to GDP, interrupting the required energy flow from that reaction. Actin isn't normally produced, and the result is a cell that turns flabby and somewhat amorphous. The cell doesn't know up from down. Most importantly, the borders between cells erode. With the trauma of these changes, the cells turn on their self-destruct mechanism, apoptosis, and die.

The rounding up and death of the cells lining the bowel results in the leakage of fluid, which ends up in the colon and is the source of diarrhea. Just how much is related to the extent of the damage. Some patients have only a day or two of loose stools, and others have a profound case of a dozen or more watery bowel movements daily for a prolonged period.

The changes and death of these intestinal cells command an immune response. Innate immunity processes begin very soon, mainly by the release of the neutrophil attractant interleukin 8 (IL-8). IL-8 stimulates the attraction of neutrophils, which flood into the area. Three symptoms and findings are then apparent: (1) diarrhea; (2) white blood cells (neutrophils) in the stool and bloodstream; (3) fever. Of course, C diff isn't the only organism that can produce these findings— identifying either the toxin or the genes that make it confirms the diagnosis of a C diff infection. About 20% of C diff strains do not produce toxin and therefore are not a threat. Merely identifying the organism, as one would do for *Salmonella*, is not enough to confirm a diagnosis.

The presence of copious numbers of white blood cells and the formation of fibrin and other cellular waste products may result in the formation of a white film covering parts of the bowel. It is only loosely attached and can be easily removed using a cotton swab. Since it looks like a membrane but really isn't, it is assigned the name pseudo membrane. The more severe form of C diff infection with the formation of a pseudo membrane is termed pseudomembranous colitis.

Having a C diff infection can be a temporary inconvenience, or it can take your life. It's that broad a range. Just what determines the extent and duration of the disease has not been determined. In most cases, merely discontinuing the antibiotic results in a cessation of symptoms in a few days. Some patients, though, have diarrhea that persists either constantly or intermittently for months, even years. It can be a life-altering experience. In some cases, the entire colon becomes toxic and extraordinary methods such as colectomy (removal of all or part of the colon) are required to save the patient's life. Even then, some patients die of the disease.

Most bacteria capable of producing toxins don't make them all the time. The genes responsible for toxin creation are suppressed until they are needed. The initiating factor is usually some sort of stress, and one of the most important of these is bacterial overpopulation. Bacteria have an interesting set of chemicals that warn them if their numbers are too large. They send out a protein with a very short half-live, fractions of milliseconds. If there aren't many bacteria in the immediate area, the protein breaks down, and nothing happens. The more bacteria present, the more likely one of these proteins will attach to another bacterial cell of the same species, and a chemical chain reaction results in a couple of things: the cells greatly slow down their growth rate, entering what is known as their stationary phase of growth, and, if able, they begin to produce toxin. The toxin production helps them carve out new food sources to enable their already burgeoning population to expand.

So, to produce toxin, C diff needs to have an unfettered ability to grow and reach a very high number of cells in the bowel. The main instigator of this is an antibiotic that kills off its competitors for nutrients. Just about all antibiotics can, at times, do this, but some do it better than others. Most bacteria in the bowel are anaerobic, so antibiotics that kill anaerobes are best at enabling the proliferation of C diff. The antibiotics clindamycin, levofloxacin, and third-generation cephalosporins, such as ceftriaxone, have a track record of preceding C diff infections. But they are not the only ones.

The tragedy accompanying a C diff infection can be shown in a most unfortunate case history. A 71-year-old woman, let's call her Beverly, was admitted to a major hospital for a routine hip replacement. Beverly was a very socially active woman and was deeply involved in her family, especially her grandchildren. Married to a prominent member of the legal profession, her family was quite well off financially. She was in overall good health, exercising regularly and eating well. She was a non-smoker and drank alcohol only on social occasions. Not only was her health good, but her spirits were also. Many people liked and respected her; she was known for her quick wit and generosity.

Beverly was admitted for her routine hip surgery. She had no physical complaints or problems at the time of admission. An hour before surgery, as is routine for orthopedic procedures, she was administered a dose of the antibiotics cefazolin and vancomycin intravenously. (Single IV doses of broad-spectrum antibiotics like cefazolin are routinely given shortly before surgery to prevent infection. Vancomycin is commonly added in orthopedic procedures to help prevent infection with methicillin-resistant *Staphylococcus aureus*, or MRSA. They are discontinued after the procedure).

226

The surgery went well, with no technical problems or complications. Following two days' recovery, Beverly was scheduled to be discharged to her home. Her daughter was to spend a week with her until she could get around independently. But on the morning she was to be released, Beverly developed the classic symptoms of lower urinary tract infection, frequency and burning. A quick urinalysis performed in the lab showed she had a urinary tract infection, and she was placed on the antibiotic levofloxacin, pending the result of the urine culture. To be safe, she was to now remain in the hospital until the UTI cleared up.

But she got worse. Four days post-op, she developed a 103° fever and diarrhea. At first, the diarrhea was just a few loose stools, but it soon developed into watery diarrhea with around a dozen bowel movements a day. Her peripheral white blood count was 15,600, much higher than expected with an uncomplicated lower UTI. A lab test for the presence of C diff toxin was positive, and the diagnosis of *Clostridium difficile* infection was established.

Then the worst-case scenario: Beverly was diagnosed with a distended colon, an emergency. Her entire colon was removed, but even that wasn't enough. She died a day later, despite the best medical treatment available.

While extreme, this case points out the many problems surrounding the pathogen *Clostridium difficile*. Beverly came into the hospital as a relatively healthy woman, but during her stay, she contracted two infections due to her medical procedures: a urinary tract infection and C diff. In most cases, both are easily managed, the former with the administration of antibiotics, the latter by their cessation. When C diff persists, it can usually be successfully treated with the antibiotic Fidaxomicin. Oral vancomycin can also be given. Unfortunately, despite appropriate antibiotic treatment, in some cases, diarrhea persists over many weeks, sometimes longer. Rarely, the toxin release and effect are so profound that cases like that presented here can occur.

Clearly, the way to halt C diff infection is to eliminate the toxin or the organism that produces it. It sounds simple, and there is precedent here with toxigenic diseases such as tetanus and diphtheria. But using an antitoxin in the bowel has not worked out to date. Like other bacteria, C diff is susceptible to antibiotics, but it makes spores that are unaffected. When the antibiotic fades away, the C diff spores germinate into vegetative cells, and they get a head start on the competing bowel flora. C diff can be an on-again-off-again infection, appearing and receding over a prolonged period.

One approach to treating C diff infections has been administering large quantities of benign bacteria, which can compete with C diff for nutrients in the bowel. Termed **pro**biotics, as opposed to **anti**biotics, these live organisms are generally taken by mouth with the intent that they will take up residence in the bowel. The efficacy of this procedure is complex and not easily discernable since there are so many variables. How many probiotic organisms survive the stomach and small bowel and take up residence in the colon? How good are they out-competing C diff? C diff feeds mainly on short-chain peptides, about 5-8 amino acids in length. If the probiotic organisms feed on other substances, they don't offer much competition for nutrients. There are around a thousand species of bacteria in the gut. Do any of them make an antibiotic-like substance that can inhibit the growth of the probiotic bacteria? These and other questions are tough to answer. While the theory of probiotic therapy makes sense on paper, it hasn't worked out too well for treating C diff infections. In the cases where it has seemed to have worked, one must remember that spontaneous remissions occur, so attributing the cure to the probiotic is unclear.

Along with probiotics (living organisms) is the concept of **pre**biotics, or nutrients supplied to allow for the luxuriant growth of gut flora, including probiotics organisms. We might think of prebiotics as lawn food, the fertilizer you put on your grass to allow it to flourish. In the microbiology lab, culture media is supplemented with nutrients for bacteria to feed on and grow, and prebiotics do the same, except within our bodies. Of course, our gut flora normally feeds on the same stuff we do, and not all bacteria metabolize different nutrients in the same way. Like probiotics, then, the efficacy of prebiotics is challenging to evaluate, especially when looking at millions of people with different diets and normal gut flora. In some cases, pro- and prebiotics may work very well; in others, they may not.

The practice of surgery is well known for its abhorrence of bacteria. The operating room is as free of germs as human hands can make it. Attending personnel are covered in sterile garments from the tops of their heads to their feet. Every instrument is scrupulously sterilized before being placed on the operating room tray. So it is a bit strange to encounter a surgical procedure that deals directly with the deliberate administration of living bacteria into a patient. Fecal microbiota transplant, or FMT, is a last resort measure to treat people with a serious and prolonged C diff infection experience. Fecal material is usually taken from a patient's family member who is known to be free of viral infections such as HIV and hepatitis and implanted into the C diff-infected patient by either colonoscopy or nasogastric tube. Cure rates over time have been quite good with this procedure, often over 90%.

The hardship of a C diff infection became more problematic with the emergence of a particularly nasty strain, BI/NAP1/0. First observed around the year 2000, these strains present several challenges that routine "garden variety" strains do not. (NAP refers to the location where it was first found and the technique used to describe it, North American pulse field. It is also known as PCR ribotype 027 and restriction endonuclease analysis type 1, or B1. Quite a list; most just call it NAP1).

For one thing, the NAP1 C diff strain is resistant to the antibiotic levofloxacin (Levaquin) and therefore survives better than its competitors when a fluoroquinolone antibiotic is used. (Levofloxacin is a commonly prescribed antibiotic, as is its sister drug, ciprofloxacin, or Cipro. Resistance to one yields resistance to the other). Also, the organism's gene that normally suppresses the expression of toxins A and B is damaged and fails to function, so the toxins are expressed in greater quantities. As if that weren't enough, these strains of C diff have incorporated a third toxin, called the binary toxin, which seems to enhance virulence. The presence of a hyper-virulent strain can cause more severe disease, as well as predispose to recurrences.

There have been some reports of community-acquired C diff infections, usually associated with antibiotic use for an unrelated infection, but most cases are hospital-acquired. C diff is the most common hospital-acquired infection, affecting over 200,000 patients annually, with over 12,000 deaths in the United States. The annual cost of treating C diff patients runs into hundreds of millions of dollars in the United States alone. But the numbers don't reflect the misery and negative quality of life impact this organism inflicts. For technical reasons, the organism *Clostridium difficile* has been reclassified to the new genus *Clostridioides*. Whatever you call it, it is a scourge that continues to harm our most vulnerable.

Chapter 16
Milk Bugs

Defense avoidance
And lifestyle alterations.
Cunning predators.

Brucella is a bacterium that can exist in two very different worlds. One day it may be soaking up some sun on a blade of grass in a field. The next it can be inside a macrophage floating along in an animal's bloodstream. It's equally at home in either condition. Humans are not the natural host for the organism; grass-eating animals such as sheep, goats, cattle, and camels are. But we can easily become infected with *Brucella* by consuming dairy products or contaminated meat. The organisms are incredibly tiny, and it only takes a few dozen bugs to infect us. If left untreated, the infection may take decades to resolve, and its effects can be life-altering.

Macrophages of all types and descriptions are designed to efficiently kill and remove bacterial invaders. They also play the vital role of digesting the beast and displaying little parts of it on its surface to initiate the process of acquiring sustained immunity to the organism. Through eons of trial and error, *Brucella* has achieved the power to circumvent the macrophage's operations and direct its activities. It literally seeks out and enters the cell designed to kill it.

When it comes to devouring and killing microbial invaders, one might say there are two types of cells in the body: professional and nonprofessional. The pros are the macrophages and neutrophils, endowed with many weapons to carry out the mission. But many other cells in the body, though they primarily carry out different functions, may nonetheless aid in repelling microbial invaders. The epithelial cells, the cells lining the outside of our organs, have this capability. There are several ways these non-professional cells aid in our defense.

Most microbes cannot pass through the cell's outer membrane when they encounter a cell. If there is no receptor to accommodate the microbe, it just drifts away. However, some microbes have an accommodating molecular appendage on their surface. Like a hacker getting into a computer system, the microbe has the correct "password," or molecular structure, corresponding to the receptive molecule on the cell's surface. The host cell membrane, where the microbe attaches, often disengages from the rest of the membrane and surrounds the bug. Following a series of reactions, this tiny bit of membrane-encircled microbe is incorporated into the host cell. This structure is known as a phagosome, a little "jail cell" the host sets up to encase invading microbes, just like the professional cells.

Residing within all nucleated mammalian cells are small vacuoles containing digestive enzymes. Known as lysosomes, these digestive vacuoles clean up regular activity within the cell, a process known as autophagy or "self-eating." Their role is essential, keeping the cell environment clear of toxic products. When needed, the lysosomes of non-professional cells can be pressed into service just like the granules of neutrophils. They don't have the many different anti-microbial substances that are within the neutrophil granule, but their digestive enzymes are usually enough to do the job of killing the invader. The lysosome fuses with the phagosome, and the microbe is in real trouble.

On the surface of most nucleated mammalian cells are very long molecules that extend from the outside of the cell down quite deep into the inside. They serve as signaling devices, beginning the process of alerting a full range of cells and molecules of the innate immune system to the presence of an invader. They bear one of the strangest names in biology, Toll-like receptor, or TLR. First discovered by a team of workers in the lab of German researcher and Nobel laureate Christiane Nusslein-Volhard, the name reportedly comes from the exclamation by the workers on the discovery of the molecule in fruit flies, "Das is ja toll!" or "That's great!"

Humans have ten types of Toll-like receptors in our cells, numbered TLR-1 to TLR-10. Most project into the environment, but a few are entirely within the cell. Each one has a receptor for a molecule unique to a microorganism. These microbial molecules are known as PAMPS or pathogen-associated molecular patterns. Microbes have specific surface structures that are unique to them, structures that we don't have. For instance, Gram-negative bacteria have lipopolysaccharide (LPS) in their cell walls, and we don't have cell walls, let alone LPS. TLR-4 is set up to combine with LPS.

Each of the ten TLRs combines with a specific microbial surface molecule. When it does, the entire TLR molecule starts to wiggle and change, and the part deep within the cell's interior changes its shape. If another TLR of the same type is also activated externally (for instance, two TLR-4s), the deep sections of their respective molecules sort of wiggle into each other and combine. The bottom part of the TLR extends down into the cell. It's known as the Toll-interleukin-1 receptor domain, TIR. When this TIR end of the molecule becomes activated with another like it, a molecular chain reaction begins, ending with the activation of a vital molecule called Nuclear Factor kappa B, or NFκB.

We have hundreds of genes on our chromosomes that are covered up and not allowed to be transcribed and translated into the substances they hold the code for. Releasing these substances regularly would create havoc within the body. But when a microbial invader attacks, these gene products must be produced and released. A crude analogy would be unlocking an armory when a town is being attacked.

Nuclear Factor kappa B's mission is to effectively remove the molecules blocking the genes that code for important signaling molecules and allow the cell to produce them. The result is the synthesis and release of substances like tumor necrosis factor alpha (TNF-α) and other cytokines. It's the cell's 911 call, resulting in a significant inflammatory reaction.

Sometimes, the production of inflammatory cytokines is poorly controlled. A stimulatory effect stays turned on, and cytokines are produced over an extended period. The triggering event, whether it be a microbial invasion or an autoimmune reaction, stays active, and the cytokine production spigot remains open. Some medications are designed to reduce cytokine production and relieve symptoms. Unfortunately, they can also reduce the immune system's response against microbes.

Review of reactions to activate cytokine release:
1. TLR contacts a unique part of invading microbe.
2. More than one of the same type of TLR begins to wiggle and shake.
3. The cellular ends of the TLRs (the TIR region) are now active.
4. The TIR initiates a series of chemical reactions of several resident, formerly inactive molecules.
5. Following this chain reaction of molecules, NFκB is activated.
6. NFκB makes its way to the host cell chromosome.
7. After the reaction on the genome by NFκB, the genes coding for several inflammatory cytokines are unsuppressed and free to be transcribed, resulting in the creation and release of molecules responsible for a vigorous immune response.

There are several detection and gene activation pathways in addition to Toll-like receptors. They work similarly, with unlocking suppressed genes as the goal.

Cells invaded by microbes are programmed to begin a process by which they kill themselves, the action known as apoptosis. Better to let one easily replaceable cell perish than have it serve as a factory for producing pathogenic microbes. The enzymes inside the cell responsible for the destruction are known as caspases. (The term "caspases" comes from the fact that the active part of the molecule is cysteine, starting with "c," and it attacks regions of molecules that contain aspartic acid, the "asp"). Caspases aren't just floating around randomly destroying enzymes but are present in a non-active form known as procaspases. When the signal is given, the procaspases aggregate and their proximity leads to their activation. Once the process begins, there is no turning back. The cell has hit the self-destruct button.

These three activities, destruction of the microbe within the phagosome, molecular signaling to the immune system, and self-destruction, are usually more than enough to prevent microorganisms from gaining a foothold. But the clever little *Brucella* has found a way around it.

Brucellae have developed a way to combat the defense put up by the epithelial cells. The organisms have a protein on their surface which is recognized by a receptor on the epithelial cell's surface. Contact between the two initiates the envelopment of the organism by the host cell's membrane and the bug's entry into the cell's interior inside the phagosome.

At that point, the game is on. The attachment of lysosomes results in the killing of most brucellae within the phagosome. But a few, probably less than 10%, start cranking out several protein products designed to get around the cell's destructive artillery. The primary weapon brucellae possess is called the "*virB* operon."

Bacteria have a lot of genes in their DNA that they don't express. Why produce some material that is not immediately needed but requires much energy to make? Sitting out in the environment soaking up some rays doesn't require the presence of *virB*. But being inside a phagosome about to be digested by a lysosome demands a certain sense of urgency.

virB refers to the virulence genes of *Brucella*. It is not just one gene but a whole bunch of them linked together, coding for at least 15 different proteins, each of which profoundly affects the host cell's metabolism. An essential product of the *virB* operon is a very large complex structure called the Type IV secretion system, or T4SS. After it is produced, T4SS inserts itself into the phagosome membrane encapsulating the organism. It then allows for the excretion of the various virulence products of the *virB* genes into the host cell's cytoplasm.

A couple of the proteins produced from the *virB* operon interfere with the ability of the lysosome to merge with the phagosome and kill the *Brucella* within it. Others enable the organism to direct the phagosome to the cell's endoplasmic reticulum, where the microorganisms can multiply unmolested. Others interfere with the molecules that carry the signal from the TLR's TIR domain to the activation of NFκB, thus mitigating the cell's production of chemical messengers to the immune system. So, with the activation of the genes of the *virB* operon, including the very important Type IV secretion system through which they can escape, tiny little *Brucella* can take over and redirect many of the host cell's defense mechanisms to suit its own purposes. They also produce a protein that interferes with host cell apoptosis, forcing the invaded cell to stay alive.

The organism still wouldn't last too long if it had to remain within sedentary epithelial cells. So they have evolved to infect the professional phagocytes, most notably the macrophages, in much the same manner they infect the non-professional cells. Once inside a macrophage, they use it as their private taxicab, traveling around the bloodstream and exploring various tissues and cell types.

One cell type they seem to prefer is the osteoclast that surrounds bone. Osteoclasts are merged macrophages–multiple cells come together to form one giant cell with multiple nuclei. Their job is to balance out the effects of their neighboring osteoblasts, which create bone. The osteoclasts break down the bone and resorb the calcium using their lysosomal acids and enzymes. Large macrophages are irresistible for the circulating *Brucella*, which enter the osteoclasts and divide. That is probably one reason patients with brucellosis often have such horrific pain associated with bone and joints.

Brucella prefers cells of the placenta and breast in their natural animal hosts. That way, they can be excreted outside the body and re-infect other animals. If they stayed inside one animal all the time, they would eventually die with it, and they would not be able to perpetuate themselves.

Humans are not a preferred host animal for *Brucella*; we are an accidental side trip they take when we drink the milk or eat the cheese that contains them. But our cells and immune system are closely allied to their natural hosts, so the infections they set up in us are similar.

Brucella has several unique biologic features that help make it an extremely resourceful pathogen. Compared to other bacterial pathogens, *Brucella* is very tiny. Comparing it to *Salmonella* or *E. coli* would be like comparing the size of a submarine to a battleship. Laboratory workers sometimes have trouble seeing the organisms under the microscope because they are so small. "Grains of sand" has been the usual characterization of their appearance. This small size may aid their invasion of epithelial cells and macrophages.

Brucella also has a prolonged generation time. Other pathogens, once they get going, can reproduce every 20 minutes or so, creating many organisms in just a few hours. But *Brucella* takes around 16 hours to generate a new cell. Perhaps by having such a slow rate of metabolism, they can defer some of the host's actions directed at them.

Another feature of the organism is its ability to survive in the environment for prolonged periods. Perhaps it's their small size, but they can live out in the open spaces for days, just waiting for that goat or cow to munch on the blade of grass they happened to land on.

Despite their small size and prolonged generation time, *Brucella* is highly infective to humans. Just a few dozen organisms are all that is needed to set up an infection, one of the lowest infective doses for any pathogenic bacterium. Laboratory workers are especially at risk of becoming infected. Infection in the U. S. is rare, and lab workers are not used to seeing *Brucella*. While working with the bug, they may inadvertently infect themselves.

Four species of Brucella can cause disease in humans, but two predominate. They are the cow species, *Brucella abortus,* and the goat and sheep species, *Brucella melitensis.* The other two, *B. suis* and *B. canis,* are much less commonly seen in humans.

The disease and the organism were first described on the island of Malta, which lies about 50 miles south of Italy and 200 miles north of Libya. Historically, one of the principal industries of Malta was goat herding. In the late 1800s, there was an outbreak of brucellosis among the herd animals on the island. British military workers described the disease and named it "Mediterranean Fever."

Major-General Sir David Bruce was the first worker to isolate the causative agent in culture. He called it *Micrococcus melitensis.* The organism is very tiny and appears round, so he thought it was a coccus. The "melitensis" part comes from the Greek name for Malta, *Melita,* which comes from the Greek word for honey, one of the island's bountiful products.

There are three main reasons brucellosis is a rare disease in the U. S. and other developed countries: vaccination of farm animals, pasteurization of dairy products, and serologic testing of livestock.

There currently is no vaccine for brucellosis that is approved for humans. It is okay to vaccinate farm animals, but it is not all right to vaccinate humans with the same material because, bluntly, if a few cows get sick or even die from vaccination, we can accept that. For humans, there needs to be a certain threshold of safety that current vaccines don't meet. Work is being done on a human vaccine, but the most effective one is an attenuated live vaccine, and there is a real risk that it could revert to a pathogenic type and end up giving you a full-blown case of brucellosis.

The current vaccine most used for the cow disease caused by *B. abortus* is a live, attenuated strain called S19. It's been around for over 100 years after being discovered by accident. It is given mainly to female animals because it can cause tissue damage in males. Some females will occasionally develop the disease as well.

An important way of controlling the disease is serologic testing on many animals if the disease is suspected. Animals giving a positive serology can be removed from the herd and slaughtered, mitigating the chances of spreading the organism to other animals. One drawback of the S19 vaccine strain is that it gives a positive serology, even years after it is given. One cannot tell if the animal tested is harboring *Brucella abortus* or if the positive serology is from its previous vaccination. Additional, more complicated testing must be done.

The vaccine strain for goats and sheep is *Brucella melitensis*, Rev.1. It was first developed in the mid-1950s. It is also a live attenuated strain that can occasionally infect humans and gives a positive serology test.

There is currently no approved vaccine for *Brucella suis* or *Brucella canis*. The little piggies and puppies have to fend for themselves.

The currently available vaccines have shortcomings. Much work has been done to develop a better one, but things get very complicated when dealing with an intracellular pathogen. You can't just kill the organism and inject it into a person or an animal, as was tried shortly after the organism's discovery. Researchers have tried many different formulations involving portions of the organism, but nothing has been proven satisfactory. So, we're still using vaccines developed many years ago.

Because of Brucella's low infective dose and ability to survive in nature for long periods, it has been developed as a possible biological weapon. In fact, it was the first pathogen that the United States Defense Department developed in the days after World War II when there was concern that the Soviets were also actively working on biological weapons. While the organism doesn't usually kill, it can leave a victim very sick and require prolonged antimicrobial therapy. The organism exists primarily inside the body's cells, so getting the right antibiotic to the organism may be tricky. Treatment takes about a month, and there are a significant number of treatment failures. While the use of biological weapons is now forbidden by international law, the fact is there are about 500,000 cases of brucellosis naturally occurring in the world every year, and it is not out of the question that people resigned to employing such a weapon could harvest organisms in some remote part of the world. The results of its calculated use could be dire.

On the surface, *Listeria monocytogenes* isn't at all like *Brucella*. For one thing, it is Gram-positive, so it possesses a very different cell wall. It's also much larger, has flagella that make it motile, and grows much faster. But it does share some similarities, giving us a very good example of what is known as convergent evolution. That is, its life cycle mirrors that of *Brucella*. It is a tough, hearty little beast that can live for days in wide-open spaces, and it can dwell inside an animal by invading its macrophages and other cells. Like *Brucella, Listeria* has a "trigger," a protein that, when activated, transforms the bacterial cell from one that thrives in the external environment to one that rapidly adapts itself to life within a host animal. It's called PrfA.

Listeria has several attachment proteins on its surface that allow it to enter the host cell after it bumps into it. Mammalian cells, unlike the outside environment, are rich in glutathione, and that seems to be the substance to which PrfA reacts. Once exposed to glutathione, PrfA acts like a zipper, unleashing the genes already present on the Listerial chromosome, enabling them to be transcribed and their protein products enabled. Like *Brucella*, this set of about 15 previously suppressed proteins enables *Listeria* to circumvent the host cell's defense mechanisms and exist with impunity within the macrophage or other cell designed to kill it.

Listeriolysin is the first protein to become active once the organism is inside the host cell. Like all engulfed microbes, the organism is encased inside a phagosome, awaiting the arrival of a lysosome. When the lysosome merges with the bacteria-containing phagosome, the death of the microbe is imminent. Listeriolysin breaks down part of the phagosome membrane, enabling the bacteria to escape before the deadly lysosome hooks on. The organism is then free to roam around the host cell.

Key to the activity of *Listeria* inside the macrophage is its ability to take over part of the actin proteins and use them like little propellers to go gliding through the cell. In the outside environment, *Listeria* has flagella located at one end. The flagella are shut down inside the macrophage, and movement is turned over to the actin proteins. This allows the organism to go directly from one cell to another without ramping up the immune system.

An interesting characteristic of *Listeria* is its ability to alter itself according to temperatures. Refrigeration is used to preserve foods, but *Listeria* not only survives refrigerator temperatures, but it also multiplies. Cheese with only a few organisms will have a lot more if left in the refrigerator for several days or weeks. At the other end of the temperature spectrum, flagella production is shut off at higher temperatures, and the organism becomes non-motile.

Unlike *Brucella*, *Listeria* is not rare in developed countries. It's quite a common bug. It is most likely found in dairy products, especially soft cheeses, but it is common in lunch meats and some produce. That's because *Listeria* colonizes the bowels of mammals. Like *E. coli*, *Listeria* is eliminated with fecal waste from farm animals and can follow a similar pattern of occurrence in various foods.

The obvious question is, if Listeria is so common and an effective pathogen, why aren't more cases of it seen clinically? Annually in the U.S., about one to two thousand cases of listeriosis are reported. Most cases are serious, sometimes fatal, but of limited scope, despite the relative abundance of the organism. One reason is that not all strains of *Listeria monocytogenes* are created equal. There are 13 recognized strains of *Listeria*, but only 3 (4b, 1/2a, and 1/2b) are pathogenic for humans. If we have *Listeria* in our food, it may not be a potentially dangerous strain. Also, *Listeria* is very susceptible to acid. It dies if the pH drops below 5.5. Stomach acid is normally much below that. For the organism to make it through the stomach, the individual potentially infected must consume very large amounts of the organism, over 10 million bugs. Even though the organism grows at low temperatures, that's a very high infective dose. Food containing the proper strain would have to be left out at room temperature or warmer for prolonged periods. Or, of course, the infected patient may have reduced stomach acid, which can occur when taking antacids.

Even though the organism possesses mechanisms to help it avoid the immune system, it is not foolproof. Its intracellular habitation reduces the effectiveness of complement, antibodies, and neutrophils, but it is still vulnerable to macrophages. Macrophages (those that are uninfected) can destroy an infected cell and the bacteria along with it. TNF-α is a great help in directing this destruction of infected cells. Once free of the dying host cell, *Listeria* is fair game for passing members of the innate immune system and is quickly disposed of.

An intact immune system is necessary to take care of *Listeria*. Those most vulnerable to infection are people whose immune systems are compromised, either by a disease condition or therapy. One group of people with a reduced immune system is women in their third trimester of pregnancy. Adding to their vulnerability is the organism's propensity to infect the placenta. Like *Brucella*, it has a great affinity for the cells of that organ, and once attached, it is hard for wandering macrophages to enter the placenta and dislodge it. The baby is at significant risk since its immune system is not developed.

Another organ *Listeria* has a great attraction for is the central nervous system, especially the meninges. Meningitis is the most common infection caused by *Listeria* other than those in the placenta and babies. Meningitis is most common in people with immune systems that are not functioning properly.

Sometimes, elderly people with no known immune deficiency become infected.

Brucella and *Listeria* are two organisms associated with contaminated milk, but there are others. *Mycobacterium tuberculosis*, usually the bovine strain *M. bovis*, can be found there, as can *Salmonella*. Pasteurization and refrigeration are highly effective tools in limiting the number of infections from dairy products.

Chapter 17
Toxic Assault

Powerful poisons,
Homeostasis distressed.
Tremendous pain lurks.

Bacteria can invade our bodies and make us sick in several ways. Some directly enter our cells and reproduce inside them. Some invade and disorient the cells designed to kill them, the macrophages, lymphocytes, and neutrophils. Others enter the body but don't enter our cells, growing in the surrounding fluids and spaces, employing several devices to thwart our immune system. Some organisms are with us continually, situated in relatively peaceful coexistence, until our immune system breaks down in some way, allowing them the opportunity to advance into an infectious stage.

Some bacteria have acquired the means to make poisons, altering the metabolism of our cells. These poisons are called toxins, and since they are released from the bacteria that produce them, they are called exotoxins, *exo* meaning "outside" or "exterior." In this group, we find some of the deadliest organisms known. The organism that produces the toxin is quite docile and ordinary. But the poisonous protein they manufacture is deadly.

Tetanus

For centuries, one of the great horrors of warfare was a scourge that came after the battle. Glaring wounds often became infected with bacteria that caused a foul, decaying, wretched episode. Pain and terror were immense; quite often, there were more deaths from infected wounds after the battle than from direct combat.

But the most feared post-traumatic disease was due to a silent killer that usually crept onto the scene almost innocently and without notice. But it resulted in a disease so terrifying that the mere mention of its name sent a sense of horror throughout the community. The disease was tetanus, and the suffering was unimaginable.

The word tetanus comes from the Greek *tetanos*, meaning "taut" or "stretch." Most of us have had what is commonly called a "Charley horse," a prolonged contraction of a voluntary muscle of the leg, usually with significant pain. (The term Charley horse may have come from a baseball player in the 1880s named Charley Radbourne, nicknamed "Old Hoss." Apparently, he got a cramp in a game, and the name stuck). Of course, cramps pass after a few minutes and leave no aftereffects. Imagine, though, excruciating cramps, not just in the leg but all over the body. And they don't stop after a few minutes but recur indefinitely. Their intensity is much more than the simple Charley horse type. That's tetanus, perhaps the most painful and horrifically debilitating infectious disease.

Hippocrates, or one of his acolytes, gave a good description of the disease in ancient Greece, including the observation that it occurred several days after a flesh wound. A profound depiction of tetanus came from the early neurologist Sir William Gowers in 1888: *"Tetanus is a disease of the nervous system characterized by persistent tonic spasm, with violent brief exacerbations. The spasm almost always commences in the muscles of the jaw and neck, causing closure of the jaws* (trismus, commonly called lockjaw), *and involves the muscles of the trunk more than those of the limbs. It is always acute in onset, and a very large proportion of those affected die."*

Of course, tetanus is not confined to the battlefield. Many have been afflicted after incurring an injury doing everyday chores. The organism responsible for the toxin production, *Clostridium tetani,* is found in dirt everywhere. It is a common inhabitant of the intestinal tract of animals such as horses and cows, so fields rich in manure are especially at risk for harboring the disease. The "rusty nail" adage doesn't hold unless, of course, the nail happened to be sitting in dirt or manure.

The first realization that a bacterium caused tetanus came from a Japanese bacteriologist, Shibasaburo Kitasato, who worked in Germany in 1889. He showed conclusively that the disease resulted from a toxin produced by the organism. Around the same time, Emil von Behring showed that a toxin caused diphtheria. Shortly thereafter, it was discovered that after injecting an animal with a toxin, the serum of the immune animal could be injected into those recently sickened, and the toxin-induced disease could be significantly reduced. This helped give rise to the scientific discipline of serology and immunology. In 1923, it was discovered that by taking purified tetanus toxin and exposing it to formaldehyde, its ability to act in the body was curtailed, but not its ability to induce immunity. With the introduction of a vaccine, tetanus could be truly contained.

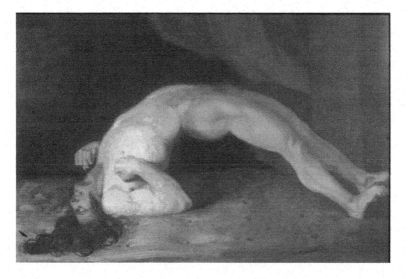

One of the most striking medical paintings of all time, "Tetanus Following Gunshot Wounds" by Sir Charles Bell.
Sir Bell was a physician as well as an artist. He captured many of the features of tetanus, including the fixed jaw, arched spine, rigid fingers, and extended and separated legs. The horror of the disease is overwhelming. (LOC)

Clostridium tetani is a rather large bacterium, usually staining a deep purple on Gram stain. However, older organisms tend to lose this feature and may stain variably or pale red like a Gram-negative rod. A characteristic trait is the position of the spore. Members of the genus *Clostridium* form spores within their cytoplasm, and when the mother cell dies the spore is released. The spore will develop into a vegetative bacterium when environmental conditions are accommodating. Each species is unique in the position of the spore, either central, between the middle and the end of the cell (sub-terminal), or

245

terminal. *C. tetani* forms its spore at the very tip of the cell, the terminal position. Because of this, it is often described as having a "tennis racket" appearance. Not many clostridial species do it this way, so seeing a sizeable Gram-positive rod with terminal spores on a Gram stain is highly suggestive of the organism's presence.

But the mere presence of the organism in a wound isn't enough to establish a diagnosis of tetanus. It's the toxin that matters.

Our muscles receive electrochemical signals from the brain and spinal cord. A nerve that serves a muscle has its cell body in the spinal cord. The neuron has a long extension, the axon, that traverses bodily tissues and comes very close to the muscle it acts on. On the other end of the cell body, opposite the axon, are several tree-like extensions of the cell known as dendrites. The dendrites receive the necessary electrochemical signals from the brain to instruct the motor neuron and excite its activity. In a matter of microseconds, the muscle responds to the signal.

Situated next to the motor neuron are two other types of neurons that give it signals. One is for excitability, the other for inhibition. Both are necessary. The excitability neuron releases the chemical acetylcholine into the very narrow space, or synapse, between its axon and the dendrite of the motor neuron. This signal tells the neuron to fire. The inhibitory neuron also releases chemical substances into the synapse. Its chemicals are the amino acid glycine and gamma-butyric acid, commonly called GABA. GABA and glycine have the opposite effect of acetylcholine. They raise the threshold of acetylcholine necessary to get the motor nerve to fire. We might think of the excitatory neuron as having the impact of a "hair trigger" on a gun. Just touching it slightly makes it go off. The inhibitory neuron makes the reaction more definite, requiring a higher amount of acetylcholine to get the motor neuron to fire. Without the inhibitory neuron and its GABA and glycine chemical signal, the motor neuron doesn't know when to quit and keeps firing. It is the inhibitory neuron, specifically the GABA/glycine portion of it, that the tetanus toxin disables. The motor neuron doesn't get the signal to slow down; it just keeps sending the signal for the muscle to contract.

For tetanus to occur, several circumstances must be present, beginning with a wound to the flesh accompanied by dirt and/or manure. The wound must become necrotic, cut off from blood supply with substantial tissue death. The spores of *Clostridium tetani* use this dead, oxygen-free tissue to develop into growing, vegetative cells. The spores do not make and release toxin; only the vegetative cells do. The bacterium must have a suitable environment of dead tissue to grow and create its sickening brew. Often the wound is apparent, but sometimes it can seem relatively minor, such as a puncture by a rose thorn. There are some cases in which the wound is not apparent at all.

Clostridium tetani makes two toxins. One, called tetanolysin, destroys local tissue and allows the organism to have a better growth environment. The main tetanus toxin is known as tetanospasmin. The genes for producing it are not carried on the organism's main chromosome but on a separate strand of DNA known as a plasmid. Not all strains of *Clostridium tetani* manufacture the toxin; those that lack the plasmid don't. When it gets rolling, the toxin is produced in one very long strand, which is then released from the bacterial cell. We don't know just what the toxin does for the organism in its natural habitat, but they make a lot of it. By weight, the toxin produced can be as much as 10-15% of the weight of the organism that produced it.

Shortly after the toxin is released from the cell a bacterial enzyme sitting nearby cleaves the long nascent toxin molecule into two parts, one about twice the size of the other. These two pieces don't drift apart; a single disulfide bond links them. The individual proteins do, however, rearrange themselves in new three-dimensional shapes to carry out their functions. The two sections have different duties. The bigger piece, the B fragment, is designed to attach the toxin complex to a receptor on the nerve cell and allow cell penetration and migration. The smaller strand, known as the A fragment, is the business end of the toxin, attaching to and disabling a vital part of the inhibitory neuron.

After its release from the bacterial cell and subsequent cleavage, the toxin floats around the surrounding tissues. The bloodstream picks some up, and some diffuse through the local tissue milieu. The long chain is designed to attach to the terminal portion of a motor neuron, which readily binds to it and absorbs the entire complex into the nerve cell. The toxin is now primed to do its worst.

Clearly, tetanus is a unique and complicated disease. We don't "catch" it from another person, we don't ingest it, and we don't inhale it. We get it by having a cut on our skin contaminated with dirt or manure. The injury must destroy enough local tissue to allow the anaerobic organism to grow unimpeded by our innate immune system. The strain of *Clostridium tetani* present must contain the plasmid that codes for the toxin, produced as one long strand. That long strand is cleaved outside the bacterial cell by an enzyme produced by the organism, forming a two-part molecule. The large fraction amounts to a vehicle carrying the smaller active toxin through neural membranes and up the axon channel.

Clinically, tetanus can be conveniently classified into four types of disease. The toxin action is the same for each, but the different clinical presentations reflect the site of infection and the host factors involved. Usually, the time it takes from the initial injury to the first appearance of symptoms determines the prognosis of the disease: the shorter the time, the more severe the disease, and the worse the prognosis. A short time is about ten days.

The most severe form of the disease is generalized tetanus, which begins around the face and mouth with two classic symptoms: a peculiar type of "smile," and lockjaw. The "smile" is not that at all, but the spasmodic contraction of the muscle system around our mouth, the orbicularis oris. The medical term is *risus sardonicus*, or "sardonic smile." Lockjaw, or *trismus*, is the contraction of the masseter muscle, producing the classic symptom. In severe cases, there is flexion of the arms and extensions of the legs, along with abdominal rigidity. The pain is intense and unremitting. Patients do not lose consciousness. Sometimes the upper airway may be obstructed, or the diaphragm may be thrown into muscular contraction, leading to a fatal result. Generalized tetanus may take up to two weeks to progress depending on how much toxin is present. Recovery takes about a month.

A less aggressive form is localized; the only muscles affected are nearby the predisposing wound. Usually, this form is self-limited, but sometimes it is the first sign of a much more severe disease. Similar to the localized form is the third form, cephalic, where the wound is on the head. Chiefly affected are the cranial nerves, with symptoms displayed in the mouth and facial areas.

The fourth type of tetanus affects newborns, invariably the result of contamination of the umbilical stump. Babies at first show general weakness and failure to nurse, followed by rigidity and spasms. Sadly, over 90% of newborns with tetanus die from the disease or from sepsis associated with other organisms invading the umbilical stump. If the mother is adequately immunized against tetanus, the disease will not likely occur.

For millennia, humans have suffered from the horrible effects of tetanus. After the cause of the disease was discovered in the late 19th century, progress was made toward treating and eradicating it. The first breakthrough came in the form of passive immunity, in which serum from an animal that had been given the toxin and thereby contained antibodies to it was administered to a person potentially exposed to the organism. In theory, this makes a lot of sense.

Tetanus is such a dangerous and unusual disease that it is impossible to set up experimental criteria to test human therapies. Field trials are the best way evidence may be gathered to accept or refute treatment. Ethically, researchers cannot deliberately infect a person with tetanus, then give them serum from an immunized horse and see how it goes. There normally are too few cases of naturally occurring tetanus, so appropriate field trials in humans are difficult to achieve.

But such a situation for testing hyper-immune tetanus antitoxin presented itself during World War I. Known as the "war to end all wars," in 1914, millions of men were exposed to conditions that favored exposure to the tetanus bacillus and its horrific effects. The armaments of the time were more advanced than had ever been used before, with bullets, shrapnel, and other debris flying everywhere at a furious pace. The battlefields employed were mainly farmland, with fields liberally treated with manure from cows or horses. And the battle scenes were primarily trench warfare, where soldiers spent months in intimate contact with dirt, and proper hygiene was unavailable.

Indeed, during the first few months of conflict, cases of tetanus appeared at an alarming rate. With the fog of war, highly accurate information is elusive, but the best statistics gathered at the time showed a high rate of tetanus among the wounded. Britain declared war on Germany on the 4th of August 1914. The first major offensive of British troops entered Belgium on August 18th, and fierce fighting began shortly thereafter. German records show that between that time and October 31st, 27,677 soldiers were wounded in battle. Of those, 1,744 developed tetanus, an extremely high number for what is usually a rare disease. Mortality attributed to tetanus was over 75%. British records were similar. One German nurse, Henriette Riemann, wrote, *"in the earth, which bears this bacillus, is the smallest, most cruel, most malicious weapon of this war."*

By mid-October, German and British medical teams initiated widespread treatment with hyper-immune anti-tetanus serum. All wounds contaminated with dirt or manure, or those with wounds that penetrated clothing (in other words, most of them), were to be treated. All medics carried ampules of the serum, and soldiers were inoculated at the time of injury on the battlefield or in service hospitals. Medics also carried ampules of iodine to be applied to the wound's surface to aid in killing bacteria introduced.

The results were amazing. The number of tetanus patients dropped precipitously. The British reported no cases of tetanus from 12,00 wounded soldiers who were inoculated for two months after introducing the passive immunity order. In a similar period before the serum was used, there were 27 tetanus cases from 998 wounds.

When used properly and in a timely way, hyper-immune serum made a huge difference in preventing the onslaught of

250

tetanus in individuals at high risk. But the technique was not without shortcomings.

When made in an animal, the antibody is a foreign substance to a human and is treated as such by the immune system. Passive antibodies to tetanus injected into a person last only several days, a week at most, so at least three injections spaced a week apart are necessary for an effective treatment. A single injection often didn't get the job done. Some individuals are hyper-allergic to the serum of some animals and can go into a severe, life-threatening anaphylactic reaction. In 1914, these reactions were often fatal, as they didn't have the chemical therapy (epinephrine) available today. Another adverse reaction, discovered in 1906, is called serum sickness. It is also an allergic reaction, although not as severe as anaphylaxis. Patients usually get diffuse rashes, muscle aches, headaches, and perhaps fever, which generally subsides after about a week. It is due to a generalized reaction against several animal serum proteins.

No doubt there were some cases of death due to hypersensitivity to horse serum and many cases of serum sickness. Just as war has collateral damage, indiscriminate use of horse serum given prophylactically is bound to cause some cases of moderate to severe side effects. In war, sometimes the options are limited. Using tetanus hyper-immune gamma globulin on the wound's initial presentation saved many more lives than it cost, not to mention the incredible suffering from the disease.

In 1923, the discovery of the tetanus vaccine revolutionized the battle against the dreaded disease. French veterinarian and biologist Gaston Ramon discovered that the toxin could be inactivated by formaldehyde but still retain its ability to induce immunity. Another Frenchman, P. Descombey, a student of Ramon, developed the formula to produce it in safe quantities and determined its dosage. With some refinements, it is the vaccine we use today.

One of the ironies of tetanus infection is that we don't naturally produce antibodies against the toxin, even when there is a full-blown generalized disease. It is so potent that it doesn't take very much toxin to make us ill, and it quickly enters nerve cells after it is produced, protecting it from the T- and B-cells needed for antibody production. Vaccination with the toxoid does protect us, but it must be done correctly, as the culprit is a protein, not a whole bacterial cell or a virus. It usually takes at least three vaccine injections to initiate immunity. Unfortunately, that doesn't last more than ten years in many people, so we need to get a tetanus vaccination shot every ten years. If a person can't remember their last tetanus shot after sustaining a significant cut or deep tissue injury, it is highly advisable to go ahead and get one. It can't hurt, and it may save a life. Tetanus takes at least ten days to develop, so giving a tetanus vaccination shortly after injury allows plenty of time for adequate antibody protection to develop.

Thanks to vaccination, tetanus is a rare disease in the developed world. Unfortunately, it still occurs in undeveloped countries, no doubt the result of poor or non-existent vaccination programs. Tetanus has been called "the inexcusable disease," as the vaccine is readily available, is very safe, and is relatively inexpensive. We'll never be free of tetanus; the organism is everywhere. It is not communicable and has a very specific pathogenesis. Its prevention is a no-brainer.

Botulism

As opposed to muscle-contracting tetanus, the disease botulism involves muscle relaxation. Instead of going into protracted spasms, muscles affected by the botulism toxin become flaccid (pronounced "flassid), unable to move. While one of the early signs of tetanus is trismus (lockjaw), an early sign of botulism is slurred speech because the muscle of the tongue is unable to move. The presentation of the two diseases could not be any different.

But the causes of them are very similar. Tetanus and botulism toxins are remarkably similar in their formation and action on nerve cells. Both start as a very long polypeptide that gets sliced by an enzyme into two sections: the large carrier part and the smaller active one. A single disulfide bond joins the two, so they travel together, the larger one attaching to receptors allowing the smaller, active toxin to gain entrance. Both act on receptors found exclusively in neurons. The neuronal receptors, though, and the clinical symptoms are different. Both toxins are extremely powerful, and often deadly.

Botulism has been around for millennia, but the first inkling of its source came in the early 1820s from a very unusual German fellow, Justinus Kerner. Best known as a poet, author, and purveyor of the arts, Kerner was also trained as a physician and worked as what we would now call a public health investigator. Botulism usually occurs as food poisoning: somebody makes a contaminated food product, and in a short time, several people who consumed the food become extremely ill. It's hard to miss. Kerner found out what each ill person had eaten, found the shared link, and deduced the cause. He also described the pathology of the disease, noting that the motor nerves are much affected, but mental faculties and sensory nerves are left untouched. He reported that the toxin is formed under anaerobic conditions and that only minute quantities are needed to elicit disease. He even mentioned the possibility that one day the botulinum toxin could be used therapeutically, a truly prescient observation for the 1820s.

The word botulism comes from the Latin word for sausage, *botulus*. The saying has it that we may enjoy eating sausage, but we really don't want to see it being made. That process of making sausage, whatever it entails, is ideal for creating botulinum toxin: an encased amount of protein developing in an environment free of oxygen. Just a little dirt is all it would take to introduce the spores of the soil-dwelling, spore-forming organism *Clostridium botulinum* into the mixture, and, voila, the toxin is produced. Of course, botulism is not confined to sausage. Any process which gives suitable conditions, such as canning, can allow for the growth of the organism and the production of its deadly toxin.

Despite the similarities in chemical structure and activity, there are some notable differences in the toxins of tetanus and botulism. The former is generated within the dead tissues of a wound after the organism is introduced. It takes at least ten days for it to be noticed. Botulism toxin is pre-formed in a food product and eaten. The symptoms are apparent soon afterward. Tetanus occurs in individual cases; botulism usually involves several people. But both are potentially deadly and result from toxins that directly damage neurons.

Because it is a large molecule with a specific receptor, tetanus toxin can only enter the neurons preceding the motor neurons, which signal the inhibition of muscular contraction. Due to its large molecule section, botulism toxin can only enter the motor neuron near the end of the axon. The botulism toxin targets the vesicles containing acetylcholine, the chemical that goes from the neuron to the muscle, signaling it to contract. Like tetanus toxin, botulism toxin attaches to and inhibits a molecule in the cell membrane allowing the acetylcholine to escape. There are several of these acetylcholine-containing vesicles. Which are attacked depends on the botulism toxin type. Since acetylcholine is blocked from escaping and migrating to the muscle, the activation signal is not received, and muscle contraction does not occur.

Unlike tetanus, which has only one type of toxin, there are several different types of botulism toxins. Conveniently labeled by letters, the two most commonly affecting humans are the A and B types. Occasionally E is involved in human disease, and even more rarely, F. Types C and D affect animals exclusively, while G is not known to cause disease in animals. The difference in the botulism toxins is in the smaller, active portion of the toxin and its ability to bind portions of the membranes of the motor neuron axon. They differ antigenically so that an antibody to one does not bind to another type.

Like tetanus, the first signs of botulism occur in the face and mouth, with other muscles involved later. The affected neurons can eventually regenerate more acetylcholine vesicles and their attachment sites, making the disease reversible. It takes about a month or two. The real danger in the first day or two is the toxin binding to the throat and diaphragm muscles, inhibiting the patient's ability to breathe. If a respirator is available, the gravest danger can be ameliorated, although some patients show some sequelae after recovery. Sometimes the damage is psychological.

In developed countries, botulism is a very rare disease. Modern processes of canning and other food preparation methods have all but eliminated it as a cause for concern. Even if a case slips through, usually with home canning, the food product is so foul smelling and full of gas that any thinking person would not for one minute consider consuming it.

Botulism toxin is the most potent poison known to man. A single molecule will stop a neuron from working. Toxins are measured by a number called Lethal Dose 50, or LD50. It is approximately the quantitative amount of poison required to kill half of the test subjects. The LD50 for strychnine is 2 milligrams of poison per kilogram of the person's body weight. For botulism toxin, it is .00001 milligrams—quite a difference.

Botulism toxin is ingested, and the entire human population is vulnerable to its actions. Because of this, it has been developed as a bioweapon. Treaties have banned its use, but it's not very hard to manufacture and could be produced in high quantities and potency. A major factor mitigating the natural consumption of botulism toxin is the wretched smell of the food product, which by its very nature is spoiled and often full of gas. Purified botulism toxin does not have this characteristic, so all a perpetrator must do is implement a way to introduce it into food. Given its potency, it doesn't take much.

Diphtheria

Everybody gets a sore throat. Many viruses that infect the upper respiratory tract cause inflammation of the pharynx with resultant redness and pain. Worse than that is infection by *Streptococcus pyogenes,* or Group A strep, commonly called strep throat. The toxins produced by that organism may result in enlarged tonsils and pus formation. The pain of streptococcal infection is usually more than that caused by viruses. Occasionally the streptococcus bacterium deeply invades the local tissues and causes abscesses, but most infections, like the viruses, are of limited duration and severity. Still, sore throat can be a significant illness, at times incapacitating.

But the viral and streptococcal infections pale compared to diphtheria, a disease that has plagued humankind for centuries. One might say that diphtheria is "the mother of all sore throats." Thankfully, it has been nearly eliminated in developed countries, although it is still very much alive in some parts of the world.

Diphtheria is caused by a small, rather non-descript little Gram-positive rod, *Corynebacterium diphtheriae*. The name comes from *korynee*, Greek for "club," a description of the organism's appearance on Gram stain, and the Greek word *diphthera*, which means "leather hide," describing the gross appearance of the pseudomembrane which covers the throat during the disease. Like tetanus and botulism, it is caused by a toxin released by the bacterium, not the organism itself. This bacterium happens to inhabit the upper respiratory tract, as opposed to the wounds of tetanus and the food products of botulism. Strains of *Corynebacterium diphtheriae* that do not produce toxin are of no consequence. They are entirely avirulent, that is, unable to cause infectious disease. But when the toxin is produced, it's a whole different story.

The fascinating thing about the toxin of *Corynebacterium diphtheriae* is that the bacterium does not produce it. It is the product of a virus, called β-phage, that invades and inhabits the bacterial cell. The virus incorporates itself onto the bacterium's genome. When the DNA of the bacterium is copied in the usual way, the toxin encoded in the virus is produced and escapes. When the bacterium colonizes the upper respiratory tract, as most do, it settles in, and the toxin is produced as part of the organism's normal metabolic functions. The result for the affected individual is disastrous.

Microbes of all sorts make chemical compounds that destroy or inhibit other microbes. The mold *Penicillium* makes a compound that interferes with the manufacture of cell wall material of some bacteria, stopping or inhibiting their growth, thus creating a better environment for the mold to flourish. We've discovered this compound, named it penicillin, and use it to combat microbes. It is called an antibiotic, and there are others. We have discovered and manipulated a few to our advantage, using a substance made by a microbe to fight off another microbe. Diphtheria toxin is just such a compound, but it works in reverse: the microbe makes a substance that acts as an antibiotic against humans.

Diphtheria toxin is one of the most studied molecules in all of nature. Its entire amino acid composition is known, as is its three-dimensional shape. Even though the organisms are not related, the toxin of *Corynebacterium diphtheriae* is generally of the same construction as that of tetanus and botulism: A large portion of the toxin serves as a carrier of the smaller, active toxin. The large portion attaches to the host cell and allows for entry of the business end of the molecule. Antibiotics such as gentamicin and erythromycin inhibit protein synthesis in bacteria. Diphtheria toxin inhibits protein synthesis in humans, with similar fatal consequences. It's the bacteria's version of an "antibiotic against humans."

Since the organism colonizes the throat, most of the toxin is concentrated there. Symptoms begin innocently enough, usually about two to four days after we acquire the organism. Like cold viruses, diphtheria is spread from person to person by respiratory droplets (coughing and sneezing). The disease first presents as a "scratchy" throat and nasal congestion, perhaps with a low-grade fever. It feels like an ordinary common cold, but it doesn't take long for the trouble to begin. The first sign is a white coating over the tonsils and perhaps the uvula. In another couple of days, this white creeping crud called a pseudomembrane spreads over the entire throat area, beginning as white, then turning a dark, ugly gray. The pseudomembrane is made up of lots of dead epithelial cells killed by the action of the toxin. It also contains lots of fibrin, dead white and red blood cells, and anything else that gets trapped in the growing web.

The pseudomembrane presents the most immediate danger, especially to young children. As it works its way down into the larynx, or if it breaks off and is aspirated, it can clog the respiratory passages and lead to suffocation. If good medical care is available, the patient can be placed on a respirator, or in some situations, a tracheostomy can be performed to allow breathing to continue. But in poor, rural areas of the world, those options don't readily exist.

The toxin's action is not confined to the mouth and throat epithelial cells. Just about any cell of the body is susceptible, but outside the throat it primarily attacks the cells of the heart, nervous system, and kidneys. In the acute phase of the disease, the effect on the nerve cells around the head is of special concern. Nerves affecting breathing and swallowing can be compromised, leading to even more difficulty in respiration and the potential for aspiration of a loose piece of pseudomembrane. The symptoms of the attack on the heart come later in the disease and can result in significant heart damage, sometimes resulting in death.

The history of our knowledge of diphtheria closely parallels the advancement of our understanding of infectious diseases. The organism causing the disease was discovered in Germany in the 1880s, as was the demonstration that a toxin is responsible for the symptoms. In the early 1900s, it was shown that taking serum from a person recovering from the disease and giving it to a recently sickened person lessened the development of the disease, the first glimpse into the field of serology and immunology. The vaccine, in the form of a modified toxin, was developed at nearly the same time as the one for tetanus in the mid-1920s. Today diphtheria is a rare disease in the developed world. But it still is seen in less developed countries.

The reason diphtheria has become so rare is something of a mystery. The vaccine doesn't target the organism, only the toxin produced by a virus inside the bacterium. Theoretically, the organism *Corynebacterium diphtheriae* should be able to colonize people's throats, whether it contains the toxin-making virus or not. But that is not the case; toxin-negative strains are rarely seen. For some reason, organisms unable to generate the toxin cannot compete with other bacteria in the mouth and throat and cannot gain a foothold there. Just why is still a mystery, but the results work in our favor since there are very few carriers of the pathogenic strain of the organism.

Of course, that could change. Diphtheria, in its heyday, did not come around every year like influenza tends to do. Sometimes as many as twenty years would pass between recognized epidemics, maybe longer. Diphtheria has not disappeared from the planet, and someday it could make a comeback, perhaps in a big way. Adequate vaccinations, beginning in early childhood, are the best way to prevent such an occurrence.

Pertussis

Most of us have had a cold that lingers. Two, three weeks, maybe longer, we're still coughing and blowing our nose. Rarely do we get tested for the organism causing it because it goes away eventually, and chances are high that there is no specific treatment for it anyway. That lack of testing is one reason we don't know how much pertussis, commonly known as whooping cough, is in the community. It presents as the "cold from hell," one that makes us sicker than usual and continues to plague us for over a month. Adults rarely have a serious outcome, but it can be a very different story when it affects infants and toddlers.

The common cold, of course, is a symptomatic disease and can be caused by a couple of hundred different viruses. Sore throat, runny nose (rhinitis), cough, general congestion, maybe a slight fever. It lasts a few days to a week; then, we're back to normal. Some, either due to the nature of the virus or the patient's immune status, last longer. But all are an inconvenience rather than a major worry. Pertussis takes the common cold to a much higher level.

Pertussis is not caused by a virus but by a bacterium, *Bordetella pertussis*. *Tussis* is a Latin word meaning "cough." *Per* is also Latin and can have several meanings, but in this case, it means "intensive." Humans are the only creatures that can harbor or be infected by *B. pertussis*, and it is passed from person to person through respiratory droplets expressed during coughing. The organism does not deeply invade human cells; it merely colonizes the respiratory tract like many harmless commensal bacteria. The toxins it produces make it pathogenic, and it possesses a sophisticated mechanism to release several toxins over time.

The first step in the development of pertussis is the organism's attachment to the cells of the airway. The human trachea is not a friendly place if you are a bacterium. A lot of mucus sticks to them, and cilia on the epithelial cells are constantly beating to carry away anything caught up in the mucus. If an organism does get in there and attaches, we have a cough reflex to help propel whatever is there to the outside. To allow for this most inhospitable environment, the pertussis organism has several very large proteins that enable the bug to adhere to the human cell surface. One, called filamentous hemagglutinin (FHA), forms a rather loose attachment to the cilia of the trachea, enabling the organism to escape elimination by ciliary action and remain in proximity to the cell surface. The strongest attachment molecules of the organism are fimbriae, threadlike projections from the bacterial surface. Depending on the strain, several different ones can be produced (FIM2 and FIM3 are the most important). These form a solid adherent to both ciliated and non-ciliated cells of the trachea, and the organism locks on.

Another attachment mechanism is a protein called pertactin, usually abbreviated PRN. While not a fimbria, it is a protein that provides another solid bond of the bug to the host cell surface. Once attached, they are tough to get rid of, even with the continual beating of the cilia. The word that refers to the firmness of the attachment is avidity, from the Latin word *avidus*, to "crave." With FHA, various fimbriae, and pertactin, *Bordetella pertussis* has a very high avidity to our airway epithelial cells.

Bordetella pertussis does not invade the inside of the cell to which it attaches, as many pathogens do. Sitting outside the cell in the middle of the airway leaves them vulnerable to the immune system, both mechanical (mucus, cilia, cough) and innate (neutrophils, complement, antibody, macrophages). For the bacterium, this will not do. They have several mechanisms to deter the immune system and remain attached. They aim to reproduce and spread from person to person, continuing the species. Their ability to inhibit the immune system is part of their plan. The high avidity of their attachment is one means of circumventing the mechanical forces designed to eliminate them. They also possess the chemical means to help ward off the innate immune system components.

The "first responder" to the attached *Bordetella pertussis* is the complement system, which is, of course, found in serum, but is also abundant in mucus secretions. Complement greatly assists neutrophils and antibodies in capturing and destroying invading bacteria, and it can directly damage and destroy the pathogen.

Complement is a powerful weapon against invading microbes, but it's also potentially destructive to human cells, not a good thing. Thankfully, our cells possess molecules that destroy complement components when they contact the host cell membrane. Incredibly, *Bordetella pertussis* has a system of molecules, most notably one known as Vag8, that can strip a complement-inhibiting protein from a human cell and use it for its own good. When Vag8 is active, C1, the first member of the complement cascade, cannot be converted into C1q, short-circuiting the entire complement system. Essentially, the bacterium steals a molecule from the surface of our cells and uses it to repel our attack on it. Clever.

Bordetella pertussis has several other complicated mechanisms designed to thwart complement activity, thereby ensuring its more prolonged survival in the human host. The first line of defense, complement, is much less active than it is designed to be, giving the microbe a leg up.

If you are a microbe, the next order of business is to eliminate, or at least mitigate, the host cells designed to attack you, macrophages and neutrophils. Macrophages are constantly wandering through the airway lining, ready to pick up any type of debris that comes their way. They also have the mechanisms to signal the immune system to deploy more help to the area, including more neutrophils, complement and other serum molecules, and the various types of T and B lymphocytes. The main toxin of *Bordetella pertussis*, pertussis toxin (PT), has an inhibitory effect on the macrophages, rendering them much less a threat. The specific mechanism it uses against macrophages effectively quells their activity, both phagocytosis and signaling.

The activity of neutrophils in the area is also reduced, not directly but by indirect methods. When a pathogen is detected in our tissues, chemical signals are sent to release more neutrophils from the bone marrow and attract them from nearby blood vessels into the affected area. Pertussis toxin reduces both tools by counteracting the chemical signals designed to make this happen, and neutrophil incursion into the infected area is significantly reduced.

Without our benefit of complement, macrophages, and neutrophils early in the infection, *Bordetella pertussis* gains a foothold on the cells lining our trachea and can set up a progressive infection.

Bordetella pertussis makes other toxins besides pertussis toxin. A very important one is adenylate cyclase toxin or ACT. It is a very large toxin with a short half-life, so it doesn't move very far from the organism once released. Its action is directed mainly toward macrophages and neutrophils that come into the area close to where the bacteria reside. It enters the phagocytic cell, then converts ATP into cyclic AMP. This reaction effectively halts the ability of phagocytic cells to kill the invading bacteria. We can think of the actions of PT and ACT as a one-two punch: The pertussis toxin mitigates the arrival of phagocytic cells, while the adenylate cyclase toxin, along with PT, kills the few that arrive on the scene. Together, the two toxins allow for the persistence of the organism at the infection site, the trachea and bronchi.

One reason the symptoms of pertussis are so severe is the presence of a toxin called tracheal cytotoxin, or TCT. Unlike the other toxins, which are made inside the bacterial cell and then released, TCT is a permanent structure of the organism's cell wall. All bacteria have it because it is a vital component of the bacterial peptidoglycan, which forms the wall's rigid backbone. Most bacteria have an enzyme that firmly attaches TCT to a section of peptidoglycan in the bacterial cell wall. TCT is needed to construct more cell walls as the bacteria grow. Not so *Bordetella pertussis*. It lacks the controlling enzyme, so its TCT is released into the local environment. Our cells are equipped with sensors to detect the presence of bacterial cell wall material, so this stuff sends the response into full operation. One chemical our cells produce to help kill invading bacteria is nitric oxide (NO). It is probably induced by interleukin 1, produced because of all the TCT floating around. Because of the abundant *Bordetella* cell wall material, our cells make much more nitric oxide than would normally be produced with other bacterial infections. Unfortunately, nitric oxide kills our cells too. The primary victims of this attack are the ciliated epithelial cells of the airway, especially the trachea. The result is the build-up of mucus, dead cells, and other gunk in our airways. Without the reliable rhythmic beating of cilia, much of the mucus and debris created locally remains in the airway, inhibiting breathing and initiating a cough reflex to remove it. Pertussis toxin then flows down to the underlying tissues, killing many of the cells there. All this local damage results in fluid release from the surrounding blood vessels, causing edema that further constricts the diameter of the airway. The combination of the debris build-up and the edema makes for a perilous situation for young children; the effects are sometimes fatal.

Infection with *Bordetella pertussis* gives us a reduced number of macrophages and neutrophils. But it has the opposite effect on our lymphocytes. They are created in great numbers in the bone marrow and flood into the lymph nodes around the trachea and bronchi. In the peripheral blood, the pertussis patient has an elevated white cell count, but, in contrast to most other bacterial infections, the predominant white blood cells are lymphocytes, not neutrophils. In fact, in a patient with a persistent cough and a peripheral count of over 10,000 lymphocytes, a diagnosis of pertussis can be confidently made.

Bordetella pertussis differs considerably from other bacteria that commonly infect the human respiratory tract. Three important ones, *Streptococcus pneumoniae, Haemophilus influenzae,* and *Staphylococcus aureus*, are readily visualized under a microscope in a Gram-stained preparation from a representative sample. They also grow readily on culture plates commonly used in clinical microbiology laboratories, taking a little less than a day for typical colonies to be observable. *Bordetella pertussis* is much different. That organism, a tiny Gram-negative coccobacillus, is not easily seen directly in clinical material, especially if the disease has progressed for several days, as it usually does before medical attention is sought. It doesn't grow on common laboratory media, requiring its own unique blend, and it takes almost a week to grow out, not just a single day. *Bordetella pertussis* is not seen on a routine laboratory bacterial culture.

Scientists looked in vain for the causative organism of pertussis throughout the 1890s. The first to recognize the organism were two Frenchmen, Jules Bordet and Octave Gengou, in 1900. They were somewhat lucky because they saw

263

it on a Gram-stain preparation from some sputum from a 5-month-old girl sick with the disease, which is not an easy accomplishment. It took them another six years to develop a culture medium that would support the organism's growth, using the starch of potatoes as the medium base, supplemented with blood. They didn't have to look far for clinical material to test the culture plate; Jules Bordet's son Paul was ill with the disease.

Bordet and Gengou didn't stop with the description of the pathogen. They attempted to produce a vaccine, but it didn't work very well. It would be another 43 years before a successful one was developed. But they did describe a toxin produced by the organism, one they called dermonecrotic toxin (DNT). When pathogenic strains of the organism are grown in culture, the crude culture broth, when injected into a laboratory animal, produces skin lesions. We now know this dermonecrotic toxin is similar in its action to the toxin produced by the intestinal pathogen *Clostridium difficile*. Its action disrupts the formation of structural proteins inside the target cell (mainly the so-called rho proteins), leading to cell death. Just which cells and tissues DNT specifically targets is not known, but when acting in concert with the organism's other toxins, it adds to the bug's disruptive force.

It's somewhat unfortunate that pertussis is commonly called "whooping cough." In some ways, that may trivialize it; the word "whoop" has several connotations. But there is nothing trivial in how the organism infects and injures patients, especially the young. In pertussis, the word "whoop" comes from the sound made on inspiration during a coughing fit, a pernicious feature of the disease. The most malicious symptom of the disease is called a paroxysm (from the Greek *paroxysmos,* meaning "irritation" or "exasperation"). It is a coughing fit that is a hallmark of the disease. Paroxysms can last for several minutes. Some people get it so bad that coughing may mechanically injure them, such as a pulled back muscle or rib injury. Most of the cilia lining our airways are non-functional, so the only way we can clear the debris clogging it is to cough it out. And the cough can reach epic proportions.

Besides the organism's several exotoxins, each bacterial cell contains the classic endotoxin typical of all Gram-negative bacteria. Our immune reaction to the endotoxin gives rise to fever and muscle aches. We feel just plain lousy for the duration of the disease, which, unfortunately, takes several weeks, sometimes months. The Chinese once described it as the "cough of a hundred days."

It would be nice if we could just take an antibiotic for a few days and be done with it. After all, it is caused by a bacterium, and the organism is exquisitely susceptible to the common antibiotic erythromycin in the test tube. Unfortunately, this is another area where *Bordetella pertussis* differs from other bacteria. Unless treated very early in the disease, antibiotics have little effect on the patient being treated. They may reduce the patient's ability to spread the disease to others, but there is only minor, if any, relief for the one afflicted.

The diagnosis of pertussis is enigmatic as well. A simple Gram stain of expectorated or aspirated material from the airway rarely shows the organism. It does not grow on ordinary laboratory culture media, so the physician ordering the culture must designate a pertussis culture using culture plates like Bordet-Gengou or Regan-Lowe agar. The organism is killed if the swab obtaining the specimen is cotton rather than dacron. The pertussis organism takes about a week to grow, so other bacteria that grow more quickly can overwhelm the culture media. All this means that pertussis is not easy to diagnose, and in many cases, it is missed.

Today's diagnostic method of choice is a molecular genetics test that detects a portion of the organism's DNA. Known as polymerase chain reaction (PCR), the test can detect the organism's presence with greater sensitivity than culture. The results are usually available in a day or two rather than a week.

The first half of the 20th century had to be very frustrating to doctors when it came to pertussis. The cause of the disease was known, and it should have been a relatively simple matter to develop a vaccine to prevent it. Just grow the bacterium in culture broth, kill it, then inject some of it into the child to be vaccinated. Sounds simple. But, alas, it wasn't to be. Pertussis makes several toxins, but they are denatured with the demise of the bug. *Bordetella pertussis* is a Gram-negative organism, and therefore contains the hallmark constituent of all such bacteria: lipopolysaccharide (LPS). Present in all cell walls of Gram-negative bacteria, LPS contains Lipid A, a very potent toxin, and it is not denatured by killing the organism. Our immune cells are primed to detect and combat Lipid A whenever it is encountered. Lipid A attaches to Toll-like receptor 4, which is present in all our cells. Macrophages are specially equipped to handle it. Once detected, a chain reaction occurs within the cell, enabling nuclear factor κ B (NFκB), signaling macrophages and other cells to turn on their cytokine-producing machinery. The result is a potent release of cytokines such as tumor necrosis factor-α, Interleukin-1β, Interleukin-6, and others, collectively making us feel sick. Fever, muscle aches, listlessness, and maybe a headache. Giving someone an injection of killed *Bordetella pertussis* also gives them a small dose of Lipid A, along with the repercussions.

Small quantities of Lipid A are usually tolerable and don't make us very sick. A little discomfort of a day or two isn't too high a price to pay for long-lasting immunity to a wretched disease like pertussis. But just how much is a "small dose"? Unfortunately, a small dose of Lipid A also means a small dose of the killed organism, and here again, *Bordetella pertussis* proves to be a conundrum. It takes many organisms to initiate an immune response, even when an adjuvant is given. The more organisms you give, the more Lipid A you give, along with its symptomatic sequelae. It took several decades to figure out the proper dosage, but administering whole cells of Gram-negative bacteria was never the ideal option.

The first step toward developing a vaccine for pertussis that didn't have the nagging side effects of the whole cell preparation came from the Japanese researcher Yugi Sato and colleagues. In the early 1980s, they prepared cell wall fragments that lacked Lipid A but contained pertussis toxin. It worked. Japan went to it as the vaccine of choice for pertussis, and other countries followed. Since then, other preparations have been developed, all based on parts of the organism but lacking Lipid A and its toxic effects. The most important fractions of the vaccine are the organism's attachment structures, plus pertussis toxin. If it can't attach and hold on, it can't infect, and antibodies the vaccine induces block the attachment points. It is known as the "acellular" preparation. Since the pertussis vaccine is usually administered in combination with diphtheria and tetanus in the DPT formula, it is now known as DTaP, with the lower case "a" standing for acellular, concerning the pertussis component.

Before the use of an effective vaccine, pertussis showed a cycle of epidemic outbreaks. The disease would come around every three to five years, mainly striking young children and babies. Presumably, older patients had previously encountered the organism and were much less susceptible. Pertussis still shows this cyclic pattern, but the affected patients include the young and the older. The acellular vaccine has done much to reduce the side effects of vaccination. Still, it may be that the immunity it imparts doesn't last as long as the whole cell preparation or natural infection.

Bordetella pertussis isn't known to naturally inhabit animals besides humans. Just where it goes between epidemics is anybody's guess. There could be a carrier state of some magnitude, but it is very difficult to detect. It's hard enough isolating and identifying the organism during acute disease; it's impossible to detect a few relatively dormant critters just hanging on, not causing any trouble. The toxins of *B. pertussis* are contained in a segment of its DNA strand known as the Bvg (*Bordetella* virulence gene). The organism can turn off all its virulence factors as environmental conditions change and enter a non-virulent phase. It happens all the time to organisms in laboratory culture. Organisms that are continually passed on culture media go from a silver, hemolytic colony (often described as "drops of mercury") to a white, chalky non-virulent phase. Finding itself in a human airway, conditions are right for it to activate its Bvg genes and become virulent again. Exactly what this has to do with the 3-5 year period of epidemics is unknown.

Pertussis is a serious disease. Because of vaccination, we in developed countries no longer fear it, as did past generations. But it used to be a serious killer. In the pre-vaccination era, it killed more young children than measles, scarlet fever, diphtheria, polio, and meningitis combined. Worldwide, it is estimated that there are over 20 million cases of pertussis every year, with at least 160,000 deaths, most of them young children. In the U.S., there are reportedly about 50,000 cases per year, but given the difficulties of diagnosis, especially in adults, there are undoubtedly many more.

Cholera

Just as we all get a common cold occasionally, we also encounter bouts of diarrhea. And, just as pertussis takes the common cold to another level, infectious diarrhea can occur in an extreme form—the disease cholera is debilitating and often fatal. Fortunately, cholera is extremely rare in developed countries because of adequate sanitation. Unfortunately, it continues to plague lesser developed nations, sometimes mercilessly.

The history of the word cholera is interesting. It comes from the Greek *khole*, meaning "bile." Bile was one of the ancient "four humors" of blood, phlegm, black bile, and yellow bile, which were associated with air, water, earth, and fire. Bile has a bitter taste and was thought to be associated with anger and irritability. The original term cholera referred to a state of rage and extreme agitation. The disease we now call cholera was associated with this state of disposition, as if the "yellow bile" became out of balance. Of course, bile has nothing to do with the disease cholera. A toxin-producing bacterium that lives in water does.

The history of discovering the microbial cause of cholera is also fascinating. One of the great and often-told stories of medical history is the inquiry by physician John Snow into the episode known as the "Broad Street Pump," the first well-documented attempt to track down the source of an infectious disease.

Born in 1813, John Snow grew up poor and was constantly exposed to dirt, grime, and filth. Without scientific foundation, he believed these conditions predisposed people to diseases. He became enamored with cleanliness, both in

268

personal hygiene and food and drink, ideas that weren't popular at the time. In fact, they sounded downright strange and were subject to ridicule. He was brilliant and received his medical degree at the age of 18 in 1831. Around that time, cholera emerged in England, though it is a disease usually found only in very warm climates.

Without proper sanitation, cholera spreads rapidly and with devastating consequences. Thousands of Englanders died of the disease. In 1854, there was a severe cholera epidemic in the section of London known as the Soho district. Many people of all ages and socioeconomic statuses were sickened; hundreds died. Dr. Snow lived a short distance from the Soho area, and he made it his mission to investigate the outbreak and test his theory, published a few years before, that cholera was not caused by "miasmas," or bad air, as was commonly believed, but was due to some toxic substance in drinking water. Nobody believed him, of course. He couldn't say what this toxic substance was and what it did to you. Without the scientific foundation, he worked alone, often the subject of derision and contempt.

Being the scientist he was, he went about the investigation methodically. He interviewed many medical workers and private citizens, establishing the residence of each person who had cholera in the area. He got a grid map and plotted every known case. He checked not just who contracted the disease but, equally important, those who didn't and where they got their drinking water. Dr. Snow worked exhaustively to complete his inquiry, and his results from several lines always took him back to one point: the pump from a water well on the corner of Broad and Cambridge Streets in the Soho district. In short, whether they lived in the area or not, people who drank water from the pump got cholera. Even if they lived in the area, people who didn't drink from the Broad Street pump were cholera free. The evidence was overwhelming, and irrefutable. The local politicians weren't convinced, given the lack of scientific knowledge at the time and the fact that to admit the accuracy of Dr. Snow's theory was to acknowledge that fresh drinking water in the city was exposed to raw sewage. Still, they complied with the recommendation to dismantle the Broad Street pump. People had to secure their water elsewhere.

Immediately, new cholera cases ceased–a dramatic occurrence, to say the least.

In all, over 600 people were thought to have died from their exposure to the water from the Broad Street pump. It's impossible to know how many lives John Snow saved following his actions. Still, certain is the fact that a new method of disease investigation, what we now call epidemiology, had its beginnings in the 1850s around a water well near the corner of Broad and Cambridge streets in the Soho district of London.

John Snow was best known in his day for his work with anesthetics, mainly ether and chloroform. His "day job" was as an obstetrician, and he incorporated the new drug discoveries into his practice. Indeed, Queen Victoria, with the birth of her eighth and ninth children, allowed the use of anesthetics on herself, giving credence to the controversial technique. Dr. Snow never married and died of a stroke at the age of 45. Today, some refer to him as the "Father of Epidemiology."

In 1854, Italian physician and anatomist Filippo Pacini made another major discovery on the disease cholera. Dr. Pacini was blessed to have a very good microscope for the time, one that he helped make himself with an achromatic lens made by Giovanni Amici, one of the top lens makers of that period. (An achromatic lens is a double lens, two lenses glued together to bring the light of different wavelengths, primarily blue and red, in synchrony to remove the aberration or fuzziness of the image). Mostly he used his microscope to study human tissue, a discipline we know today as histology. When the cholera pandemic of the mid-19th century struck Italy, he examined the intestines of corpses of victims of the disease. While doing so, he noticed a tiny cell found only in cholera victims. When looked at in the live state, the organism seemed to vibrate; what we now know was because of its very active polar flagellum. He named the tiny creature *Vibrio*, from the Latin *vibrare*, to "vibrate." He published his results and became the first to record the observation that a microorganism can cause human disease.

Snow and Pacini made remarkable discoveries; both were way ahead of their time. They were superb researchers and rigorously employed the scientific method to make discoveries that, even in their embryonic form, created the foundation for the fields of epidemiology and bacteriology.

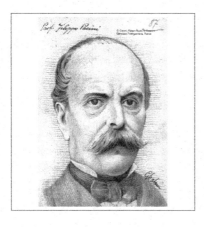

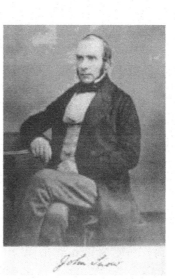

Unknown to each other, Filippo Pacini (L) and John Snow made extraordinary discoveries into the nature of the disease cholera in 1854. (LOC)

The disease they described, cholera, probably originated in the Indian subcontinent. There are references to such a disease in Sanskrit from the 5th century B.C., but ancient references have yet to be found in European literature. It likely spread from India and surrounding territories by trade, slowly at first, then more vigorously with the development of more advanced forms of transportation. Beginning in 1817, there have been seven recognized pandemics of cholera. The one arriving in Europe during the 1850s was the third pandemic (1846 until 1860). It was also the first to reach South America, most notably Brazil.

Vibrio cholerae is a unique organism as the cause of human disease because it doesn't normally inhabit mammals. It is a water organism colonizing microscopic aquatic creatures like copepods, zooplankton, shellfish, and plants. It is salt

271

tolerant and can live in both fresh and brackish waters. The organism can readily adapt to its surroundings. When the water is warm and its preferred hosts are plentiful, it reproduces and spreads rapidly through the water using its vigorous flagellum. When conditions change, it can go into a dormant state, altering its genetic output to down-regulate genes favoring the aggressive form and up-regulate genes favoring a latent existence. As in other bacteria, viruses often invade *Vibrio cholerae*. They can carry genetic information with them (transduction). It is also adept at picking up genetic material from other organisms in its environment and incorporating it into its genome (transformation). These genetic alterations have led to many variations of the organism. Over 200 different biotypes of *V. cholerae are* known, but only two are pathogenic for humans.

All Gram-negative bacteria have a complex structure in their cell walls known as lipo-polysaccharide. The inner lipid part, lipid A, is a toxic substance common to all Gram-negative bacteria. Extending out from lipid A are two sets of carbohydrates. The one adjacent to lipid A is a core carbohydrate common to all members of a bacterial genus. All species of the genus *Vibrio* share the same core carbohydrate. Attached to the core carbohydrate and extending into the exterior is another carbohydrate commonly known as the O antigen. About twenty different sugars can be arranged in numerous fashions, usually from three to five repeating units. The sugars of the O antigens of bacteria are unusual, with some not seen elsewhere in nature. Examples are aquebose, tyvelose, and colitose. This gives a wide diversity to the number of O antigens that exist. One species, *Vibrio cholera*, has over 200. The O antigen is part of bacterial communication with the outside. It is the substance that often contacts human and other cells. It is also the target of antibodies directed against the organism and, in some cases, can interfere with complement activity. Some O antigens are more adept at these functions than others.

For *Vibrio cholera*e, the O antigen types that can cause cholera are types 01 and O139. None of the others can. Even types 1 and 139 are not always pathogenic; they must possess the genetic material to produce a toxin. This genetic material comes from a virus (a phage) that invades bacteria and incorporates itself into the organism's genome. Known as the CTXϕ phage, it is the only source of the toxin of cholera. (ϕ is the Greek letter phi, which rhymes with pie). Strains of the organism that don't have the phage are non-toxigenic, even if they are type O1 or O139. It's reminiscent of the phage that infects *Corynebacterium diphtheriae*, rendering an otherwise innocuous organism pathogenic.

Humans are not the natural environment for the water bacteria *Vibrio cholera*. The organism fortuitously possesses an O antigen that enables them to adhere to the epithelial lining of the intestine, but they are still very susceptible to stomach acid's effects. It takes a lot of organisms in drinking water, probably a few hundred thousand, to set up an infection. Most are killed in the stomach, but with a heavy inoculum, enough make it through to the intestine to initiate an infection. People with lower amounts of stomach acid, such as those who take antacids, are more vulnerable. In many developing countries, much of the population is infected with a stomach bacterium, *Helicobacter pylori*. This organism makes an enzyme that produces ammonia, reducing stomach acidity. People harboring *H. pylori* are also more vulnerable to lower doses of *Vibrio cholera*. Also, people of blood group O contain a receptor on their intestinal walls enabling greater adhesion of *V. cholera*, making them more vulnerable. (Blood group O is not related to the O antigen of the bacteria).

Once the organism successfully passes through the stomach and enters the small intestine, it adheres to the cells of the lining. The organism does not enter the cell to which it attaches but begins producing a toxin that does. Like other toxins, the one made by *Vibrio cholera* has two parts: a large B segment that transports the smaller A component, the active portion. The B segment attaches to the cells lining the small intestine and is actively transported into the cell. Once inside the cell, the A segment breaks away. The A segment is comprised of two parts, A1 and A2, which then divide, leaving the A1 toxin ready to act.

All our cells are equipped to ensure the proper handling of salt content. As many schoolchildren know, our bodies are about 60% water. It's not fresh water, but salt water with lots of solutes. Our cells have systems to control the amount of salt they contain. The chief means of doing this are chloride channels, literally holes in the membrane through which chloride ions may be actively pumped. The chloride must be actively pumped out by the action of proteins, activated by chemical signals from the outside environment. Chloride ions are transferred into and out of the cell to achieve the correct balance. It is a two-way system. The chloride pump is controlled by G-proteins in the cell membrane and activated by converting GDP to GTP. It is at this point where cholera toxin operates. By interfering with the action of the G proteins, ATP is converted into cyclic AMP, the activating factor for the chloride pump. Unlike the natural system, cholera toxin doesn't receive chemical signals to shut down, so it is locked in the "go" position.

After activation by the cholera toxin, chloride ions are continually pumped out of the cell. Wherever chloride ions go, sodium and potassium ions go. And wherever the salt goes, water follows. In the case of cholera, it is lots of water expelled from all the cells lining and surrounding the intestine, flooding the intestine with fluid. This is the source of the diarrhea of cholera, water flowing into the intestine from local tissues to dilute the salt content produced by the one-way action of the toxin-induced chloride pump.

The effect of the disease cholera on humanity has been incalculable. We all must drink water to live. If the water is contaminated with toxigenic *Vibrio cholerae*, disaster ensues. Cholera is undoubtedly an ancient disease, but the first Western descriptions of its devastating effects emerged from Portuguese, Dutch, English, and other explorers of India in the 16th century. Massive numbers of dead were described in the Ganges and other Indian rivers, so many that it was impossible to bury all the dead promptly. In more modern times, there have been seven recognized pandemics. The more that travel developed, the further the pandemics spread. The 7th and current cholera pandemic began in 1961, caused by the El Tor strain. It spread throughout developing countries, many lacking good sanitation to prevent the disease. People can asymptomatically carry *Vibrio cholerae*. With world travel as common and efficient as it is, cholera can suddenly occur without warning in places that have not encountered it in many years. An example is Haiti in 2010, a Caribbean Island that had not had the disease in many years. They suffered a severe outbreak affecting over 500,000 people.

A fascinating theory holds that a serious genetic disease, cystic fibrosis, has persisted in humans because the heterozygote stage renders the individual less susceptible to the ravages of cholera. Cystic fibrosis is a disorder in which the chloride pump is damaged, so the mucus in the lungs is not properly diluted. It is very thick and gummy, and lung congestion results. About one in 20 Caucasians carry a single gene for CF, a very high number for a potentially fatal disease. The heterozygote state does not give the symptoms of CF; only receiving genes from both parents gives the symptoms of cystic fibrosis. Having only one gene, the heterozygotic state, has been shown in laboratory animals to give the patient a significantly reduced reaction to cholera toxin, allowing that person to survive an attack. The theory (and it is still a theory) is similar in concept to the sickle cell gene, which renders a person more resistant to falciparum malaria in the heterozygote state.

The toxin-producing *Vibrio cholerae* mimics several other toxigenic organisms: it is an environmental bacterium like *Clostridium tetani* and *Clostridium botulinum*; it produces its toxin as the result of a virus (phage) that inhabits the bacterium, like *Corynebacterium diphtheriae*; it makes a toxin that catalyzes the conversion of ATP to cAMP, like the ACT toxin of *Bordetella pertussis*.

Other organisms besides those mentioned here produce toxins of various sorts, giving rise to various illnesses, some very serious. Just how toxins in bacteria evolved is a mystery, as is knowing whether they primarily were selected for their attack against mammals or other animals, or their attack against other microbes.   They have profoundly affected human health throughout the ages and will continue to be a threat.

Chapter 18
"The Scourge of Armies"

Depraved conditions.
Pediculus arises.
The mass murderer.

During World War II, two doctors in Poland pulled off one of the most successful and elaborate hoaxes ever described in medicine. They saved thousands of lives, alleviated horrible suffering, and were unsung heroes in times of great tribulation. They also raised a serious question that is still debated in courses on medical ethics.

The disease typhus has been known since ancient times. At least, we think so. The symptoms are not specific, and descriptions of an epidemic of the disease may describe another ailment. In more modern times, in the last 200 years, it has become apparent that typhus is indeed a scourge. Often, more soldiers died of typhus in wars than died from armaments. Famous examples are Napoleon's misadventure in Russia and the immense mortality of the disease in World War I. Millions died. When World War II began, the German military was very mindful of the threat of typhus on military operations and avoided it at all costs.

Dr. Eugene Lazowski had been imprisoned in a German concentration camp. Somehow, he scaled a wall undetected, sneaked a ride in a horse cart, and made it back to his hometown of Razwadow, Poland. There he worked as a physician for the Polish Red Cross.

Dr. Lazowski was familiar with a test commonly done to diagnose typhus. Fortuitously, Proteus OX19, a bacterium unrelated to typhus, contains an antigen identical to one found in the typhus organism. The typhus organism is difficult to cultivate and harvest antigens from. But using dead Proteus OX19 as an antigen will give a simple, highly specific test for antibodies to the typhus organism, confirming a diagnosis. Mix a sample of the patient's serum with Proteus OX19, and if it agglutinates, the test shows the patient has an antibody to typhus. It is called the Weil-Felix test, named for the individuals who happened to discover it during the First World War. Proteus

OX19 is unremarkable, possibly occasionally causing a urinary tract infection. But its strong serologic resemblance to the typhus organism has given it a certain amount of fame.

The German military greatly feared typhus and shunned any area known to harbor it. Dr. Lazowski, and a colleague, Dr. Stanislaw Matulewicz, set a plan in motion to establish their town of Razwadow, Poland, as the typhus capital of the region. Taking killed cultures of Proteus OX19 and injecting it into patients gave a positive Weil-Felix test for typhus, even though the patient didn't have the disease. It was merely a cross-reaction. The two enterprising doctors convinced the Germans that Razwadow was a hotbed of typhus by fudging their records and getting positive lab tests. Accordingly, the Germans avoided the area like the plague. It is estimated that the two doctors saved around 8,000 people from harsh imprisonment, perhaps death.

As ingenious as the plan was, it does raise a serious point. The doctors did not inform their patients that they injected them with the killed organism. They couldn't risk detection; revealing it to anyone would jeopardize the plan. While benign, Proteus OX19, like all Gram-negative organisms, contains the endotoxin Lipid A, and it can make one feel quite ill with chills and fever for a couple of days before spontaneously resolving. Patient permission was not sought, nor was the patient informed.

In today's world of seemingly endless consent forms and HIPAA regulations, it seems incongruous that a physician would administer something to a patient without their knowledge or consent. But this was Poland in World War II. Doctors Lazowski and Matulewicz felt obliged to seek the greater good, ethical considerations aside.

The name "typhus" is a bit unfortunate since it is sometimes confused with another serious disease, typhoid. The source of the two diseases is not at all similar, one originating from the bite of a louse, the other from consuming contaminated food or water. The name "typhus" comes from the Greek *typhos*, meaning "foggy" or "hazy." It is a general description of the patient's mental status while in the full throes of the disease. But while unrelated, the two diseases often are found in similar circumstances: filth, deprivation, and the breakdown of hygiene. Both have had profound consequences on the human condition.

The discovery of the agent of typhus was not easy, mainly because the organism causing it is so odd. It's a bacterium, but not one we can see on a Gram stain or culture plate. Like viruses, the organism only reproduces when inside an animal cell, but unlike viruses, it has its own enzymes, ribosomes, and cell wall. They are bacteria. Eons ago, the organism entered the parasitic state, infecting insects. Somehow, through many trials and errors, the bug could infect insects and mammals, including humans. We now know of many related organisms causing different diseases, all going by the genus name of *Rickettsia*.

An extraordinary scientist elucidated a vital part of the nature of these organisms in the early 1900s. It wasn't typhus he was working on at the time, but a related disease, Rocky Mountain spotted fever (RMSF). Still, the work opened the investigative channels to uncover the cause of one of the great scourges of humankind. The scientist's name was Howard Taylor Ricketts.

Dr. Ricketts was born in a small town in Ohio. He received his college degree from the University of Nebraska, then his medical degree from Northwestern University. His chosen area of specialty was pathology, but he always had a yearning for investigative work, mainly in infectious diseases. He had studied in Europe for one year under some of the top scientists in the field, and in 1906 he set out to explore a perplexing disease in the state of Montana, about as far as you could get from the intellectual centers of Vienna and Paris. In Montana, the disease was known as "a blight of the Bitterroot," after the name of the location where it was mostly found. In 1902 two researchers from the University of Minnesota, Louis Wilson and William Chowning, made an important observation on RMSF, noting it resulted from tick bites. Infectious diseases spread by insects were well known then, with diseases such as malaria fully described. However, most agents of insect-borne diseases known at that time were parasites. Other than bubonic plague being spread by fleas, bacteria were not thought to be spread this way.

In 1906 Dr. Ricketts came to Montana to study Rocky Mountain spotted fever. He was meticulous in his work and made some astute observations. He confirmed that a tick spread the disease, and showed that the organism was not a parasite but a "filterable agent." The organism's identity would have to await further investigation, but Rickett's work laid the foundation for a panoply of discoveries on the agents of infectious diseases. Unfortunately, while Dr. Ricketts was working on typhus during an outbreak in Mexico City in 1910, he contracted the disease and died from it. He was 39 years old. Before his death, he discovered that human lice spread typhus, and the organism was similar to the one that caused Rocky Mountain spotted fever.

Another fascinating scientist in the history of the discovery of the etiology of typhus was Stanislaus von Prowazek. Descended from Czech peasant stock, Prowazek was not a medical doctor but a zoologist and naturalist. He received his Ph.D. in 1899 and began a whirlwind career working with numerous exotic diseases in different parts of the world. His travels took him to Java, Rio de Janeiro, Samoa, Saipan, North Africa, Turkey, and several European areas. His studies mainly concerned parasites and protozoa, emphasizing infectious diseases. In 1915 he and a colleague, Henrique da Rocha-Lima, were sent to investigate a typhus outbreak in a Russian prisoner-of-war camp near the Polish border. Dr. Prowazek and Dr. Rocha-Lima both contracted typhus, and Dr. Prowazek died from it. Dr. Rocha-Lima recovered and went on to describe the bacterial cause of the disease. He named the organism for his deceased colleague, Dr. Prowazek. The organism is known as *Rickettsia prowazekii*.

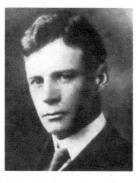
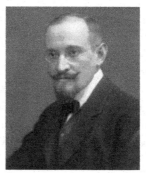

Howard Taylor Ricketts (L) spent several years living in an army tent in Montana, working on the cause of Rocky Mountain Spotted Fever. He later died of typhus while working in Mexico. Stanislaus von Prowazek (R) was a zoologist who traveled the world describing parasites and their vectors. While working with typhus he contracted the disease and died. The organism causing the disease, Rickettsia prowazekii, is named for Dr. Howard Ricketts and him. (LOC)

Rickettsia prowazekii is a well-adapted organism. It is what is known as an obligate intracellular bacterium. It cannot reproduce and grow outside of the cells of an animal. Its range of hosts is broad, but the insect for the disease typhus is the body louse, *Pediculus humanus humanus*. The body louse differs from head lice, *Pediculus humanus capitis*. Body lice dwell only on filthy clothing, not skin, while head lice live in human hair. It is only the clothes-dwelling body louse that carries the organism causing typhus. (*Pediculus* is the Latin word for lice. The name of the genus was assigned by Carl Linnaeus in the 18th century).

Unlike many other insect vector diseases, the introduction of the organism causing typhus does not come from the insect's bite. Instead, the organism grows in the midgut of the louse and is expelled from the insect by defecation. The bites of many lice cause itching, and when scratched small openings occur in the skin allowing the organism in the louse feces to enter the body. It doesn't sound like a very efficient way to spread the disease, but hundreds of lice can infest a single person, and each louse takes a blood meal several times a day. It has been reported that when a person has a fever, the lice don't like it, fall off, and can then infect another person. Simply washing the clothes in warm water with soap is enough to destroy the lice, but even that simple act is not possible in some conditions of deprivation. *Rickettsia prowazekii* does not form spores, but it does enter a state of dormancy that allows it to remain viable in louse feces for months. It can't reproduce, but it can still infect.

After entering the body, the organism has several proteins on its surface that allow it to attach to several types of human cells. But it prefers the cells lining the inside of blood vessels, the vascular endothelial cells. Aiding the attachment and penetration into the endothelial cell is an outer membrane protein (Omp). Members of the *Rickettsia* genus have two Omps, labeled A and B; *R. prowazekii* only contains the OmpB, but it's enough. After entering the human cell, the organism is trapped inside an endosome, but it quickly jumps into action. The dormant phase of the organism "wakes up" and starts to reproduce. It expresses many enzymes that allow it to survive and thrive inside its human host cell. It first makes an enzyme that will enable it to escape the endosome before the lysosome hooks on to kill it. The enzyme the organism uses to break up the host membrane around the endosome is phospholipase D, found commonly throughout nature, including in human cells. Soon after entering the host cell in an endosome, the organism produces proteins like phospholipase D and many others it needs to escape the endosome and grow inside the cell. They are released through a secretory channel produced inside the endosome. It also makes enzymes that destroy the host cell's autosomes, ensuring it can reproduce unmolested. It even makes enzymes that destroy caspases, the apoptosis agents, so the host cell must stay alive and serve its uninvited intruder.

Many intracellular pathogens hijack the host cell's actin system to help it navigate toward the outer reaches of the cell so that it can escape and invade other cells. *Rickettsia prowazekii* doesn't take over the actin. It simply reproduces in massive quantities inside its helpless host cell, using the host cell's chemical resources of amino acids, carbohydrates, and nucleic acids to grow. Once it reaches very large numbers inside the cell, the host cell bursts, and the bacteria escape. They can either proceed to nearby endothelial cells to reinfect, or be carried by the bloodstream to cells far away. Once the process starts, it quickly spins madly out of control.

With its OmpB protein, the liberated *Rickettsia prowazekii* can now infect many different types of cells throughout the body, including the brain, liver, and kidneys. The endothelial lining of blood vessels remains a favorite target. At this stage of the infection, the organism is already in its vegetative state and doesn't have to spend time changing from the dormant phase. Phospholipase D and the other destructive enzymes are being manufactured at a high rate, and millions of organisms are being produced.

Much of the damage done to the body is the destruction of blood vessels. Clots form, fluid is leaked, and the normal state of the vascular system is disrupted. When the damage is done to the blood vessels of the lungs and brain, severe, often fatal, symptoms appear.

Because the organism is primarily a pathogen that invades cells and is not prominent in body fluids, cellular immunity is of vital importance. The body makes antibodies, but getting them inside the cell to attach to the organism is not easy. Instead, immune cells are summoned to attack the host cell harboring the bacteria. A critical factor in this effort is interferon-gamma (IFN-gamma), which signals natural killer lymphocytes and monocytes to become engaged in the battle. During the conflict, many cytokines of an inflammatory nature are released, including the potent interleukin-1β, IL-6, and tumor necrosis factor-alpha (TNF-α).

The results of the infection and subsequent immune response are the many symptoms of typhus. The list of fever, rash, severe headache, and muscle aches doesn't tell the story of this intense disease. It typically takes about 8-10 days for symptoms to begin. The fever is very high, and it alternates with chills. The headache is excruciating, and many patients experience delirium. The muscle aches, or myalgia, are also severe. In parts of Africa, the illness is called *sutama*, the local description for the crouching position some of the infected assume to alleviate some of the pain. The rash typically appears on the abdomen about four days after symptoms begin. It is due to the bacterial invasion of the endothelial cells lining the skin's tiny blood vessels, with the subsequent arrival of macrophages and lymphocytes. Other symptoms, not specific, often include cough, red eyes, dry tongue, and constipation. Symptoms can last two weeks. Death occurs in about one in eight of those afflicted.

The organism causing typhus is not subtle. It doesn't appear to do much to inhibit the immune response. It is so efficient in invading and replicating that its sheer numbers overwhelm the body's defense mechanisms, and the resultant cytokine storm produces great damage and symptoms. Because it lacks a cell wall typical of other bacteria, the typhus organism cannot be successfully treated with antibiotics that target that site, like penicillins and cephalosporins. Thankfully, most strains of *Rickettsia prowazekii* are very susceptible to the tetracycline class of antibiotics. Doxycycline, the long-acting formulation, is most often prescribed, and if treated early enough, most cases resolve with little permanent damage. But when proper medical attention is unavailable, typhus is a serious, often deadly, disease.

Because typhus is an intracellular disease, there are some instances in which it can persist in a patient. Perhaps it is because the organism reverts to the more dormant form it exhibits in insects, but it is well known that cases of the disease can become active after several years of quietude. Known as the Brill-Zinsser disease, it is the recrudescent, or re-emerging, form.

Body lice transmit epidemic typhus. There is also an endemic form transmitted by other insects, usually fleas. The organism causing it is a member of the genus *Rickettsia*, but it is the species *typhi*, not *prowazekii*. *R. typhi* is a more benign organism, but the disease is still significant. A rather famous outbreak occurred in the Los Angeles California Civic Center in the last few months of 2018. Rats had invaded the building, carrying their fleas with them. The fleas carrying the typhus organism became embedded in the carpeting, and several employees were infected. Rat control is very important in preventing endemic typhus.

Chapter 19
Sucker Punch

Cool, refreshing stream
High in the fresh mountain air.
Giardia lamblia's home.

The symptoms and causes of many infectious diseases are often straightforward. Description of the disease comes first. Some diseases share symptoms and must be differentiated. Then there is the identification and characterization of the infectious agent. Sometimes it isn't too difficult to find and identify the culprit. If we look at typhoid fever, the first step was to distinguish it as a unique disease, then isolate and identify the typhoid bacillus. Most other diseases are the same–define the disease, describe the pathogen. But with some diseases, the organism is elusive and evades detection, and many years of searching are needed to find the organism responsible.

In the case of one common disease, the straightforward approach didn't work too well. The organism we call *Giardia* has been known to exist for a very long time. Reportedly, Antonie van Leuwenhoek, the first to visualize tiny creatures with a microscope, described it in his own stool specimen. That was in the 1660s, over 350 years ago. The organism, a single-celled animal that's easy to see with a good microscope, was fully described in the late 1800s. But its role in disease, now indisputably accepted, was debated for nearly a century.

Part of the confusion over *Giardia*'s role in disease is due to the organism's variability and different immune responses in those infected with the organism. When we get typhoid bacillus, we're sick. Some can carry it without symptoms, but, for the most part, there is no doubt about the illness. With *Giardia*, though, illness doesn't always follow infection. Many harbor the organism in their intestines with no symptoms whatsoever. Some are only mildly ill. Some get very sick indeed. With intestinal disorders in general, the cause is often elusive. Many cases of acute diarrhea, presumably caused by a microbe, go undiagnosed. Just tough it out, and the ailment is likely to go away. So seeing *Giardia* trophozoites or cysts in a stool specimen for many years raised the question: is it the

Giardia causing the ailment, or is it some other non-identifiable cause? The subject was hotly debated. Even the creature's name has been disputed, with some preferring the species name *lamblia,* others *duodenales,* and others *intestinalis.* That discussion still goes on.

Today, the role of the little flagellate we call *Giardia* as a cause of an intestinal disturbance is no longer a matter of debate. The parasite can be carried within a person with no or few symptoms. But sometimes, the disease it causes can be quite serious. Malabsorption, diarrhea, weight loss, lethargy. Those are the main symptoms of those afflicted in more developed countries. Giardiasis can be devastating when combined with other conditions, such as parasite infestation and poor nutrition, which is often the case in less developed countries.

The genus name comes from a French zoologist, Alfred Mathieu Giard. The species name *lamblia* is derived from the Czech scientist who first described it in scientific literature. It seems appropriate that the parasite's name has undergone numerous changes through the years because its discoverer also underwent several name changes. Wilhelm Lambl spoke and published in several languages, including German, Czech, Russian, Polish, Italian, and French. He would often publish with a spelling of his name suitable to the language used. A very learned man, Dr. Lambl traveled and researched thoroughly around the countries of eastern Europe, and he became the chief pathologist at several prestigious hospitals. He first described *Giardia* from the stool of a 5-year-old child in 1859, naming it *Cercomonas intestinalis.* Dr. Giard later added a great deal to knowledge of the parasite's life cycle. The proposed name of the organism was bandied about for several years, and many variations emerged, but it was eventually changed to honor its two discoverers, *Giardia lamblia.* Today there are two synonymous species names, *duodenales* and *intestinalis,* but it's the same organism.

Giardia exists in the external environment as an oblong cyst. When the organism leaves the body, it does so in the cyst form to make it resistant to the harsh external environment. The cysts are remarkably resilient. They can last in still water for several months, provided the temperature doesn't rise too much. We get sick from *Giardia* by drinking water containing cysts, and it doesn't take much. Just a few dozen cysts will be enough to infect. Once the organism goes through the stomach acid, the cyst wall is ripped away, and the parasite emerges. It is a one-cell creature, but it has a lot of organelles. For one, it has four pairs of flagella, eight in all, to help it scoot around. It has a distinct type of motility, resembling a "falling leaf." It has not just one but two nuclei. Perhaps the parasite's most significant asset is a large, conspicuous disk on its bottom, or ventral, side. It looks like a suction cup, the kind of thing you press on to get a hook to stick to a window. Whether there is any suction involved is unknown, but it is with the ventral disk that the creature attaches to the wall of the upper small intestine, either the duodenum or the jejunum. It hooks onto the lining of the intestine, and it won't let go. Once established, it starts to feed, then reproduce.

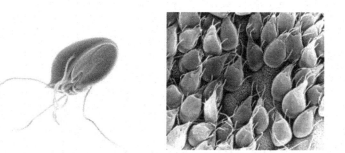

Left, Giardia trophozoite showing ventral disk and flagella. Right, confluent growth of Giardia covering intestinal lining. (PHIL)

Giardia feeds at the expense of the intestinal lining, causing damage. The organism produces two sets of enzymes to steal nutrients from the host cells. The first are proteases that break down the host cells' mucin lining. These proteases damage the host cell surface, allowing nutrients to flow out for the parasite's nourishment. The second set of proteins it produces are called tenascins. Our cells have various types of these to manage the adherence of one cell to another. Some help the epithelial cells stick together; others drive them apart.

Giardia manufactures the kind that leads to the lack of stickiness between cells, further releasing nutrients to engulf.

This release of nutrients from the host cells needn't be too traumatic. If everything goes well, the parasite and the host can get along without much damage. In such cases, the symptoms of the disease usually aren't too bad, or aren't noticed at all. But with all these nutrients flowing out of damaged cells, it creates an opening for other organisms in the area, namely bacteria. Just which bacteria have access to it depends on which bacteria are present in the individual's gut microbiome. Some bacteria are by their nature inflammatory, others much more benign. A good part of the progression of the disease depends on which bacteria are present and how aggressive they are.

Another factor in the disease progression is the number of parasites covering the intestinal wall. *Giardia* is such a good progenitor that the upper intestine is crammed with masses of the little devils in a short time. They adhere to the intestinal wall's cells, forming a film. This mass of parasites can interfere with the physiology of the intestinal wall, blocking the absorption of nutrients and altering the normal functioning of the area.

All this activity obviously will catch the attention of the immune system. One of the chief defensive measures against an organism like *Giardia* is the release of secretory antibodies, IgA, into the area. When coated with antibodies the parasites cannot function properly, and their elimination is imminent. To overcome this, *Giardia* has devised an ingenious scheme. It changes its surface antigens. When an antibody to one surface protein is formed and begins to attach, the organism develops another one not recognized by the antibody. A different antibody must be created, buying the parasite more time. *Giardia* can make many other surface proteins, so the game goes on with the result of the organism establishing a long-lasting infestation.

The organisms receive some signal, possibly the attachment of antibodies, which induces them to begin turning into cysts. The cysts have a hard shell covering, allowing them to pass through the intestinal tract and into the environment. They can persist for quite a long time, especially in cooler temperatures. It only takes a few dozen cysts to set up an infection in a new host.

There are many different species and strains of *Giardia* and many different hosts that can be infected. Fortunately, the strains that infect domestic animals, such as dogs, do not infect humans. For some reason, those that infect beavers do, so that is one reason it's not a good idea to drink mountain stream water. Beavers (or other humans) may have pooped in the water upstream, and the cysts are viable. One nickname for the disease is "beaver fever."

The organism of *Giardia* was discovered in the late 1800s, but it wasn't until 1981 that the World Health Organization recognized it as a pathogen of humans. Finding the organism in a stool specimen does not mean the person is sick. There are so many variables, such as the host's immune status, the strain of infecting organism, and the strains of extraneous bacteria that may cause a secondary infection, that the disease progress cannot be predicted. For those who do become ill, the symptoms are variable. Some have mild discomfort, perhaps bloating, belching, flatulence, mild diarrhea, or constipation. Some become quite ill, with severe cramping, marked diarrhea, and weight loss. Weight loss is connected to the malabsorption of nutrients, especially fats and vitamins. Loss of appetite also factors in. The disease can proceed for several months, and a twenty-pound weight loss is not unheard of. The condition needn't be life-threatening for those previously healthy with access to good nutrition. But the effects of a *Giardia* infection can be devastating for those in impoverished countries who don't have access to good nutrition and have other parasitic diseases. In children, it sometimes means stunted growth and physical and mental abnormalities.

The diagnosis of giardiasis is made by laboratory testing. Several tests are available. The tests detect the organism in a stool specimen. Since the cysts are passed intermittently, it's necessary to collect multiple specimens over several days.

Standard treatment for giardiasis in developed countries has traditionally been the anti-microbic metronidazole, commonly called by its original trade name Flagyl. (Flagyl and alcohol don't get along well together; a patient taking Flagyl should avoid alcohol).   There are other related drugs (nitroimidazoles) that can also be used. Usually, just a few days of treatment and you're as good as new.

Chapter 20
Freeloaders

Slimy, crawly pest
Always take, but never give.
Disgusting helminths.

The word parasite has many connotations. It comes from the Greek, meaning one who eats at another's table. Many think of a parasite as a particularly useless person, sponging off another's largess. Biologically, it means any organism living on or in another organism, obtaining its nutrients. That covers much ground, including bacteria and fungi. In medicine, parasite usually refers to animals that invade, whether a single cell or massive. While an invasive bacterium is technically a parasite, the term in medicine is usually reserved for animal cells that invade us. They range in size from very small to very large.

Parasites have been associated with human beings since there were human beings. All mammals have them. Some, like the Plasmodia that cause malaria, the Trypanosomes that cause Chagas' Disease and African Sleeping Sickness, *Giardia*, *Toxoplasma*, and others, are tiny and cannot be seen with the naked eye. Helminths, commonly called worms, are much bigger but have a massive range. Some are quite small, some only a few millimeters in length, while others are large, tapeworms being the prime example. There are many helminths. Most dwell within our intestinal tract, but some like to live in other areas like the urinary tract or the lungs. Fortunately for most people in developed countries, helminths there are rare. Few of us have to go to the doctor to get ourselves or our children "de-wormed." But that's not true in some of the poorer countries, as parasitic loads can sometimes be overwhelming and impart a terrible burden on the individuals infested as well as the society and economy.

The words "infect" and "infest" are often confused, as are "infection" and "infestation." To infect means that a pathogen has invaded tissues and thereby caused them harm. For instance, a microbe that enters intestinal cells with a resulting inflammatory reaction is said to infect. The word infests means that an organism is present on the surface, sometimes in large numbers, but does not directly invade the tissues. Lice living in the hair is a good example of an infestation. When describing parasites, the term infest is usually used by convention, although there are many times the word infect would be more appropriate.

The word "helminth" comes from the Greek word for worm, *helmins*. The term refers to a broad range of free-living and parasitic creatures. The parasitic worms that affect humans are divided into three distinct groups. The **nematodes** have an elongated cylindrical body, looking much like the worms you see crawling around your garden. They are often called roundworms. The name derives from the Greek word for thread. The **trematodes** are the flukes or flatworms. They have external suckers to attach themselves to surfaces. The name comes from the Greek word for holes. The **cestodes** are the tapeworms, long segmented worms with tiny heads for attachment. The name comes from the Greek word for belt.

We don't "catch" helminths from another person, at least not in the usual way. Each has a rather elaborate life cycle, so rather than picking them up from another person as we do with a respiratory or intestinal infection, we usually get helminths from the environment. The worms can often be found in a large percentage of the population, but that usually reflects a common source, such as contaminated water or soil. Most don't reproduce inside of us, so the number of worms we get often depends on how much source material the person is exposed to and how many infective units, usually eggs or larvae, are contained.

Parasitology is a fascinating field with all sorts of creatures involved. Many parasites must travel through an intermediate host, such as a snail or a fly, before getting into a human. Quite often, the human is not the primary host, just one that happened to be there as the parasite was trying to get into another animal. Sometimes multiple animals can be invaded. In this review, we will focus on just a few organisms to explore how each can overcome the host's immune system and enable itself to become established and persist.

Parasites are foreign invaders, and it is the duty of the immune system to get rid of them. Over the eons, a very complex set of chemical signals and cellular actions developed to do just that. In brief, the body has specialized cells called mast cells situated at regular places. They serve as sentinel beacons. Starting out in the bone marrow as part of the myeloid line, like neutrophils and macrophages, they travel through the bloodstream and eventually enter the tissues. They localize at strategic locations, like under the skin, in the lung tissue, in the underlying layer of the gastrointestinal tract, and near lymph vessels. When activated, they go into hyper-drive, emitting several inflammatory chemicals, including histamine, tryptase, heparin, leukotrienes, and prostaglandins.

Histamine is a small but mighty molecule with several functions, but an important one is dilating blood vessels to allow the influx of immune cells and chemical mediators. Histamine also promotes the activity of several different kinds of immune cells, enhancing their activity.

Tryptase is a member of a group of chemicals known as proteases. It is there to literally help destroy some types of human tissue, namely the connective tissue matrix, to allow easier migration both in and out of immune cells and chemical agents. A little collateral damage is acceptable when faced with an invader hell-bent on taking over.

Heparin is an anticoagulant, a chemical that slows down the clotting of blood and serum. When released from the mast cell, its presence helps ensure greater flow into the infected area of essential cells and chemicals, like the role of tryptase.

Leukotrienes are similar in function to histamine, only they are bigger and badder. They perform several roles, including dilating blood vessels and signaling several immune cells and chemical agents.

The prostaglandins are like the leukotrienes. Both are made from the same chemical stock, a lipid situated in the cell membrane. The term prostaglandin was coined in the 1930s by Swedish chemist Ulf von Euler, who discovered it in semen. Thinking the prostate gland produced it, he named it so. We know now that there are four different chemicals of the prostaglandin class, and a wide variety of human cells produce them. Similar in function to the leukotrienes, the prostaglandins pack quite a punch. When we take an aspirin or an Advil, we are really trying to knock down the COX enzyme leading to prostaglandin creation. While they are most useful in helping us ward off various infectious organisms, including parasites, prostaglandins cause several untoward side effects, including pain. We have a love-hate relationship with the prostaglandins.

Mast cells have all this potent chemical weaponry packed inside. So does a similar cell, the basophil, which we can think of as a "mobile mast cell." Strategically placed in the body, mast cells attract a wide variety of immune cells, each with its own destructive power. Mast cells prepare and clear the local tissues for their inward migration and tissue mobility. Clearly, this all must be tightly controlled. We can't have all these destructive chemicals released by chance. Animals can accept a bit of tissue damage temporarily in the fight against intruders. But we can only take so much.

The trigger as well as the safety of the mast cell is the antibody class known as IgE. There are five classes of antibodies, all made by the B-lymphocytes. IgE is the least common type found. IgE has a great affinity for mast cells. Like all antibodies, there are two ends to the molecule, the constant region, known as Fc, which is the same for all IgE antibodies, and the longer variable portion, which is different and unique to each antibody. Mast cells have on their surface a chemical receptor known as $F_{\epsilon\epsilon}R1$. It strongly binds the F_c portion of IgE to the mast cell, whether it is bound to an antigen or not. If it is unbound, the mast cell is inactive, but if the IgE antibody is bound to an antigen, such as a little piece of a parasite, the mast cell becomes highly activated, literally bursting and releasing chemicals from both its granules and its membranes. The result is a rapid inflow of cells, such as neutrophils, macrophages, and killer lymphocytes, all programmed to take out the invader.

An especially powerful cell when it comes to parasites is the eosinophil. Produced in the bone marrow as part of the myeloid line, eosinophils contain a chemical known as major basic protein (MBP). This chemical is highly toxic to several parasites and is an indispensable weapon in the anti-parasite fight.   When an invading parasite has been encountered, chemical signals sent to the bone marrow stimulate the production of a large number of eosinophils. A high eosinophil count (often called "high eos") in a blood sample is often an indication of a parasitic infection (but not always).

Interestingly, these cells and chemicals designed to thwart the invasion of parasites, mast cells and their contents, IgE, and eosinophils, are the same cells and chemicals responsible for the reactions we have in allergies. The immune system at the local level treats a bit of pollen, animal dander, or some other material as if it were a parasite. Of course, there is a lot more pollen or other allergens than there are parasites, and the reaction to them is far more robust, giving the very unpleasant symptoms of allergy, whether in the respiratory tract, digestive tract, or the skin.

Certainly one of the most successful human parasites is the nematode *Ascaris lumbricoides*. It is estimated that several hundred million people, possibly as many as a billion, are infected by this slithery roundworm. It is found mainly in tropical areas with high temperatures and moisture levels. Despite some rather formidable obstacles, it is exceptionally adept at infecting people. After mating with a male, the females lay their eggs in the intestinal tract. The fertilized eggs are then expelled with feces. The egg has a rigid lining, protecting it from the elements. They can last in the soil for several months. Once the egg hits the ground, the larva within begins to grow. When a human comes along and gets the larva-containing dirt in their mouth, usually by eating something associated with it, the larva inside its protective egg covering travels through the acid-filled stomach into the small intestine. There the larva hatches from the egg and immediately invades the intestinal lining. The active, wiggly little larva penetrates the intestinal lining, enters the bloodstream, and travels to the liver. Sometimes it causes some damage there, but the liver is not its final destination. It re-enters the bloodstream and settles in the lungs. After more molting steps in the lungs, the mature larva gets into the trachea, makes its way into the mouth, and is swallowed to re-enter the intestine. Quite a complicated journey, and it takes quite a few eggs to be consumed to make sure at least one gets through, but get through they do as their infective success rate indicates.

When the worm reaches the small intestine a second time, it settles down and begins to grow. Then they look for a mate. After mating, the females start to lay eggs and are absolutely prolific. They must be when you consider the odds of one reaching a human host and going on to maturity.

There are many obstacles for the *Ascaris* worm to overcome. Survival inside the egg in the environment, getting into a human host, surviving stomach acid and bile, making its way into the liver, then the bloodstream, then the lungs, getting coughed up and then swallowed, and again surviving stomach acid and bile. They also have to prevent themselves from getting digested by intestinal tract enzymes. And, of course, they must circumvent the many weapons of the host's immune system. Quite a gauntlet, but after thousands of years, billions of trials, and billions of errors, they have become an extremely successful parasite.

One thing they mustn't do is kill or seriously injure their host. If the host dies, the parasite dies with it. In this, they are also very successful, as most people infected with *Ascaris* aren't aware they are carrying the worm inside them. Trouble can arise when there are too many worms, obstructing the intestinal tract. Sometimes the immune system overreacts, making the patient allergic. But the parasite and host usually reach a state of near equilibrium, and the infection goes unnoticed. *Ascaris* don't produce new worms inside the host, and their life expectancy is from one to two years, so if the individual is not re-infected, the condition clears itself in that time.

To resist digestive enzymes and acids, *Ascaris,* both adult and larval forms, has an outer protective coating rich in collagen. Adults don't attach to the lining of the small bowel, so many of the host's immune system's weapons are thus neutralized. They "swim against the tide" so they don't get swept away by the movement of the bowel. They don't give off toxins or enzymes that might be destructive to the lining of the intestine, so they don't elicit a significant inflammatory

296

response. In a routine situation, they just sit in the small intestine, gobbling up any nutrients they need.

They also have sex—and a lot of it. The female worm is about twice as long as the male, about ten inches versus around six, although there is quite a range in size. The female can store over 20 million eggs in her uterus and lay up to 200,000 daily. With the odds against successful maturation in a new host so great, this abundance of fertilized egg production is necessary. The laboratory observation of the characteristic eggs of the worm in a stool specimen is the most common way of diagnosing the infection.

With all these creatures meandering around the body and going through larval molts along the way, the host's immune system is alerted. Molecular patterns on the parasite and damaged tissue along their route stimulate immune system activity. But, like all parasites, *Ascaris* has means of dealing with the immune response and reducing its effectiveness.

Two of the body's immune suppression messengers are interleukin-10 (IL-10) and Transforming Growth Factor-β (TGF-β). When we have an inflammatory response, it has to stop sometime, and the healing process is allowed to begin. IL-10 and TGF-β are instrumental in this function. Also, interferon-gamma may play a role. In a complicated process, *Ascaris* secretes proteins that up-regulate the anti-inflammatory cytokines, putting a significant damper on the immune response. As the larvae make their way through the body and eventually settle in the small intestine, the immune response to it is scaled down, and the worm can avoid being attacked and gobbled up by macrophages. The chief antibody response is IgE, which pokes holes in the invading beast. The creation of IgE is impaired. Also, the maturation of dendritic macrophages and the presentation of antigens on MHC-II are diminished, so fewer antibodies are produced, and the cellular response is much less than usual.

It is not in the best interest of the worm to damage the animal it is invading. It wants to prevent its own demise, but it needs the host to provide it with nutrition and a safe environment. So the production of anti-inflammatory cytokines is not excessive, lest the host be laid susceptible to some other pathogen, be it bacterial or viral. Through evolution, the worms have become quite good at producing just the right amount of immune suppression.

One of the biggest problems with *Ascaris* infestation is asthma. The part of the immune system that attacks parasites, such as IgE, eosinophils, and mast cells, are the same ones that produce allergic reactions, such as asthma. Quite often, the only symptom a patient notices when infected by a few worms is asthma, not intestinal symptoms. When many worms are present, sometimes a very curious thing occurs. A patient with asthma due to another cause finds their symptoms ameliorated. The immune-suppressing proteins from the invading *Ascaris* reduce the allergic immune response, relieving asthma. For this reason, the proteins of helminths are being studied as a possible treatment for asthmatic patients.

Ascaris lumbricoides is a very common invader of humans. It has been known for a long time and was once prominent throughout humanity. The scientific name was given to it by the father of scientific names, Carl Linnaeus, in the 1700s. Today most people in developed countries are not infested by worms, and for that, we must be truly grateful. While not usually a serious threat to our lives, they can impair one's life quality, especially for children, robbing the victim of adequate nutrition. Sometimes, when they are present in high numbers, they can block the bowel and give rise to a life-threatening condition. They also reside right at the very top of the "gross" scale, as anyone who has seen one of these creatures squirming around in the toilet will testify. (Sometimes, a patient in the ICU, unconscious and off food for a while, will have an *Ascaris* crawl out of them in search of food, either out their nose or anus). Poor sanitation is the main thing standing in the way of an *Ascaris*-free world.

A potentially serious helminth infection in humans are hookworms. There are two species, the so-called Old World and New World varieties, *Ancylostoma duodenale* and *Necator americanus*, respectively. While the eggs of the two species are indistinguishable, the Old-World species is larger and has a shorter life span, one or two years versus three to five. The name "hook" worm comes from the slight hook-like appearance of the head where it attaches to the body. One could also make a case for the "hooks" on the worm's head that allow it to attach to the intestinal lining, although they are teeth and plates. It is estimated that over a billion humans are infected with hookworm. The infection often goes unnoticed, but sometimes there can be marked iron deficiency anemia since the creatures feed on blood from the vessels of the small intestine. The amount of blood one worm takes daily is small, only a tenth of a milliliter, but if the infestation is substantial, especially in children, the symptoms can be life-altering.

Like *Ascaris,* the hookworms lay eggs that contain larvae. Once it gets into the soil, the larva hatches from the egg and begins a series of molts. The first form is the rhabditiform larva. (From the Greek *rhabdo,* meaning "rod"). The rhabditiform larvae are not infective. They undergo a couple of molts in the soil to become filariform larvae. (From the Latin *fila,* meaning "thread"). These are the infective forms, and they slither their way to the top of the soil. When a barefoot human traipses through the area, they are poised to strike by latching onto the unsuspecting victim's foot or ankle. From there, they work their way through the skin, eventually into a blood vessel, and are carried to the lungs. Here the hookworms' journey somewhat resembles the path used by *Ascaris,* working their way into the trachea and mouth, from whence they are swallowed. From there, it is just a matter of the filiform larvae attaching themselves to the small intestine's lining and establishing a new home.

Hookworms are the ultimate bloodsuckers. Every day they drink their fill. They aren't very big, just a few millimeters, so they don't take too much. If there are only a few of them, we don't even know they are there. But when one gets a heavy load of them, trouble, mainly in the form of iron deficiency anemia, can ensue. It is particularly dangerous in young children.

The immune system can easily detect the creatures and should be able to take the invaders out. But hookworms, like other successful parasites, have developed means to reduce the ferocity of the immune response and ensure their survival.

The most immediate problem for hookworms is that they live in the digestive tract, where enzymes to digest food are present. Examples are trypsin and chymotrypsin. There are others. To protect itself, the hookworm secretes enzymes that destroy the host digestive enzymes, thus becoming far less susceptible to their action. Just how much this loss of digestive juices affects the host's nutritional status is a question, but it probably affects children the most. Hookworms produce a substance that induces T-lymphocytes to destroy themselves through apoptosis. Just what that substance is remains to be elucidated, but the T-cell response to the worms' presence is reduced.

In most infectious diseases, the neutrophils circulating in the bloodstream are given a signal to adhere to the wall of a blood vessel near the infection site, then migrate post-haste to the center of the infection. Hookworms produce a substance that significantly reduces the number of neutrophils adhering to the blood vessel wall, thus reducing the number of them gathering at the site where the worms have attached, generally scaling down the inflammation surrounding them.

Dendritic cells play a major role in directing the immune response against an invader. When an infection occurs, the damaged human cells secrete a substance known as matrix metalloproteases (MMPs) that are tasked with repairing the damage. These molecules also attract more dendritic cells to the scene. Hookworms secrete a substance known as tissue inhibitors of metalloproteases (TIMPs) that attach to the MMPs and significantly lessen this activity.

There are other ways hookworms that invade us can modulate our immune response and thereby help ensure their survival. The fact that they can remain intact in a human host for several years and produce millions of eggs is testimony to their success.

Whipworms are bizarre creatures. They are nematodes with cylindrical bodies, but they look very different from most worms. About an inch and a half long, one end is very narrow, the other bulging. They are well-named as they look very much like a bullwhip. Their scientific name, *Trichuris trichiura,* was assigned by Carl Linnaeus in 1771. The name derives from the Latin *trich,* meaning "thread or hair." The odd thing about them is that the thin end is the head, and the bulge is the tail end. The head burrows into the wall of the large intestine, and the worm remains planted in a stationary setting. The tail end stays outside the intestine wall, floating free in the intestinal lumen. They reproduce sexually, which means a male and a female must somehow get their rear sections together.

Like all nematodes, they are prolific egg layers, and contaminated soil from human feces is their chief vehicle for re-infecting another host. Unlike *Ascaris* and hookworm, they don't pass through another body part after being ingested. When eggs are deposited in the soil, the developing larva is infective after a couple of weeks. After the eggs containing the developing larvae are ingested, the egg hatches in the colon and the developing worm embeds itself in the mucosal lining. It prefers the area known as the cecum, the section of the large intestine adjacent to the small intestine. It produces an enzyme to allow it to penetrate the tissue, and the cells of the intestinal lining then fuse around it. It takes about three months after ingesting eggs for the worm to become embedded in the intestine.

This lifestyle presents two immune system-related problems for the worm. One, of course, is the presence of the worm in such intimate contact with the intestinal lining. The other is the presence of large numbers of bacteria which, with the bowel lining penetrated, have a direct channel to invade the host's tissues. Both are designed to put the immune system on high alert, and inflammation at the site of penetration and implantation is expected. To overcome the wrath of the immune response, whipworms have developed a means of quelling the immune response, mitigating its ferocity to the point that most people infected by whipworms are oblivious to their presence.

Whipworms secrete a large amount of a substance commonly found in human tissue, prostaglandin E2 (PG-E2). It has been found in experiments to alter the immune response by changing the function of CD4 lymphocytes from the Th1 type, typically found in acute bacterial infections, to the Th2 type, usually seen in parasitic infections. Because of this, there is a lot less production of the inflammatory cytokines interleukin-1, interleukin-6, and tumor necrosis factor-α, resulting in a muted response to the bacteria in the area. In addition, the tissue in the infected area is less damaged, so less oxygen is released. This means that the type of bacteria present are mostly the more docile anaerobic variety, not the more invasive facultative enteric Gram-negative rods like *E. coli* that can live in the presence of oxygen. Because the inflammatory response is muted, the epithelial cells surrounding the head of the worm quietly form a tunnel around it, forming a tight seal.

The other way whipworm modulates the immune response is by significantly raising the level of interleukin-10, the cytokine that down-regulates immunity. Even though the immune response is of the Th2 variety, which usually increases the worm-antagonistic response of eosinophils and IgE, releasing IL-10 minimizes the reaction. Somehow, over time, worms and the host's immune system have each acquired a level of comfort to prevent the demise of each.

While most infestations with whipworm are benign, some are not. Patients can experience severe indigestion, diarrhea, anemia, and fatigue. In extreme cases, especially in children, there may be rectal prolapse.

Many other helminths parasitize humans; discussing them would require a college course in parasitology. Many have a fascinating lifestyle, employing some rather exotic intermediate hosts on their way to their main prize of the animal they are designed to infest. Much of the world's population is plagued by these creatures, sometimes several in one individual. Often their presence is not readily felt, reflecting the parasites' elaborate means of subduing the host's immune system. But some infected people are symptomatic. There is a broad range of symptoms for each organism and patient. Things can get a whole lot worse when a patient has several different organisms.

Several helminths and other organisms are part of a group of pathogens known as the "Neglected Tropical Diseases," NTD. They generally affect the world's poor and don't receive the attention that other diseases, such as HIV/AIDS or malaria, receive. Many of the NTDs are treatable at low cost, and improvements in sanitation and hygiene would greatly help in their elimination.

Much notice has been lately directed to the helminths' immunomodulatory effect and the resultant reduction of symptoms in several autoimmune diseases and hyperimmune conditions. Deliberately implanting live worms in patients to reduce their symptoms is a bit drastic, and side effects are certainly possible. But isolating the molecules secreted by the creatures and using a purified form of them to curtail specific immune reactions is a possibility. It is currently being explored vigorously in research centers.

Chapter 21
The Kiss of Death

Revolting creatures,
Penetrating predators.
Resident for life.

The kissing bug is one of the most poorly named animals in all creation. The moniker makes you think of some cute little creature like a ladybug or a butterfly. Soft, carefree, and life-enhancing, the name kissing bug is all joy and felicity.

Not even close. Better, it went by its other name–the assassin bug. This repulsive bloodsucker is about as ugly as they come and twice as mean. They creep around at night when you're asleep and "kiss" you with their pincers, then suck your blood until they become so bloated they can barely walk. To add insult to injury, they defecate into the wound they created, then waddle away. The name kissing bug comes from their preference for soft skin like lips and eyelids. To awaken in the middle of the night with one of these little monsters crawling around your face is like a glimpse into hell itself.

Despite the loathsome insult of their bite, that's not their real damage. It's what they leave behind that really gets you: the metacyclic trypomastigotes of *Trypanosoma cruzi*, the cause of South American trypanosomiasis, better known as Chagas Disease.

Many insects can do us real harm, not by their direct bite but by the pathogenic organisms they harbor and spread. At the top of most people's list would be the mosquito, well known to infect humans with malaria, West Nile virus, yellow fever, dengue, and many other viruses. Then there is the tsetse fly, which spreads a cousin of Chagas disease called African sleeping sickness. The sand fly harbors and spreads Leishmaniasis, the Asian rat flea is infamous for spreading bubonic plague, and ticks are responsible for several diseases, including Lyme disease, Rocky Mountain spotted fever, and Ehrlichiosis. Lice are also on the list, giving us maladies like typhus and trench fever. Thankfully, the bed bug, so common in many areas of the world, is not known to harbor and spread infectious diseases.

The term we ascribe to an insect that spreads an infectious disease is vector. It comes from the Latin *vehere*, which means "carrier." Some vector-borne diseases can be prevented by breaking the infection cycle. If no humans are harboring the pathogen to be carried by the vector, no transmission can take place. We have no malaria in the United States, even though we have mosquitoes capable of transmitting the disease. There aren't any humans infected with malaria to serve as index cases.

The exceptions to this epidemiology rule of thumb are infections like Chagas disease. That's because the trypanosomes causing the disease are found in animal species other than humans. If a kissing bug bites an infected goat, for example, it can next bite and infect a human. In fact, hundreds of animals can be infected by the organism and bitten by the bug, giving a seemingly endless cycle of infection.

Kissing bugs are known by a couple of scientific names. The family name is *Reduviidae*, and the subfamily name is *Triatominae*, often referred to as reduviids or triatomines. The locals call them "vinchucas." Also "barbieros," or "barbers." This family has over 7,000 known species, many of which can harbor trypanosomes. But to infect humans, the insects must dwell in a habitat accessible to humans and harbor the trypanosome species capable of causing human disease. Only three genera of the creature are commonly found here: *Triatoma, Rhodnius,* and *Panstrongylus*, with the first two being by far the most common.

Ancient triatome bugs dwelt in forested areas. They fed on all sorts of animals, primarily mammals like raccoons, opossums, rats, or anything else that happened to come along. They need blood to survive. About an inch long, they have a long proboscis, essentially a spear that emerges from their head designed to penetrate a victim and facilitate the sucking of blood. And they've got the blood-sucking down to perfection. The proboscis is equipped with both an anesthetic and an anticoagulant, so you don't hurt too much, and the blood flows freely. The bugs are nocturnal, usually attacking the victim animal at night, and quite often the victim doesn't know what hit 'em.

The bugs are absolute gluttons, taking as much as twelve times their body weight of blood. They take so much that they must defecate so they can waddle away. One blood meal is enough to sustain them for several months.

As human populations encroached into the wild areas inhabited by the kissing bugs, a few species adapted to the huts and shanties and began feeding on humans. They hide in the crevices and crannies of walls, floors, and ceilings, with ceilings being their favorite hangout. Many species of kissing bugs live in the branches of dead palms, so the thatched roof of a village hut would be a ready-made habitat.

The kissing bug antennae are equipped with a heat sensor so that it can pick up a sleeping person from across the room. They also can detect insect pheromones, so if a person has had some insects on their body recently, their position is also picked up for that. So, we have these heat-seeking, pheromone-sniffing creatures wandering around your hut at night, waiting for the first opportunity to crawl up to your face and suck your blood.

As if that weren't enough, they have another feature that makes them even more sinister. They have wings. Not for flapping like a butterfly or moth, but for gliding and soaring, mostly down from their perch on the roof. They can also glide from hut to hut or from hut to an animal enclosure and back again if the winds are right and it's not more than about 50 meters away. So, they are voracious and mobile, a very scary vector indeed.

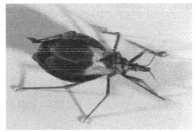

The kissing bug, Triatoma, is the vector for Trypanosoma cruzi, the agent of Chagas Disease. (PHIL)

But it's the payload the creatures carry that is the scariest part. The infective organism is known as *Trypanosoma cruzi*, a member of a microscopic family of parasites that have been infecting animals for over a hundred million years. The genus name *Trypanosoma* comes from two Greek words, *trupanon,* meaning "borer," and *soma,* meaning "body." They look like a corkscrew. Trypanosomes and their relatives are located worldwide and infect everything from invertebrates to humans, and they usually do so with great efficiency. In most humans, the infection is relatively mild and self-limited, but the disease progresses to a fatal outcome in some cases. The determination of the disease progression after infection depends on both the parasite and the host. They engage in a fascinating chemical warfare battle: the host uses the components of the innate immune system, and the parasite circumvents that system.

The trypanosomes belong to a group of organisms called the kinetoplasts, from two Greek words, *kinetikos,* for movement, and *plastos,* meaning anything formed or molded, usually referring to a cell. The kinetoplast is an organelle that is all about energy production. It derives from mitochondria, the energy-producing units of eukaryotic cells. The trypanosomes depend on their flagella to propel them around their environment, and the kinetoplast provides a constant stream of energy. Comparing a kinetoplast to a mitochondrion is like comparing a Corvette Stingray engine to a lawn mower. The kinetoplast is packed with power, and the flagellum can propel the organism around its environment at a very high rate of speed.

A flagellum is a whip-like structure that beats through a liquid environment at a furious pace, allowing the organism to move. They are found in both prokaryotic and eukaryotic organisms. The proper scientific term in prokaryotes, such as bacteria, is flagellum. In eukaryotic organisms, such as trypanosomes, the appropriate term is mastigote, from the Greek *mastix,* meaning "whip." Most often, the whip-like appendage is called a flagellum wherever it is found, but the term we use to describe the stages of the Trypanosomal life cycle uses the proper scientific designation, mastigote.

Trypanosoma cruzi has distinct stages in its life cycle, all ending with the suffix mastigote. The "epi" mastigote is the stage found in the kissing bug. The "trypo" mastigotes are found in the patient's bloodstream. The infective form of the parasite, that is, the form between epimastigote in the kissing bug gut and trypomastigote in the blood, is the metacyclic trypomastigote. The metacyclic form enters the patient's skin and penetrates down to the deeper tissues. Finally, the "a" mastigote, which lacks a flagellum, is found inside the human host cell.

So, it starts as an epimastigote in the insect, which matures into the metacyclic trypomastigote, which enters the human body. That one develops into trypomastigotes in the bloodstream. After the trypomastigote enters the cell of the host animal, it transforms into the amastigote stage. Then, after replication in the human host cell, it's back to the trypomastigote form and into the blood. Following a blood meal, it's off to the epimastigote in the bug.

After the trypomastigotes enter the kissing bug following a blood meal, they enter the insect's midgut. The organism doesn't want to move around too much in there, so the kinetoplast migrates away from the flagellum to the other side of the nucleus. This presumably supplies less energy to the flagellum and slows the organism's movement. From there, the epimastigotes migrate to the bug's rear and mature into the metacyclic trypomastigote stage, ready for action when the bug poops it out.

From the trypanosome's perspective, there are a few obstacles and challenges to be addressed if it is to be a successful parasite. These things have been around for hundreds of millions of years, so they have it down by now. The major challenges:

1. Entering the host
2. Making it into the circulatory system
3. Surviving in the circulatory system
4. Getting out of the circulatory system and into the tissues
5. Entering the host tissue cell where it can replicate
6. Getting out of the host cell and back into the circulatory system
7. Re-entering cells to replicate again
8. Re-entering the kissing bug

In getting into a new host, the trypanosome is at the mercy of the kissing bug vector. In the wild, the kissing bug can either take a blood meal from the host or be eaten by it. Since the trypanosomes can enter the host through the intestinal tract, the organism can enter through the skin or the intestines. Since most humans don't dine on kissing bugs, the chief means of human infection is by way of the skin, usually the face. Humans can, however, be infected by consuming bug poop mixed in with their food if it contains trypomastigotes.

Kissing bugs prefer soft skin, so they zero in on the lips and the eyes. One very reliable sign that the bug has paid a middle-of-the-night visit is a marked swelling on the patient, usually coming up about a week after the bite. The swelling is known as a Chagoma, the "Chag" from Chagas disease, the "oma" from the fact that it resembles a tumor. If the eye is swollen, the condition is referred to as Romaña's sign. Romaña's sign, usually seen in children, is the classic diagnostic hallmark of acute Chagas disease. Seeing a symptomatic child with it in an endemic area pretty much makes the diagnosis of acute Chagas.

Trypanosomes need help from the human host as well as the kissing bug. The African form of trypanosomes, *Trypanosoma brucei*, causes African sleeping sickness. It's injected into the body with the bite of a tsetse fly. They mature in the tsetse fly's salivary gland and are ready to go once the fly bites a human. *Trypanosoma cruzi* does it from the other end, maturing in the kissing bug's hindgut, so it's harder for them to enter a host. The kissing bug's bite makes the area itch, and scratching the site of the bug bite greatly facilitates the trypanosome's entry. The salivary form of development seen in the African trypanosomes is called, conveniently enough, *Salivaria*. In the hindgut forms, like Chagas disease, it is called *Stercoraria*. Even though the two parasites look identical under the microscope, there are significant differences in their biology and development.

The trypanosomes deposited on the skin after defecation are not very great in number. People who count such things have found that only a couple of hundred metacyclic trypomastigotes are viable after the event. How many enter the body is anybody's guess, but it is probably measured in the dozens.

Once the trypanosomes enter the skin, there's little subtlety about them. They just burrow down. They have a corkscrew-like shape, a flagellum for propulsion, and that turbocharged mitochondrion we call a kinetoplast for energy, and they just grind on in. A squamous epithelial cell is about 100 microns in diameter, while the trypomastigote is only about 1/5th its size, so they have quite a bit of work to do. After getting through the skin, they make their way through the basement membrane and enter the bloodstream directly or through a lymphatic channel. It takes a few days to get into the blood.

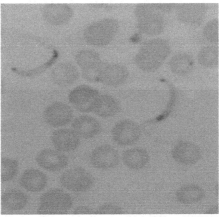

Two trypomastigotes in a blood film. (PHIL)

Complement is one of the first immune defense systems the tiny parasite is likely to encounter on its journey through the skin and in the blood. Complement is not one molecule but a system of around 30 proteins that act in a cascade-like action. (See Chapter 8). Once the first one becomes activated, it turns on a second, which turns on a third, and so on, through number 9. All must work in concert and harmoniously for the system to work effectively.

Complement classically relies on antibodies to assist it in engaging the invading organism, but there are two alternative pathways independent of antibodies that are also effective.

A group of "reconnaissance" proteins constantly circulating in the blood are the ficolins. They don't bind to antibodies, but molecules commonly found on the microbe's surface. There are two ficolins associated with the complement system, L-ficolin and H-ficolin. These two proteins bind to *Trypanosoma cruzi* trypomastigotes and initiate the complement reaction.

The ficolins carry around a protein known as MBL-associated serine proteases or MASP. The MASP just hangs around, not doing anything until the ficolin attaches to its target on the parasite's surface. Then it springs into action. After receiving a signal from the ficolin to become active, MASP changes its shape when complement factor 4 (C4) bumps into it. C4 also changes its shape and splits off a smaller piece. This allows complement factor 2 (C2) to bind. The combination of these two components, activated C2 and C4, forms an essential enzyme, the C3 convertase. Following this reaction, microbe-killing machine C3 is activated.

Once formed, the C3 component of complement splits into two parts, C3a and C3b. C3a departs and serves to attract other members of the immune system to the battle scene. C3b is highly destructive to microbes. Its killing power, a thioester bond, is sequestered while it floats around in the serum, but the combination of complement factors C2 and C4, which create the C3 convertase, enables its destructive power.

C3b is produced by the dozens, if not hundreds, of molecules, resulting in many membrane-craving proteins attaching to the microbe's surface. Damage to the organism is considerable, and lysis and death may result just from that attack. But the C3b isn't the whole complement package. Other microbe-destroying compounds, C5b and MAC, become activated later in the complement cascade.

So, the trypomastigote that enters the body is faced with a considerable obstacle right off the bat. Complement takes no prisoners. Also, there usually aren't that many trypomastigotes to begin with, as they depend on the bug pooping and the patient scratching. But the creatures have had over a hundred million years to figure out how to evade the complement onslaught.

This immune system modulation is one of the secrets of their success.

One of their biggest weapons is "complement C2 receptor inhibitor trispanning," which goes by the much easier-to-remember acronym CRIT. CRIT is abundant on the surface of the metacyclic trypomastigotes, but it is not formed on the epimastigotes in the kissing bug. There is no need to waste energy expressing it where there isn't any complement. In the animal body, CRIT on trypomastigotes is a virtual C2 sponge. It sucks up complement factor 2 from the serum, depriving the growing C3 convertase of this vital ingredient. The result is that the C3 convertase isn't abundant, and not much C3b is produced. Hence, not much C5b or MAC is made either.

They also have a protein that can rip apart much of the C3 convertase that forms. It goes by two names, GP160 and CRP (complement regulatory protein). Thus, the C3 convertase cranking out C3b and C3a to confront the trypomastigote is muted, as is the inflammatory signaling designed to call in reinforcements.

A fascinating *Trypanosoma* anti-complement molecule is one that we have ourselves. It's called Decay Accelerating Factor, or DAF. In humans, it sits on cell membranes and picks apart C3 convertase so our cell membranes aren't inadvertently destroyed by the powerful C3b. The trypomastigotes have the same molecule! The DNA of the gene that makes it is remarkably similar in humans and trypanosomes, so it was either human DNA incorporated into the Trypanosome genome or confluent evolution. Either way, it's another effective line of defense against complement by the parasite.

After entering the body, complement isn't the only host defense system the organism encounters. Early on, the trypomastigotes are met headlong by the body's main sentinels, the macrophages, which eagerly engulf them in a phagosome. In the natural scheme of things, a toxin-containing lysosome will join the organism-containing phagosome. This phagosome-lysosome merger is the beginning of the end for most organisms. The lysosome contains a lot of toxic material, and the bug is dead tout suite.

But *Trypanosoma cruzi* hasn't been around for millions of years by being defenseless. It has developed mechanisms to counteract the macrophage's highly developed, effective systems. For one, they like being inside the vacuole. The presence of the lysosome doesn't kill them; it activates them to create their own little enclosure, called the parasitophorous vacuole, or PV. Being in the PV signals the trypomastigote to begin the maturation process and enter the amastigote stage.

The macrophage contains on its surface signaling Toll-like receptors that activate a series of molecules which end in the activation of nuclear factor kappa B (NFκB). Once activated, the NFκB migrates to the host cell nucleus, where it acts to release the previously sequestered genes that code for a bunch of defense molecules, including interferons and interleukin-12. By doing so, the entire immune system is alerted, and the remaining invading organisms are effectively shut down.

A remarkable trypanosome defense mechanism is a protein known as cruzain. This little sharpshooter is essential for the parasite's success. Without it, the organism is annihilated in a very short time. It is a proteolytic enzyme, also known as a protease, because it cleaves and destroys specific proteins. (It is pronounced cruz ay' –in. Proteases usually end in the suffix – in, like trypsin, pepsin, or papain. The cruz part is obvious). The protein it inactivates is, not surprisingly, NFκB. So, the signal to the nucleus to begin releasing all its immune firepower is suppressed, and the parasite can carry on its business right in the middle of an intact cell.

Cruzain potentially damages other proteins in the host cell, so the parasite doesn't release it into the cell's cytoplasm. It keeps it attached to its outer cell membrane, kind of like a sidearm. The NFκB gets attached to the parasite membrane, and the cruzain just knocks it out.

Trypanosoma cruzi can invade many tissue cells. When first observed in the 1930s, it was felt there were two forms of cell invasion: direct invasion, where the trypomastigote bulls its way in using its powerful propulsion, and vacuole invasion, where the host cell surrounds the organism with a vacuole and incorporates it into its cytoplasm. Some remarkable early film

313

shows the trypomastigote slithering its way into a host cell, seemingly backing up the first hypothesis. But we know now that the invasion of the host cell involves the formation of a vacuole, the creation of which the trypomastigote initiates.

The trypomastigotes have many proteins on their surface that can attach to a wide range of cells. That's not true of all organisms. Many pathogens can connect to only a few cell types, some to only one. We call this phenomenon "tropism," or an organism's affinity for one cell type. For instance, malaria parasites invade only liver cells and red blood cells, depending on the stage of their development. Giardia attaches only to the cells lining the upper part of the small intestine.

But the trypomastigotes of *Trypanosoma cruzi* can seemingly attach to just about any tissue in the body. They can attach to both human and non-human mammalian cells. To do this, an organism must have the correct "key" to each individual cell type.

All our cells have an outer plasma membrane. Protruding from the plasma membrane surrounding the cell, predominantly lipid, are many different individual substances, such as proteins, carbohydrates, glycopeptides (a combination of protein and carbohydrate), and others. These substances are unique to each cell type, depending on their function. So, a muscle cell will have a unique set of molecules on its surface, an endothelial cell has its own, etc. A parasite wanting to attach and eventually enter a cell must have a "key" molecule that will fit into one of the molecules on the host cell's surface, allowing its entry into the cell. Some only have one or a few. The trypomastigotes of *Trypanosoma cruzi* have evolved a vast number of molecules on their surface that bind many different receptors on many different cell types.

Trypanosomes have some attachment molecules that are stronger and more accessible than others. They are particularly good at entering macrophages, muscle cells, and the nerve cells that innervate them. They are especially good at entering smooth muscle and cardiac tissue.

On their cell surface, trypomastigotes contain an interesting enzyme called trans-sialidases, or TS. Many of the molecules on the surface of human cells are covered by a small carbohydrate coat. Think of it as the little rubber thing on the end of a folding chair leg or a cane. Nine different carbohydrates can serve here, an important one of which is sialic acid. Sialic acid is unusual because it contains nine carbon atoms instead of the typical six. It is present on a lot of human cell surfaces. To make sialic acid, various proteins are made by a complicated array of genes. *Trypanosoma cruzi* lacks these genes and cannot produce its own sialic acid. So, it does what any parasite would; it just steals it. It has on its surface an abundance of the trans-sialidase enzymes that take the sialic acid from the host cell surface and translocate it to its own surface proteins. This masking device makes the parasite protein appear human to the immune system, enhancing its immune system avoidance.

Trypanosoma cruzi has many mechanisms to thwart the immune response mounted against it. None of its tools are foolproof, but each is successful enough for the parasite to carry on its life cycle within human cells.

The prefix "a" means without; the term mastigote is the animal version of flagella, so the term amastigote means "without flagella." It is the form the parasite assumes to reproduce once it's entrenched within the host cell. Amastigotes are little round-looking bodies, just a couple of millimeters in diameter. They still have something of a flagellum, a tiny little spike that protrudes, but it doesn't wiggle.

The amastigotes have an enzyme, TcTox, that can rupture the membrane of the cell's vacuole that encases them. They then sit out in the cell's cytoplasm for a short time but quickly make their own encasement, known as a pseudocyst. It is within this pseudocyst that replication takes place. It takes about 24-36 hours for the pseudocyst to form and cell division to begin. The amastigotes reproduce by binary fission, and it takes about 14 hours to complete the cycle. When enough amastigotes are present, they usually mature into trypomastigotes. After reaching a critical mass, the pseudocyst ruptures, and the trypomastigotes (along with some immature amastigotes and epimastigotes) are released, first into the cell's interior, then outside the cell. From there, they enter the blood to be picked up by a hungry kissing bug or infect another of the body's cells.

Much of the pathologic trouble for humans resides in this amastigote stage within the cell. While most amastigotes reproduce and give rise to daughter cells that mature into traveling trypomastigotes, some don't. They just stay in an arrested stage within the cell, sometimes for years, lounging around in their little pseudocyst. Pathologists can see them under their microscopes when looking at stained preparations of infected tissues.

The arrested development in the amastigote stage gives the organism an advantage in the wild. Humans are accidental hosts; trypanosomes are much more common in the cells of wild animals. While organisms can invade almost any tissue, they specialize in invading macrophages and muscle fibers. The macrophages help them by carrying them around the body. When residing in muscle tissue, the organism benefits if a predator eats its host. The amastigotes are infectious, even if in the arrested, pseudocyst-residing state. They can infect the predator through its intestinal tract, and the life cycle begins anew. This way, it doesn't have to exclusively depend on kissing bugs sucking up organisms from the blood, either free-floating or within macrophages. They have a backup system in place.

A problem for humans is that the immune system is activated when the creatures dwell within our muscle fibers for extended periods. Severe illness results. There are two theories on what happens, and they are not mutually exclusive. The first is the straightforward explanation that all the cellular abnormalities summon the killer and helper lymphocytes, and the resulting inflammation is eventually harmful and destructive.

A second possibility, which is difficult to prove but is nonetheless provocative, involves the organisms' array of DNA in its kinetoplast. All animal cells have mitochondria for energy production. Mitochondria are each equipped with their own unique DNA. The kinetoplast is an enormous mitochondrion with its own DNA and then some. One of the more fascinating structures in all biology is the DNA arrangement in the kinetoplast of trypanosomes and related organisms. The DNA exists in a series of circles resembling crop circles or delicate lace. There are two arrangements, the maxi-circles and the mini-circles—the maxi-circles code for the business of the kinetoplast, producing its proteins. The mini-circles code for nucleic acid that apparently guides the execution of the functions of the maxi-circle-derived RNA and the proteins produced. The visualization of electron micrograph images of these things is truly remarkable. They are not found anywhere else in nature, only in the kinetoplasts of these organisms.

The interesting feature of the kinetoplast DNA relies on some good evidence that the mini-circle DNA can be inserted into the genome of the host cell's DNA. It's difficult to prove the result of this phenomenon, but there are a few possibilities. One is that the inserted parasite DNA can block some of the host's genes and thus alter its response to the invader's presence. Another possibility is that the parasite DNA inserted into the host's chromosome from the mini-circles is transcribed, and proteins are produced. These proteins may then migrate to the cell's surface and give the immune system a signal that the cell is foreign, even though it is, in fact, native. The immune system attacks it as if it were a foreign tissue, much like it attacks a tissue transplant. The result is tissue rejection.

This latter observation happens in terminally ill patients with Chagas' disease. The muscle tissue most invaded is the heart, and the changes to the heart over time resemble those seen in tissue rejection. The cardiac myofibrils are slowly destroyed, with accompanying swelling. There is also often a marked effect on the heart's conduction system, leading to pronounced arrhythmias. Death often results.

It's pure speculation, but based on some evidence, one can build a very interesting case about the nature of tissue invasion by *Trypanosoma cruzi* and its means of propagation. If there is an advantage to the organism that a predator eats its host, it would be in the trypanosome's best interest to damage its host to ensure it gets eaten. By invading and damaging muscle tissue, including the heart, the host would be weakened and much more vulnerable to predation. The parasite could infect the next animal without relying on the kissing bug. Inserting its DNA into the host's chromosome and producing proteins that incite the host's immune system to attack and damage itself would be one way to accomplish that. It doesn't make much sense when

317

applied to humans, who are seldom prey, but rats, opossums, and the like are—an intriguing theory.

Chagas disease kills about 20,000 people yearly, nearly all in South America. Over 90% of the deaths are due to heart failure. It's hard to say with any precision because of the nature of the affected population. Still, about 10 million people are most likely infected with the agent of Chagas disease, *Trypanosoma cruzi*. As with many infectious diseases, there is a wide range of symptoms, ranging from asymptomatic to death. It's difficult to say how many patients are without symptoms in the early stages because most infected people live in areas lacking quality medical care and diagnostic capabilities. Many don't even have access to a doctor. The unassailable diagnostic sign in endemic regions is the chagoma, or Romaña's sign, a painless swelling around the eye. The other common symptoms of acute illness are all non-specific: fever, muscle aches, and perhaps a headache. Without laboratory confirmation, the diagnosis is elusive.

Many infected have a limited course, with the disease not detectable after about a month. But there is the ominous "indeterminate" stage. One just doesn't know if the parasite is hunkered down inside the body's tissues, avoiding the immune system, awaiting its time to emerge. It usually takes years, perhaps even decades, to do so. By far, the heart is the most affected organ, with about 95% of chronic Chagas disease patients showing cardiac pathology. It is usually heart failure that leads to death. On average, a person infected with *Trypanosoma cruzi* has about nine years less to live than an uninfected person of the same socioeconomic background. There is no cure for the disease, and treatment is only palliative. Heart transplant has been tried but with limited success.

Another complication of chronic Chagas disease is megacolon. The smooth muscle lining of the bowel is infected. Thus there is marked swelling and decreased bowel motility. Patients sometimes don't have a bowel movement for weeks, resulting in bowel perforation, with resultant peritonitis and sepsis. Without heroic medical intervention, death is usually the result.

Chagas disease is named for the doctor and scientist who discovered and described it, Carlos Ribiero Justiniano Chagas. Even though a disease bears his name, most people have no acquaintance with the man or his work—such a pity. Chagas was a brilliant, dedicated researcher, and one of the notable oversights of history is that he never received a Nobel Prize for his contribution to modern medicine.

Dr. Chagas was born on July 9, 1879, in the town of Oliveira, Brazil, in Minas Gerais, a few hundred miles north of Rio de Janeiro. The name minas gerais translates to "general mines" in Portuguese and was so named because of its heavy mining industry. His family was prominent and well-recognized; his ancestors had emigrated to this region of Brazil in the mid-1600s. They owned a coffee farm and were looked on with much respect by the townspeople. Unfortunately, Carlos' father died when he was four years old, leaving his mother a twenty-four-year-old widow with four young children. When he reached school age, Carlos was enrolled in a Jesuit-run boarding school, where he resided until he was 14. Upon his mother's insistence, he entered the School of Mining Engineering in Ouro, Puerto, to become a mining engineer, the most probable path to a comfortable income and lifestyle.

During his first years at mining school, Carlos became ill and had to withdraw to recuperate. He stayed at the home of an uncle, a physician. During this quiescence, he discovered his true calling. Despite his mother's objection, he transferred to medical school in Rio de Janeiro and graduated at the top of his class in 1902. He did his thesis on malaria, a blood-borne parasite.

The top medical researcher in Brazil then was Oswaldo Cruz, who was quite young, only seven years older than Carlos. He saw great potential in the young physician. He invited him to join the research team at his facility, Manguinhous Institute, a first-class research center dedicated to alleviating the rampant infectious diseases in their country. Carlos gave it much consideration but decided instead to strike out on his own as a physician and worker in sanitation and hygiene.

In the early 1900s, a brilliant physician in an impoverished area had much to ponder. One could diagnose and treat individual patients as well as possible. But it was apparent that without proper sanitation and hygiene, the diseased patients would keep coming, with no end in sight—like being on a treadmill. Carlos Chagas was motivated by his family's deep roots in the country and the national pride that goes with that. He intensely desired to do all he could to reduce the tremendous burden of diseases rampant in his country.

At the time, shipping companies avoided much of Brazil because of the genuine worry of contagious diseases and their vessels' crew members' exposure to them. This added to the impoverishment of the community. Carlos was determined to wear several hats: personal physician, epidemiologist, political adviser, and researcher. He was very good at each.

To sharpen his medical skills, he first took a position at a hospital in Rio de Janeiro, where he worked for about a year. In 1905 he was offered a position with the Santos Docks Company in Sao Paulo, a construction firm building port facilities. Malaria and yellow fever were severe problems in the area. Mosquitoes spread both diseases, a fact Dr. Walter Reed proved during the building of the Panama Canal in 1901. Dr. Chagas was familiar with a chemical agent derived from chrysanthemums, pyrethrum, that can significantly inhibit mosquitoes. Some can no longer fly, and females are inhibited from biting. He employed this natural chemical agent in workers' homes and residents in the dock working area. It was a great success; malaria and yellow fever cases decreased dramatically. The following year Dr. Chagas joined the Institute of Oswaldo Cruz.

In 1909 the Brazilian government attempted to complete a railroad line from the Amazon to Rio de Janeiro. Like in the experience of the Panama Canal, work had to be systematically halted because of the tremendous toll of mosquito-borne diseases. Because of his earlier success, Dr. Chagas was deployed to the town of Lassance, a community about 350 miles from Rio. Lassance was small but vital to the project. Because of its geographic location, it was the hub of railroad construction activity, and controlling malaria and other diseases was crucial.

To say the facilities used by Dr. Chagas at Lassance were austere would greatly understate it. He used an abandoned boxcar for two years as his office and research center. Sweltering heat and uncomfortable accommodations were the rules rather than exceptions. But he persevered.

The mission was to diagnose and control mosquito-borne diseases. But Dr. Chagas was intrigued by an insect he encountered in this little back-water town. The locals called them *vinchucas* or *barbieros,* also known as "the bloodsucker." It was well known to suck blood and was easy to discern by its bloated body after a blood meal. Mosquitoes can spread diseases by feasting on blood; could the same precept apply here? He and his associates had seen some cases of patients with symptoms of an acute febrile nature distinct from malaria and yellow fever. He decided to study it further.

In examining the midgut of the bugs, he was astonished. They harbored a parasite that strongly resembled the agent of African sleeping sickness. He took material from some of the bugs and caused a disease similar to what he had observed in humans by administering it to laboratory animals. He then did detailed studies on the insect and the parasite and called the organism *Schizotrypanum cruzi*, honoring his mentor. The genus name was later changed to *Trypanosoma*. He uncovered two vital pieces of the disease puzzle: the agent and the vector. The final piece was presented to him one day as a little three-year-old girl, Berenice.

On April 23rd, 1909, the little girl's parents had brought her to see the doctor because she had a fever and muscle aches and was very listless. Also very noticeable was a swelling on her face around her eye. Her illness did not fit the pattern of malaria, but no other diagnosis was apparent. Dr. Chagas had a blood sample taken and did a routine examination for the parasite that causes malaria, *Plasmodium vivax*. He didn't see that, but what he did find astounded him: the trypomastigotes he had observed in the midgut of the kissing bug! Here it was, the first objective evidence in a human of the disease American trypanosomiasis, now called Chagas disease after its discoverer.

Being the careful scientist he was, Dr. Chagas investigated many more cases of the disease and recognized the

321

two forms of its presentation: acute and chronic. He described 27 cases of the acute form and over 100 of the chronic. He had discovered and described, by himself and with the help of immediate co-workers, the agent of a human disease, the insect vector, and the disease itself. He meticulously worked up each one and presented his findings to the world in a classic paper in 1909: *New Human Trypanosomiasis: Studies About the Morphology and Evolutive Cycle of Schizotrypanum cruzi, Etiologic Agent of a New Morbid Entity of Man.*

Dr. Chagas' friend and mentor, Oswaldo Cruz, died of kidney failure in 1917 at age 44. Dr. Chagas became the head of the Research Institute (now known as the Oswaldo Cruz Institute) and Director of the National Department for Public Health. He remained in those positions until his death in 1934 at age 55. During his tenure, he worked to alleviate suffering from many infectious diseases, including Hanson's disease (leprosy), tuberculosis, influenza, sexually transmitted diseases, and many others. His legacy is enormous.

Carlos Chagas received many awards, including the prestigious Schaudinn Prize for pioneering work in protozoology and tropical medicine, election into the National Academy of Medicine, and honorary doctorates from several universities, including Harvard. The one prize that eluded him was the Nobel. Although nominated twice, he was passed over.

Oswaldo Cruz perhaps best summed up the work of Carlos Chagas on the disease American trypanosomiasis: *"The discovery of the disease is the most beautiful example of the power of logic in the service of science. In biological sciences, never such a complex and brilliant discovery had been made, and, what's more, by a single researcher.*

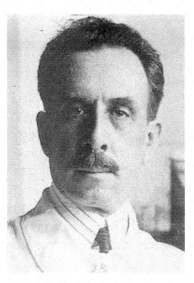

Carlos Chagas (LOC)

Unfortunately, despite all our knowledge, the infection known as Chagas disease still plagues us today. It is estimated that 20,000 people die of it every year, and over 10 million are currently infected. Currently, there is no effective treatment or cure.

Chapter 22
"Bad Air"

Nocturnal vermin
Within insect Trojan horse.
Spreads worldwide terror.

A well-worn adage states "the best things come in small packages." The wisdom of that opinion is certainly debatable, but the antithetical statement that the *worst* things come in small packages is hard to dispute. A case in point is the lowly mosquito, a troublesome little pest that shows up uninvited at the most inconvenient times. They sure don't seem like much of a threat, about a quarter inch long and weighing around 10 milligrams. But mosquito bites result in more deaths per year than all the lions, tigers, and bears combined. And by a lot. Every year over 400,000 people die because of an infection incurred by a mosquito bite. Some estimate that half of every human being in history who has died has done so due to diseases incurred following mosquito bites. That's another statement whose accuracy may be contentious. Indisputable, though, is the tremendous effect mosquitoes and their bites have had on the health of people around the world since ancient times.

The word mosquito comes from the Spanish. In Latin, the word for fly is *musca; in* Spanish, it's *moska.* So mosquito is "little fly." They've been around seemingly forever. Author Michael Crichton used the image of mosquitoes attacking dinosaurs as the foundation for the theory of his fictional book "Jurassic Park." They've certainly been around as long as humans and have adapted themselves very well to their unwelcoming hosts.

An individual's personal relationship with mosquitoes is variable. Picture a man and his wife sitting comfortably in their backyard around sundown. Suddenly, slowly at first, then in greater numbers, the mosquitoes arrive. The man notices them very little, just brushing them aside with little care. The woman, on the other hand, is entirely enveloped by them and has no recourse but to dash inside as fast as she can. There was something about her that the mosquitoes found attractive, while the male not so much. Theories abound. Carbon dioxide exhalation, body temperature, pregnancy, and blood type have all been suggested—also genetics, skin microbiota, perspiration, diet, and alcohol intake. The list is long. Just what it is depends on the mosquito species and probably several factors. But ultimately, mosquitoes will bite anyone, even though it's some more than others.

It is only the female that bites. Since they fly, mosquitoes need a lot of energy to help propel their wings, which they get by feeding on fruits and nectar. That's all the males need. But the females produce and lay eggs. So while they need the energy-yielding plant food, the eggs developing inside the female mosquito need protein and iron. Blood, of course, has both. So she bites through the skin of an animal to get it.

Not many people think about mosquito saliva, but it's actually quite a wonder. In it are over a hundred proteins. Most of them have functions that aren't known, but some are pretty remarkable. Since they are protein, some of them are allergenic. This is obvious when you see different people a day or two after the same mosquito species has attacked them. Some have little or no noticeable signs; others have large, red, inflamed welts in multiple places. These are most likely not due to a direct intoxication of the mosquito saliva left in the bite but the immune system's over-exuberant reaction to it.

One of the most intriguing facts about mosquito saliva is its direct effect on the immune system. Studies have shown that some salivary proteins can alter the ratio of the type of T-lymphocytes present, increase the amount of the inflammation-reducing cytokine interleukin-10, and alter the amount and ratios of other cytokines as well. It's been demonstrated experimentally that some alphaviruses cause more serious diseases in laboratory animals when introduced into the animal by mosquito bite along with its saliva than when administered merely with saline. A subject of continuing investigation is how this immune modulation affects disease initiation and progression and which diseases are most impacted. But there is little question that there is much more to mosquito saliva than is currently known.

Mosquitoes have been remarkably successful in the big scheme of things. Flying around for millions of years, they inhabit every part of the globe and can be found on some of the highest mountains and in the deepest caves. They are classified in the Order *Diptera*, from the Greek *Di*, or "two," and *petrous*, "winged." The Family is *Culicidae*, which is from the Latin *Culex*, meaning gnat. There are 112 genera of mosquitoes and over 3,000 species, 176 of which are found in the United States.

Mosquitoes grow in four stages, egg, larva, pupa, and adult. The female lays her eggs most commonly in still, fresh water, but they can be laid out of water. Eggs are very resilient. They usually hatch in the warm summer months. But when environmental conditions aren't optimal, they can remain dormant for many months until temperature and water content conditions are suitable for their hatching. Even the larvae and adults can survive the cold winter by going dormant.

The larvae need air to breathe, so they remain on the water's surface, feeding on microorganisms in the water. Like a snorkel, they have a small tube extending to the surface to obtain air. Larvae undergo several molts as they grow. In the pupa stage, there is no eating, but they still breathe oxygen. After a few days, the adult mosquito emerges.

Three genera are important vectors for disease transmission: *Anopheles, Aedes,* and *Culex. Anopheles* is the only one that can transmit malaria, while *Aedes* and *Culex* can transmit viruses. Bacteria and fungi are not known to be transmitted by mosquitoes but are found in other insect vectors.

Culex is found throughout the world. They are most associated with polluted water rich in organic material. They are carriers of the viruses West Nile and several others that cause encephalitis and are vectors of parasitic filarial worms by carrying microfilariae.

Aedes is a major transmitter of viral diseases throughout the world. The list of viruses it carries is ominous: Yellow Fever, all four types of Dengue, Chikungunya, and Zika. Of all the mosquitoes, *Aedes* is the most "domesticated." It prefers humans to get its blood meals and is found in and around human habitats. While most mosquitoes feed in the evening, *Aedes* is active all day long, giving it a wide range of victims. *Aedes* is

Greek for "distasteful" or "unpleasant." The species causing most of the trouble is *Aedes aegypti.*

The genus name *Anopheles* is the Greek word for "harmful" and "useless." This one genus of mosquitoes has caused incalculable human misery. It can transmit some viruses, but it is infamous for being the only mosquito that can transmit malaria. Its geographic range is global, and it is indeed a very hearty little creature, able to withstand a wide range of temperatures. There are over 450 species of *Anopheles*; about 30 of them can transmit malaria to humans.

The recorded history of malaria goes back thousands of years, with writings from India, China, Mesopotamia, and Greece showing a strong likelihood of a substantial presence of malaria in many cultures worldwide. Some historians make a solid case that the introduction of malaria into Rome from Africa was a major factor in the Empire's downfall. Many other tales relate to how malaria quite possibly altered history.

The name malaria comes from the Italian words *mala,* or "bad," and *aria,* or "air." Other words to describe it were ague (acute fever), miasma (pollution or defilement), and paludism (swamp or marsh). The disease most probably originated in Africa in non-human primates then spread to humans and accompanied them as they spread around the world, taking the mosquitoes with them. It most likely spread to the Americas with the opening of trade, particularly the slave trade. The mosquitoes could easily have traveled to the New World in the water containers on the ships and the parasite in the bloodstreams of the native Africans and crews.

The 1880s and 90s were a time of great advancements in understanding the causes of infectious diseases. Pathogens were being discovered at a rapid rate, and information was shared liberally between scientists. But the cause of one of the most terrible diseases in the world escaped discovery. At the time, severe diseases were found to be caused by bacteria: cholera, typhoid, diphtheria, etc. It was assumed that a disease like malaria, with profound chills, fever, and rigors, would also be caused by bacteria. Parasites were not known to cause acute febrile illness. The ones recognized were the helminths, the large worms. The thought that an animal parasite could cause a disease like malaria didn't seem at all possible. So all attention was given by the top scientists of the day to discovering the bacterial cause of malaria.

One worker took a different approach. Charles Louis Alphonse Laveran was a physician in the French military. His father and grandfather were both men of medicine, and his mother's father and grandfather were prominent in the French army. After serving in the Franco-Prussian war, Dr. Laveran was posted in Algeria, where he could first-hand examine the blood of a nearly unlimited number of malaria patients. Though his microscope was crude and able to magnify to only around 400x, he described in some detail the presence of tiny crescent-shaped creatures that appeared protozoal, not bacterial. He noted in many a tiny pigment, which we now know to be a breakdown product of hemoglobin that the organism secures from the infected red blood cells.

Dr. Laveran's description and theory of malaria's cause were initially met with great skepticism, but other scientists confirmed his findings. Of great help was the use of aniline dyes, especially those developed by Dimitri Leonidovitch Romanowsky in the early 1890s. Romanowsky's stains were particularly effective in showing the components of blood. We still use the Wright and Giemsa stains, developed from his original. In addition to blood cells, they also show in great detail all the stages of the malarial parasite. Meanwhile, the Carl Zeiss Company developed a high-powered lens that, using a clear oil to reduce refraction of the image, could magnify 1,000 times, giving a much better look at the tiny microbes. With Laveran's initial discovery and the confirmation achieved by better staining and microscopic technique, it was firmly established that malaria was indeed caused by an animal, albeit a tiny one, known as a protozoon.

The means of acquisition of the disease was as perplexing as its cause. The two obvious ways of getting an infection are food and water or inhalation. But all efforts to demonstrate these means of transmission met with failure. Mosquitoes had been associated with malaria for hundreds of

328

years, but just how was mere speculation. Some thought it might be drinking water in which mosquitoes had died. Others offered the idea that the wind carried dead dried-up organisms to people in the area who breathed them in. Of course, no credible evidence was ever presented for these or other theories.

One theory was that the mosquito wasn't just a passive carrier of the organism but a vital part of the malarial organism's life cycle. A prestigious investigator of tropical medicine working in England, Patrick Manson, became intrigued by that possibility and, along with some Italian workers, set about the task of discovering this possibility. While carrying on his medical practice in London, Manson engaged a British Army physician named Ronald Ross to carry out the investigation in the field. Ross was stationed in India and began the work in 1895.

Ross was a military officer first, a malarial researcher second, and the two careers often conflicted. He was also given to writing a novel and some poetry, which didn't help the malaria investigative cause. His early work involved looking at mosquitoes such as *Culex* and *Aedes,* which don't spread malaria. So after dissecting over a thousand mosquitoes over two years, nothing was learned, and the effort seemed fruitless. But one day, he happened to encounter an *Anopheles* mosquito which did indeed have evidence of malarial parasites in its abdomen. Just like that, the first inkling of the spread of the disease became known. Through diligent work, he and other workers, mostly the Italians, showed conclusively that Anopheline mosquitoes not only transmitted the disease from person to person but were critical to the pathogen's reproduction and infectivity.

Laveran and Ross were awarded the Nobel Prize in Physiology or Medicine for their work.

The third very important part of the natural course of the disease to be discovered is what happens after the organism enters the body following a mosquito bite. It was known that the organism travels around the body in the bloodstream, making the patient ill while it multiplies in the red blood cells, then is picked up by another mosquito in which it undergoes sexual reproduction. The cycle is begun anew with another bite. But the incubation time following the bite is around two weeks. What happens to the creature during that time, after the invasion, and before it starts invading the red blood cells? The question eluded researchers for decades.

Unfortunately, a grave mistake was made early in investigating the organism's pathogenicity, and the wrong course was pursued for many years. A very influential German scientist, Fritz Schaudinn, described and published in 1903 what he claimed to be a direct observation of the malarial sporozoites, the infective units spit out by the mosquito, directly invading red blood cells in the bloodstream. This was held as truth for forty years until 1948, when scientists working at, appropriately, the Ross Institute for Tropical Medicine in London, showed conclusively that the organisms invaded the liver after inoculation and developed there for two weeks before proceeding to enter the bloodstream to infect red blood cells.

Today, students reviewing the life cycle of malarial parasites are given a very concise informative diagram of the events, usually in circular form. Little do many realize the painstaking, often dangerous, work that went into discovering these relatively simple facts. It took over a half-century by some of the world's great scientific minds. It's not as simple as it looks.

The name assigned to the malarial parasite of humans is *Plasmodium*, which derives from the Greek words *plasma* and *ode,* which mean "molded" or "formed," and "like." There are five recognized species of humans, with two predominating, *Plasmodium vivax and Plasmodium falciparum.* Two other less common species are *P. malariae* and *P. ovale*, and a fifth rare species of *P. knowlesi.* All have the same general life cycle, which is carried out in three stages:

Mating and growth in the mosquito abdomen
Development in the cells of the human liver
Development in the bloodstream

The mosquito provides the parasite double service. For one, they suck blood from the victim and bring it into their bodies along with the malarial parasites. In the mosquito abdomen, the sexual forms of the parasite, the male and female gametes, unite, giving the embryonic form of new organisms. These take a few weeks to develop. They then proceed to the mosquito's salivary glands. The embryonic organisms in the mosquito are known as an ookinete, which comes from Greek words meaning "mobile egg." (The word ookinete is an odd one, with about a half dozen possible pronunciations. Two are accepted, o uh kin EET, and o uh KINE eet). The ookinete is mobile by a flagellum, and it works its way up the mosquito's gut as it matures, the embryo growing inside it. When it reaches the mid-gut, the ookinete turns into a cyst. Again, the creatures inside are growing, and when the cyst is ripe, they burst out and "swim" to the mosquito's salivary gland.

These slithering little creatures are known as sporozoites. The spore part comes from the Greek word meaning "seed," and the "zoite" suffix indicates that they are indeed animals. While considered spores, they sure don't look or behave like fungus or bacterial spores that come to mind. They emerge from a cyst, and like a typical spore, they seek a place to implant and begin growing, but they are actively motile and are powered by a dynamic energy system. With many of them in the mosquito salivary gland, they are ready for the next part of the journey.

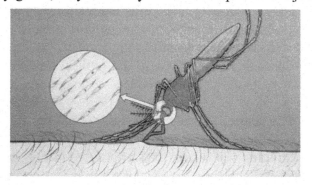

Sporozoites are inoculated into the skin with the saliva of the female mosquito. (PHIL)

The sporozoites look like tiny worms, and they have the means of a rather forceful movement, described as gliding motility. The number of sporozoites introduced into the skin by the mosquito varies, anywhere from a dozen to over a hundred. When taking a blood meal, the mosquito must first inject an anticoagulant present in its saliva, and it is with this injection act the sporozoites are pushed out.

When injected by the mosquito into the skin of the unfortunate human victim, the sporozoites begin a downward sojourn until they reach a blood vessel. Some will encounter a macrophage in the skin and be eliminated; some will enter the lymphatic system and make their way to a lymph node, also most likely to be eliminated. But those that reach the blood will eventually find their way to the liver.

The liver is the body's only organ in which sporozoites can carry out their early mission. To ensure they get there, they have a protein that can detect that they are in the right place. They even can travel right through the Kupffer cells, the resident macrophages of the liver, to get to the liver cells, known as hepatocytes. The sporozoites have on their surface a protein (circumsporozoite protein, CSP) that allows them to attach to a receptor on a liver cell that is the same one that receives high-density lipoprotein-bearing cholesterol. Once attached, they penetrate the cell. At that point, the infection has taken root.

When inside the liver cell, the sporozoite is encased in a parasitophorous vacuole. Inside this membrane, it is free to begin reproduction. It also emits proteins that prevent the host cell from undergoing apoptosis, thus maintaining its source of sustenance. The type of malarial reproduction in the liver cell is binary fission, as one cell splits into another, which in turn continues dividing. It's similar to the replication of bacteria. The number of malarial cells produced in the single liver cell inside the vacuole is impressive, over 30,000. Because the splitting of a single one is the means of making this many daughter cells, the term **schizont** is applied. The Greek word for "split" or "divide" is *skhizein*. It is often used in English as the prefix schizo-. Each tiny member of the enormous schizont is given the term **merozoite**, the "mero," taken from the Greek word *meros,* meaning part or share. The same terms are applied to the parasite when they are in the bloodstream.

332

At a certain point, the burden of these rapidly growing merozoites overwhelms the liver cell. One side of it opens, and a vast number of merozoites come pouring out into the bloodstream. They make it to the lungs. There, a capsule surrounding the cell is removed, and they are freed into the bloodstream. From there, entering a red blood cell is a simple matter.

Malarial merozoites have a front and back end. On the front end, they have attachment and red cell penetration devices that easily allow them to enter the red blood cell. Once inside, they begin to gather nutrients from hemoglobin. At this stage, the merozoite has become a trophozoite, the actively feeding stage. Trophozoite comes from the Greek word *trophe,* meaning "nourishment." After it has been well fed, the trophozoite begins the division process anew, forming another schizont, this time in the red blood cell. The number of merozoites making up the red blood cell schizont is nowhere near the number seen in liver cells, anywhere from 6 to 36, depending on the species. (Counting the number of merozoites is very useful in the laboratory for identifying the malarial species present). Just like in the liver, each little organism is termed a merozoite. At maturation, the red blood cell bursts open, and the merozoites come pouring out, each capable of infecting another red blood cell.

The merozoites do not spend much time exposed to the circulatory system. It takes less than a minute for one to enter a red blood cell, and there is no limit to the number of cells that may be infected.

This cycle keeps getting repeated. The tiny merozoites quickly adhere to and enter red blood cells, and the red blood cells get ripped to shreds as the dozen or more newly created merozoites exit. Depending on the malarial species, it takes a few days for the red blood cell growth phase to progress.

The symptoms of malaria are mainly due to the inflammatory cytokines, especially tumor necrosis factor-α (TNF-α). The induction of chills, fevers, and rigors is primarily the result of the monocytes of the blood encountering fragmented red blood cells as well as the occasional merozoite and releasing potent inflammatory cytokines.

The bodily organ tasked with removing defective red blood cells is the spleen. The spleen becomes greatly overworked with the tremendous number of defective red cells, often resulting in marked swelling. An enlarged spleen, known as splenomegaly, is one of the hallmarks of malaria.

This cycle of malarial merozoites being released, re-infecting, then again being released goes on for some time, often a couple of weeks. For some reason that is not understood, some of the merozoites do not re-infect another red blood cell after their release but instead mature into either a male or female gametocyte. When a mosquito comes along and takes a blood meal from an active malaria patient, the merozoites it picks up are irrelevant. For the parasite, the only things that matter at this point are the gametocytes that will go on to come together in the mosquito's gut to produce the ookinete, potentially leading to another person becoming infected.

It's no wonder it took about 50 years to discover this elaborate life cycle of *Plasmodium*. So many invasive steps, organism transformations, maturation, and transmission cycles that one gets mixed up just thinking about it. But the entire process has been going on successfully for millennia and is just as vigorous today as it was in ancient times.

A major obstacle to any invading microorganism is the host's immune response. The human immune system is amply equipped to combat invading organisms with weapons such as complement and other serum proteins, phagocytic cells, cytotoxic lymphocytes, antibodies, and apoptosis. Clearly, though, the *Plasmodium* causing malaria gets through, often in no small way. Massive numbers of parasites circulate in the body when the disease is at its apex, sometimes taking weeks for the infection to clear. Sometimes the disease progresses almost unnoticed, with few symptoms, while the disease is profoundly debilitating to many. Some patients, especially pregnant women and children, die.

One of the organism's advantages is its quickness. They don't stay exposed in the tissues or bloodstream for long. Being intracellular pathogens (they reproduce inside a living cell), they are protected in their habitat in two ways. One is in the liver, where they form a parasitophorous vacuole (PV), a membrane surrounding them, while they form a schizont. The PV cannot unite with the liver cell's lysosome, so the parasites can develop inside the cell with impunity. *Plasmodium* also prevents the host liver cell from killing itself through apoptosis, but other cellular functions are carried on near-normal, not to alert any natural killer lymphocytes.

The cell for their asexual reproduction is the circulating red blood cell. These cells lack nuclei, so there is no signaling to the genome to release cytokines or other signaling molecules. RBCs are not attacked by natural killer lymphocytes or cytotoxic CD8 or T-helper CD4 lymphocytes. Damaged RBCs are removed from the circulation, mainly in the spleen and liver, but the parasites have found a way around that.

When a red blood cell floats through the spleen's red pulp, it must be skinny and pliable enough to pass through. The spleen effectively removes, disables, and recovers RBCs that don't measure up. On a routine basis, this usually means RBCs that are too old. It's a common, necessary procedure. A red blood cell infected by *Plasmodium* is not likely to safely make it through the spleen, so one species, *falciparum,* the deadliest malarial parasite, has a solution: don't circulate through the spleen. *P. falciparum* manufactures at least three proteins expressed on the surface of the red blood cell it is infecting. They cause the RBC to adhere to various surfaces, including the endothelial lining of small blood vessels, other red blood cells, and some types of lymphocytes.

By attaching to the lining of venules, the organism inside its host red blood cell is not swept along with the circulation. It just stays in one place as it matures, forming its schizont. Other red blood cells are infected when the schizont bursts and the merozoites are released. They circulate, but some make it through the spleen because the red cell deformity is not advanced in younger infected cells. This adhesion is the reason for the peculiar, characteristic fact about falciparum malaria: in the peripheral blood, only the early ring forms (single merozoite) stage is seen, not the more mature trophozoite and schizont stage.

Other red blood cells are another surface the falciparum adhesion molecules can stick to. The result is a clump of RBCs known as a rosette. The formation of a rosette serves two purposes for the parasite: the cluster will get stuck in the small venules, preventing circulation through the spleen, and it also provides protection from complement and phagocytes attacking the infected cell. Having all these normal but stuck RBCs around it shields the parasite's surface proteins from recognition by members of the immune system.

Malarial parasites, of course, depend on mosquitoes to assist them in propagating the species. Sometimes the mosquitoes aren't there, either because of the weather or another reason. The adherence proteins may help the parasite "hide out" in the host for a prolonged period and produce gametocytes at a low level for a while, at least until the mosquitoes return.

Plasmodium feeds on the hemoglobin of the red blood cell that it invades. The hemoglobin is broken down into two major components: globulin, the protein portion, and heme, the iron-containing section. The protein portion is digested into its component amino acids. The heme portion presents a problem. *Plasmodium* doesn't use all of it, so the excess is freed during the infection. It is toxic and must be taken care of. The organism has the means to aggregate the free hemoglobin into insoluble crystals, called hemozoin, which can float free to be picked up and metabolized by monocytes. This is beneficial to both the parasite as well as the host. In some heavy infections, however, especially those caused by *Plasmodium falciparum,* the release of heme is not controlled, and there is considerable tissue damage to the host, particularly the kidney. The result is a condition known as "blackwater fever," a lurid description of the color of the urine. Often, this condition is fatal.

The serum aggregate of proteins known as complement is an important deterrent to many potential invading organisms, including *Plasmodium.* It is a potent weapon, and when unleashed, it can destroy any type of cell, including our own. To prevent self-destruction by the highly detrimental complement component C3b, we are equipped with an influential protein known as Factor H. It is a regulator protein that associates itself with human cell surfaces, rapidly deactivating the destructive portion of complement. Some malarial parasites have created their own version of Factor H, thus rendering themselves much less vulnerable to complement's destructive powers.

Several chemical compounds have been discovered and modified through the ages to combat malaria. The first was quinine, derived from the bark of the cinchona tree of South America (Chapter 4). Quinine had its problems, notably unreliable dosages in the early days and toxicity, but it was a reasonably effective drug for hundreds of years. In the 1930s and 40s great effort was made to find an alternative to quinine, or at least modify it to give it a more standard dose and reduce its toxicity.

Quite a few drugs were developed, most of them variations on the chemical structure of quinine. The one that has survived is chloroquine and its close modification, hydroxychloroquine. They are still used effectively today, particularly for prophylaxis, although drug resistance by parasites has become a significant problem. Heme, the iron-containing part of hemoglobin, is toxic to *Plasmodium*. That's why it goes to great lengths to detoxify it by converting it into large hemozoin crystals. Chloroquine, an alkaline compound, enters the food vacuole where heme metabolism occurs, preventing hemozoin formation. The build-up of free heme is toxic to the organism. Drug resistance in the parasite is probably due to the inability of chloroquine to attach to and enter the food vacuole or an efflux pump developed by the organism to excrete it.

Another important anti-malarial drug has a fascinating history, just as quinine does. The sweet woodworm plant *Artemisia annui* has been used for thousands of years in traditional Chinese medicine. Known in China as Qinghao, it was mentioned as an anti-malarial drug in the *Handbook of Prescriptions for Emergency,* written during the Eastern Jin Dynasty, 317-420 A.D. During the Vietnam War, malaria was a severe problem for all involved, and chloroquine resistance by the pathogen was becoming commonplace. The Chinese government enlisted Dr. Youyou Tu, an expert in traditional Chinese and Western medicine, to seek alternative therapy. Dr. Tu and her colleagues made a thorough search of over 2000 Chinese herbs as well as a study of ancient writings. They came up with what we now call Artemisinin. After experimenting with extraction techniques, the drug in a relatively pure form showed itself very effective in curing acute malaria patients. Various chemical modifications to the core molecule have yielded several effective drugs, which are prominently used today.

The mode of action of Artemisinin has been hard to pin down, but it appears to resemble that of chloroquine, that is, disruption of the formation of hemozoin by the parasite with the resulting killing of the organism. Unfortunately, as with other anti-malarial drugs, resistance has shown up in several endemic areas.

Malaria due to *Plasmodium vivax* and *P. malariae* sometimes manifests with a delayed liver stage. Called hypnozoites, the merozoites do not emerge from the liver cell early in the disease but can exist in a dormant state, free to enter the bloodstream later. The drug primaquine is often included in the regimen when treating either of these two species, as it is effective against hypnozoites.

Malaria has been a scourge of humanity for thousands of years. Despite our extensive knowledge of the life cycle of the parasite and the availability of anti-malarial drugs, it remains a problem for about 40% of the world's population. Hundreds of millions are sickened yearly, and over half a million, primarily pregnant women and children, die. After World War II, the United States embarked on an ambitious program to eradicate malaria from its shores. Patients with the disease were put in strict isolation to keep them away from mosquitoes and given chloroquine to rid them of the parasite. Extensive mosquito-infested areas were sprayed with DDT to vastly decrease the mosquito population. It worked. Today malaria is not seen in the United States, despite the presence of Anopheline mosquitoes. When the mosquitoes take a blood meal, there are no *Plasmodium* gametocytes for them to take up. The cycle has been broken. Now, many mosquitoes are resistant to DDT, which in many areas is a banned substance, and many organisms are resistant to chloroquine and artemisinin, so this technique is no longer possible.

Developing a vaccine for any microbe is difficult, but making an effective one for parasites is even more challenging. For malaria, the organism undergoes numerous biological changes, and knowing which stage to target is not easy. In the early 2020s, a vaccine was introduced against *Plasmodium falciparum*, the species with the highest mortality rate. When in the sporozoite stage, the one that enters the body from the mosquito and enters the liver cells, there is a protein on the parasite, circumsporozoite protein (CSP). It attaches to the receptor on the liver cell and enables the parasite to enter. By adding a portion of CSP to an inactive hepatitis B virus, antibodies are formed to CSP, and the activity of the sporozoite is greatly diminished. An adjuvant was added to boost the immune response. In addition to the B-lymphocyte response creating antibodies to CSP, there is also a vigorous T-cell response, with killer lymphocytes primed to eliminate the liver cells that harbor the invasive sporozoites.

While early vaccine trials have been promising, malarial parasites are notorious for mutating and developing resistance to chemical agents. It remains to be seen if they can show similar resistance to the vaccine. CSP is highly conserved, and if it is to function correctly for the parasite, it may have to remain unchanged. Time will tell.

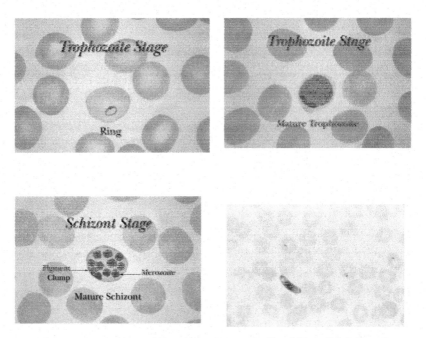

The maturation stages of Plasmodium as seen in blood films. Top left, early trophozoite after the merozoite enters the red blood cell (ring form); Top right, mature motile trophozoite preparing to enter schizont stage; Bottom left, schizont showing discreet merozoites; Bottom right, gametocyte. Gametocytes are seen outside RBCs. Species is usually determined by counting the number of merozoites in schizonts. P. falciparum does not display mature trophozoite or schizont stage in peripheral blood specimens. (PHIL)

Chapter 23
Out of Africa

Sickest of the sick,
Wretched beyond description.
Interferon thieves.

Microorganisms constantly mutate and assimilate new genetic information, so it is not unusual for one to occasionally change the animal it infects. Most of these crossovers occur with little notice. Either the newer version of the bug is ill-adapted to prosper in the new host, or the infection is very mild or not even noticed. Occasionally, however, the "Big One" hits. Most earthquakes can only be detected by sophisticated seismic equipment, but when a devastating one occurs, there is no missing it. So it is with some diseases caused by an infectious agent that crosses to a new host. While most are benign, sometimes the result is catastrophic. Bubonic plague, smallpox, coronavirus, and influenza are thought to have originated in animals and then jumped to humans, with horrific consequences.

The term viral hemorrhagic fever (VHF) is broad, with the keyword being hemorrhagic. The bleeding is not caused by direct invasion of the virus but rather by a generalized disruption of the integrity of the vascular and coagulation systems brought on by an over-enthusiastic immune response. The bleeding may be into the tissues or, in severe cases, escape from the body. Such hemorrhages are a grave sign, and death usually ensues. All viral hemorrhagic fever cases are acute.

There are three main groups and one lesser group of viruses that can cause a case of hemorrhagic fever. All are RNA viruses. Ebola and Marburg viruses belong to the group known as the filoviruses, "filo" coming from the Latin *filum*, or thread, because of their appearance under the electron microscope.

A second major group is the flaviviruses, from the Latin *flavus*, meaning "yellow." The name comes from the common name for one disease caused by the group, yellow fever. This group has many members, the most recognizable being yellow fever, dengue, West Nile, and Zika. There are over 60 different flaviviruses in all. All are carried by insects, primarily mosquitoes, some by ticks, so the name often applied is "arbovirus," or arthropod-borne virus. Yellow fever and dengue most likely crossed the Atlantic to the Americas during the slave trade, while West Nile and Zika may have crossed the ocean on a modern-day jet airliner.

A third virus group responsible for acute hemorrhagic fevers is known collectively as the Bunyavirus family. Some of the more generally recognized members of the group are the Crimean-Congo virus, Rift Valley Fever virus, La Crosse, and Hantavirus. All are associated with rodents and are transmitted by insects, usually mosquitoes and ticks. The name Bunyavirus comes from Bunyamwera, an area in Western Uganda where the virus was first isolated in the early 1940s. While not as prevalent as the flaviviruses, the Bunyaviruses can also cause severe disease, including viral hemorrhagic fever.

The arenaviruses are the fourth group of viruses capable of producing hemorrhagic fevers in humans. They are rare, usually associated with rodent droppings, and apparently not transmissible human-to-human. Like the other hemorrhagic fever viruses, they greatly reduce the amount of interferon the infected host produces. Lassa fever virus is the most well-known of the arenaviruses.

Ebola. The Legbala River is a relatively small body of water in the Democratic Republic of the Congo in Central Africa. About 160 miles in length, it feeds into the major Congo River. The European name for Legbala became Ebola. Regrettably, the name of this peaceful and beautiful river has evolved into a word synonymous with horror and death. Just like the river's setting in deepest, darkest Africa, the virus causing the disease is one of mystery and intrigue.

By their very nature, viruses are very specific for the cells they infect. On their surface is a protein that will attach to one, and only one, receptor on a cell. The rabies virus will attach to only nerve cells. Hepatitis viruses have a specific receptor on liver cells. Ebola virus, though, can attach to several different types of cells, whether liver, kidney, skin, intestinal or other, so it can gain entrance to a wide variety of tissues throughout the body. Its favorite targets are the very cells that are meant to kill it, the macrophages. Whether monocytes in the bloodstream or the macrophages or dendritic cells of the tissues, the Ebola virus forms a firm attachment to them and invites itself inside. The result is catastrophic.

After the virus enters, the macrophage, like all cells of the body, releases several cytokines. Most are inflammatory, like interleukin-1β, IL-6, tumor necrosis factor-α, and others. They have many functions, but they significantly increase body temperature, muscle aches, and blood vessels' porosity. A small amount of cytokines is not dangerous, but the damage is profound when they are released in large quantities. The macrophages cannot destroy the Ebola virus, which emerges after replicating. One thing they can do, though, is to send out molecules to attract other macrophages, giving newly made virions a new host cell to invade. This results in an expanding cascade of more cytokines, and the integrity of the blood vessels is soon challenged. With the pronounced inflammation, fluid, including blood, starts leaking out of blood vessels into the surrounding tissues. In many cases, it gets entirely out of control.

The dendritic macrophages' job is to pick up the invading virus, digest it, display various molecules of the virus on its surface (encased on MHC molecules), then transport the goods to the nearest lymph node. The lymphocytes with the correct receptor for the viral protein displayed will activate and initiate acquired immunity. The Ebola virus, however, has other ideas. It contains a protein, one we call VP-35 (short for viral protein-35), that prevents the maturation of the dendritic macrophage so that the entrails of the virus are not displayed on the dendritic cell's surface. Hence the presentation of the viral protein to lymphocytes does not occur, and immunity is significantly mitigated.

The coagulation system is an integral part of our physiology that is upended during an attack by the Ebola virus. Made up of many components, coagulation plugs leaks in blood vessel walls. The coagulation cascade kicks into high gear with the release of large amounts of cytokines during monocyte and macrophage invasion and the subsequent leakage of blood vessels. Clots are formed throughout the body, sometimes within the blood vessels themselves. This is called disseminated intravascular coagulation, or DIC, a very serious situation. Many of the blood clotting factors are used up in the process. Clotting factors are manufactured in the liver, but, as fate would have it, the Ebola virus can infect liver cells, shutting down the manufacture of fresh clotting factors. Not enough clotting factors are available to plug blood vessel leaks. The result is uncontrolled bleeding into tissues, sometimes through skin openings. The leaking blood contains the virus, one means for person-to-person spread.

The filoviruses, Ebola and Marburg, can enter a broad range of cells in the mammalian body. The flaviviruses go them one further. They can infect several cells of humans, mosquitos and ticks, and non-human animals. The attachment protein for the flaviviruses is known as the E-protein, and it does its best work on cells of the lymphoid tissues. After entering the body through a mosquito bite, the virus is taken up by a dendritic macrophage and transported to a nearby lymph node, where it can enter lymphocytes. The virus replicates in the lymphocytes, eventually bursting the host cell to enter the bloodstream. From there, it circulates throughout the body and ends up in select places depending on the virus. Yellow fever virus goes to many places, but it is primarily attracted to the liver, and the dengue virus similarly travels to numerous locations. They both can cause viral hemorrhagic fever. West Nile and Zika gravitate to the central nervous system.

Our chief defense against invading viruses is interferon production, particularly the α and β varieties (Type I). Interferons are not always present in the body; the genes responsible for their production are blocked. When an invading virus is detected, a series of chemical reactions occur, resulting in nuclear factor kappa B (NFκB) taking the cap off the interferon genes and allowing them to be expressed. Interferons don't kill the invading virus directly but instead travel to nearby cells, instructing them to protect themselves from the virus. Once incorporated into a cell, interferons are responsible for releasing hundreds of anti-viral proteins. For a virus to succeed, it needs to reduce the impact of interferon on its reproduction. The Flaviviruses are masters of this.

344

Flavivirus is an RNA virus. Most RNA viruses have some feature that distinguishes their RNA from human messenger RNA, and that difference is enough to trigger the cascade of reactions that unleash interferons. But flaviviruses' RNA is indistinguishable from the human type. After the virus enters the cell, its RNA is released, and it travels to the ribosomes to be copied just like a routine human messenger RNA does. This can significantly delay the production of interferon.

As the copying of viral RNA proceeds, differences do appear, and the interferon production mechanisms begin, albeit delayed. Flaviviruses have a second means of curtailing interferon production, however. They have proteins that can prevent the activation of several molecules in the interferon-enabling cascade. Viral protein NS5 is especially good at this. They even have some proteins that can actively destroy the precursors to interferon, thus reducing its amount.

Dengue. Dengue (pronounced deng-y, the u is silent) is a potentially severe ailment observed in many world areas. It's been found in over 100 countries. The name probably comes from the Swahili term for it, "Ka-dingo pepo," meaning "cramp-like seizure caused by an evil spirit." It may be that Spanish explorers adopted the name from that. A vivid name for the disease is attributed to American physician Benjamin Rush in the 1780s, who used the descriptive moniker "break-bone fever." The muscle and joint pain can be so severe that it feels like your bones may break.

Clinically, dengue is an odd disease. Odd in that when the virus first infects a person, they usually don't become very ill. They may have a little discomfort, but it is often not enough to seek medical advice. The real trouble begins after a second infection. The severe symptoms are a result of an over-vigorous immune response.

There are four different types of the dengue virus. Types 1 and 2 predominate. The virus infects the cells of the mosquito that carries it, *Aedes aegyptii*. *Aedes* has two features that make it especially troublesome. It is "domesticated" in the sense that it is well adapted to humans and our environment. The other is that it is an active feeder during the day, so many people are potentially exposed to bites.

Dengue virus makes ten proteins. Three are on the surface, giving the virus its structural integrity. The other seven are non-structural and located in the virus's interior. One of these non-structural proteins, NS-1, is responsible for many people's severe reactions after getting infected.

The virus releases NS-1 during infection. It gets into the bloodstream and circulates throughout the body. It has a strong affinity for the cells of the endothelium lining of blood vessels and attaches to them. Upon the first infection, the immune response to the virus is typical: antibodies are made to the proteins making up the viral core and the free-floating NS-1 protein. The virus and NS-1 are cleared in a short time, usually without much harm to the patient.

Trouble occurs when the patient is infected a second time with another type of the virus. Say the initial infection was with type 1. Antibodies are made to its core proteins as well as to NS-1. If the individual is infected a few years later with type 2, the immune reaction to the core proteins is a matter of routine; antibodies to type 1 do not protect against type 2. But the NS-1 proteins of types 1 and 2 are antigenically the same, so the immune system is locked and loaded to react to NS-1. The problem is that there is so much NS-1 produced during the second infection, and the immune system is primed to take it out, and there is a tremendous immune overreaction. NS-1 is attached to the inner lining of blood vessels, and antibodies bind to it at that place. The result is a deterioration in the integrity of the blood vessel lining with resultant leakage. As in Ebola infection, the result is sometimes viral hemorrhagic fever, a very serious condition.

The range of symptoms displayed in a dengue infection is wide. Many patients display mild to moderate reactions, but some are severely affected. The genetics of both the patient and the microbe, the strain of the virus, the timing of the initial infection, and the amount of virus injected by the mosquito all play a role.

Yellow fever. The yellow fever story is one of the most epic sagas in medical history. A flavivirus originating in Africa was brought to the New World by sailing ships and their crews and became endemic in tropical and subtropical areas. For centuries the virus and its mosquito vector proliferated across North and South America, leaving death and suffering in its wake.

The name yellow comes from the jaundice most patients display. Many called it yellow jack because ships coming into a port from an infected area had to fly a yellow flag. (Ships flags were called jacks). The name of the viral genus, *Flavivirus*, comes from the Latin word for yellow.

Unlike dengue, yellow fever makes a person ill on first exposure to the virus. It hits like the proverbial "ton of bricks." Chills followed by severe fever and rigors, intense back pain, severe headache, nausea, vomiting, and general muscle aches. The fatigue is profound, with most patients unable to move around for days. Not all people go on to such extreme symptoms, but about half of those who do die.

For centuries people speculated on the cause of yellow fever. The most common explanation was that fomites like blankets and clothing transmitted it. In the 1880s and 90s, it had become apparent to scientists that bacteria were the cause of infectious diseases, so it was logical to think that some undiscovered bug caused yellow fever. Despite a vigorous search, one was not found. At that time, viruses were not detectable.

Walter Reed was an Army doctor who had been stationed at multiple locations during his service. In the late 1890s, he was stationed in Washington, D.C., and worked at Johns Hopkins Hospital. In 1898 Dr. Reed was assigned to investigate an outbreak of yellow fever at a U.S. garrison in Cuba, known as a hotbed of the disease. One theory of insect transmission appealed to him, and with colleagues' assistance, Dr. Reed proved the vector to be a mosquito. The virus does not naturally infect non-human animals other than some higher primates, so some workers volunteered to be bitten by infected mosquitoes. Some became very ill, and a few died.

For many years, researchers worldwide sought to find the agent of yellow fever and develop a vaccine for its prevention. The virus is hazardous to work with, and many workers died after being infected with it.

In the late 1930s, a vaccine was finally developed. Most of the credit goes to Max Theiler, a native of South Africa who worked at the Rockefeller Institute in New York. Dr. Theiler passed the virus through mouse brains until an attenuated strain was achieved. The vaccine strain, 17D, is still used today. Because of its discovery, millions of lives have been saved, and countless millions spared the torment of this relentless disease.

Yellow fever virus is unique among the flaviviruses in that it primarily infects humans and a few advanced primates. After entering the body by mosquito bite, it is transported by macrophages to the lymph nodes, where it infects lymphocytes. After entering the bloodstream, the virus, with its unique surface E protein, attaches to several human cell types, with the cells of the liver predominating. Infected cells rapidly die, and a cytokine storm ensues, with consequent systemic inflammation. As with all flaviviruses, the interferon-suppressing non-structural protein 5 (NS5) greatly enhances viral virulence.

West Nile. There are over sixty known flaviviruses. Some exclusively infect non-human animals, some only humans and higher primates, and some infect a wide range of animals, including humans. West Nile virus mainly infects birds. It was considered a non-descript virus of minor importance in remote areas of Africa for a long time. A few reports of the virus' presence in Israel and Romania were considered one-off events. But one day in 1999 in New York, a bird fell out of the sky, dead. Then more birds. And more. The proprietors at the Bronx Zoo revealed that several zoo birds suffered the same fate. After laboratory testing, the infectious agent was identified as West Nile virus. Not long after that, the virus was discovered in birds in many different areas.

Initially, the public reaction was benign ambivalence. Too bad birds are dying, but we humans are not affected. Sadly, it was not to be. West Nile virus infects a few animals besides birds, and unfortunately, that includes humans. Horses are also on the list, and some higher primates can also be infected. Humans and horses are not where the virus wants to be. The number of virions in the bloodstream is small, so when a mosquito takes a blood meal, there isn't enough virus to get sucked up into the mosquito, and the virus stays with the mammal host, a dead end.

The mosquito that harbors the West Nile virus and serves as its vector is a member of the genus *Culex*. There are many species in the *Culex* genus, but only a few bite birds as well as horses or humans. How much West Nile virus is present in a geographic area depends on several factors. The mosquito species, the number of infected birds, the strain of the virus, and the environmental conditions all play a role.

Our skin is a marvelous barrier to infectious diseases. Not only is it a great physical barrier, but it also contains cells that act as sentinels when a microbial invasion occurs. Two important cells in the skin are the dendritic macrophages (Langerhans cells) and the cells that manufacture keratin (keratinocytes). West Nile virus readily enters both cells, and the cytokine signaling begins. Since the virus is injected with the bite of a mosquito, the insect's saliva can play an important role in the early reaction to infection. Some mosquito saliva can reduce the immediate immune response, often by reducing the activity of local mast cells in their attempt to attract additional virus-fighting immune system responders.

The dendritic macrophages carry the virus to the nearest lymphoid tissue. West Nile virus can replicate inside the macrophage, increasing its numbers. When in the lymphoid tissue, the virus infects the lymphocytes, which then carry it around the body. Especially vulnerable is the central nervous system, as the lymphocytes can cross the blood-brain barrier and introduce the virus into that area. Several clinical manifestations can be seen, including symptoms that resemble Parkinson's disease, those that mimic poliomyelitis, and those that look like meningitis and encephalitis. Recovery often takes several weeks. Unfortunately, some patients are severely affected and show neurologic signs for an extended period.

Usually, West Nile virus is not a serious infection. Many who are infected show either no symptoms or very few symptoms. Those who display the worst symptoms are usually aged or have a previous compromising condition. It does not cause hemorrhagic fever, but its involvement in disease can devastate some people.

Zika. Zika is a flavivirus that, like West Nile virus, has a predilection for nerve cells. It also had a rather dramatic introduction to world attention when it appeared in clinical situations around the 2016 Olympic Games in Brazil. Until then, it was obscure, even though it was first described in the late 1940s in Africa. The name Zika comes from the name of a forest in Uganda, where it was discovered. Unlike West Nile, which is spread by *Culex* mosquitoes, Zika is spread by mosquitoes of the genus *Aedes*, the same that spreads dengue. Zika infects mammals, including higher primates. Most people infected show only mild symptoms, if any at all. It is the fetus of an infected woman that is most at risk. The E-protein on the virus' surface binds strongly to the cells of the placenta. After entering the placenta, the Zika virus can enter the nerve cells of the developing fetus. Frequently, these infected nerve cells undergo apoptosis. The result is a malformation of the infant's brain. Stillbirth and microcephaly sometimes occur. For infected babies born alive neurologic sequelae such as epilepsy often occur.

The Bunyaviruses contain non-structural proteins that seem to interfere with protein synthesis by the host cell, thus limiting the amount of interferon that can be produced. These proteins attack host cell messenger RNA, knocking out the ability of the cell to produce interferons to signal nearby cells, allowing the virus to propagate to very high levels and giving serious disease.

In the developed world, viral hemorrhagic fever is rare, but millions of people in some areas are stricken yearly. The filoviruses, Ebola and Marburg, are transmissible person to person through body fluids, while the flaviviruses, Bunyaviruses, and arenaviruses are all insect-borne. Reducing the number of insects, mainly mosquitoes, is vital to the control of these wretched diseases.

350

In recent years, bats have become the focus of attention for their involvement in incubating and spreading sometimes deadly viruses. A few viral diseases have recently jumped from bats to humans. The Nipah virus, first discovered in 1999, causes a severe, usually fatal brain disease. It went from bats to pigs. Humans who work on farms and abattoirs in southeast Asia were the most commonly infected. (The name Nipah comes from the name of a village in Malaysia where the virus and the disease were first described). The Hendra virus was discovered in horses in Queensland, Australia, in 1994. Horses get the virus by eating feed contaminated by fruit bat saliva and droppings. It can spread from one horse to another or from horses to humans, causing an influenza-like illness with frequent involvement of deep tissues. The bat, known as the flying fox, is the host.

Other viral diseases seen in humans that are thought to have originated in bats are Ebola and coronavirus. There is strong evidence that Nipah and Hendra jumped directly from bats to pigs and horses, respectively, while the Ebola and coronavirus associations are more circumstantial. Most viral diseases associated with bats involve a jump to a non-human animal, then from that animal to humans. That makes sense because, Batman and Count Dracula notwithstanding, humans have minimal contact with bats. (A notable exception, of course, is rabies).

The obvious question is, what is it about bats and their immune systems that places them at the center of such serious viral disorders? There are around 1,500 species of bats, and considerable variability exists between them, but some fascinating facts about bat immunology have emerged.

Flying requires tremendous energy, resulting in many waste products, including oxygen-free radicals. If these accumulate, the result is a build-up of inflammatory cytokines. Such massive, chronic inflammation is detrimental to an animal, so an alternative path is needed. Bats have evolved to produce lower levels of inflammatory cytokines, such as tumor necrosis factor-α (TNF-α), than other mammals. That's good for giving them lower levels of chronic inflammation but really bad for protecting them from viruses' invasion. To compensate, many bats constantly produce low levels of interferon. In other mammals, interferons are produced in an "as-needed" fashion: only when a virus enters the body. The genes responsible for producing interferons are locked when no virus is present. However, because of their particular susceptibility to viruses, bats constantly make interferons, and they are always present (constitutive). This makes for a unique situation for many bats. Viruses can invade, but only at low levels, and they can persist in a sneaky, undetectable way. They can persist and constantly replicate in such a state, and mutations are inevitable. This is especially true if they are RNA viruses prone to multiple mutations.

Many species of bats dine on fruit, either wild or cultivated. When eating a piece of fruit in a tree, bat saliva gets on the material. If a respiratory virus infects the bat, the piece that drops to the ground is contaminated with the virus. Along comes an unwitting animal, say a monkey, palm civet, or pangolin, that eats the remaining fruit, thus infecting itself with the virus initially in the bat. If the virus cannot infect the ground animal, so be it. But if the virus can infect the ground animal, another infection begins. Rarely, the virus mutated to such an extent in the bat that it can infect the ground animal and humans. If humans eat the animal on the ground, trouble, sometimes much trouble, begins.

Chapter 24
Reverse Assault

Acquired horror.
Immune system gone awry.
Pathogens unleashed.

Notorious infectious diseases can usually be traced back hundreds, sometimes thousands of years. Descriptions and allusions to their occurrence are often documented in ancient texts, and physical evidence is sometimes unearthed by current-day researchers. Such information is by its nature speculative, but it's safe to assume that the serious infectious diseases we encounter today were present in a similar form centuries ago.

A notable exception to that general statement is the disease Acquired Immune Deficiency Syndrome, usually referred to as AIDS. Caused by the human immunodeficiency virus, HIV, AIDS was unknown before the year 1981 when the Center for Disease Control and Prevention reported in its publication Morbidity and Mortality Weekly Report the occurrence of five cases of the very rare infectious disease Pneumocystis pneumonia in five previously healthy young males from southern California. Over the next several years many more cases of Pneumocystis pneumonia along with previously rare infections like Kaposi's sarcoma, toxoplasmosis, cryptosporidiosis, and others were reported at an alarming rate. From seemingly out of nowhere this ferocious malady emerged to afflict people around the world.

HIV arose from a similar virus found in chimpanzees, simian immunodeficiency virus, SIV. It has most likely been around for millennia but confined itself to higher primates, excluding humans. During the 20th century, the virus jumped from monkeys to humans, and the previously unknown virus became a worldwide terror in the latter part of the century.

The most likely explanation for the viruses' sudden appearance is related to the changing cultural conditions in Africa over the last hundred and fifty years. Colonialization, industrialization, insurrections, wars, famine, greater mobility, and other events greatly transformed the cultural and social landscape of many countries on the continent.

The social turbulence in many areas was accompanied by famine and starvation. To alleviate hunger, bushmeat became a greater part of the diet, and bushmeat can include primates. The virus was able to jump from the blood of the dead animal and infect a cut on the knife wielder's body. It could then be spread by sexual contact. In addition to sexual spread, medical procedures undoubtedly played a role. In developed countries hypodermic needles are disposable, but in underdeveloped areas, they must be reused. If not sterilized properly the needles can transmit the virus, much like what was seen in the case of intravenous drug users. Sadly, simple medical procedures like the administration of antibiotics, vaccines, and vitamin injections contributed to the emergence of HIV. Modern means of international travel also played a significant role.

Human immunodeficiency virus, HIV, is a strange one. In the biology of advanced organisms, deoxyribonucleic acid, DNA, carries the genetic code. Its codes are transcribed to ribonucleic acid, RNA, and RNA carries out the job of messenger and transfer agent. But HIV does it backward: it is an RNA virus, but its RNA strand is transcribed to DNA instead of the expected RNA. Because of this unique phenomenon, the term retro is applied. HIV is called a retrovirus.

HIV can infect both CD4 lymphocytes, also called T-helper cells, and macrophages. Both have the receptor for HIV, the molecule CD4, extending from their surface. When HIV enters the body, it is usually in the skin or mucus membranes. There aren't many CD4 lymphocytes there, but there are plenty of macrophages, so the virus usually first enters a macrophage. The virus-containing macrophage then dutifully makes its way to the nearest lymph node, where millions of CD4 lymphocytes exist.

Most viruses have a single adhesion molecule to attach to a single receptor on the host cell. HIV has three. The first one on the virus to engage is called gp120. The primary host cell receptor for gp120 is the molecule CD4. To enter the lymphocyte or macrophage, gp120 attaches to the CD4 molecule. Gp120 then alters its shape. In doing so, it binds to a second receptor in addition to CD4. The second receptor is either CCR5 or CXCR4. (CCR5 and CXCR4 are chemokine receptors. Their role in life is to receive chemical signals from cells that have engaged a microbial predator, informing the cell they are on to become active. Ironically, the very part of the immune cell designed to signal an invader's presence is the one HIV uses to help penetrate the cell).

Once gp120 on HIV binds to both the CD4 receptor and the secondary one, its shape changes, and the virus is pulled closer to the cell surface. This signals another viral adhesin, gp41, to become active. When gp41 gets this chemical signal, the virus attaches to the host cell's membrane. The virus then enters the cell.

Once inside the cell, the HIV RNA strand gets active. In the host cell cytoplasm, it is copied to create a single strand of DNA, which then becomes a double strand, the classic DNA double helix. Special enzymes then transport the viral DNA through the nuclear membrane. Once inside the nuclear membrane, the viral DNA is integrated into a host cell chromosome. The integrating enzyme is called, appropriately, integrase. Which chromosome the viral DNA becomes a part of is not constant, but somehow the integrase is usually able to insert into a section that is active and not dormant. The fate of the virus now lies with the nuclear activity of the host cell.

After integration into the host cell chromosome, the viral DNA is transcribed and translated into protein, just like any other host cell gene. Several of the proteins produced are stuck together to form one long one, a polyprotein. These must be cut at the right places to yield individual proteins for incorporation into the new virions. A viral protein called a protease is responsible for the cutting process, nicking the polyproteins at just the right places. The viral proteins and newly formed RNA make their way to the cell membrane, the new virions are constructed, and the virus escapes to seek new T-lymphocytes and macrophages to infect. It is a highly complex process, but one that the virus has mastered. Millions of free virions are created. With all this activity, a massive number of byproducts are also produced.

Cells infected by a virus have chemical sensors letting them know something is wrong. Several remedies are enacted, with apoptosis, an organized form of self-destruction, being an important one. Another form of self-destruction is pyroptosis. With all the viral DNA and other enzymes present in the lymphocyte's cytoplasm, chemical alarm bells activate caspase-1. When caspase-1 is activated, two things happen: the infected cell begins releasing inflammatory cytokines, especially interleukin-1β, and cell death ensues. The cell death induced by pyroptosis is not as controlled as that generated in apoptosis. The word pyro refers to fire or explosive, and it is appropriate. The cell suddenly bursts, releasing the virus's proteins and DNA along with the recently formed inflammatory cytokines. This all attracts cells of the immune system, including CD4 lymphocytes.

An unusual feature of advanced HIV disease is the massive drop-off in the number of CD4 lymphocytes. Oddly, many more of these cells die than are actively infected by the virus. Normally, we have between 500 to 1200 CD4 lymphocytes per cubic millimeter of blood. With most viral infections, the total lymphocyte count usually rises. But with an untreated HIV infection, the number of CD4 lymphocytes drops. If it falls below 200, the immune system cannot function properly; the patient is immunosuppressed.

Some people are born with part of their immune system compromised by a congenital defect. Such problems usually manifest during childhood. If we make it through childhood without observable immunologic problems, we can assume our immune system is not severely damaged. With an infection such as that caused by HIV, our immune system is compromised later in life; it is acquired. When HIV began infecting people in the developed world in the early 1980s, the cause wasn't known. But it was easily seen that people with formerly intact immune systems were becoming gravely ill and dying from infections that a properly functioning immune system normally kept in check. The disease name Acquired Immunodeficiency Disease Syndrome was applied. Most refer to it as AIDS.

CD4 lymphocytes are essential in helping to control pathogenic organisms that infect inside of cells. Those

356

infections progress out of control when HIV infects without treatment. There aren't enough helper T-cells to contain the pathogen. Eight infectious diseases were observed in the early 1980s to be diagnostic for AIDS: The parasitic infections toxoplasmosis and cryptosporidiosis, the fungal diseases cryptococcosis and pneumocystis pneumonia, the viral infections caused by herpes viruses 5 and 8 (cytomegalovirus and the cancer Kaposi's sarcoma), and the bacterial infections caused by *Listeria* and mycobacteria. All these infections are caused by microbes that enter the human cell and cause an infection within. Without the helper CD4 lymphocytes, the containment of infection is highly problematic. Other infections associated with HIV infection are also seen.

Therapy for patients with an HIV infection can seem daunting to the non-specialist. Over two dozen anti-HIV drugs are available, several more are in development, and they are usually administered in combination. Some are administered by injection; others can be taken orally. Thankfully, most anti-HIV drug regimens available today effectively control the infection. Unfortunately, they don't eliminate the virus, and side effects are not uncommon.

The acronym for Anti-Retroviral Therapy is ART. The drugs developed in the early 1990s were delivered singly and came under the heading of ART. Late in the 1990s and the early 2000s, more anti-HIV drugs were available and administered in combination. This approach to therapy was called High Activity Anti-Retroviral Therapy, known as HAART.

HIV has several unique features that anti-virals can target:

1. The proteins that attach the virus to the surface of the CD4 lymphocyte.

   To enter a cell, HIV must first attach and undergo several structural changes in the adhesion molecules. Some drugs block the virus's attachment to co-receptor CCR5, and others bind to viral protein gp41, thus preventing viral penetration.

2. The proteins that incorporate nucleic acids into the growing viral-induced DNA strand in the host cell cytoplasm.

    Transcribing RNA into DNA in the host cell cytoplasm is not a natural event. It is directed by an enzyme of the virus, RNA polymerase, which constructs the nascent strand of viral DNA. Some drugs prevent the elongation of the growing viral DNA strand in the cytoplasm.

3. The protein that incorporates the viral double-stranded DNA into the host cell DNA (integrase).

    The viral DNA must be transported to the host cell nucleus and placed into an active site of a host cell chromosome. Anti-integrase drugs prevent this from happening.

4. The protein that breaks up the long strand of viral proteins and frees up individual viral proteins to form a new virus (protease).

    HIV is vulnerable in the way it constructs its proteins. Instead of cranking them out individually, it creates one long chain of proteins that must be clipped at key sites to free up each individual protein. The viral protein that chops up the long poly-protein is called a protease. The drugs that interfere with viral protease are called protease inhibitors.

Like many RNA viruses, the polymerases copying the RNA are prone to mistakes, so the DNA integrated into the host cell nucleus often has alterations. These can lead to mutations, and HIV is notorious for these changes, which can sometimes enable the virus to evade the immune system or drugs. To get around this problem, anti-HIV drugs must be administered in combination. If one of the target sites has been altered and the virus has developed resistance, chances are high that it remains susceptible at one or two other targeted sites. The use of combination therapy for HIV has proven this theory correct: the incidence of full-blown AIDS secondary to HIV infection has dropped precipitously when appropriate combination therapy is prescribed and adhered to.

Most human cases of HIV are caused by a type that is believed to have infected chimpanzees, then became able to infect humans. It's known as HIV-1. A second type was first detected in the late 1980s. Found in West Africa, it most likely was zoonotic in sooty mangabeys before infecting humans. It's known as HIV-2. HIV-1 is far more common and potentially damaging, but HIV-2 is still a threat. Some of the effective drugs against HIV-1 are much less effective against HIV-2.

The clinical laboratory is vital in the diagnosis and management of infections by HIV. Detection of viral antibodies and viral RNA assist with the diagnosis. Enumeration of CD4 lymphocytes in the bloodstream and the amount of virus present, known as viral load, are essential in monitoring the effectiveness of therapy. HIV today isn't the scourge it was when first discovered, but it can still cause irreparable harm if not effectively managed. Scrupulous diligence is necessary.

Chapter 25
The World's Greatest Unintended Consequence
The smallest virus
Causes such immense misery.
Benumbed cruelty.

Anyone who lived in the 1940s and 50s would react much differently to the word polio than someone born later. The very name of the disease is enough to elicit painful memories for those of us who lived through the epidemic. To see bright, active, happy children and young adults brought down by this mysterious ailment was something you never forget. Every community, and just about every neighborhood, was affected—a girl in your school, a boy in your Little League, your cousin's best friend. Everyone knew of someone who was stricken. History books show how the world united to fight aggression in World War II. The united fight against polio was no less compelling.

But it wasn't always that way. Before 1900 polio was a rare disease. It wasn't even called polio, but infantile paralysis. Only a few hundred scattered cases a year occurred in the U.S. in the late 1800s. In the early 20th century, a few more cases started to appear. Doctors had to consult their medical books to refresh their memories to make a diagnosis. As the years passed, more cases occurred, and small epidemics were noticed in various communities. Then, the big one, New York and the northeastern United States, 1916. Over 27,000 cases of paralytic polio were reported, with over 6,000 deaths. The pandemic had begun.

With anything so profound and sudden, wild explanations are inevitable. The most common and pernicious reasoning blamed the war raging in Europe and refugees arriving in the U.S.—"the 'foreigners' were bringing the disease to America." Open hostility toward European immigrants was not unusual, and a difficult situation was made even worse. Science wasn't much help, since a virus causes the disease, and the technology of the time had very little information on those microorganisms. The disease was thought to be infectious, but the cause and means of spread were unknown.

As time went on, the disease spread. It was mainly observed in summer, but sporadic outbreaks would occur throughout the year. Soon the entire country was affected. There was no cure.

Now that polio is under control in developed countries and its cause has been elucidated, the reason for its sudden emergence in the early 1900s has become apparent. Astoundingly, it was the introduction of sanitation.

Throughout history, the virus has been widespread. The lack of proper sanitation exposed virtually everyone to the polio virus. Water was often contaminated; there were no flushable toilets and very little running water. People would rarely even wash their hands except to remove large amounts of dirt, and folks often shared the same wash basin. The polio virus spread nearly universally, and just about everyone contracted it.

When a woman became pregnant, she had already developed antibodies to the virus, protecting her. These antibodies would go from the mother to her baby in the uterus, a process known as passive immunity. Passing these antibodies into the baby in utero makes the newborn immune to the virus for about six months after birth. Since the virus was so common, the baby would encounter it during the first few months of life and develop its own immunity while still protected by its mother's antibodies. This is referred to as naturally acquired immunity.

What changed was the introduction of sanitation. Around the turn of the century, scientists discovered the link between contaminated water and infectious diseases like cholera, typhoid, and dysentery. The introduction of good plumbing and the establishment of a public mindset about personal hygiene significantly reduced the exposure of the turn-of-the-century youngster to naturally occurring viruses. Their mother's antibodies still protected them, but those dissipated after about six months. Because of sanitary practices, the children weren't exposed to the virus and didn't develop their own active immunity. These kids grew up without naturally acquired immunity, making them susceptible to the virus. It seems ironic, but the introduction of sanitation was primarily responsible for the onslaught of polio in the modern world.

The virus that causes polio is a member of a large group called the enteroviruses. About 80 different enteroviruses are known. Some cause severe disease; others are more benign. Individual enteroviruses are made up of a core of ribonucleic acid, or RNA, surrounded by a protein wrapping. The protein coat allows the virus to attach to a specific receptor on a human cell, sort of like microbial Velcro. The virus wanders around until it finds its receptor, attaches, and the infection begins. The only thing that prevents attachment are antibodies specific to the virus, preventing its attachment.

Polio is caused by three different viruses, called simply enough poliovirus 1, 2, and 3. All three can cause neurologic disease. Resistance to one does not convey resistance to the others.

Poliovirus enters the body through the mouth, either by food or drink. The enteroviruses are very stable in acid, so they withstand stomach acid. In the days of the polio epidemics, it was commonly held that kids should avoid swimming pools, which was probably good advice, even though the virus is rapidly killed by chlorine. Once the virus enters the intestinal tract, the infectious process begins. Where it stops is nearly impossible to predict.

Which cells the polio virus initially enters is not absolutely known, but we have a pretty good idea. Experimental evidence is conclusive that the virus enters the tissues mainly through the cells lining the distal small intestine, the ileum. When we look at the landscape of the epithelial cells on this mucosal surface, it looks like a shag carpet with a few manhole covers strewn about. The "shag carpet" is the villi of the enterocytes lining the small bowel. (The word *villus,* pleural *villi,* is Latin, meaning "shaggy hair"). The "manhole covers" are the so-called M-cells, short for microfold cells. These cells lack the finger-like projections of the enterocytes. Instead, they have a very rough, convoluted surface and lay flat. They overlay lymphoid cells. Both cells contain the polio virus receptor.

Whether the polio virus enters the intestinal epithelial cell or the M-cell is not known. It could be both. There are similar receptive tissues in the mouth, and they could also enter there. However, there is no conclusive evidence that polio can be a respiratory infection. If the mouth is the source for the introduction of the organism, it must be from the food or water consumed.

The host cell receptor for the virus is a protein that is usually referred to as simply PVR, for poliovirus receptor. Its actual name is CD155. This very interesting protein has multiple uses. For one, it forms part of the "glue" that holds cells together, preventing fluid leakage. It is especially important for the tight junctions between adjoining cells. It helps form the sides of endothelial and epithelial cells. Another function is less well-defined, but given its ubiquity, it is obviously very important. Many cells of the body, not just those of the intestinal tract, express CD155 as a molecule that is anchored in the cytoplasm but extends beyond the cell membrane into the environment. It seems to act as a signal to cells of the immune system as to the health of the cell—it is over-expressed when conditions such as cancer or infection occur, letting immune cells, such as natural killer lymphocytes, destroy the cell before it gets out of control. A soluble portion of the CD155 molecule also resembles an antibody. It can break off and end up in the serum. To date, we don't know its function since it is non-specific.

The CD155 protein has three sections, or domains, outside the cell, designated D1, D2, and D3. All three types of poliovirus attach to the D1 part of the molecule. The attachment protein on the virus is a bit unusual. It is not a spike of a molecule out from the surface of the virus. Instead, it is a crevice, or "canyon," in the viral coat (capsid). The CD155 D1 molecule sticks down into the viral canyon, and the attachment is firm. The viral coat proteins break apart immediately after hooking onto its receptor. The single strand of viral RNA makes its way into the cell, then goes to the cell's ribosomes to begin transcription and the production of viral proteins.

All three of the polio types enter the cell and replicate similarly. Most of our cells contain the CD155 molecule, so poliovirus is not restricted to a single cell type like most viruses are, but they initially enter the body through cells in the small intestine.

Poliovirus is a member of the enterovirus family, which is classified as a picornavirus. "Pico" is a mathematical term meaning very small, and rna means, well, RNA. The standard measurement for the size of viruses is the number of kilo base pairs, abbreviated kb. Polio and the other enteroviruses are among the smallest human-associated viruses, at about 7-8 kb. By comparison, influenza, a negative sense segmented RNA virus, weighs in at around 12-15 kb. The leader in size is the smallpox virus, about 200 kb.

The tiny naked strand of messenger RNA from the virus is capable of great things, virally speaking. The first order of business is for it to make its way to a cellular ribosome for transcription. It carries the correct origination codes, so as soon as it meets an intact ribosome, it gets transcribed, yielding one long chain of amino acids called a polypeptide. This polypeptide is made up of all eleven virus proteins stuck together. It is much more efficient for the virus to construct its proteins this way rather than individually; it requires fewer enzymes and RNA initiation sequences.

One of the viral proteins, known as Protein 2A, is an absolute marvel. It is like the Swiss Army knife of viral proteins, having multiple uses. Its first order of business is to cleave the long polypeptide of viral proteins into individual proteins, first into four parts, then into all the individual proteins. The virus is now cranking out all its proteins using the ribosomal machinery of the cell.

The virus then must shut down the cell's ability to make its own proteins. Protein 2A is active here as well. The cell has a series of molecules that escort cellular messenger RNA from the nucleus to the ribosome and allow it to be translated to make protein. One of the escort proteins, with the forgettable name of eIF4G, is cleaved by Protein 2A, stopping the host cell's messenger RNA in its tracks so that nearly all host cell protein synthesis is shut down. The virus has now completely controlled the cell's manufacturing capability.

The ability of the viral RNA to dictate the generation of viral proteins is truly astounding. Four viral proteins are structural and used in the capsid or virus coating. Each one requires sixty copies for each new virus, for a total of 240 protein molecules. That's just for one virus. Tens of thousands of individual viruses (virions) are to be made, so the number of copies of proteins is very high. The viral messenger RNA goes about making these virtually unimpeded by the cell.

Another essential part of the virus-making operation is the production of many copies of its RNA. The virus has a positive sense variety but needs a negative sense strand to make RNA copies. A viral polymerase from among the eleven proteins takes on this task, and positive-sense RNA is manufactured from the negative-sense one. Briefly, the two form double-stranded RNA until the positive sense one breaks away. This double-stranded RNA is unique to viruses; human cells have only single-stranded RNA. Double-stranded RNA is a dead giveaway to the chemical sensors of the cell that a viral invader is present.

After several hours of viral transcription, tens of thousands of viral proteins and nucleic acid strands are made, a somewhat chaotic situation. To bring some order to the process, the virus has a protein that effectively hijacks the cellular autosomes. Autosomes are the cell's "garbage dump," small vesicles designed to eliminate cellular waste. The virus has ways of incorporating all its parts, protein and nucleic, into these autosomes for easier viral assembly. True efficiency.

The cell, meanwhile, is just serving as this little virus factory, producing tens of thousands of virions while its own business is put on hold. This cannot be allowed to go on. Human cells, both professional phagocytes and others, have a vast array of chemicals at their disposal to put an end to all of this. The very best one against viruses is called interferon.

The interferons are proteins but very small and nimble. They represent the body's best defense against most invaders, especially viruses. They don't act directly against the invading microbe like an antibiotic, but instead, they serve to alert and prime cells to make them more resistant to the microbes' invasive efforts.

There are about a couple of dozen distinct interferons, all subtypes of the three main ones, interferon-alpha (IFN-α), interferon-beta (IFN-β), and interferon-gamma. The first two, alpha and beta, are most effective in preventing viral and acute bacterial infections. Interferon-gamma is designed to enhance macrophages to rid the body of, or at least contain, intracellular pathogens, organisms such as the tuberculosis bacillus. The alpha and beta interferons come into play for viral infections like polio. The alpha and beta interferons are called type 1; interferon gamma is type 2.

Once an invader like a virus enters the host cell, it activates at least two different molecules that send signals to the cell's nucleus and alert it that trouble is afoot. One is called the Toll-like receptor (TLR), and the other RIG-I-like receptor (RLR). (Humans have 10 TLRs, six in the cell membrane and four inside the cytoplasm. Each detects different groups of microbes. RLRs are inside the cell and are specific for viruses). The molecules within these two groups are constructed to detect a part of the microbe that is different from human. Double-stranded RNA is a good example. Activating either TLR or RLR initiates a chain reaction of intracellular molecules that releases chemical agents that migrate to the cell's nucleus to unlock the genes that code for interferon. The DNA coding for these small proteins is unleashed, and messenger RNA is dispatched to the ribosomes to produce them. It is really an elegant system.

The interferons are powerful medicine. While they don't directly kill the invader, they have the power to help protect virtually every cell in the body from further attack. Our cells are rich in interferon receptors, and when a flood of interferon is released, all our cells go into protective mode. Once cells are activated by interferon, viruses do not as easily cross into them. When they do, they are met with an onslaught of anti-viral proteins and defensive mechanisms, preventing their reproduction. The infected cells are much more likely to send chemical signals to their surface, instructing killer lymphocytes to destroy them before they become virus factories. After the release of interferons alpha and beta, virus reproduction goes way down, even before the onset of acquired immunity and the release of specific antibodies.

There is a downside to interferon release, however. It makes us feel sick. The fever, muscle aches, headaches, diarrhea, mucus release, and the like do not come directly from the presence of a virus. It is due to the body's response to the viral invasion in the form of interferons and cytokines like tumor necrosis factor-alpha (TNF-alpha). The untoward release of large amounts of interferon can bring about a significant amount of tissue damage. Its storage and release must be carefully guarded.

About one hundred and fifty genes code for interferons and similar proteins the body uses to fight off invading microbes. Because of the damage they can cause, they are sequestered; there is a chemical overlay of the DNA section on which the genes reside. It's like locking up armaments in an armory until you are sure you really need them. When the cell is under attack, a chemical signal is sent from the cytoplasm through the nuclear membrane and into the DNA region. This signaling molecule unlocks the protective overlay of the section of DNA harboring these important genes. The interferon and cytokine genes are then copied, and messenger RNA is sent to the cell's ribosomes to be decoded and the proteins made.

The defense system is very sophisticated and highly developed, but there is a vulnerability in the scheme that the polioviruses have exploited. Both the signaling compounds going into the nucleus and messenger RNA bearing the coding for the proteins coming out must pass through a channel in the nuclear membrane. There are three protein parts of these channels: the structure of the channel (or pore), the proteins that anchor it to the nuclear membrane, and the proteins needed to escort the signal proteins into the nucleus and messenger RNA out. It is this set of escort proteins that the poliovirus attacks so that very little can get into the nucleus and very little out. It's like a burglar who cuts the alarm and phone lines while inside the building, cutting down communication.

The nuclear transporting proteins are severed by poliovirus protein 2A, the same one that is used to chop up the viral polyprotein and shut down cellular RNA transcription. Without chemical communication with the nucleus, the host cell's ability to produce proteins is significantly curtailed. This includes the manufacture and release of interferon. The virus has completely controlled the cellular apparatus and can propagate without interference.

The amount of virus produced in a single cell is amazing. Over a hundred thousand new viruses can be made in a relatively short amount of time. Each virus has a coat of 240 proteins plus its RNA payload. Upon release, each of these can infect other cells, either close by or in some remote area of the body.

The release of all those newly made polio virions from the cell is made possible by a protein similar to Protein 2A: Protein 2B. This enzyme increases the permeability of cellular membranes. Just a few don't have much of an effect, but when they are produced by the tens of thousands, their development reaches critical mass, and the host cell's membrane bursts, releasing the virus.

Once released from the host cell, the virus has three directions it can go. One is to infect nearby cells, creating many more virions. The second is to enter the lumen of the bowel and be excreted with the infected person's stool to perhaps infect another individual. Thirdly, they can passively diffuse into the deeper tissues to eventually be picked up by lymphoid tissues and make their way into the bloodstream. All three occur, and how much of each seems to depend on random chance.

The virus greatly curtails the body's immediate immune response, but the response is not zero. A small amount of interferon is always made, and a few lymphocytes are activated. However, so much virus is made that its elimination is substantially delayed, allowing the poliovirus' presence in the body to continue for some days.

The first phase of viral infection is usually not accompanied by symptoms in the patient. The symptoms of fever, muscle aches, diarrhea, and the like are created by the body's immune response to the virus, not the local damage the virus causes. But these immune response symptoms are greatly mitigated by the activity of viral proteins, so we can excrete rather large amounts of the virus without knowing we are infected. This can go on for some weeks. One reason polio is so infectious is that asymptomatic carriers outnumber sick ones.

Around 70% of people infected with the poliovirus have this asymptomatic type of infection. Once infected, even without symptoms, we become immune for life to the infecting strain. However, being immune to one type of polio virus does not confer immunity to the other two types.

The virions that enter the circulation are randomly carried around the body, but they tend to eventually enter the tissues of the reticuloendothelial system, organs such as the spleen, liver, and bone marrow. The initial entry of the virus into the bloodstream is called a viremia, the "vir" part from virus, the "emia" from the Greek *haima*, meaning blood. The poliovirus in the blood at this stage of the disease does not result in very profound symptoms, perhaps just a mild fever. This stage is referred to as minor viremia. About 25% of polio-infected patients display this condition only. It is called abortive poliomyelitis.

In most cases, once the virus enters the tissues of the reticuloendothelial system, its days are numbered. These organs are rich in anti-viral immune cells, aided by complement, interferon, and other cytokines, as well as newly formed IgM antibodies to eliminate the virus. It is not understood why it happens, but in a few individuals, less than 5% of those infected, the virus isn't stopped at this stage. Maybe infected individuals didn't mount enough of an interferon or antibody response. At any rate, the tissues of the infected organs all contain the poliovirus receptor, CD155, on their surface and, therefore, can become infected. If this happens, there is a massive release of the virus, many of which enter the bloodstream for a second time, known as a major viremia. If this happens, the patient becomes very ill. High fever, prostration, rapid pulse, profound muscle aches. Following major viremia, the virus can enter the central nervous system.

Poliovirus is not the only member of the enterovirus group that can enter the central nervous system. In fact, most cases of viral meningitis (usually called aseptic meningitis because it doesn't involve bacteria) are caused by an enterovirus. Aseptic meningitis is usually not a life-threatening disease. The patient feels terrible for a few days with headaches, fever, and perhaps some disorientation, but symptoms usually resolve without requiring intensive medical intervention.

Some, probably the majority, of polio victims having central nervous system involvement have this self-limited meningitis, much like that caused by other enteroviruses. It generally lasts a few days to a week, and the patient recovers completely. Most enterovirus meningitis cases do not require hospitalization—just a spinal tap to send fluid to the lab to confirm the diagnosis and some palliative care.

In all these conditions, the poliovirus does not differ significantly from other enteroviruses: many cases of asymptomatic infection with a few considerable illnesses, to even fewer with a limited form of meningitis. But then there is the bad one: paralytic polio.

The nerves that signal the movement of our muscles, the motor neurons, originate in a portion of the spinal cord called the anterior, or ventral, horn. The similar structure on the back, or dorsal side, is called the posterior horn, which functions in a sensory capacity. When the poliovirus makes it into this area, it can only infect and damage the neurons of the anterior horn, the motor neurons. The sensory nerves of the posterior horn are not involved. The reason for this needs to be clarified. Perhaps the motor neurons contain more of the poliovirus receptors than the sensory neurons.

The motor neurons are composed of cells commonly called gray matter because of their color, which occurs because their axons are mainly unmyelinated. The white matter has mainly myelinated axons and appears white. The Greek word for "gray" is *polios*, and their word for spinal cord, or marrow, is *myelos*, hence poliomyelitis.

For many years, there was debate and uncertainty about how the polio virus entered the anterior horn motor neurons. Was it from the bloodstream after the virus had caused a major viremia, or did it enter at the tip of the axon, where it meets the muscle? The two are not mutually exclusive, and both may occur. The axons of motor neurons do not contain ribosomes for the virus to replicate. However, they have a "transportation system," which allows for the carriage of material back to the cell body in the anterior horn, the part of the cell where the virus can replicate. The proteins dynein and kinesin attach to and move proteins and tiny organelles around the axon, dynein going from the distal axon to the cell body, and kinesin the other way. It is certainly possible that poliovirus may enter the neuron at the junction of the muscle and the axon, encase itself in a small autosome-like structure, then be pulled back to the ribosome-containing cell body for replication, with the resultant cell-destructive consequences. It has been known for some time that if an individual suffered a muscle injury coincident with the onset of polio, the injured muscle was commonly the first one affected, suggesting the virus may jump from the infected injured muscle to the adjoining neuron.

The paralysis that ensues is what is known as flaccid, that is, limp or lacking firmness. The word flaccid, which may be pronounced in two ways: "flak-sid" or "flass-sid," comes from the Latin *flaccus*, meaning flabby. The sensory neurons are not damaged, so the patient can feel the affected limb but cannot move it because of the damaged motor neurons. The number of motor neurons involved and the muscles they innervate occurs randomly, although the legs are often the most commonly affected. Paralysis almost always occurs while the patient is febrile; when the fever stops, so does the progression of neuronal involvement. Once that happens, it is a waiting game. Most patients recover at least part of the function of the paralyzed limb; others do not. If the muscular damage has not abated after about a month, the chances are it will be permanent.

Even worse than the paralytic form of the disease is bulbar. The "bulb" refers to the medulla oblongata, the bulb-like portion of the spinal cord connecting it to the brain. It contains the cranial nerves, and it's usually the ninth and tenth cranial nerves that become involved. These control the pharynx and larynx, among other things, so swallowing and breathing are impacted, making bulbar poliomyelitis life-threatening. 5% to 35% of paralytic polio cases also involve the bulbar form. The lungs themselves and the diaphragm and intercostal muscles are not affected. Usually, the damaged cranial nerves recover within a week to ten days, but respiratory assistance and intravenous feeding are required to get over the immediate crisis.

In summary: the polio virus enters us through our water and food. It primarily infects us through the cells lining the distal small intestine, the ileum, although it may enter through similar cells in the mouth. The virus binds to the polio virus receptor, CD155, a long three-headed molecule. One part of it, the D1 portion, extends into a crevice in the protein coat of the polio virus. This triggers the break-up of the coat and the injection of the positive-sense single-strand of RNA into the cell. This viral RNA is decoded by a ribosome in the cell, yielding one long chain of the virus' eleven proteins, all stuck together. One of the viral proteins, 2A, breaks off and cuts free the other 10. Host cell protein synthesis is cut off by the action of Protein 2A, damaging one of the cell's proteins necessary for RNA transcription. The chemical signals warning of the microbe's presence are usually sent from the cytoplasm to the nucleus. But the polio viral protein 2A significantly interferes with this process, and the manufacture of cellular proteins, like interferon, is much reduced. Protein 2A takes out the molecules that escort these chemical signals and host cell RNA through the nuclear membrane. The virus normally develops in the cell's autosomes.

After reaching a critical mass, the assembled virus escapes, numbering in the tens or hundreds of thousands. Some enter nearby cells, others are eliminated in the stool, and some make their way into the bloodstream, causing a minor viremia. When these blood-borne virions reach the tissues of the reticuloendothelial system, like the spleen, liver, and bone marrow, they are usually destroyed. But in a few individuals, they multiply to reach new high levels and are released into the bloodstream, giving a major viremia. They can then reach the neurons of the spinal cord's anterior horn and cause neural damage. Some enter the ninth and tenth cranial nerves causing problems in the pharynx and larynx, including swallowing and breathing.

The time frame for the progression of symptoms varies, but typically is:

Incubation time for the virus, from presumed first contact to excretion of the virus in the stool, is three days.

Abortive poliomyelitis, characterized by fever, perhaps a headache, vomiting, and listlessness, 5-6 days after presumed first contact.

Non-paralytic poliomyelitis, similar to meningitis caused by other enteroviruses, occurs around a week to ten days after exposure.

Paralytic and bulbar polio take place 12-15 days after exposure.

There is no specific anti-viral treatment for the poliovirus.

One of the more excruciating parts of polio is the "waiting game" that accompanies the paralytic and bulbar forms. Some patients displaying these symptoms recover most or even all of their muscular activity after a week to ten days of paralysis. Some don't, although polio's bulbar form usually reverses if the patient can be kept alive. If the paralytic symptoms don't subside after a month, the chances are high that the damage is permanent.

A condition known as the post-polio syndrome is an interesting sequela of patients who have recovered some or all their muscular function. It occurred in about 20-30% of paralytic polio patients years after the initial disease. It presented as a gradual onset of weakness, pain, and fatigue in the muscles initially involved in the disease. Neither the virus nor antibody to it is found, so the most reasonable explanation is that the neurons that took up the job of innervating these damaged areas become overworked with age and give out. The condition is not usually severely disabling but can impact the quality of life.

A device that came to symbolize polio was the negative pressure respirator, better known as the iron lung. Today we use the positive pressure device known as a ventilator, in which a tube is inserted into the airway, and air is pumped in. But in the 1930s and 40s, there was a real problem of pulmonary infection after intubation, and there were no antibiotics to treat pneumonia and possible sepsis. Most polio patients with bulbar disease would recover the ability to breathe independently after a week or two, and the iron lung was a safe way to pull them through the crisis without risking serious infection.

The prototype iron lung was developed by two scientists at Harvard, Philip Drinker and Louis Agassiz Shaw, in 1927. It consisted of two vacuum motors pulling air out of the chamber. Doing this also pulled the air out of the patient's lungs. After each cycle, air rushed back into the chamber, filling the vacuum and expanding the lungs. The machine was calibrated to cycle about 15 times per minute but could be adjusted. Various modifications of the original version were developed. Still, the cost of the machines (about $1,500, nearly the price of a new home in those days) and their distribution were always a problem. During spikes in the number of seriously ill patients, it wasn't unusual to have a shortage of machines. Difficult decisions had to be made.

Another "symbol" of the polio era was not a machine, but a person, Sister Elizabeth Kenny of Australia. She was not a Catholic nun, as the "Sister" title might imply, but a nurse, albeit without formal training. The term "sister" was frequently used in British and Australian hospitals to refer to the head nurse of a unit, what we might call a charge nurse today. Elizabeth Kenny was very proud of the title when it was bestowed on her because she didn't have much formal education and learned the nursing profession the hard way: through many years of arduous work and on-the-job training.

Elizabeth (Lisa to her friends) Kenny was born in 1880 in Warialda, New South Wales, Australia. Her father was an immigrant Irish farmer; her mother was a local. At a young age, she took an interest in nursing and learned from any who would allow her to accompany them. Eventually, she possessed enough knowledge to treat patients independently, often riding alone on horseback to see patients, usually for no fee. By 1910, at age 30, Elizabeth Kenny was a very talented, knowledgeable nurse, though she had no degree to hang on her wall.

In 1911 a few cases of a mysterious illness affecting children appeared in New South Wales. It was new to Elizabeth, but upon corresponding with Dr. Aeneas McDonnell, a physician in Toowoomba, the diagnosis of infantile paralysis

374

was suspected. He instructed her to treat the patients with hot cloth "fomentations," a mixture of ointments and other potions. The few patients she had all recovered. It left an indelible mark on her.

In 1915 Elizabeth enlisted in the Australian Army Medical Service and was assigned to a troopship treating injured military personnel being transported back home. She remained in military service in this capacity until 1919. She was given the title "Sister" for her exemplary nursing service.

During the 1920s, she continued her nursing career in Australia, spending most of her time with traumatic injury cases that needed rehabilitation. She also treated polio patients. By this time, the polio epidemic was expanding, with many more patients presenting for medical treatment. Ms. Kenny continued to employ her heat and passive movement method, similar to what she would use on a traumatic injury. This ran counter to the accepted theory of the day, which called for immobilization of the affected area with splints and braces to prevent the onset of a skeletal deformity. She was very good with her patients, both children and adults. The kids just loved her, and the parents had many of their fears and anxieties relieved. She exuded an air of confidence and understanding, sometimes lacking in other healthcare professionals. Her reputation grew and spread.

Her supporters said that Elizabeth Kenny's methods were superior to that used by the conventional medical practitioners of the day. People swore that her methods led to a more rapid and complete recovery from the paralysis of polio. Even patients who had been affected for some time maintained that her methods led to at least some recovery. She was confident in her methods and sought to persuade the medical establishment of its success. But, for several reasons, her supplications usually fell on deaf ears. In some cases, there was even open hostility.

One area in which Ms. Kenny was decidedly wrong was her conviction that polio was a muscular disease and that it should be handled in much the same way as a traumatic muscle injury. She was not trained in the formal medical arts. Whether she was aware of the pathology studies showing damage to the anterior horn motor neuron as opposed to the muscle itself, we don't know. But when medical doctors hear a nurse expounding on treatment while professing a "fact" they know to be incorrect, they tend not to listen. Then there are generally three types of patients afflicted with the paralytic form of the disease: those who recover entirely after a week or two, those who don't recover at all, and those who recover some muscular ability over time. One cannot predict the outcome when the patient first presents for treatment, and the question always arises: did the treatment in the first week or so really speed recovery, or was it just the natural progression of the disease? Since paralytic polio only affects humans, there is no way to do animal experiments to find out. The results, by their nature, are merely intuitive. It is not unlike the arguments one hears for alternative therapies today: was it the herb, supplement, or practice undertaken, or something else? The placebo effect, perhaps?

Nevertheless, Sister Elizabeth Kenny's methods and reputation grew exponentially. People came from all over the world to her Australian clinic, and she eventually visited England and the United States, where she was awarded many honors. Hollywood even made a movie about her, "Sister Kenny," starring Rosalind Russell.

Besides treating polio patients, Sister Kenny was known for treating debilitating wounds and developed many effective therapies. In 1927 she introduced the Sylvia ambulance stretcher, designed to reduce trauma during medical transport. (It was named for the first person transported on it). Some regard her as one of the founders of physical therapy.

Sister Kenny contracted Parkinson's disease in 1951, retired to Toowoomba, Australia, and died about a year later. She never married, and despite her fame and hard work, she never made much money. She sincerely desired to help those in need—a remarkable woman.

Of course, when someone today thinks about people and polio, the name Jonas Salk is the first, and sometimes only, name that comes to mind. Iron lungs and physical therapy were beneficial aids in treating afflicted persons, but the ideal is not to get the disease in the first place. Vaccines and their effectiveness had been known for some time, since 1800, in fact, in the use of the smallpox vaccine. By the late 1930s, several vaccines were widely available, including those for diphtheria, tetanus, typhoid, and others. Directly treating a virus with an anti-viral agent, as an antibiotic treats a bacterial infection, was out of the question. The only medical approach to eliminating the threat of the disease was the employment of a suitable vaccine.

Two schools of thought prevailed on vaccine development in the 1940s: live, attenuated strains given in the same manner as a natural infection but unable to induce disease, and "killed," or inactivated virus injected into the body. Emotions ran high on both approaches. In the case of a "killed" virus, can we always be sure it is really "dead?" Are viruses alive in the first place? They can't reproduce on their own, and without a cell to invade and do their metabolism, they just sit there. The inactivation of a virus by chemical agents may result in a virus that may still be viable under certain circumstances, or the inactivation process alters its chemical structure to make the antibody response irrelevant to the actual wild-type virus. For live, attenuated viruses, the potential problem lay in the possibility that a suitable type would never be found, or the attenuated type could revert to the wild type and initiate the disease.

Journalists and historians tend to focus on a particular individual when a remarkable feat is accomplished. Edward Jenner is commonly referred to as the conqueror of smallpox, and Alexander Fleming the discoverer of penicillin. They deserve great praise, but others were involved in their breakthrough discoveries. Many of the local farmers in Jenner's time were well aware that milkmaids who got "the cowpox" on their hands were immune to smallpox. Jenner listened to their tale, tested it, then wrote a letter to London's Royal Society about his results. He had the wherewithal to test and reports his findings, but the actual discovery of the process lay with others. Fleming did indeed observe and test the ability of "mold juice" to kill bacteria. Still, the discovery lay dormant in his lab until Ernst Chain and Howard Florey at Oxford did the work to make penicillin a usable pharmaceutical product.

Jonas Salk certainly deserves the accolades that have been his through the years. But we mustn't forget those whose work preceded and accompanied his to make his accomplishment possible. The existence of three distinct types of poliovirus was confirmed by the work of John R. Paul and James Trask in 1931. The three types were initially called Brunhilde (type 1), Lansing (type 2), and Leon (type 3). They also confirmed that polio was an enteric infection. Albert Sabin and Peter Olitsky were the first to successfully cultivate the polio viruses in cell culture, using human embryonic neuronal tissue, in 1936. Until then, it was impossible to grow the virus in artificial culture. Unfortunately, this cell line was difficult to perpetuate and maintain. The enormous breakthrough by John Enders, Thomas Weller, and Frederick Robbins in 1949 led to the polio virus's cultivation in non-neuronal cell lines, which led to the ability of Jonas Salk to do his work. Until then, one couldn't get enough virus from cell cultures to produce enough to do vaccine experiments. The work of Enders, Weller, and Robbins allowed this to happen. They were jointly awarded the Nobel Prize in medicine in 1954 for their work.

Jonas Salk's inactivated vaccine was first tested in 1954. All three types of the polio virus harvested from monkey kidney cells were mixed in about equal quantities and inactivated by suspending them in formalin (dilute formaldehyde). About 1.6 million children from the U.S., Canada, and Finland were enrolled in the field trial. Some got the inactivated virus, some got a placebo (saline injected into the arm), and some got nothing. This was the most extensive field trial of a vaccine in history. The number of children in the trial was so large because the number of paralytic polio victims in an infected population was small, less than 1%, and it was necessary to vaccinate a vast number of children to give a result with statistical relevance. The trial was a great success, and the vaccine, with great fanfare, was approved for use in the United States in April 1955.

The success of the use of the vaccine was unmistakable. In 1954 the incidence of paralytic polio was 13.9 cases per 100,000 population. By 1961 that number had decreased to 0.8 cases per 100,000. There was no question that the vaccine was working, but there were problems. The most obvious one was the "Cutter incident," which occurred in 1955. The Cutter Laboratories in California contracted to make large amounts of the polio vaccine. Unfortunately, the vaccine it produced was defective, with significant amounts of virus remaining viable. Injecting this live virus into the arms of susceptible children was a catastrophe. There were a reported 260 cases of paralytic polio and ten deaths. Either the vaccine preparation had too much foreign material in it, or some of the viral particles clumped, shielding them from the action of the formaldehyde. A second filtration step was soon added, and ensuing preparations were non-infectious, but the "Cutter incident" lives on in vaccine infamy.

One of the problems with the early polio vaccines was the source of the cells to cultivate the virus in the laboratory. The cell line that worked best was that taken from the kidneys of monkeys, especially rhesus macaques from south and central Asia and green monkeys from west Africa. Making a million doses of the polio vaccine took about 1500 monkeys. That's a lot of monkeys, and they were usually taken right out of the jungle. There was always the worry that even though they looked healthy, there could still be something wrong with them, and, sure enough, it was discovered a few years after vaccine production began in full force that some of the imported monkeys were infected with a virus called a polyomavirus (that's POLYOMA, not polio). Its official name is Simian vacuolating virus 40, but most refer to it as SV40. It is a circular double-stranded DNA virus that replicates mainly in the infected cell's nucleus. The virus usually stays attached to the nuclear material of the cell it infects, although sometimes it escapes, killing the cell it resided in.

There has long been concern about what a virus like this could do to a human. It was estimated in 1960 by Ben Sweet and Maurice Hilleman that about 10-30% of people given the polio vaccine had also been injected with the SV40 monkey virus. Usually, the virus sits on the nucleus and does nothing, but there is always a chance it can become active and cause some type of cancer. There is a human counterpart to SV40, the JK and BK viruses. They are pretty common, but neither does much unless the infected person becomes immunosuppressed by HIV infection or immunosuppressive therapy. Perhaps the SV40 virus acts in the same way. Today's cell lines for producing the polio virus for vaccines are laboratory cell lines, not wild type, so they don't contain any viruses other than the one being cultivated.

Another drawback to the Salk vaccine was that the virus was inactivated and administered intramuscularly, certainly not its usual means of entering the body. The immune system to combat foreign organisms consists of two cell lines, the B-lymphocytes and the T-lymphocytes. The B-cells make the antibody, and the T-cells enhance antibody production and are primarily responsible for immune memory. The IM administration of a dead organism usually stimulates only the B-cells. Also, a single injection may fail to elicit an appropriate B-cell response, so more shots, usually three, must be administered to ensure a good antibody response. In addition, a shot to "boost" the immune response, commonly called a booster shot, should be given 4-6 years after the first series of shots. If only the B-cell line was stimulated initially, the immunity might wane after a few years. The booster shot reactivates the antibody manufacturing cells and helps ensure long-lasting immunity. All of this presupposes that a parent will dutifully bring their child to a doctor or clinic to get the shots.

Even in the 1950s, it was well recognized that live, attenuated (altered) viruses and bacteria give a more effective and longer-lasting immunity. The problem is coming up with one that is safe. Researchers of the time often engaged in rather heated, sometimes rancorous, debates on the correct approach to a polio vaccine: chemically inactivated or live attenuated. The first to appear was Dr. Salk's inactivated vaccine in 1955. Six years later, the live, attenuated trivalent vaccine of Dr. Albert Sabin became commercially available in the United States.

Dr. Sabin was from Poland, born there in 1906. His family emigrated to the United States when he was 15, and he received his medical degree from New York University in 1931. He immediately began his polio research. One of the leading philanthropic organizations of the 1930s in the battle against polio was the Rockefeller Institute in New York. He joined that organization in 1935 and left a few years later to work at the

Children's Hospital Research Foundation in Cincinnati, Ohio. There, he and colleagues were the first researchers to grow the virus in neuronal tissue, and he confirmed that polio was an intestinal virus. During World War II, he was in the U.S. Army and helped develop vaccines for several tropical diseases.

The attenuated polioviruses that Dr. Sabin and his team developed could enter the host cell and multiply, just like the wild-type virus. Virus production in the cell, however, was limited. The alteration to the virus lay in the part of the virus that attaches to the host cell ribosome, the so-called initiating sequence. With an altered amino acid in the initiation sequence, the strength of the attachment to the ribosome, known as avidity (from the Latin *aviditatem*, or "eagerness"), was much reduced. Instead of producing hundreds of thousands of viral copies, only a few hundred were produced. The Protein 2A content was much reduced, so it was not nearly as active, especially on the nuclear membrane. The process of chemical signaling and interferon production took place close to normal. As a result, the T-cell line and the B-cells were activated, and a robust, long-lasting immunity took place. All three types of polio were included in the vaccine, as the Sabin team discovered attenuated types for each.

The live, attenuated vaccine is clearly superior to the inactivated injected form. Only one dose is needed, and repeat clinic visits are not necessary. Also, while not present in copious amounts like the wild type, the attenuated virus is shed in the stool and can still be spread from one individual to another. When immunizing populations where reaching everyone is not likely, the vaccine can still be spread from person to person, inducing immunity like the wild type but without the disease.

Developing an attenuated strain takes years, and a lot of luck. Put simply, you just keep passing the virus through cell cultures or a test animal over and over until you can detect a product that doesn't infect as strongly. You keep passing that one until the virulence is reduced even more. It can take hundreds of passages, and there is no guarantee of a suitable outcome. Working with material supplied by other workers, Sabin's team developed attenuated viruses for all three types.

Even though the new live strains looked promising, they still had to be tested. Since the inactivated poliovirus was so commonly administered in the U.S. in the preceding years, another naïve population had to be enlisted. A study involving about 26,000 children was conducted in Cuba in 1962, but more data was needed. Sabin was from Poland, and he had made the acquaintance of a highly respected Russian virologist, Mikhail Chumakov. Dr. Chumakov was a fascinating individual. In his early days as a researcher, he worked with a Siberian virus known as tick-borne fever, which is caused by a virus related to yellow fever and dengue. He became accidentally infected, resulting in his going blind and being paralyzed on one side. Despite this, he continued as a high-level research scientist and made several important discoveries.

Even though the relationship between the U.S. and the Soviet Union at the time was poor, the two eminent scientists convinced the Soviet government to allow the wide-scale testing of Sabin's live vaccine strains. Over 2 million children were vaccinated, and the results were all they had hoped for. The live vaccine was soon approved for use in the U.S.

There's one problem, though, and it's big. All three vaccine strains can spontaneously mutate back to the wild-type form, causing full-blown polio, either in the person receiving the vaccine or someone unfortunate enough to come into contact with the vaccinated person's excrement. The initial mutation is in only a single nucleotide on the viral RNA: In poliovirus 1, the adenine at position 480 is altered to guanine; in poliovirus 2, the guanine at position 481 is changed to adenine, and in poliovirus 3, the cytosine at position 472 is changed to uracil. It only takes a random mutation of one of these single nucleotides to have the virus revert to wild type, a situation calculated to occur once in every 750,000 viral replications.

So the risk is relatively straightforward: one can immunize 750,000 people and run the risk of creating at least one case of polio, or immunize no one and run the risk of a full-blown polio epidemic. In the U.S. and other developed countries, as polio started to wane due to vaccination and herd immunity, the oral vaccine was discontinued, and only the inactivated, injected vaccine was recommended. In remote, undeveloped countries, the oral vaccine was continued because of its ability to often reach unvaccinated members of a household or community.

The good news is that poliovirus 2 is now considered extinct in the wild. It has not been detected since 1999; in September 2015, it was declared eradicated. Poliovirus 3 is most likely gone as well, having last been detected in a patient in November 2012; it was declared eradicated in 2019. That leaves only poliovirus 1 in the wild.

One could logically ask why polio vaccination is still recommended for children in the United States and other developed countries. The disease hasn't been detected in these countries in decades. We have other vaccines that are not routinely administered unless travel is involved. For instance, there are very good vaccines against typhoid and yellow fever, but they are not given to everyone, just those traveling to a country where the disease is endemic. Why polio vaccine for everyone? The answer, of course, has to do with the biology of the disease. Many more people infected with the virus are asymptomatic carriers than those with symptoms. A person traveling from an endemic area to a non-vaccinated one could easily, but unknowingly, carry and therefore spread the virus. Without herd immunity present in the community, it could be really bad. Several Public Health labs in the U.S. routinely test raw sewage for genomic evidence of poliovirus. Although no cases of poliomyelitis have been seen, the labs report the presence of the virus. It's not extinct.

Polio is a fascinating disease, from the biology of the virus taking over a cell and evading the immune system, and humanity's efforts to control and eradicate it. Given its sudden emergence as the unintended consequence of the introduction of general sanitation, one cannot help but ponder what other disease agents may be lurking. Polio isn't the only enterovirus. There are over 70 viruses in the family, and some have shown a predilection for the central nervous system. Viral meningitis is the most obvious, but two strains, D68 and A71, have given some children classic myelitis symptoms. They apparently are contracted through the respiratory route, giving rise to what appears to be a common cold, then progressing to involve the anterior horn cells. The condition is called acute flaccid myelitis, or AFM. To date, these have been rare, but with a simple mutation here or there, things could get a lot worse.

Chapter 26
Mind Control

Rabere, Rabhas
Creeps up the nerve-cell highway.
Bullet to the brain.

Fred Gipson was an American journalist who grew up on a farm in Texas in the early 1900s. The first part of his writing career was devoted to newspaper reporting, but in the 1940s he began writing short stories, eventually novels. He had several published, but his most memorable work was the book "Old Yeller," the story of a stray dog a Texas pioneer family adopts in the mid-1860s. The book won the prestigious Newbery honor and was made into a successful motion picture by the Walt Disney Company in 1957.

While growing up in Texas hill country, his grandfather told Gipson a story about a dog that was attacked and bitten by a wolf, then went on to contract the dreaded disease rabies. This incident stayed with him and became a central part of the book "Old Yeller." Fortunately for most of us, the fictional story of Old Yeller and its dramatic depiction in the film is the closest we will ever get to this most horrible disease. Modern practices of vaccination and animal husbandry have seen to that. But in some parts of the world, rabies is still a scourge, just as it has been for millennia.

For some serious infectious diseases, the torment comes from the physical manifestations of the ailment. In rabies, while the physical pain is formidable, the horrific nature of the illness is the mental terror accompanying the physical signs, including fear, panic, and the frightening reality that another entity controls our thoughts. The rabies virus makes its way into the victim's brain and objectively redirects their thoughts to suit its own needs. It directs the infected person to bite other people. This is true of animals as well as humans. The rabies virus spreads through the introduction of infected saliva into another mammal's body, and it can alter the mind of the host animal to achieve its purpose.

In "Old Yeller," two portrayed facts tell a lot about the disease. The ailment is called hydrophobia, the fear of drinking water or other fluid. Another classic sign is "foaming at the mouth." The two are related because the inability to swallow causes the symptoms. Swallowing water cannot be controlled, and it is likely to "go down the wrong pipe" directly into the lungs. The infected individual is acutely aware of this and avoids drinking fluids, including their saliva, which appears as "foam" as it collects around the exterior of the mouth.

The other is that the locals recognized "hydrophobia" in the area, referring to the siting of several animals diagnosed as rabid by their characteristic wild, savage, out-of-control appearance. This behavior is typical of the infected animal or person and foreshadows the unique symptom of the disease, the overwhelming urge to bite. In Old Yeller's tale, the mention of local hydrophobia comes up several times, and the index case is a wolf that suddenly appears on the scene of the ranch where the family lives. Wolves were known to avoid human camps and communities, but this one came in and attacked. Old Yeller rises to the occasion and saves the family but becomes infected. The wolf's strange actions, going decidedly against its nature, raise high suspicion that he was rabid. As is the case today, Yeller was put into quarantine and checked daily for symptoms. When they unmistakably appear, he must be put down, sadly, by the 14-year-old boy who loves him, as the father is away. For the boy, Travis, it is an unenviable rite of passage.

Rabies is an ancient disease, one affecting animals primarily, humans incidentally. It may be the first infectious disease for which the epidemiology was fully known to ancient people: an animal that has the disease bites another animal, and that animal or human becomes rabid. The infected animal's wild, deranged behavior is usually unmistakable, and infected animals need to be destroyed before they can spread the infection. The first known writing about rabies comes from ancient texts from the Middle East in the area we now call Iraq. (It is sometimes referred to as Mesopotamia, *mesos*, meaning in the middle or between, and *potamos,* or river; between the Tigris and Euphrates rivers). In the mid-1940s, a pair of tablets from the area, written about 4,000 years ago, were recovered from a site about 30 miles northeast of Baghdad. They were a set of laws from the community of Eshnunna and are known as the Laws of Eshnunna. The laws are written in a very simple form, as if they were meant to be memorized. One of the laws states, *"If a dog becomes rabid and the ward authority makes that known to its owner, but he does not watch over his dog so that it bites a man and causes his death, the owner of the dog shall pay forty shekels of silver; if it bites a slave and causes its death, he shall pay fifteen shekels of silver."* (The word for "rabid" can also be translated as either "furious" or "vicious." As a reference, the near-contemporary Code of Hammurabi states that a small boat costs two shekels, so 40 or even 15 must have been a tidy sum).

The first reported description of rabies transmitted by a dog's saliva is attributed to the Roman scholar Celsus in the first century AD. He also recommended a cure, holding the patient underwater. The logic behind such a remedy escapes us today, but it may have sounded like a good idea at the time. Without knowledge as to the microbial cause of the disease, much assignment for the nature of the condition went to supernatural causes, often something akin to demonic possession. Numerous incantations and ceremonies were developed to dispel the disorder, and some may have seemed effective to those present at the time. The fact is, being bitten by a rabid dog doesn't mean a bitten person will develop rabies. The bite must be deep with enough tissue damage to introduce the virus. Wounds that bleed excessively are more likely to expel the virus, lessening the chance of infection. It's also possible the dog was just plain mean, not rabid, so no virus transmission occurred. If a preventative measure had been taken, it may have seemed effective, and its tale of wonder spread.

Besides the supernatural, there was historically a school of thought that the dog's saliva was poisoned, like that of a poisonous snake or insect. There were "cures" proposed for that as well, such as a preparation from the skull of a hanged man, cutting out a portion of the patient's tongue, various poultices and herbal dressings, and hanging a calcified hairball from the stomach of a ruminant (known as a "madstone") around your

387

neck. A phrase that survives today, but in an entirely different context, is "the hair of the dog," short for the original "hair of the dog that bit you." It refers to the thought that "like cures like" (the Latin phrase is *Similia similibus curentur*): placing hairs from the animal that bit you on the wound so rabies would not ensue. Today, of course, it refers to taking a drink of the alcohol that caused a hangover, hoping that a small amount of the drink will relieve the pains brought on by the large amount.

Clearly, none of the historic remedies had any effect on the unfortunate rabies victim. Even today, there is no cure for a person who develops the disease. One procedure that was a somewhat effective attempt at preventing the disease immediately after the bite is cauterization, using a red-hot iron to kill the tissue in and around the bite site. The procedure is first known to have been proposed by the Greek physician and pharmacologist Pedianius Dioscorides, who lived in Asia Minor and had close ties to the Romans. He wrote the time-honored volume *De Materia Medica*, a series of books containing information about herbal and other treatments and remedies. It remained "in print" for over 1500 years, and the cauterization technique for the prevention of rabies following an animal bite became something of a standard procedure. Getting one such burn is horrifically painful, but rabies victims are usually bitten several, sometimes dozens of times. The pain and horror of this preventative treatment are indescribable, but the other option was most likely an even worse death. Today we have very effective vaccines available, and the lag time from the bite to symptoms of the infection is at least a month, so there is time to administer vaccination soon after the rabid bite, a much better idea than burning flesh. But once the disease takes hold, the mortality rate approaches 100%. At one time, euthanasia, by smothering the victim between two mattresses, was a not uncommon practice once the symptoms were in full severity.

The origin of the term rabies is interesting. Interesting in that the two languages to which it may be ascribed are not related. The Latin term *rabere* means to "rave" and would seem to be the logical source of the term rabies. But there is a Sanskrit word, *rabhas*, which means "violence." Perhaps there was a confluence of terms during cultural interaction through early trade routes. The Greek word for madness is *lyssa*, which has become the technical name of the genus of the virus causing the disease, *Lyssavirus*.

It seems appropriate that the deadliest infectious disease is caused by a virus that physically resembles a bullet. The virus can enter the body in several ways, but in the vast majority of cases it enters by way of an animal bite introducing viral-containing saliva into the wound. The deeper the wound, the better for the virus. After a few weeks, the virus enters the axon of a nearby neuron, attaches itself to the internal transit system of the nerve cell, and progresses rather rapidly to the body of the nerve cell located in the spinal column. It can enter either motor or sensory neurons. From the spinal cord, it makes its way into the brain, then proceeds to infect an enormous number of brain cells, yielding a very high number of virions. Next, it progresses down a neuron into the tissues of the throat area, especially the parotid (salivary) glands. The activity in the brain results in the production of more virions and a profound effect on the infected person or animal's thought processes. Namely, the infection causes the infected individual to have an overwhelming desire to bite another creature. There are also changes in the mental status of the infected individual. Death nearly always ensues. One might say that rabies, with the shape of the virus, is like a "bullet to the brain."

The rabies virus contains only five proteins, plus its genetic material in the form of single-stranded RNA. The key to the virus' profound ability to infect and kill is a remarkable substance, the G-protein. (The G stands for glycoprotein, a combination of sugar and protein). It is present as the "fuzz" that projects out from the virus's surface. The G-protein is remarkable in that it is responsible for not just one but several vital operations in getting the virus into and through cells and into the brain. It also is chiefly responsible for reducing the immune system's response to the invasion of the virus.

After entry into the body of the victim, the virus enters muscle fibers near the bite. Entry into the muscle cell is facilitated by the G-protein, which binds to a receptor on the outside of the cell. The virus is then actively transported into the muscle cell and resides inside an endosome. Because of the change in pH from neutral outside the cell to acid inside, the shape of the G-protein changes, allowing the virus to adhere to the endosome's membrane, causing the endosome to break apart and release the virus into the cell's cytoplasm. During this process, the virus disassembles, and its RNA is released and available to be copied by the host cell's ribosomes. Rabies virus RNA is "negative sense," so it has to be copied by its own polymerase to make "positive sense" RNA, which is able to bind to ribosomes and produce protein.

The rabies virus is a marked exception to the aphorism "more is better." While very efficient at making copies of itself within the host cell, it is designed to curtail its numbers: enough to get the job done, but not too many to trigger the death of its host cell or signal the immune system as to its presence. Rabies is a "stealth" virus, creeping inside peripheral neurons until it reaches its targets, the brain and the salivary glands. Rather than acting like a powerful infantry, marching along with a great show of force, it assumes the role of a small unit of commandoes, much smaller in size but highly efficient and capable of great destruction.

After replicating and producing suitable numbers in the muscle fibrils, the virus escapes into the space (synapse) between the muscle cell and the adjacent neuron. It then binds to a receptor on the neuronal surface and enters the neuron's axon in much the same way it entered the muscle cell, using the G-protein. After entering the nerve cell axon, it attaches to the "fast-track" transport system, which carries molecular material from the axon's tip back to the nerve cell body in the spinal cord. Tetanus and botulism toxins utilize this same mechanism of transport.

Again, the G-protein is responsible for this adhesion and transport. While the explanation is not clearly known, the virus can speed up its transport up the neuron, proceeding more rapidly than usual. It still takes a while, with an estimated rate of about 3 millimeters per hour. Axons can be up to a meter long, so it can take a couple of days for the virus to journey to the spinal cord. But being inside a cell protects the virus from the antibodies, macrophages, and lymphocytes the immune system uses to detect and eliminate invaders.

After trekking up the nerve cell's axon to the spinal cord, the virus enters the neuron cell body, replicating as it did in the muscle fibrils. Again, the number of virions produced is minimal, resulting in three favorable outcomes for the virus. First, the infected cell is much less likely to destroy itself through apoptosis. Apoptosis is often precipitated by viral proteins bumping against the cell membrane. Since there isn't that much G-protein to adhere to the membrane, the apoptosis signal is not easily sent. Second, the chemical signals that are usually sent to the host cell genome to produce interferons α and β are muted, so very little of that protective substance is produced and transferred to nearby cells. This allows the virus a smoother trip along the neurons of the spinal cord on its journey to the brain because each cell on the way is more receptive to its entry. Third, chemical distress signals normally sent to the cell surface to alert natural killer lymphocytes are muted, and the cell appears perfectly normal and is spared. These three abilities of rabies, keeping the host cell intact, reducing interferon production, and mitigating against host cell destruction by killer lymphocytes, allow the rabies virus to trudge along nearly unmolested en route to its ultimate destination, the brain.

After entering the brain, the virus no longer relies on the nerve cell transport system to carry it along. It is free to enter any and all of the brain's nerve cells. And it does. Virtually every cell in the brain is infected during a typical case of rabies, with obvious devastating consequences. The virus is especially good at infecting brain cells of the amygdala, the hippocampus, the thalamus, and the hypothalamus, key members of what has been called the limbic system. Just why it seems to strike these areas so virulently isn't known; they rest on the top of the brain stem, so ascending viruses will likely encounter this area of the brain first. Perhaps these cells have more receptors on their surface for the virus to latch onto. Whatever the reason, attacking these specific areas results in marked behavioral changes. The infected patient becomes openly hostile and combative. They are also restless and agitated, and small sounds or other stimuli can send them into a hyperactive state. There is also the overwhelming urge to bite someone. Paranoia is extreme, and patients lash out at the slightest thing in fear for their lives.

Meanwhile, the virus has infected brain neurons and neurons leading away from the brain and into the peripheral tissues. It becomes especially concentrated in the parotid, or salivary, glands. The mouth and throat muscles become paralyzed, and there is a loss of control over swallowing. Hence, the onset of hydrophobia and "foaming at the mouth." This all plays into the virus's plan, enabling it to spread to another individual so it may propagate itself.

The symptoms of rabies were elegantly chronicled by the eminent British neurologist Sir William Gowers, referred to by some as the founder of the science of neurology. Between 1886 and 1888, he wrote a classic two-volume reference, *Manual of Diseases of the Nervous System*. It is still used in some form today. In his chapter on rabies, he was very clear and thorough in his description:

> *"Early symptoms show some discomfort about the throat, and occasional sense of choking, or a little difficulty in swallowing liquids. The attempt to drink occasions some spasms in the pharynx, which increases in the course of a few hours, and spreads to the muscle of respiration, causing a short, quick inspiration, a "catch in the breath." This increases in severity to a strong inspiratory effort, in which the extraordinary muscles of respiration, sterno-mastoid, scaleni, etc., and even the facial muscles take part; the shoulders are raised, and the angles of the mouth drawn outwards. As the intensity of the spasm increases, so does the readiness with which it is excited. It may be caused by a mere contact of water with the lips, and a state of cutaneous hyperaesthesia* (increase in sensitivity of the sensory organs) *develops, so that various impressions, so that a draught of air, which normally excite the respiratory effort,*

bring on the spasm. The mere movement of air caused by raising the bedclothes may be sufficient. The patient is often unable to swallow the saliva, which is usually abundant and viscid, so that it hangs about the mouth and is expelled with difficulty. Vomiting is common. The spasm attacks are very distressing to the patient; the mental state which they occasion increases the readiness with which they are produced; in some cases, the mere sight of water or the sound of dropping water will cause an attack. It may even be excited by visual impressions that cause a similar sensation, as the reflection from a looking glass or a strong light. The sufferer's horror and dread of these excitants becomes intense. Thus the disturbance in the act of swallowing liquids, which constitutes the first symptom and keynote of the disease, spreads on the one hand, to mental disturbance, and on the other to extensive muscular spasm. In each of these directions further symptoms develop. The spasm, at first confined to the muscles of swallowing and respiration, spreads to the other muscles of the body, and the paroxysms, at first respiratory, afterward become general, and assume a convulsive character, although still excited by the same causes. The convulsions may consist of general muscular rigidity. Actual delusions occasionally supervene, and there may even be wild delirium. The mental derangement is most intense during the paroxysms of spasms, and the frenzied patient may spit his saliva at those about him, and often attempts to bite them with his teeth, making occasional strange sounds in his throat which have been thought to resemble the barking of a dog."

After several days of this horrible experience, the patient invariably lapses into a coma and dies. Once the disease enters this late symptomatic stage, there is no cure. The patient may be placed in an induced coma in developed countries, but death is still inevitable.

The description above is known as "furious" rabies. In about 25% of cases, the disease takes another path initially, causing general paralysis. Why the disease progresses this way is not known, but just as with furious rabies, paralytic rabies results in death.

For thousands of years, the fight against rabies was a losing one. Like in the novel *Old Yeller,* destroying an animal suspected of having the disease was the only recourse, along with cauterizing the wound(s). Most people were painfully aware of the consequences of a bite by a rabid animal, and one can only imagine the horror felt if a member of your family were bitten. For thousands of years, rabies plagued not only humans but their livestock, creating terror and sometimes food shortages, even though the disease was not primarily human or domestic animal by nature. People lived close to the land, and the wild mammals that inhabited it were continually subject to becoming infected by the very efficient and lethal rabies virus.

German physician Georg Gottfried Zinke presented in 1804 the first scientific evidence of what was suspected for centuries, that the saliva of an infected animal spread rabies. He took the saliva from an infected dog, injected it by syringe into a healthy dog, and produced the disease. He also produced the disease in rabbits by the same method. An enormous breakthrough came in 1882 when French veterinary microbiologist Pierre-Victor Galtier injected rabies-laden saliva into sheep, but not into their skin. He injected it into their veins. Much to his surprise, this did not give them rabies. On the contrary, it protected them from the virus he subsequently inoculated into their skin. Galtier's research laid the groundwork for the historic discovery made a few years later, a vaccine against the dread disease.

Many people consider science boring—repetition after repetition, written in words that resemble a foreign language. But sometimes science can present compelling, suspenseful, emotional dramas that rival the best of books, plays, or motion pictures. Such was the case with the development of the first anti-rabies vaccine by a team led by Louis Pasteur in 1885. Pasteur, of course, was familiar with the smallpox vaccine, which used a virus that was similar but different from the one that caused the severe disease. He himself had produced a vaccine protective against chicken cholera bacteria (now called *Pasteurella multocida*) and the often-fatal animal bacterium *Bacillus anthracis*, the cause of anthrax. He used old, dried-out cultures of chicken cholera bacteria. And he and grew the anthrax bacterium at higher and higher temperatures. In both situations, the microbe was changed or "attenuated." This way, they could be inoculated into animals without causing the disease but still inducing the formation of immunity. (The word attenuate, meaning to weaken or lessen, comes from the Latin *tenuis*, to "make thin"). By 1885 Pasteur had made two other extremely important discoveries: gently heating wine and beer to prevent spoilage (later called Pasteurization), and isolating diseased silkworms from healthy ones to allow the more abundant formation of silk, a major industry in France at the time. In doing all this, he gained notoriety and was well-known to the average Frenchman. Arguably, his greatest accomplishment was still to come: developing a vaccine for the terrifying disease rabies.

Pasteur hypothesized that a changed microorganism similar to but distinct from the disease-causing agent could induce immunity but not cause the disease. He sought to produce such a change in the microorganism responsible for rabies. The animal model he used was the rabbit, in which it was possible to induce rabies by injecting them with rabid dogs' saliva, as Zinke showed many years before. As one can imagine, rabid rabbits are much easier to work with than rabid dogs. Since rabies takes a long time to develop when it is injected into muscles, Pasteur short-circuited the natural route by injecting the material directly into the rabbit's brain, a technique called trepanation. Rather than waiting months to harvest the virus, it could be done in a few days. When injected this way, the virus spreads through the rabbit's brain and into its spinal cord. This was the objective of Pasteur's investigations. He harvested the spinal cord of the dead rabbits and put each into a sealed container containing a tiny bit of potassium. The potassium removed the water from the air, giving a dry environment. By experiment, Pasteur found that rabid rabbit spinal cords dried this way were not infectious after about two weeks. Those freshly put into the dry air containers were highly infectious for one to two days. There was a clear spectrum, showing more virulence with shorter time periods and little or no virulence after two weeks, with time periods in the middle showing some but markedly reduced ability to infect.

The work was arduous, and it was dangerous. Imagine being assigned the job of securing saliva from a rabid dog. When the test animals were inoculated, the virus was just as virulent as the wild type, and any slip-up in handling the animals would be deadly. And not just a simple death, but a brutal, torturous one. Pasteur, of course, gets the credit for the theory and the experiments, but the nameless laboratory assistants who did the work also deserve much adulation.

The telling experiments began once the attenuated virus was obtained in ground-up rabbit spinal cords. Fifty dogs were immunized, first by giving them two-week-old, or non-virulent, spinal cord material. A few days later, more material was given, this time from material that was thirteen days old. Then twelve-day-old material, and so on, down to spinal cord material only a couple of days old. The dogs were observed for two weeks, and none developed rabies. Then the real test: the fifty dogs were each inoculated with fresh saliva from rabid dogs. Much to the elation of the Pasteur team, none of the dogs developed rabies. All were immune.

Alsace, France, is a picturesque area in the mountain region bordering France, Germany, and Switzerland. It is on the western bank of the Rhine River, and the area's culture shares the traditions of both French and German history. Known for its lush valleys and scenic mountains, the quaint Alsatian region and lifestyle are the stuff of tourist brochures and quiet getaways. In 1885 it was part of Germany. In this quiet mountain area began one of the epic tales of medical history.

One morning in early July 1885, Alsatian baker Joseph Meister sent his nine-year-old son, also named Joseph, to a neighboring village to get yeast from the brewery there. From out of nowhere came a large, viscous dog, clearly mad, who caught and attacked the helpless boy in the most savage fashion. A policeman shot the dog. Joseph received 14 severe wounds from the dog, whom neighbors saw and clearly identified as rabid. The dog's owner, Monsieur Theodore Vone, knew his dog had recently changed dramatically and thought him rabid. Joseph's wounds could be bound up and possibly healed, but the boy's parents knew they were not the primary concern: the dog was rabid, which was a death sentence for their young son—a most horrible one at that.

The town physician, Doctor Eugene Weber, came to treat Joseph's wounds that evening, about 14 hours after the attack. He treated them with carbolic acid and sutured those that he could. Dr. Weber was honest and blunt in his conversation with Joseph's parents. While not every bite by a rabid dog results in rabies, many do, especially when there are multiple wounds. The prognosis was grave.

Some locals had heard reports, even way out here in the far reaches of the German/French countryside, that scientists in Paris were working on a preventive cure for rabies. The dog's owner, Monsieur Vone, had stopped by a pub on his way home after visiting Joseph's family, and he listened intently as the conversation centered on the Paris scientists' work. He rushed back to the Meister home to relay what he had heard. Without hesitation, Mademoiselle Meister took her son on the three-hundred-mile train ride, even though she didn't know anyone in Paris and didn't know the name of the scientists. The dog's owner accompanied them. When the mother and boy arrived in Paris, she immediately went to a hospital, explained her situation to a doctor, and inquired about the scientist working on rabies treatment. The doctor knew right away about the work of Pasteur and his associates and escorted them to his laboratory. It was July 4, 1885, when the Meisters met Louis Pasteur.

In the 19th century, there were no government oversight committees on medical treatments as we have today. Doctors and scientists were guided by their sense of ethics and morality, and therapeutic trials were based on what was seen as the wisest options available. Pasteur listened intently and with sympathy to the tearful woman explaining her son's situation, but he was naturally concerned. His treatment had successfully prevented rabies in dogs, but the jump to humans, using a known killer virus, was disturbing. What if the virus wasn't fully attenuated and injected directly into a human? Certainly, it would mean a horrible death to the injected individual. Pasteur would have preferred more animal trials and time to evaluate the data, but the case before him couldn't wait. Young Joseph had already received a death sentence and was likely to die a wretched death. One prominent physician-scientist in the laboratory, Emile Roux, reportedly refused to participate in the therapy on ethical grounds. Pasteur reluctantly decided to go ahead and allow the administration of his anti-rabies emulsions.

> *"As the death of this child appeared inevitable, I decided, not without deep and severe unease, as one can well imagine, to try on Joseph Meister the procedure which had consistently worked in dogs."*
> *—Louis Pasteur*

Pasteur was not a medical doctor. A physician was required to oversee the injections, and two volunteered, Drs. Alfred Vulpian and Jacques-Joseph Grancher. On July 6th, young Joseph received his first injection, material taken from a 15-day-old emulsion of a rabbit spinal cord. Over the following ten days, Joseph received 13 doses of younger and younger emulsions. At ten days, he received an emulsion that was only two days old, clearly enough to induce rabies.

Waiting can be excruciating, especially when the outcome may be horrific. But after two months, it became clear: Joseph Meister was rabies-free! The treatment had been a tremendous success, and the world was on its way to at least partially containing this most terrible disease. Much work remained to be done to advance from these crude beginnings, but the prophylactic rabies treatment performed in Paris in July of 1885 was one of the great accomplishments of human history.

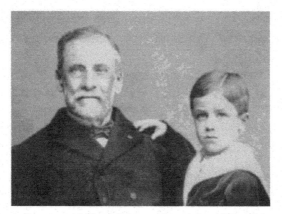

A photo of Louis Pasteur and Joseph Meister. Joseph would spend the rest of his life working as a janitor a the Pasteur Institute in Paris. He died tragically in 1940. (LoC)

Of course, scientific experiments need to be confirmed, and another case presented in October of the same year. Fifteen-year-old Jean-Baptiste Jupille was tending sheep in the farming community of Villers-Farlay in eastern France, not too far away from Alsace. He was also watching over five young children. A rabid dog appeared, threatening all, but Jean-Baptiste threw himself into direct contact with the dog, fighting it until the children could run away. He sustained multiple deep bites in his act of heroism, and his future was in grave peril. But he was able to travel to Paris to receive the new therapy at the Pasteur Institute, and, like Joseph Meister, his life was spared.

Word of the success of the post-exposure rabies treatment traveled fast. Soon bite victims from all around Europe were coming to Paris to be treated. Nineteen people traveled from Russia after being attacked by a rabid wolf. This created an enormous problem, as the vaccine material was in short supply and was very difficult to make. Also, it didn't travel well and could not be shipped to remote locations, requiring bite victims to make their way to Paris. Adding to the difficulty was what is known today as the "worried well." Not every dog that bites a person is rabid, and not every wound from a rabid animal will result in rabies. Given the limited supply of vaccination material, difficult decisions had to be made based on the time elapsed from the bite, the nature of the wounds, and the veracity of accounts as to the condition of the animal involved. But the workers in Paris did the best they could, and in one year after the first trial, over a thousand patients were treated with rabies post-exposure treatment. Most survived, although there were a few deaths.

Following the dramatic success of the Pasteur rabies treatment in Paris, clinics sprang up worldwide. Elie Metchnikoff led the first one in Odessa, Ukraine, in 1886, with many to follow. Some were directly associated with the Pasteur Institute in Paris, but many were not, though they still carried the name.

Advances to the treatment came incrementally, with the most significant breakthrough at the hands of a British doctor, David Semple, who served as a lieutenant colonel in the British army in India. In 1911 he perfected the means of giving live rabies virus to rabbits, letting them develop the disease, then harvesting their brains with the intact virus. He killed the virus by subjecting the "brain soup" to phenol. This created a vaccine that could be stored and transported and didn't have the chance of giving a patient rabies instead of preventing it. Later the virus was grown in sheep instead of rabbits. To be effective, the Semple vaccine had to be administered by injection into the patient's abdomen, a painful event. And one shot was not enough; a half dozen injections were necessary. The fact that the patient was receiving not just a killed virus but emulsified sheep brain was a big concern, as a few patients developed a hyperimmune disease. It was better than the original rabies post-exposure prevention, but it was clearly not ideal. Still, the Semple method was the preferred rabies prevention therapy for nearly half a century.

In the late 1950s, scientists at the Eli Lilly pharmaceutical company succeeded in growing the rabies virus in duck eggs. That freed the vaccine of most contaminating material. More recently, the virus has been successfully propagated in cell culture, and it can now be administered with very few side effects. The current regimen for people exposed to a suspected rabid animal in developed countries is straightforward. The virus and the infection it causes are unique, so preventative therapy must be tailored to combat the disease most advantageously. Nothing in medicine is one hundred percent effective, but the current therapeutic regimen is reliable for the most part.

The rabies virus, known technically as *Lyssavirus*, does not normally enter the bloodstream. In fact, it doesn't enter body cavities or intercellular spaces. During its early phases, it enters muscle cells, then jumps to neurons. Unlike most viruses, it doesn't produce large quantities of itself while reproducing. It makes just enough to get its travel job done, and until it gets into the brain, very few virions are loose in the body. Thus, the immune system doesn't encounter the virus enough to build an immune response. The virus proceeds to the brain by traversing the synaptic spaces, a very small area, and traveling up the nervous system, moving from one cell to another. The synaptic space for us is very small, but it is quite a distance for a tiny virus. The synaptic space is the only location where the virus is exposed to the immune system and its many weapons. Cellular immunity is ineffective since the virus is very good at suppressing the host cell's signaling and self-destructing mechanisms. Humoral immunity, antibodies produced by B-lymphocytes, is the only effective means of thwarting the virus' advance. Flooding the synaptic space with antibodies prevents the viral G-protein from adhering to its nerve cell receptor, and the virus cannot advance.

Since the virus normally doesn't inhabit areas in the body that would illicit contact by dendritic cells or lymphocytes, antibody production is minimal to non-existent. Indeed, people with full-blown rabies don't have their own naturally occurring antibody until it's too late. It is only in the very late stages of the disease, when death is imminent, that antibodies produced by the patient begin to appear, too late to do any good.

Following the bite of a dog or other animal that may have rabies, the wound(s) must be thoroughly cleansed. Soap and water are a good start, along with an antiseptic. Povidone iodine has proven effective. Topical antibiotics, of course, do no good for rabies since a virus causes it. Still, other diseases may occur following a dog or cat bite, and a topical antibiotic would be useful in preventing them.

The key to preventing the onset of rabies after the bite exposure is to get as much antibody into the patient as possible. This is done by two means: Administering an antibody already made in another person or animal (passive immunity), and administering large quantities of dead virus to stimulate the patient's immune system to stimulate a strong response (acquired immunity). For passive immunity, the so-called hyperimmune serum is administered on the first day of treatment, preferably in the vicinity of the bite wound. The dead virus-containing vaccine is administered over a period of several days. The two injections must be given in different parts of the body, as the pre-formed antibody would quickly inactivate both itself and the dead virus if given in close proximity. In the days of the Semple vaccine, the one using killed virus mixed with the brains of infected sheep, the inoculation had to be given into the abdomen over the course of around seven injections, a very painful process. Today, the virus is prepared in cell culture, and it usually only takes four injections into the arm, and they are relatively pain-free. The Centers for Disease Control in the U.S. recommends that the vaccine be given on days 0, 3, 7, and 14.

The prevention of rabies by this method is unique. The disease incubation time is so long that it is preferable to quarantine the offending animal for ten days to determine its status before initiating treatment. But that still leaves enough time to begin therapy. If the animal remains healthy, there is no need to proceed. If the animal is unavailable or is determined to be rabid, the vaccine is given in a short time. For most other diseases, multiple doses of vaccines are administered over months, often years. With rabies, it's four doses in just two weeks. The plan is to induce the formation of much specific antibody in a short amount of time.

The diagnosis of rabies is usually very easy or very difficult. It's obvious when the patient is known to have been bitten by a rabid animal and goes on to display classic symptoms. It is difficult if the animal bite is not apparent. In the developed world, most rabies cases arise from the bite of a mammal other than a dog, such as a bat. The disease may take months to develop, and the patient may not comment on the event, especially if it's a child. In such cases, the diagnosis is problematic.

In the early stages of the disease, the virus can't be cultured or detected by molecular methods from easily obtainable specimens like blood or spinal fluid. It doesn't induce antibody formation early in the infection, so serology to detect antibodies is fruitless. No known chemical substances can be detected in the blood or other body fluids that can serve as a marker to raise suspicion about the presence of the virus. And early abnormalities of vital signs are non-specific.

In 1903 an Italian pathologist, Adelchi Negri, reported finding material within the brain cells of dogs that had died of rabies. The material was seen as round, red-staining (acidophilic) dots about the size of bacteria. They were only seen in cases of rabies, and for a good part of the 20th century, these Negri bodies, as they came to be called, were a diagnostic hallmark of rabies. For a long time, there was debate about what Negri bodies were. Dr. Negri insisted they were a tiny parasite that caused the disease. Others maintained that was not the case, as the agent was filterable, that is, able to pass through a very tiny sieve. These "filterable agents" were later called viruses, and the Negri theory of a parasitic cause of rabies was erroneous. Nevertheless, finding Negri bodies in biopsy and autopsy material was a useful diagnostic tool for many years.

(It is interesting to note that another scientist, American Dr. Anna Wessels Williams, also discovered the cellular inclusions of rabies around the same time as Dr. Negri. But since the Italian scientist published his data first, they came to bear his name. Dr. Wessel's staining technique, though, is the one that became the standard).

Today we have a much better technique for diagnosing rabies, the fluorescent antibody test. Antibody to rabies is attached to a molecule that will fluoresce when exposed to ultraviolet light. When the suspected infected cell is flooded with this agent, the antibody will adhere to the virus and be seen under a fluorescent microscope. Detecting the Negri body is very suspicious for rabies, but false negatives exist. The fluorescent antibody test is much more sensitive and specific. It is the method of choice today. Unfortunately, both tests require cellular material obtained by either biopsy or autopsy. Quite often, the diagnosis comes too late.

Other infectious diseases can result from a dog bite or exposure to dog saliva. The most common is the bacterium *Pasteurella multocida*. The organism was first described by Louis Pasteur as the cause of fowl cholera and was the organism he attenuated to induce immunity in chickens. While more common in house cats, *P. multocida* often exists as normal bacterial flora in the dog's mouth. It doesn't make the dog sick, but when transferred to a human in an open wound, the bacteria can set up an infection within the bite area. The wound becomes inflamed and red, often draining pus. It is usually cured with appropriate antibiotics. Less common is the human infection caused by the dog bacterium *Capnocytophaga canimorsus*. While less common than *Pasteurella multocida*, it is often more serious. It usually doesn't infect people with intact immune systems but those with underlying medical problems. Alcoholics are the most vulnerable, as well as the elderly. The organism doesn't have to enter the body by a bite. Sometimes the dog merely licking the individual is enough. The organism can cause sepsis, and vigorous antibiotic therapy is required.

Both organisms are bacteria, and neither is related to the virus rabies. As with rabies, proper cleansing and decontamination of the wound, if there is one, is important to ward off a possible infection.

To many in the developed part of the world, rabies is a remnant of a bygone era. We read about it in stories or see a newspaper account of a rare case being described somewhere in a rural area. Unfortunately, though, rabies is by no means extinct. The World Health Organization reports at least 55,000 cases of rabies occurring in humans annually, all fatal. Many of the afflicted are children. That's the number officially reported. Undoubtedly, many cases in rural areas of underdeveloped countries go unreported. Part of the reason for the virus' persistence in causing human infections is the cost of vaccines. Costs vary over time, but some approximations:

The Semple vaccine, prepared crudely in the brains of sheep or goats, costs about $5 per course of post-exposure treatment. The vaccine is administered abdominally and is quite painful. This is the vaccine most used in underdeveloped areas of the world.

The human diploid cell human vaccine used in the U.S. costs about $500 per course. It is administered in the arm and feels like any other shot.

Access to good medical care is also essential, of course. Proper cleaning and disinfecting of a wound are essential in preventing rabies and more common bacterial infections. Many people in the world don't have access to even that.

Most people wish for a dignified death. Perhaps a quiet room in our home, with family and friends in attendance. The horror of rabies steals that away. Death from rabies is inevitable, and its terror is unrelenting. Fear, anxiety, paranoia, and combative behavior. Hardly the makings of a peaceful death. In developed countries, it is possible to induce a coma so that the patient slips away quietly. But rabies is a dreadful curse in areas without access to quality health care. With control measures well known, it is a very sad affair.

Toxoplasmosis

While dogs are the notorious carriers of rabies, their fellow domestic animals, cats, have their own mind-influencing infection. Toxoplasmosis is a parasitic disease not restricted to felines, but the organism must find its way into a cat to reproduce sexually. Quite commonly, the creature makes its way into a human and sets up residence. Most of the time, its presence within us is subtle and goes unnoticed. In some individuals, however, the infection can become severe, sometimes resulting in death.

We might think of rabies and toxoplasmosis as representing the yin/yang of infectious diseases. Rabies is the "yanger," controlling the infected person's faculties, overpowering the helpless victim, with death inevitable. Toxoplasmosis (just plain "Toxo" to the cognoscenti) is far more passive, usually invading without symptoms, surviving

405

unnoticed in the infected person's tissues for years or decades. Its effect on the mind is also not apparent but tends to give a bias or nudge toward certain behaviors rather than a shove.

If we accept that a "good" parasite doesn't want to damage its host and can successfully invade a wide range of animals, Toxo is at the top of the list of successful parasites. It is estimated that it has been around for not just thousands of years but millions. It has become adept at interacting with the body's immune response so that it can coexist in harmony with the animal body in which it resides. If the immune system of its host doesn't function properly, then overt disease occurs. But in most infected people, the parasite exists in several tissues, including the brain, with no apparent ill effects.

The parasite *Toxoplasma gondii* was first described in two very different parts of the world in 1908. In Tunisia, French workers Charles Nicolle and Louis Manceaux found it in a hamster-like rodent that dwells mainly in dry, rocky areas, the gundi. The gundi is a quiet, nondescript creature of no particular importance, but for some reason, researchers examined the tissues of one and found the parasite. They had no clue about the parasite's importance and thought it to be an entirely different genus, *Leishmania*. Upon further review, they realized it was a newly discovered parasite and named it for its shape and the animal in which it was found: *Toxon*, from the Greek meaning "arc" or "bow," and *plasma*, meaning "shape" or "mold." The species name *gondii* is the Latinized version of the rodent's name. At nearly the same time in Brazil, Alfonso Splendore, working in Oswaldo Cruz's lab, described the same organism in a rabbit, although he didn't give it a name. Related to parasites such as malaria, Toxo is very small and spends most of its life residing inside the cells of animals it infects.

After its discovery, *Toxoplasma gondii* resided in obscurity for several decades, relegated to a few dust-gathering scientific journals. In the 1930s, it was discovered in the body of a newborn baby girl, who died about a month after birth. Several other cases of neonatal disease were described in the ensuing years, but the organism was thought to be a very rare, albeit serious, pathogen.

In the 1950s, the life cycle of the organism was worked out. It's rather complicated. *Toxoplasma gondii* can invade just about any warm-blooded animal, including birds. Still, the only place it can undergo sexual reproduction is in the lining of the small intestine of cats. All cats: lions, tigers, bobcats, jaguars, and house cats. Something about that environment allows them to mate, and remarkably, they have evolved chemical mechanisms to allow themselves to end up in a cat's tummy. After mating, they produce a round cyst, technically called an oocyst (pronounced like oh-uh-cyst). As with many parasites, the oocyst gets pooped out, sits around in the soil or other environmental site, then gets consumed by an unsuspecting animal. If the animal is a cat, then the process is repeated. But if, as is likely, the foraging creature is another warm-blooded animal, then the parasite goes to "plan B." The viable entity inside the oocyst is a tiny, slithering creature known as a sporozoite.

After hatching from the oocyst, the sporozoites invade the intestinal epithelial tissues. The sporozoite of *Toxoplasma* is similar to the sporozoite of malaria. It doesn't have a flagellum for propulsion but manages to wriggle around the tissues until it contacts a cell receptor that will accommodate it. It then pushes itself into the hapless host cell, taking a bit of cell membrane with it to form an intracellular vacuole. The parasite manages to prevent the adhesion of the cell's killing lysosomes, so it is free to exist unmolested inside this parasitophorous vacuole. Inside the vacuole, the tiny worm-like creature divides into several others.

Reproduction isn't sexual; that can only take place in the intestine of a cat. The reproduction is asexual, kind of like cloning itself. After a while, there are so many of these tiny sporozoite-like creatures that they burst open the host cell and escape. At that point they are no longer called sporozoites but are referred to as the more mature tachyzoites. (The term *tachy*, referring to fast, comes from the Greek "tachus," meaning swift).

The released tachyzoites stream around the body in all directions, and they can enter the blood. This is where big trouble can arise. If the person who got the parasite is pregnant, the tachyzoites can enter her placenta and infect the developing fetus. The baby's immune system is not mature enough to combat the parasite, and severe complications may result. Not all babies infected display symptoms, but for those that do consequences of congenital infection can be severe. The clinical manifestations are many, including an eye infection, chorioretinitis, which can lead to severely blurred vision or blindness. Some develop epilepsy. Mental and psychomotor retardation is seen, as the parasites can infect the brain. Infected babies may also display anemia, jaundice, rashes due to low platelet count, hydrocephalus, or diarrhea. There are several others, ranging from temporary to severe and life-impacting. Children infected *in utero* don't always display symptoms soon after birth but may still go on to develop disease some years later.

It is well established that a significant factor influencing the baby's infection is when the mother becomes infected. If she has had the parasite before becoming pregnant, there is little threat to the baby. Her immune system can contain the organism and it doesn't get into the placenta. The woman who encounters *Toxoplasma* for the first time after becoming pregnant is the most likely to have trouble. The stage of the pregnancy when the parasite is acquired often determines the outcome. If the infection occurs during the first or second trimester, trouble is much more likely. Those acquired in the third trimester usually show no symptoms, although some of these children develop disease months or years later in childhood.

The wandering tachyzoites of *Toxoplasma,* of course, pose a threat to adults. Having these tiny creatures coursing through our bodies willy-nilly cannot be allowed. Fortunately, our immune system is up to the challenge, and in relatively short order, the tachyzoites are removed from open spaces within the body.

There are many modes of attack by the immune system against invading parasites. Soon after the organism is detected, chemical signals are sent out to alert the range of cells and molecules needed to do the job. Two of the most important signaling molecules are cytokines, interleukin-12 (IL-12), and interferon-gamma. As with any infection, antibody production is part of the defense, but most important is cellular immunity, involving lymphocytes and macrophages. This is because the parasite has a highly refined ability to enter many different cells of the host's body and sequester itself in a sort of hibernating state, away from the action of the body's humoral defenses. Tachyzoites can enter just about any cell in a few seconds, encasing themselves with the host cell membrane. If they continue to burst out of the host cell in the usual fashion, they will soon be gobbled up by macrophages and neutrophils, bringing their work to an end. But the parasites can enter a state of quiescence, content to remain within the protective confines of the host cell it invaded.

Surrounded by the protective membrane of the parasitophorous vacuole, *Toxoplasma* forms a cyst. This cyst can inhabit the tissues for decades. If *Toxoplasma* were in the tachyzoite stage inside the cyst, it wouldn't last long. So they convert to a much more sluggish, slow-developing stage, the bradyzoite. (While *tachy* means "swift" or "rapid" in Greek, *brady* means "slow"). The bradyzoites metabolize. They just do it at a much-reduced rate. Eventually, as circumstances allow, they can break out of their cyst and revert into the tachyzoite form. It is our immune system that prevents this from happening. If the immune system works in good order, the encased parasite is no threat to our health.

Interleukin-12 is an essential signaling molecule for our immune system. Each type of microorganism elicits the release of a chemical signal unique to its biological form. *Toxoplasma gondii* is an intracellular parasite, so (IL-12) is the first and foremost cytokine released. There are several functions of IL-12. One is to help ensure the activation of naïve lymphocytes into the CD4 helper type. Important is the differentiation of these CD4 types into the T-helper-1 (Th_1) type, which are the primary helpers in combating intracellular parasites. When the tachyzoite of *Toxoplasma gondii* enters a cell and becomes encased in its parasitophorous vacuole, the cell harboring it releases copious amounts of IL-12. This stimulates the creation of active CD4 lymphocytes of the Th_1 class, and the body's assault on the parasite is set to begin in earnest.

Macrophages are powerful killing machines. Whether they be the wandering macrophage or the dendritic type, they are our primary defense against parasites that invade a cell. Also helpful are natural killer lymphocytes and neutrophils, but the macrophages take center stage. Because of their tremendous killing power, macrophages are routinely in a minimally active state and must be activated to achieve their full killing potential. That's where the helper lymphocytes come in. When a CD4 lymphocyte of the Th1 type bumps up against a macrophage containing a parasitophorous vacuole containing *Toxoplasma*, it gives the macrophage a clear signal to activate its major killing apparatus.

The immune system also employs several other microbe-containing strategies. Still, the main one is the activity of CD4 lymphocytes of the Th1 class and their ability to ramp up the killing power of the macrophage or other cells containing the parasite. The importance of this function is evident in people who lack a pool of active CD4 lymphocytes, most notably individuals infected with the human immunodeficiency virus, HIV. Thanks to our T-helper cells, most people infected with *Toxoplasma gondii* don't even know they have it. But the results are devastating for those whose CD4 lymphocytes are not functional. In those cases, the parasite is not contained and runs wild throughout the body in its tachyzoite state, rather than being encysted inside cells in its bradyzoite state. The most notable symptoms involve the brain, heart, and lungs. Death is the usual outcome.

(When acquired immune deficiency syndrome, or AIDS, was first described in the early 1980s, symptomatic toxoplasmosis was one of the defining diseases. Others were pneumocystis, cryptococcosis, Kaposi's sarcoma, *Mycobacterium avium* infection, cryptosporidiosis, *Candida* esophagitis, and cytomegalovirus infection. They were highly suggestive of the presence of the condition. All are common organisms, usually of little or no consequence to humans, thanks to our immune system. But when the number of CD4 lymphocytes is reduced, as they are in an HIV infection, the result can be catastrophic).

410

Toxoplasma gondii has been around for millions of years and has learned a few tricks. One is quite extraordinary. Many organisms that successfully infect us have discovered ways to circumvent our immune system. They may produce a protein or two that binds to one of ours, effectively short-circuiting the chain reaction of molecules that lead to the production of an antimicrobial arsenal. The better an organism can cut off or interrupt the immune response to itself, the better a pathogen it tends to be. Amazingly, *Toxoplasma gondii* has survived as a highly successful pathogen because it has done the exact opposite. Rather than shutting down the immune response to itself, it takes measures to stimulate it. While inside a host cell, it manufactures a protein called GRA24. Remarkably, GRA24 travels to the host cell DNA and binds to a receptor, p38 MAPK, that goes on to unlock the genes responsible for the production of interleukin-12 and other inflammatory cytokines that have the direct result of killing, or slowing down, the growth of the parasite. The attachment of GRA24 to the receptor on human DNA is very strong, in fact, stronger than the body's stimulatory molecules. And once it locks on, it stays there. The chain reaction of IL-12 is steady and prolonged. The organism is taking measures to ensuring that the body's immune system is very good at its own containment..

At first glance, the parasite's enhancement of the immune system toward its own demise seems like a one-way ticket to extinction. But *Toxoplasma* knows precisely what it is doing. A "good" parasite doesn't want to kill its host. It simply dies with it. What suits it better is a steady state in which it can survive without much damaging its host. By enabling the creation of cytokines designed to stimulate the immune response against itself, *Toxoplasma* helps keep the host animal alive while allowing itself to exist in the encysted, bradyzoite-dominating form. This works very well in the parasite's favor. Remember, its ultimate goal is to end up in the intestine of some sort of cat. If it dwells within an animal's muscle, brain, or other tissues, and a cat eats that animal, it fulfills its destiny. Humans are not the targets of *Toxoplasma*. We are accidental hosts. Since it can't choose which animal it will infect, it takes a "shot-gun" approach and, in so doing, helps to achieve its own purposes.

While embedded in their intracellular "cocoon," the encysted bradyzoites of *Toxoplasma gondii* are not very active, but they're not dead. They still metabolize. And one of the products of their metabolism is a type of molecule known as a catecholamine. Most people have heard of the most famous catecholamine, epinephrine, also known as adrenaline. But there are others. A very important one in brain function is dopamine, a neurotransmitter intimately involved in sending chemical signals from one neuron to another. Dopamine works in several ways, including regulating movement, learning, sleep, memory, attention, and mood. It is carefully controlled, and imbalances in our dopamine levels can significantly alter our health. The most notorious example of that is Parkinson's Disease.

A common nickname for dopamine is "the feel-good hormone." That greatly oversimplifies its function, but it gives some insight into how our dopamine level can affect our behavior. And interestingly, it is the level of dopamine that is part and parcel to the scheming of *Toxoplasma*.

Mice have an innate fear of cats. And for a good reason. Just the smell of cat urine makes a mouse high-tail it in the opposite direction as fast as possible. Even mice that have never seen a cat, let alone been chased by one, are repulsed by cat urine odor. In one experiment, mice raised in a cat-free lab for over 20 generations innately feared anything to do with cats. But when mice are infected with the cysts of *Toxoplasma*, it all can change. In one fascinating experiment, *Toxoplasma*-infected mice were given a choice of bedding containing the scents of four animals, including a cat. Instead of avoiding the bedding scented with cat urine, the infected mice preferred it over the others, including the one scented with the urine of another mouse. Mice not infected with *Toxoplasma* behaved as expected and impulsively shunned the aroma of cats. *Toxoplasma gondii* cysts altered how the mice behaved, even to the point of putting their lives in danger.

Toxoplasma gondii has not just one but two genes that code for the formation of dopamine. That compound is instrumental in influencing function and behavior, so it seems likely that the parasite has evolved a means of bettering itself by influencing the behavior of its animal host. When exposed to cat urine, the strange action of mice and rats attests to that. It begs the question: are humans infested with *Toxoplasma* cysts affected in some psychological way? Do they think or do things they may not otherwise do because of the presence of the parasite, especially when it encysts in the brain? It's a fascinating hypothesis, but the answers are not unequivocal. *Toxoplasma* is present in about a third of the world's human population, so if it impacts behavior, it could have significant consequences. But the answers are elusive and often subject to interpretation.

Much of the work on the psychological effect of *Toxoplasma gondii* on humans has come from the Czech Republic. Dr. Jaroslav Flegr has published several works in which he raises the speculation that the organism can manipulate thought or behavior. Mice lose the innate fear of cats. Dr. Flegr postulates that a similar loss of fear may occur in infected humans. Rather than initiating a condition, current thought holds that the parasite "nudges" a person toward behavior that may not be in their best interest. If a person is suicidal, it may just push them over the edge. If a person is a reckless driver by nature, the person may take even more risks behind the wheel. There is some evidence that reaction times are slowed in the infected person, possibly contributing to the greater chance of accidents. In one survey, women rated men according to their physical attraction. The men harboring *Toxoplasma* scored significantly higher than men who did not. (Perhaps it was because of higher levels of testosterone).

Much work has been done on the relationship between the severity of schizophrenia and the presence of *Toxoplasma* in the patient. Studies have shown that people with the genetic makeup to develop schizophrenia often develop a more severe case when they also have a positive serologic test for the presence of Toxo. The question of other neurologic maladies, such as Parkinson's and Alzheimer's, is being investigated. In some countries, well over half the population is known to have *Toxoplasma* by serologic testing. Might the parasite's heavy load influence that culture's general behavior? Perhaps males tend to be more aggressive and females more submissive. Questionnaires given to small samples of individuals suggest that such may be the case, but much more work is required.

The lack of information on the parasite's presence in the brain complicates the evaluation of *Toxoplasma's* effect on human behavior. Dopamine does not cross the blood-brain barrier, so if it is elevated dopamine levels that are causing behavioral tendencies, it will follow that it must be produced by organisms residing in the central nervous system. Diagnosis of toxoplasmosis rests on finding antibodies to the parasite in the blood, which doesn't tell us if the organism is present in the brain or, if so, how many. Such information is only available at autopsy after the person dies, not in studies of large populations being screened.

It's fascinating work, and someday there may be definitive answers, but today it is primarily academic. There is no effective cure for toxoplasmosis when it exists in the encysted stage. Even if it is shown conclusively that a person's schizophrenia is made much worse because of the parasite's presence, very little can be done about it.

The laboratory test to detect toxoplasmosis is analysis for antibodies to the parasite in the blood (or sometimes spinal fluid). The first reliable test developed has remained the gold standard for serologic testing, the Sabin-Feldman Dye test. The "Sabin" in the name is the same Albert Sabin who contributed much to developing the live polio vaccine. In the late 1940s, he and Dr. Feldman found that if you took living *Toxoplasma gondii* tachyzoites, exposed them to serum containing antibodies, and added some complement, the tachyzoites were killed and could not absorb the common laboratory dye methylene blue. If an antibody was absent, the dye easily stained the parasite. It's a reliable test, but clearly, it cannot be run routinely given the need to cultivate living tachyzoites. Many other serologic tests have been developed, and which one is used depends on the clinical presentation. Tests are available to determine whether a pregnant woman has been recently exposed to *Toxoplasma*, if a newborn baby has been exposed, if an immunocompromised patient has an acute infection, and several others. A pathologist examining tissue samples can also visualize the parasite in several ways. It helps if the clinician gives the pathologist a hint that toxoplasmosis is a possible diagnosis.

Toxoplasmosis is a unique parasitic infection, one that has been associated with humans probably since we started walking the planet. The organism has adapted magnificently to reside within the person it infects, usually with no ill effects noted. Its ability to create a fine-tuned balance with its host and potentially influence the host's behavior makes it a most interesting organism. Scientists are still discovering its many talents.

Chapter 27
Kid's Stuff

Koplik's spots sighted.
Super spreader Morbilli
Has become entrenched.

"Full many a gem of purest ray serene
The dark, unfathom'd caves of ocean bear:
Full many a flower is born to blush unseen,
And waste its sweetness on the desert air."
                    -From "Elegy Written in a Country Church-Yard"
                    By Thomas Grey

Full many brilliant, resourceful scientists labor unceasingly in the quest to better the plight of humanity. Alas, only a few are acknowledged and remembered by history. Many are familiar with the names of Louis Pasteur, Edward Jennings, Alexander Fleming, and Jonas Salk, even if it was just to remember them for a social studies quiz. But many others have labored tirelessly and unyieldingly to help humanity rid itself of horrible diseases and suffering. Put the name of a Persian from the 9th and 10th centuries, Abu Bakr Muhammad ibn Zakariya al-Razi (known in the West as Rhazes), and a Dane, Peter Panum, who lived a thousand years later, on your social studies test, and it's a good bet that few would get the correct answer. But they both contributed greatly to the world's understanding and approach to medicine and disease, enabling future generations to develop treatments that benefit us today. Worlds and centuries apart, these two remarkable physicians illuminated facts about a disease that has infected humans mercilessly for at least a thousand years, rubeola. Most of us recognize it by its common name, measles. Their work was invaluable for that disease and trendsetting in the foundation of medical practice.

Rhazes was a true master. He was born in 865 AD in the foothills near present-day Tehran and spent most of his life there. At an early age, he studied music but later became interested in alchemy, philosophy, and medicine. Because of his gifts for learning and teaching, his reputation spread throughout the country, and he became famous in several fields, especially for his knowledge of medicine. Rhazes was a prolific writer, and his works were copied on a large scale and distributed widely. Since many were translated into Latin and Greek, he was considered his era's leading researcher and instructor.

Rhazes wrote over 200 volumes, a phenomenal number for his time, but his greatest influence came from his medical books. In them, he described a philosophy unknown at the time, the use of scientific logic to reach conclusions. He was reportedly the first physician to separate patient groups into two sets, one receiving a treatment, the other not, then evaluating the technique's usefulness. This is so commonly done today that none questions it, but it was unheard of in the ninth and tenth centuries. He wrote a book called *"For One Who Is Not Attended by a Physician or a Medical Advisor,"* a volume for the poor and ordinary citizens, the first of its kind. One of his greatest influences was distinguishing smallpox from measles, which up until his time, had been considered varied forms of the same disease. Though Middle Eastern, Rhazes' influence over Western medicine for the next thousand years was profound, not only for presenting medical facts and successful treatments but in the scientific approach to what was before mainly in the spiritual and superstitious domain.

The study of infectious diseases (or most diseases, for that matter) isn't conducted in a tightly controlled laboratory setting but in the real world with all its confusing extraneous, and sometimes complicated, factors. But in 1846, the embryonic period of the science of infectious diseases, an ideal situation for studying an infectious disease presented itself. It was an outbreak of measles on the Faroe Islands, located midway between Norway and Iceland. The Faroes were uniquely sequestered: the locals stayed confined to their island habitat, and strangers rarely ventured in. It was isolated for many years from outside influence, except for the occasional seaman or traveler passing through. When measles struck the island, the population was naïve to the virus; all inhabitants were susceptible. It provided the perfect opportunity for study. The Danish Ministry of Health dispatched Dr. Peter Panum to the islands to evaluate the measles epidemic and report his findings.

Dr. Panum and his team studied the natural history of the disease, including incubation time, duration of illness, and lifelong immunity. Dr. Panum undertook his task with alacrity and made many astute observations about the disease, which he published in a treatise titled *"Observations Made During the Epidemic of Measles on the Faroe Islands in the Year 1846."* The work was extremely important in describing the disease, especially its spread, when very little was known about the subject. It laid the groundwork for others to make similar observations about other diseases. John Snow is generally considered the father of epidemiology, but Panum's work preceded his by eight years.

Even though the people and physicians of olden times didn't understand the microbial cause of infectious diseases, they recognized, in a general way, their transmission from the infected person to the non-infected. The term "social distancing" was not used, of course. Still, through word of mouth, medical observance, and in some cases, governmental laws (as in the case of quarantine), most people knew to avoid those ill and showing overt signs of an illness. Measles was such a disease. The problem, of course, is that the disease can be spread before the hallmark signs are noticeable. Workers like Rhazes and Peter Panum laid the groundwork for a scientific approach to the field of epidemiology and the betterment of public health.

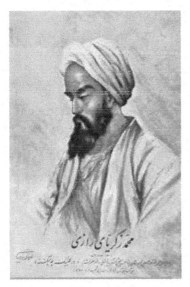

Abu Bakr Muhammad ibn Zakariya al-Razi, known to Westerners as Rhazes, was a brilliant physician, researcher, and author who influenced medicine for nearly a millennium. (LOC)

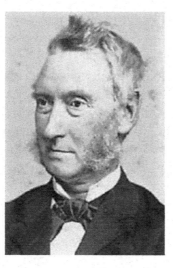

Peter Panum was a Danish physician and researcher credited with describing in detail the spread of measles in 1846. He helped lay the groundwork for the field of Epidemiology. (LOC)

Humans are the only creatures that can contract measles, but other animals have diseases caused by closely related viruses. Most dog owners know they must get their pet shots for the disease distemper, even though few actually know what distemper is. It's a disease similar to measles, at least the virus causing it is. When exposed to the distemper virus, most dogs become very ill, and some die. Sickened dogs run a very high fever, have runny noses, and develop profound diarrhea. They are listless with a reduced appetite. There is no cure for distemper, merely palliative care. Domestic dogs aren't the only members of the canine family that are vulnerable to the virus: wolves, foxes, and coyotes all can show the same symptoms. The range of animals susceptible to measles-related viruses doesn't stop with canines. Skunks, raccoons, large wild cats, and sea mammals such as dolphins have their own strains of a closely related virus that can make them seriously ill.

A cattle disease caused by a virus of the same type is of particular interest to humans. Although unknown to today's layman, the name rinderpest would strike horror into people hundreds of years ago. We humans have a list of diseases that can be catastrophic: plague, smallpox, cholera, typhoid, typhus.

419

Cattle had rinderpest, which to them is equally devastating. Nearly 100% of a herd can be wiped out once the infection sets in, with no cure once an animal is infected. Some speculate that rinderpest was the biblical fifth plague of ancient Egypt, wherein the livestock was felled. Symptoms vary with the strain of the virus, but typically there is a sudden onset of high fever, lethargy and loss of appetite, nasal and eye discharge, and rapid, labored breathing. The mouth's discharge turns bloody and necrotic, and the animal develops profuse diarrhea. Most animals die within 6-9 days following the onset of symptoms.

Fortunately, thanks to vaccination, rinderpest is extinct in farm animals today, but the history of the virus is of profound importance. (The name comes from the German word for cattle, *rinder*, and *pest* is short for pestilence). Molecular genetic evidence shows that measles, which affects only humans, originated from the virus that causes rinderpest. Some time ago, maybe as short as twelve hundred years, there was a mutation in the virus, allowing it to "jump" from cows to people. It has been firmly associated with humans ever since, leaving a path of destruction and horror in its wake.

The measles virus is technically classified as *Morbillivirus*. The "morbilli" part of it has an interesting history. Diseases often go by different names depending on time and place. Measles and smallpox have some notable similarities and were thought to be related for centuries. Smallpox was once known by the Latin name *morbus*, meaning disease. Measles was thought to be related but not as serious and was assigned the moniker *morbilli*, or smaller disease. The viruses causing smallpox and measles are entirely different, but based on symptoms alone the designation made sense, and the ancient term for measles remains as the name of the viral group.

Around the early 14th century the term measles was first used. It probably arose from the Latin *misellus*, meaning "wretched" or "miserable." The proper technical term today for the disease is rubeola, from the Latin word for red, *rubeus*.

Morbillivirus is a member of a viral family known as the Myxoviruses. Myxo is from the Greek word for "mucus" or "mucin." Mucin is a protein on the surface of red blood cells to which these viruses attach, causing the RBCs to clump (agglutination). The large group is broken down into two main types, Orthomyxovirus, or "true" Myxoviruses (the primary member here is the influenza virus), and Paramyxovirus, or "alongside" the true virus. Paramyxovirus includes many members, including the measles virus. All Myxoviruses are single-stranded RNA and have a wide range of host animals.

The invasion and infection by the measles virus is a paradox. It is acquired through the respiratory tract, but it is not a traditional respiratory virus. It initially invades lymphocytes and other cells that are part of the immune system, not the cells lining the respiratory tract. The virus does an excellent job suppressing our immune system by invading and killing the cells designed to repel it, activated lymphocytes and dendritic cells. And yet the body can still mount a vigorous immune response to eliminate the virus and establish the immune memory needed to prevent it from ever attacking again. There also is a great disparity in the mortality rate the virus leaves in its wake. There are credible reports of very high death rates in some populations and situations, sometimes reaching 20%, while the mortality rate is low in developed countries of the modern world. Such is the nature of this most unusual viral predator.

The measles virus is a relatively simple appearing creature, small and mostly spherical. It has a single strand of RNA, which is tightly wound in protein. Its coat contains two proteins, F and H, which allow the virus to attach to and penetrate a host cell. Just below these, forming the outer core, is a matrix protein, designated M. Altogether, the virus produces eight proteins.

After entering a susceptible person, the virus is encountered by dendritic macrophages, which carry it to nearby lymphatic tissue to begin building immunity to the microbe. But a funny thing happens during the journey to the lymph tissue: the viral attachment molecule H is strongly attracted to a protein on the surface of activated lymphocytes, CD-150 (also referred to as SLAM, short for signaling lymphocyte activation molecule). Lymphocytes begin their life's mission being naïve, non-specific, and awaiting chemical instructions on how to develop. Once a lymphocyte, either a T-cell or a B-cell, engages the appropriate foreign material, it becomes active and produces on its surface this CD-150 protein. By bearing it, the cell is constantly exposed to supporter cells that signal it to stay alive. Without it, the cell would die off as most naïve lymphocytes do. Keeping these activated lymphocytes alive is vital to immunological memory. If they are lost, they take with them the ability to mount a vigorous immune response when a pathogen is encountered for a second time.

By invading through the portal of the CD-150 protein of activated lymphocytes, the measles virus invades and kills the cells we need to protect us against previously encountered invaders. This, of course, leaves us vulnerable in the weeks and months following measles infection, and often the disease's fatal outcomes are due not directly to the measles virus, which is usually controlled, but by the secondary invasion of a pathogen we are no longer able to easily fend off.

Lymphocytes are mobile, of course, and they can travel to all parts of the body, taking the measles virus with them. As the virus hatches out of its host cells, millions of virions are released throughout the body, leading to a massive cytokine response by macrophages and dendritic cells. This cytokine release gives rise to the symptoms characteristic of measles, starting with the "three C's": cough, coryza (runny nose), and conjunctivitis (red, watery eyes). It takes about twelve days, give or take a couple, for the symptoms to manifest. Late in the incubation is the prodromal period, in which the symptoms begin appearing. At first, it looks like a common head cold, but over the next few days, the symptoms are anything but common—most patients, usually children, experience profound muscle aches, prostration, and fever. The fever can be severe, often reaching 106°F. Fever this high sometimes leads to seizures. These symptoms persist for up to a week. The patient is indeed very ill; some require hospitalization. Not long after the onset of fever, the rash appears, first appearing on the back of the neck, then spreading to the trunk, and then to the limbs.

The word pathognomonic comes from two Greek words, *patho*, or "disease," and *gnomonikos*, or one who "knows or judges." In medicine, the word (pronounced: pathhog-no-

MON-ic) is usually used to describe a sign or symptom that secures the diagnosis. In the case of measles, the pathognomonic symptom is Koplik's spots, small whitish spots usually on a reddened background found on the inside of the cheek, adjacent to the second and third molars. They are named after Henry Koplik, an American pathologist who first described them in 1896. (Others claimed to have described them before Koplik, but they were named after him, and so it stands). The spots are rather subtle, and a healthcare worker would likely have to suspect measles and look for them with a flashlight. They appear about two or three days before the rash and are usually gone by the time it appears.

The reason for Koplik's spots, the characteristic rash, and the respiratory nature of measles is that the virus has not one but two attachment receptors on human cells. The H protein attaches to lymphocytes, an advantageous accomplishment for the virus. But just involving itself with lymphocytes is a one-way street to extinction. The virus must get out of the host and on to the next victim (host). It does this through the second receptor, located on the surface of epithelial cells, designated nectin-4, also called poliovirus receptor-like 4, because polio attaches to the same receptor. Chemically, nectin-4 closely resembles CD150, the receptor on lymphocytes. Nectin-4 is present in all our epithelial cells, so the virus has a lot of places to go, including the skin. This attachment to the sub-layers of the skin and the immune response to it gives rise to the rash. The rash is known as maculo-papular, which is flat, red, and spreading. Pretty much the entire body, including the palms of the hands and the soles of the feet, are covered. But nectin-4 is most prominent in the epithelial cells of the respiratory tract, and that's where the virus makes its stand. With a severe cough, the virus is spread to the next vulnerable victim.

The measles virus is about the best there is at going from one individual to another. In common parlance, it's known as a "super-spreader." One person, with one cough, can spread the virus to numerous people in the same room. The infective dose for measles is very small (very few virus particles are needed to set up an infection), and millions of virions are coughed out from the infected individual. Unfortunately, the virus can cause extensive damage to the epithelial cells in the respiratory tract that it infects, leaving this area wide open for secondary infection by bacteria or other viruses. And, of course, the immune memory system has been laid low. Many of the deaths resulting from measles infection result from this immune suppression along with a secondary infection.

The measles virus is highly efficient and dynamic. It has two points of attack, activated lymphocytes and epithelial cells throughout the body. The characteristic rash that develops late in the disease epitomizes the involvement of the virus: it invades the body from the head and neck down to the soles of the feet. It's not just the skin that is involved. Just about every bodily tissue, including the brain, are vulnerable to the virus attack. Just how much damage the virus will do to any individual is unpredictable. With the suppression of the immune system and the invasion of numerous tissues, the fate of the disease is like Russian roulette. It could be a straightforward, albeit serious, viral infection that resolves within two weeks or one with a protracted or fatal outcome. There are many reported sequelae following measles, including hearing problems and deafness, encephalitis, pneumonia, and digestive problems.

Historically, there has been an extensive range of reported deaths from measles infection. In some settings, the mortality rate rivaled that of smallpox, over 20% of the population. Today in developed countries, the death rate is one in several thousand infected. One of the chief factors affecting the mortality rate is the presence of another disease or condition that leaves the patient more vulnerable to the measles virus. Known as co-morbidity, the other condition can range from malnutrition to an infectious disease. Getting hit with a rampaging virus like measles when already compromised can be a death blow.

Many bacteria can be grown in a batch of nutrients. Like organisms that grow in sour milk, some bacteria can grow in laboratory nutrients, known as culture media. The media can be carefully selected to provide just the right combination of ingredients to allow the bacterial species to prosper and grow, often displaying characteristics of its species. Viruses, however, need living tissue to reproduce and multiply. Just like the culture media required to grow bacteria, viruses have their favorite types of cells in which to grow, and choosing just the right cells for a particular virus can be challenging. Of course, the cells in the laboratory on which the virus grows must be kept alive, with special attention to preserving the cell line.

One of the pioneers in getting host cells to grow in the laboratory and finding just the right types of tissues suited for a virus was John Enders, one of the great scientific minds of the 20th century. His big breakthrough came in 1949 when he and fellow virologists Thomas Weller and Frederick Robbins got the polio virus to grow earnestly in tissue culture. This feat enabled others, notably Jonas Salk, to produce large volumes of poliovirus, disable it with formaldehyde, and create a vaccine. While Salk received most of the credit for the polio vaccine, Enders, Weller, and Robbins received the Nobel Prize in physiology in 1954 for their landmark discovery.

After the success with poliovirus, Enders turned his attention to the measles virus. Virologists had attempted to cultivate the virus for years but without success. Enders, along with colleague Thomas Peebles, worked out a system of measles virus cultivation. Enders was responsible for the lab work, while Peebles secured the specimens. Peebles traveled to several private boarding schools in Massachusetts to obtain clinical material, taking throat swabs. He then brought the specimens back to the lab, and the swabbed material was inoculated to the tissue culture plates. One of the first ones from which they cultivated the measles virus in the lab was obtained from an 11-year-old boy, David Edmonton. It was young David's virus that went on to become the measles vaccine strain, henceforth called the Edmonton strain.

After achieving the growth of the measles virus in the laboratory on human tissue cells, (tissues from discarded placentas from a nearby obstetrics unit were used), the Enders team set about the task of attenuating the virus to make it enter human cells while stimulating an immune response, but without making the person sick. It was a step-by-step process for many generations of viral passages. The measles virus only naturally infects humans and some non-human primates, but Enders was able to get it to grow on chicken embryos. This was the critical step they needed, as putting the virus into a non-hospitable environment would encourage the growth of a mutated virus instead of the wild-type one. If a virus mutates and can grow on non-primate tissue like chicken embryos, it will be selected and survive. The disease-causing strain won't be able to survive and will die out.

That's precisely what happened. After years of tedious laboratory work, Enders' team produced an attenuated measles virus that could grow on chicken embryo tissue. It could still invade human cells but in a much-reduced way. Injecting this virus into people stimulated the immune system to counter it, rendering the vaccine recipient immune, but the virus produced either no discernable disease or a very mild one. As was customary of the time (the late 1950s), the experimenters inoculated themselves and measured their symptoms and antibody response. While they all had had measles as children and were already immune, they showed that the antibody response to the attenuated measles virus was vigorous, and there were no noticeable side effects.

Of course, the live measles vaccine had to be verified for its effectiveness in the population. The researchers decided to administer the vaccine to a group of youngsters living in an institution for disabled children. Such institutions were pretty common at the time. Chosen was the Walter E. Fernald State School near Waltham, Massachusetts. The children housed and cared for there had mental or physically challenging disabilities. As happens so many times, well-meaning people can see an event in very different ways. To some, giving an experimental vaccine, a live one at that, to medically compromised children was an act of barbarism, a sure sign that the researchers considered the lives of such children minimal and expendable. The other opinion espoused by the researchers was that such children were at exceptional risk of severe complications or death should a measles outbreak occur. Since they were very confident in the vaccine's efficacy and safety, they were the very group that needed to be protected.

426

In the late 1950s, research standards weren't what they are today. Often experiments were carried out without the subjects' knowledge, or their tissues or body fluids used unknown to them. The measles research team under Dr. Enders was committed to scrupulous scientific ethics. Dr. Samuel Katz, the MD administering and monitoring the vaccine, ensured everyone involved had their parents fully informed and consent forms signed. In 1960, the experimental vaccine was administered to children in the Fernald boarding school, and follow-up studies were conducted each day. Blood samples were drawn to test for antibodies, and throat swabs were taken to search for the virus. Antibody levels were high, and the virus was undetected, a very good outcome. Based on these results, further testing was done around the United States with the same results. The measles vaccine had become a reality.

(The appropriate testing of the disabled children at the Fernald school was born out a couple of years later when a natural measles epidemic swept through the school. While recently admitted and unimmunized children became very ill with several deaths, the children given the experimental vaccine all showed no illness and no deaths).

The live, attenuated measles vaccine began to be used in the early 1960s. It wasn't perfect. Some children, maybe one or two in ten, developed some fever and discomfort a little over a week after vaccination. It was much better than wild-type measles during an epidemic, but vaccines with very few symptoms are the ideal. At Merck Pharmaceuticals, Maurice Hilleman and his crew further developed the attenuated Edmonton strain with many passages until it was more suitable than the original vaccine strain. The Merck strain has been combined with live attenuated mumps and rubella viruses to give us the present-day live tri-vaccine of measles-mumps-rubella, commonly referred to as MMR.

The alteration in the virus was marvelous. After passage through several different tissue cell lines, the chief attachment protein of the measles virus went from an affinity for the CD-150 receptor of activated lymphocytes to one known as CD-46. The latter is present in all human cells except red blood cells. The serum complement system is a potent destroyer of cells, including human. To prevent collateral carnage from activated complement, our cells are equipped with the CD-46 molecule, which effectively destroys the C3 component of complement, leaving our cells safe. At the same time, C3 does its work on invading bacteria. By attaching to the CD-46 receptor, the measles virus can still get into the host cell, but, for some reason, it is much less active, and the immune response to it is vigorous. Interferon is liberally released. The host cell undergoes apoptosis and dies, taking the virus with it. The immunized patient experiences little or no physical awareness of the virus. It's an ideal vaccine.

Another mystery of measles is how immunity to it lasts a lifetime. Our immune system has an excellent memory, but 60 or 70 years is a long time for T and B lymphocytes to hang around. The presence of CD-150 on activated cells, and its effect on memory, is helpful. Still, other infectious diseases require booster shots from time to time to keep immunity thriving. Tetanus shots, for instance, should be given every ten years or so. But immunity to measles, whether acquired naturally or through vaccination, seems to last as long as the patient. One unproven theory is that the virus is sequestered in some cells, perhaps lymphocytes, and emerges from time to time only to be confronted vigorously by antibodies, enhancing the immune response, something of a natural booster shot. Whatever the reason, the measles vaccination has been incredibly good for humanity, at least for those fortunate enough to get it.

The word "patrician" refers to a person of very good background, education, and refinement. It fits Dr. John Enders perfectly. Born into a wealthy family in Connecticut, he tried several ventures until he became enraptured by the laboratory work of his college roommate. He became a virologist and worked his way to the forefront of the development of one of the great scientific accomplishments of the modern age, the cultivation of viruses on laboratory-grown tissue cultures. Before this work in the 1940s, it was necessary to experiment with viruses strictly in animals, which was clearly a burdensome task. Ender's work led the way to the near eradication of two horrible diseases, polio and measles, and it enabled others to use his laboratory's techniques to work toward eradicating and diagnosing other pathogens. Truly an amazing accomplishment.

By his colleague's accounts, Dr. John Enders was an avuncular figure, always helpful, supportive, and encouraging. He frequently engaged in light conversation and held his employees in high esteem. The field of science can, in some ways, mimic others, with some of its members being a rapacious sort, quick to grab credit, glory, and the spotlight. This wasn't Dr. Enders, a kindly man who made some of the greatest discoveries of all time but whose name is virtually unknown to today's populace. His work has saved the lives of tens of millions of people and the terrible suffering of hundreds of millions more. He received a Nobel Prize along with Thomas Weller and Frederick Robbins in 1954, but the world owes him an even deeper debt of gratitude.

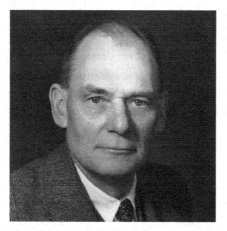

John Enders' work in virology led to the near eradication of polio, measles, mumps, and rubella in the developed world. It also laid the groundwork for the study and understanding of many different types of viruses. (LOC)

Measles is rare in the developed world. Most people today don't appreciate the magnitude of its ferocity. In the pre-vaccine era it attacked mainly children. It was estimated that by age 15, over 90% of the population would have contracted measles. Because of this, it is usually classified as a childhood disease alongside chicken pox, whooping cough, mumps, roseola, and German measles (rubella). Measles (rubeola) tends to get minimized historically. But it was, and is, a wretched disease, with a fever of up to 106° for up to a week, with seizures, hallucinations, and physical prostration. This is followed by a rash over the entire body that results in incredible itching. Add to that the suppression of the immune system for several months after the infection, leaving the patient vulnerable to potentially serious secondary infections. Measles is not, by any measure, kid's stuff.

The term herd immunity has been known to epidemiologists for many years but has become more commonly recognized in the popular lexicon in the past few years. Simply stated, infectious diseases transmitted from person to person, usually by the respiratory route, will not prosper and will quickly die out if a large percentage of the population is immune. When most of the people on the Faroe Islands had contracted measles in 1846, Peter Panum made the astute observation that the epidemic was over, and no new cases were observed. Such is the case in large cities, as the virus attacks only humans, and when all potential victims are either immune or dead, the virus has no place to go. Historically, measles came around every 2 to 4 years, when young children were old enough to be mobile and no longer protected by their mother's antibodies that they acquired in the womb.

Through much research, it has been determined that the percentage of people needed to be immunized against measles to achieve herd immunity is around 92%. That's a very high number, but one that reflects the highly infectious nature of the virus. If a mainly enclosed population does not have 92% of its members immunized, and measles is introduced, trouble, much trouble, ensues.

Chapter 28
The Black Death

From the flea's belly
To the unsuspecting node.
Purveyors of death.

Many infectious diseases have left their mark on human history, and in many ways. Some are endemic, afflicting a population segment in an ongoing fashion. Quite a few come around periodically in the form of an epidemic, sickening many in a relatively short period before fading away. Some wreak their havoc by being transported from one area of the world to another, being introduced to an immunologically naïve population. Malaria, smallpox, measles, cholera, typhoid, typhus, tuberculosis, rabies, anthrax, and diphtheria have, each in their own way, indelibly killed and sickened tremendous numbers of people and greatly influenced the course of history.

On any list of microbes that affected history, one of the most prominent is the organism *Yersinia pestis* and the disease it causes, bubonic plague. Imagine in the United States today, with its population of around 330 million, that a single organism in a couple of years killed one-third to one-half of the population, somewhere between 110 and 150 million people. That was the plague in Europe in the middle of the 14th century. Some historians claim it took 200 years for the population to recover to pre-plague numbers. The plague's appearance in Europe in such a devastating manner in the mid-1300s, at the beginning of the "Little Ice Age," tremendously influenced the course of Western Civilization's progress from the Middle Ages to Modernity. Its influence cannot be understated.

Historically, there have been three periods of the plague's appearance in the horrific form we call pandemics. The first appearance in the West was in 541 AD, during the reign of Roman Emperor Justinian I. Justinian, an extremely active ruler, earned the nickname "The Emperor Who Never Sleeps." His military exploits from his seat of power in Constantinople are the stuff of legends, and his marriage to his courtesan Theodora is the stuff of movies. But one thing he couldn't control was the bubonic plague which entered the city from the outlying areas of

Africa. It's hard enough to trace a pandemic from the Middle Ages, but describing one from the 6th century will undoubtedly be rife with speculation and extrapolation. But the plague is the most likely infectious disease to have invaded the Byzantine Empire during Justinian's reign, and it laid waste to the last resurgence of Roman power. It is said to have killed at least 5,000 per day, perhaps as many as 10,000. At least a third of Constantinople's population died. Justinian himself was stricken but survived. Things were never the same for Rome or its Empire.

The bubonic plague's introduction into Europe in 1347 is the subject of much historical discussion, given its immense ramifications. It was the second plague pandemic, and its consequences were enormous. The number of deaths, social upheaval, geopolitical realignments, and overall changes in lifestyle were profound, and many historians attribute the mid-14th century as the beginning of the transition from the Middle Ages to the Renaissance and the Modern Era.

By the 14th century, trade between East and West had been going on for thousands of years. It was mainly between India and Persia in the east, and the Middle East, northern Africa, and southern Europe in the west. There was some small trade with China, mainly in items like silk, jade, and certain spices, but the trade routes across the steppe regions of central Asia were long and treacherous.

This changed tremendously in the early 1200s with the ascendance of Genghis Khan, who united many of the tribes of the Mongols into an enormous, powerful force. By the early 1300s, the Mongolian Empire covered a vast area from China to the eastern part of Europe. With the growth of the Empire came the expansion of trade between East and West, and, as with any major disruption to an ecosystem, came new animals and organisms. Among the newcomers were Asian rats along with their fleas.

Just where the second plague pandemic originated is a matter of conjecture. *Yersinia pestis,* the bacterium causing the disease, is not a usual pathogen of humans. It infects the fleas of wild rodents, and the animals the fleas infest. The bacterium is at the mercy of the infected flea, and if the flea happens to bite a human, then that's who it'll infect. One credible-sounding theory is that the natural mammalian hosts of the *Yersinia pestis* were marmots (similar to prairie dogs) living in Central Asia's steppe areas, now Russia. As the Mongols carried their conquests west, the oriental rats came with them. The rats interacted with the marmots, and the fleas from the marmots jumped to and infested the rats. It's one theory; certainly, other explanations are just as plausible. Still, it seems most likely that the migrating Mongols brought the plague with them through the rat population that accompanied them.

Today we recognize Italy as a single nation, but in the 14th century it contained several city-states. Each had its own government, customs, and laws. One prominent city-state was Genoa, located on the coast of Italy's northwest corner, on the Ligurian Sea, not far from France. Its geographical location gave it prominence as a sea power, bringing goods from around the world to be sold into southwestern Europe. The Genoans were masterful shipbuilders and sailors, and they negotiated contracts around the known world to control seaports that could be used as trading centers. One of the cities they employed was Kaffa (sometimes spelled Caffa) on the peninsula of Crimea on the Black Sea. (Today Kaffa is known as Feodosiya). Governments in those days were subject to rapid policy changes, given the sometimes sudden changes in monarchs or rulers. The Genoans had an agreement with one of the Mongol Hordes to manage Kaffa, but in early 1343 there was bitter conflict, and under the direction of Jani Beg, the leader of the Golden Horde, the Mongols laid siege to the city. While the Mongols controlled entrance and exit from the land side, Kaffa bordered the sea, so Genoese ships could relatively easily supply the town. The siege dragged on for some time, but the Mongols gave up after a year and retreated. But Jani Beg wouldn't let the defeat go, and he and his army returned in 1345. The Mongol army was massive, but it also had a major problem. Somewhere along its march to Kaffa, it became involved with the rats that carried the fleas that carried *Yersinia pestis,* the agent of bubonic plague. As the siege began and soldiers resided in close quarters, the rats and fleas spread with impunity through the camp, and the plague struck many thousands. As one might imagine, morale sank, there were many defections, and many died. Before their retreat, the Mongols, either out of contempt or out of an act of warfare, are reported to have hurled hundreds of dead, rotting corpses over the city's walls with catapults. The terrorized Genoans hastily transported the bodies to the sea, but the damage was done.

Whether this tale is true or apocryphal, the Genoans contracted bubonic plague. Rats, of course, do not observe barriers like city walls, and they may have carried the disease with them in search of food, contaminating the city. At any rate, the soldiers and sailors returned to Genoa by way of Sicily in 1347, and the journey was one of tragedy. Most of the seamen died, and the survivors were seriously ill. They barely made it to port, and when they did, before the locals knew what was going on, the plague was introduced to southern Europe. It was in that same year that the second pandemic began, so it is easy to blame the Siege of Kaffa and the events that followed. Undoubtedly, the organism entered Europe by several routes, just as it had infected the Mongols from the north. By the late 1340s, most of Europe was engulfed in the most devastating pandemic in history.

Historians usually assign the second pandemic of the plague to have occurred from 1347 to 1352, or around five years. Certainly, the disease didn't just suddenly stop but would show up periodically for several decades. Indeed, severe disease erupted in England in 1664, and in Cologne and the Netherlands a few years later. Hundreds of thousands died. *Yersinia pestis* is a ferocious pathogen, and it alone would account for much of the deaths incurred, but the societal and psychological factors involved cannot be discounted. Panic and fear often make people behave strangely. Many fled an infected area, leaving susceptible people to fend for themselves. Northern Europe was already experiencing a significant food shortage because of the cold weather, and malnutrition was spreading throughout the continent. There are other diseases besides bubonic plague. Those, along with malnutrition, exacerbated the tragedy. People were loath to remain in a house where someone had died of the plague and would move in with friends or relatives, escalating crowding and disease exposure. *Yersinia pestis* can cause severe pneumonia as well as lymph node enlargement, and it can spread by coughing.

Looking back at the Black Death nearly seven hundred years later, we see mostly statistics and sociological impacts. Often lost is the human impact of the disease: a mother cradling her young, dying child, delirious with fever; children watching both their parents succumb in agony; rotting corpses being piled in the street for lack of workers or a place to bury them. Not every location was stricken the same. Some were infected heavily, others nearly spared. But the horror of the Black Death lived for ages.

(The term "Black Death" was not used at the time. It was assigned by historians later, probably in the mid-1700s, using the word black for the despair of death or a description of the necrotic lesions which are often a symptom of the disease).

The third pandemic of bubonic plague began in some of the smaller provinces of China in the 1860s, spreading slowly at first, then bursting on the scene in Hong Kong in 1894. Hong Kong is a seaport town, and steamships to and from there could travel long distances. Every inhabited continent was affected, but the heaviest hit was India. Death estimates are over 10 million.

The outbreak of the third pandemic of plague coincided with the dawn of scientists' discovery that microbes cause infectious diseases. Researchers didn't take long to isolate and identify the agent responsible for the plague. The bacterium was discovered around the same time by two scientists working independently, Frenchman Alexandre Yersin from the Pasteur Institute and Japanese researcher Kitasato Shibasaburo, an associate of Robert Koch. Both recovered the organism from infected individuals and injected them into healthy laboratory animals, causing them to acquire the disease. Dr. Yersin named the organism *Pasteurella pestis* in honor of his boss. Another organism was assigned to the genus *Pasteurella, P. multocida,* the cause of chicken cholera for which Pasteur had created a vaccine. The two organisms are unrelated, so in the 1970s, they were assigned different genera. The species *pestis* was assigned to a new genus, *Yersinia,* named for one of its discoverers, Alexandre Yersin.

Two years following the isolation and description of the organism, Japanese physician Ogata Masanori, working in Formosa (now called Taiwan), was intrigued by the die-off of rats just before a bubonic plague outbreak. He found the newly discovered plague bacillus in the fleas of the dead rats. He reported his findings. A year later, a French scientist, Paul-Louis Simond, an employee of the Pasteur Institute, confirmed the flea transmission and a new era of bubonic plague control was born—kill all the rats. It worked well, but not before the disease had spread to the entire world, a true pandemic.

The plague organism *Yersinia pestis* may have originated around 10,000 years ago, derived from a related bacterium that infects animals, *Yersinia pseudotuberculosis.* Another member of the genus is *Yersinia enterocolitica,* an organism transmitted to humans mostly from mice and rats. In humans, *Yersinia enterocolitica* causes a gastrointestinal ailment that can mimic appendicitis. The genus *Yersinia* belongs to the bacterial family *Enterobacteriaceae,* which includes *E. coli* and *Salmonella.* We don't know just where or just how, of course, but around 10,000 years ago, the organism now called *Yersinia pestis,* which was to become the plague bacillus, picked up some genetic material and went on its own course. The rest, as they say, is history.

The term for an infectious disease that ordinarily infects animals but can jump to humans is zoonosis, a word arising from the Greek *zoion,* or "animal," and *nosos,* meaning "sickness." The adjective is zoonotic. When an infectious disease outbreak affects many animals, the term applied is epizootic (drop the "n" from zoonotic), analogous to epidemics in humans. An epizootic often occurs parallel to a human epidemic when the disease is transmissible between species.

Yersinia pestis lives in two very different environments, an insect and a mammal. The former is, of course, cold-blooded, whereas mammals maintain a constant temperature. The organism infecting both must have a keen ability to shift its genetic expression rather quickly to allow it to survive in its animal host. *Y. pestis* does this very well, and in a very short time, it can go from flea gut to mammal skin extremely efficiently. It is pathogenic for both insects and mammals.

In the flea, *Yersinia* produces an enzyme that protects it from the digestive juices of the flea mid-gut, and it forms a biofilm that effectively blocks the flea's digestive tract. This puts the flea into starvation mode, making it feed more vigorously. When taking a blood meal from a mammal, such as a rat or human, the flea regurgitates the newly sucked blood along with a part of the *Yersinia pestis* blockage into the skin of the animal victim. This simple act efficiently introduces the pathogen to the animal host, initiating the disease path.

When *Yersinia* is introduced into the skin, it is met by two types of immune system cells. The neutrophils that exit the bloodstream and wander about the tissues are a death trap for the organism. They gobble up the bugs and digest them with impunity. The phagosome containing the organism inside the neutrophil is met with the ferocity of the phagocyte's numerous granules, and organism death ensues.

But the other cell the bacterium encounters has a much different result than neutrophils. Macrophages are designed to kill bacteria and usually do an outstanding job. But *Yersinia pestis* has a means of beating the system, and it does it with high efficiency. When taken up by the macrophage, the plague bacillus, like all organisms, is engulfed in a vacuole called a phagosome. Normally, the phagosome in the macrophage is linked up with a bacterial-killing vacuole called the lysosome; the two merge and the organism is immersed in digestive enzymes. But *Yersinia pestis* has found a way around this certain death. On its outer membrane, *Yersinia pestis* has a set of proteins called PhoP/PhoQ, a rather odd name. Together they alert the bacterium's genome that they are in a much different place than a flea's gut, and the wheels of genomic expression are set in motion. For one, the lysosome of the macrophage is prevented from merging with the phagosome, and the invading bacteria begins to replicate. *Yersinia* is a member of the rapidly multiplying family *Enterobacteriaceae,* and when it gets going, it can replicate very fast.

The microbe-bearing macrophage has two important jobs. One is to kill the invading bacteria within its phagosome. The other is to make its way to the nearest lymph node. In the case of bubonic plague, it fails dramatically in its first job. But in the second it carries out its mission admirably. While in haste to the nearest lymph node, the microorganisms within the macrophage are feverishly replicating. By the time the macrophage gets to where it's going, it is replete with viable bacteria, which have changed from when they were inside a flea.

By reaching the lymph node inside their accommodative macrophage host, the bacteria have completely transformed from flea-dwellers to mammal-dwellers. It only takes a few hours for that change to take place. If that mammal happens to be a human, so be it. Their tricks work similarly in quite a few species.

One protein the bacteria make while incubating inside the macrophage has a rather odd name, pH6-antigen, also called PsaA. When discovered many years ago, it was found only to be produced in an acidic environment, hence the pH6 part. PsaA is present as a pilus, or a tiny bit of fuzz on the bacterial surface, and its role is quite extraordinary. It binds to part of the large complex that carries cholesterol in the human body, LDL, or low-density lipopolysaccharide, sometimes given the rather unfortunate name of "bad cholesterol." pH6-antigen of *Yersinia pestis* binds to a part of LDL (apo-lipoprotein B, or *apo*-B). Doing so hides the organism from a major part of the human immune system. The organism is essentially "cloaked," as complement and phagocytes recognize the LDL portion as self and don't attack it.

The bacteria in the mammal host manufacture a capsule surrounding the bacterial cell. Called the Factor-1 antigen, or F1, the organism becomes much less likely to be engulfed by a phagocyte.

All Gram-negative organisms have a substance called lipo-polysaccharide, or LPS, in their cell walls. Also called endotoxin, it is a potent stimulator of the immune response and is usually easily recognized by the immune system. Most notably, Toll-like receptor 4 is highly attracted to it and, in concert with two other proteins, mounts a vigorous response to

438

eliminate the pathogen. Not all LPS is identical, and *Yersinia pestis* has devised a plan to maintain its necessary LPS, but at the same time avoid its detection by Toll-like receptor 4 and the immune response sure to follow. Most LPS has six acetyl groups attached, but when inside the macrophage undergoing its transformation, *Yersinia pestis* produces an LPS with only four. The result is the production of lipo-polysaccharide that eludes detection by the cells of the immune system.

The innate immune system is a powerful force against invaders, but the plague bacillus thwarts its early actions. To summarize, shortly after entering the skin of its victim through flea vomit, it avoids its destruction in the vacuole of a macrophage, transforming itself in just a few hours from an insect pathogen to a human one. Then it makes itself look like the body's own cholesterol transporter, LDL, hides its LPS from detection, and encases itself with a phagocyte-resistant capsule so that it can reproduce with very little initial resistance from the cells of the immune system. These factors go a long way in initiating the horrific infection to follow.

As if these immune system evasion strategies aren't enough, *Yersinia pestis* has the Yops. While it sounds like some disease afflicting the bacteria, Yops stands for "Yersinia outer proteins." There are several of them, and their role in life is to further impede the immune system's response to the invasion of the pathogen. Each is abbreviated Yop followed by a capital letter, like YopE or YopH. Each has a distinct, nefarious role in allowing the organism to do its worst.

Like *Salmonella, Yersinia* can inject molecules into a target cell. They form a needle-like complex, sort of like a syringe, that allows the flow of materials from the bacterial cell into the host cell. With a half-dozen Yop proteins, *Yersinia has* the right one for any occasion.

Natural killer lymphocytes are invaluable in the early stages of infection, destroying the human cells that harbor pathogenic organisms. Kill the infected host cell, and the pathogen dies with it. *Yersinia* makes YopM, a substance that can destroy large amounts of NK lymphocytes and, at the same time, reduce the amount of interferon-gamma that can be made. Without enough INF-gamma, macrophages of all stripes cannot adequately kill invaders, nor can they summon the release of cytokines that can strengthen the immune response.

Another job for some of the Yops produced by *Yersinia pestis* is disrupting the ability of phagocytes, monocytes and neutrophils, to engulf and phagocytize them. When the organism is attached, several Yop proteins are injected into the host phagocytic cell and go directly to the enzymes that provide the energy for forming actin and other molecules necessary for motility and the movement of phagocytosis. They basically paralyze the cell that is trying to engulf and digest them. The Yops also significantly reduce the production of critical inflammatory cytokines like tumor necrosis factor-α and interleukin-8, thereby tamping down what should be a vigorous immune reaction to the invading microbe.

Neutrophils are produced in the bone marrow, are released into the blood vessels, then circulate until they reach the spot where they are needed. They are "hooked" from the circulation by a chemical arm from the cells lining the blood vessel. These chemical hooks are known as ICAM and E-selectin. Two Yops, P and J, work in concert to subdue the expression of these neutrophil hooks so that not as many can enter the infected area. Also, the chemical attractant that induces neutrophil recruitment to the site of the infection, interleukin 8, is significantly reduced by the activity of *Yersinia* proteins.

One of the immune system sentinels we all have is Toll-like receptor-2. It sits atop several types of cells, but it is most prominent on macrophages and neutrophils. TLR-2 is designed to detect molecules unique to several different types of microbes, including bacteria. When it encounters a small piece of invading microbe, TLR-2 gets active and begins a process whereby the part of the DNA in the nucleus that codes for inflammatory cytokines, which was previously sequestered, is uncovered, and the molecules are manufactured. The cytokines made and released, such as TNFα, IL-1β, and IL-6, are very important in activating the immune system. *Yersinia pestis* makes a protein called LcrV (also called simply V-antigen) that interferes with the activity of TLR-2. The chemical signal meant to be sent to the nucleus to activate the release of the critical cytokines doesn't happen. The result is a muted cytokine and hence an immune response.

Invading bacteria will invariably encounter serum complement, a complicated system of over thirty molecules that act in a cascade-like fashion to assist in killing the microbe. (See Chapter 8). Whether by helping to present an antibody-bound microbe to a phagocyte or acting by itself by one of the alternative pathways, complement is a powerful force in the body's defense. *Yersinia pestis* has an outer membrane protein, Ail, that effectively subdues complement activity. Briefly, to function, the vital complement component C3 must be activated. It is a potent killing force and must be carefully controlled. Encounter with the invading microbe activates the C1 molecule, triggering a combination of C2 and C4. The active C1-C2-C4 enzyme, known as C3 convertase, has the job of activating the C3. C3 will then break into two parts, the smaller C3a portion sailing off to further activate the immune system, the larger C3b assuming the role of helping to kill the microbe and further activating the rest of the complement cascade. The Ail molecule of *Yersinia pestis* is adept at inactivating the C4 complement component, thereby preventing its hooking up with C2 to convert the inactive C3 into the active form. Obviously, without complement operating at its highest capacity, the killing of invading plague bacillus is mitigated.

Yersinia pestis is endowed with weapons that greatly damage the innate immune system of the animal it infects, whether a marmot, rat, human, or other. By evading several early response elements, whether cellular or molecular, the organism gets a rapid start in commencing its infection, something that other organisms would not be able to attain and would be repelled. *Yersinia's* chief means of propagation, going from a mammal to a flea and then back to another mammal, can only be achieved if they are in very high numbers in the host mammal's circulatory system so that when the next flea takes a blood meal, it is much more likely to suck up some *Yersinia pestis* organisms with that small amount of blood. Without having such high numbers of bacteria, the cycle would be broken, and the organism would die out.

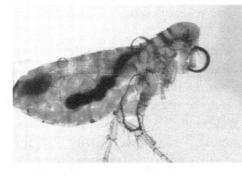

The rat flea Thrassis bacci, subsp. *johnsoni, a vector of Yersinia pestis. The dark biofilm of the bacteria is visible in the midgut. (PHIL)*

Summary of some of the means *Yersinia pestis* uses to evade or subvert the immune system:

Survive within macrophage
Camouflages itself to look like cholesterol carrier LDL
Encapsulates itself with F1 antigen, hindering phagocytosis
Reduces the number of acetyl groups on its Lipid A to escape Toll-like receptor-4 recognition
Destroys Natural Killer lymphocytes, reducing interferon-gamma release
Disrupts the cytoskeleton of phagocytes, greatly hampering phagocytosis and necessary cytokine release, such as interleukin-8 and TNF-alpha
Reduces the ability of the nearby endothelium lining blood vessels to recruit circulating neutrophils and direct them to the infected area
Interferes with the activity of Toll-like receptor-2, reducing cytokine production and inflammatory response
Disrupts activity of complement, interfering with opsonization and inflammatory response

The word bubo comes from the Greek word for groin, *boubon.* When fleas bite human adults, it is usually on the legs. Macrophages cannot kill the plague bacteria they pick up in the skin following a flea bite, but they are very good at transporting the bacteria growing inside them to the nearest lymph node. For the legs, that would be the groin or medial thigh. Somewhere in history, the term bubo came to be used for the marked swelling of these lymph nodes, along with the adjective bubonic. (The term used today for a swollen lymph node(s) is lymphadenitis). There are many diseases in which swollen lymph nodes are found, but the swollen nodes in bubonic plague are often so massive that the term bubonic is reserved for that one disease.

Fleas can bite us anywhere; other areas of the body where lymph nodes are congregated can also show buboes. The axillary region (armpit) is common, as well as the neck and chest.

Buboes can be extremely large, perhaps the size of an egg. They reportedly are incredibly painful; afflicted patients assume a guarded posture to keep from hurting. After a time, the tissue in and around the nodes dies and becomes necrotic, resulting in skin blackening. The cytokine storm that arises from the disease results in blood clots occurring within blood vessels (disseminated intravascular coagulation, or DIC), giving rise to areas of the body becoming blackened due to necrosis, especially the fingers and toes. Whether the term "black death" arose from the necrotic condition of parts of the body or the feeling of darkness and doom is hard to say. Perhaps both.

Yersinia pestis dramatically interferes with the activity of the host immune system, but it doesn't dismantle it. The organism fights more of a delaying tactic, impeding the innate immune system long enough to gain a strong foothold in its reproduction inside the body. Eventually, the immune system is strongly activated. Early in the infection, the organism is multiplying rapidly, producing enormous numbers of bacteria. As time passes, many of these bacteria die off, and the pool of dead bugs and many live ones stimulates the immune system, which, with so many bacteria in the normally sterile parts of the body, reacts with a massive response. The highly inflammatory cytokines tumor necrosis factor-α, interleukin-1β, and interleukin-6 are released en masse, and symptoms ensue.

The incubation period (from flea bite to the first symptom) is usually three or four days but can be as short as a day or up to a week. One of the hallmarks of the illness is the rapid onset and severity of the symptoms. In addition to the inflamed lymph nodes, the patient experiences sudden fever, aches, and prostration. In just an hour or two, a person feeling relatively healthy can become so ill as not to be able to move. Fever can reach 106°F, accompanied by delirium and hallucinations. Every muscle and joint in the body aches. Patients are profoundly ill and sometimes panic-stricken.

Bubonic plague-affected lymph nodes are filled with bacteria and neutrophils, which attract fluid. Invariably, some bacteria get into the bloodstream, a condition known as bacteremia, or bacteria in the blood. A more serious condition is septicemia, wherein bacteria infect the bloodstream, not just pass along in it. Septicemia with a Gram-negative organism like *Yersinia pestis* often results in a fatal condition known as sepsis. In some cases, the lymph nodes are not swollen, but the bacteria enter the bloodstream directly from the flea bite.

With bacteria in the blood, some will be introduced into the lungs. Usually, they are screened out by neutrophils, but pneumonia sets in in a few cases. Plague pneumonia is extremely serious; untreated, it usually results in death. There are two kinds of plague pneumonia, secondary and primary. In secondary pneumonia, the organisms alight in the lungs after being carried there in the bloodstream. In primary pneumonia, the patient breathes the organism in, presumably from another individual coughing out the organism. Like the bubonic form of the disease, pneumonic plague has a very rapid onset, and the patient becomes very ill. The sputum usually contains blood, sometimes in trace amounts, sometimes copious. Untreated, death occurs in a day or two.

Given that *Yersinia pestis* is such a deadly organism, it has been considered to have high potential as a bioterrorism weapon. Training a squadron of fleas to march around infecting people is not a practical idea, so alternative means of initiating an infection have been considered by people who consider such things. Aerosol release with subsequent inhalation and pneumonia seems the most obvious means of delivery.

Yersinia pestis is a member of the bacterial family *Enterobacteriaceae*, notorious for the development of resistance to antibiotics. It would not be very hard for scientists to develop strains of the organism that are multi-drug resistant. In 1995 in Madagascar, a multi-drug resistant strain of plague bacillus was isolated from a 16-year-old boy. It was resistant to streptomycin, chloramphenicol, ampicillin, sulfonamides, kanamycin, and tetracycline. It probably acquired a plasmid coding for the resistance genes in the wild, so creating such a beast in the controlled conditions of a laboratory would not be difficult.

There are two other species of *Yersinia* besides *pestis* that infect humans, *Y. enterocolitica* and *Y. pseudotuberculosis.* Both are zoonotic, but instead of usually entering the body by a bite of the skin, they enter through the consumption of food or water.

While *Yersinia pestis* burst on the scene with never-to-be-forgotten sudden horror, the awareness of *Yersinia enterocolitica* by medical professionals was far more subtle. It was introduced by way of a medium given without much thought or concern–chocolate milk. At a hospital in upstate New York in 1976, just about every day for a week, kids were coming into the emergency room with symptoms classic for acute appendicitis. Thirty-eight were admitted to the hospital, and 16 had appendectomies. The surgeons observed that the appendices appeared normal, which was confirmed by pathology. It turned out that none of the kids had appendicitis, but rather pseudo-appendicitis caused by the organism *Yersinia enterocolitica.* Upon further investigation, the source of the infections was chocolate milk served in their school cafeteria. The most likely explanation for the event was that after the milk had been pasteurized it was mixed with chocolate syrup, and somewhere the product was contaminated with rat or mouse feces containing the organism.

These non-pestis species of *Yersinia* infect as a type of food poisoning: a food product is contaminated with an animal product and then consumed. Most cases don't involve many people, often just a case or two, seemingly in isolation. The patient may present as one mimicking appendicitis or as gastroenteritis. *Yersinia enterocolitica* often invades the terminal ileus, the end of the small intestine where it meets the colon, the spot where the appendix is. It also invades lymph nodes; only these are the mesenteric nodes of the deep abdomen, so they are not visible on examination but are painful when pressed. We are lucky that *Yersinia* does not tolerate stomach acid and bile very well, and it takes a hefty dose of organisms, probably over 10 million, to infect us. *Yersinia*, like another food-borne organism, *Listeria*, grows at refrigerator temperatures, albeit slowly, so contaminated food stored for extended periods may be infectious. Diagnosis is sometimes not easily made because most laboratories don't routinely screen stool specimens for the organisms, given their rarity. The occurrence of these other species of *Yersinia* is undoubtedly higher than reported.

Yersinia pestis didn't just disappear. It is still with us, even in developed countries like the U.S. and Europe, where it is endemic in some rodent populations. The term applied is sylvatic plague, the word sylvatic from the Latin *silvaticus,* meaning "in the wild." It can occasionally make its way into a human. An example is a woman who lived in a mountainous area of California in the 1990s whose dog captured and brought home a rodent. In cleaning up the mess, the woman was infected. Prompt treatment saved her life. Thankfully, sporadic is the word we now use to describe the infection of the plague bacillus, not pandemic. Let's hope it stays that way.

Chapter 29
Biological Weaponry

Merciless killer,
And yet easily concealed.
Dust in a baggie.

People have always known that there are highly lethal diseases. While it took centuries to discover the biological nature of the causes, there was no mistaking the malignancy of some ailments. People have also been killing each other with weapons of war for a very long time. Throughout history, there have been anecdotal reports of using the former to achieve the latter. Catapulting dead plague victims over a castle wall, giving the blankets or clothing of smallpox victims to susceptible individuals, poisoning water wells with bodies of victims of some infectious disease. Such attempts were crude, "shot-in-the-dark" attempts to sow the evil miasma of the disease into the enemy. The cause of the infectious disease was unknown, but it was highly suspected that some diseases could spread.

As knowledge of microbes as the cause of disease became widely known, so did interest in their utility as a weapon. In some ways, the development of biological weapons paralleled the use of chemical weapons. World War I introduced the widespread use of chemicals such as mustard gas, chlorine, and nerve agents. Infectious agents as weapons are harder to prepare and deliver, so their use came later, but they nevertheless arrived. The first major, organized employment of pathogenic microorganisms as weapons was a truly monstrous program used by the Japanese in China before and during World War II. The horror it wrought was indescribable.

Manchuria is a large northeast Chinese province bordering Russia to the north and Mongolia to the east. For much of its history, Manchuria was inhabited by people of varying ethnicities. It was often involved in wars, either embattled itself or lending its soldiers to other countries' armies. The founders of the Chinese Qing Dynasty, which ruled China from the mid-1600s until the early 1900s, originated in Manchuria. Qing emperors ruled China until they were overthrown in 1911 when the Japanese took over the Manchurian territory. In the Manchuria region, "Manshu" in Japanese, unspeakable atrocities using biological weapons occurred.

At the center of the biological weapons operations was a prison camp known by the mundane title of Unit 731. The head of the operation was a Japanese general named Shiro Ishii. The prison camp was built in 1935, and its 150 buildings covered six square kilometers of land near the community of Pinfang. Ishii and his team used the facility for their research headquarters. The Japanese named it "Epidemic Prevention and Water Purification Department." Several high-ranking Japanese physicians and microbiologists were stationed there. In addition to Unit 731, about a half-dozen other facilities communicated with the central headquarters. It is estimated that about 10,000 Japanese doctors and scientists participated in the program. The real reason for the complex's existence was to produce and perfect the use of microbial agents in weaponry. No stone was left unturned.

Fleas were allowed to feed on animals with bubonic plague, then placed in canisters to be used as plague bombs. At first, glass was used, then porcelain was found to be better when dropped from an airplane. Cholera organisms were placed in sealed containers so troops could use them to contaminate water supplies. Anthrax spores were produced to be easily aerosolized. *Shigella,* the cause of dysentery, was grown to be disbursed in bombs or mortar shells to infect the enemy. Experiments were conducted with smallpox, as well as the transmissibility of syphilis.

From 1935 to 1937, experiments were done at various camps, with results perfected at Unit 731. There were around 3,000 captives, primarily locals of varied backgrounds: rebellious youth, old men and women, mentally ill, criminals, and foreigners. Experiments were carefully documented, and the weaponization of biological agents was perfected. No one is known to have gotten out of the camps alive. In some cases, vivisection (performing an autopsy on a live person), sometimes without anesthesia, was practiced to observe the results of infections without the "pollution" of death.

In 1937 Japan invaded mainland China, with much of the force coming from the northeast and Manchuria. The biological weapons developed at Unit 731 and other facilities were part of the invasion weaponry. The results of their release are difficult to state accurately given the fog of war, but it's safe to say at least 300,000 Chinese died due to infectious diseases released by the Japanese. Person-to-person spread is, of course, integral to many of the diseases, so the actual indirect number is undoubtedly much higher. When viewed solely from the perspective of an effective weapon, biological warfare was a success.

War crimes are punishable by death. The obvious conclusion to this unmitigated horror should have been the execution of those responsible. But the circumstances of war and international affairs are sometimes conflicting. The United States government was very afraid that the Soviet Union, bordering Manchuria, would gain access to the scientific data of the affair and gain the upper hand in developing biological weapons. At the war's conclusion, a deal was struck between the U.S. and the Japanese involved to hand over all available data, and the perpetrators would escape punishment. It was a plea bargain on a grand scale.

The Japanese took the testing, production, and utilization of microbial weapons to a high level. It did not escape the notice of other nations with the resources to explore them. During the war, the British government was convinced that Germany was developing its own arsenal of biologicals and felt compelled to develop its own program. They chose anthrax spores for testing and selected Gruinard Island, a small, deserted island off the west coast of Scotland, for the experiment. Eighty sheep were tethered to poles, and several bombs containing a highly virulent strain of anthrax spores were detonated. All the sheep died within a few days. There could be no doubt that biological material is a very effective military weapon.

Given the dramatic effect of biological weapons in World War II, the superpowers of the United States and the Soviet Union quickly established their own programs following the war. Both claimed they were afraid the other side had a vigorous program and didn't want to be left behind and vulnerable, reasoning that had a parallel in the development of nuclear weapons. Research and manufacture began slowly, then reached very high activity. All was done secretly, and public knowledge of the programs was limited.

After several decades of development, testing, manufacture, and stockpiling, both countries had accumulated vast amounts of bioweapons. Just how much is difficult to accurately say because the information was highly classified. Despite treaties avowing the discontinuation of the programs, they nonetheless persisted.

An obvious fallibility in using biological weapons is the "boomerang effect"—the attacker's troops and people can be sickened and succumb to the organism just like the opponents. The obvious exception to this rule is the disease anthrax, which isn't spread person-to-person and remains in the area where it was released. But even anthrax isn't perfect.

A tragic occurrence secondary to a bioweapons program occurred on the outskirts of a Russian city in 1979. Yekaterinburg is the third largest city in Russia, located at the foot of the Ural Mountains about 800 miles east of Moscow. (The city was named after a remarkable woman, Catherine I, who rose from a poor family in what we now call Lithuania to become the wife of Peter the Great and then the first tsarina of Russia. Following the revolution in 1917, the city was named Sverdlovsk in honor of a dignitary in the Revolution. Since the fall of the Soviet Union, the city has assumed its original name).

One day in April 1979, a worker in a factory failed to properly replace a filter on an exhaust pipe. The secret factory was manufacturing large amounts of weaponized anthrax spores. Spewing out with the unfiltered exhaust came large amounts of the deadly spores wafting about the air. Downwind from the factory, people went about their daily routines, oblivious to the event. Just how many died is the subject of much debate, as the Soviet government went into full denial mode, but it was likely at least several dozen people and many farm animals. One thing was clear: weaponized anthrax spores are deadly, even when released into the open air. The United States experienced its own confrontation with anthrax in the fall of 2001, in which a deliberate attack using letters in the mail killed five and infected seventeen others.

The word "bacillus" has something of a double meaning. The word comes from the Latin, *baculum,* which means a "staff" or "walking stick." Bacillus is a descriptive term in bacteriology, referring to a rod-shaped organism, as opposed to a round one, or coccus. But it also is the name of a genus of bacteria, *Bacillus,* a widespread group of organisms that inhabit many environments. By their nature, all members of *Bacillus* are rod-shaped spore-formers. To put it in confusing terms, "all *Bacillus* look like a bacillus, but not all organisms that look like a bacillus are *Bacillus.*" With a Gram stain, young organisms usually stain Gram-positive, but older ones may turn Gram-negative. There are over 250 species of *Bacillus*, most of which are harmless soil-dwellers. Many make and excrete toxic enzymes, but very few affect humans. Gardeners may be familiar with the organism *Bacillus thuringiensis,* commonly called Bt, which produces a potent insecticide against a wide range of insects. The species *B. cereus* and *B. subtilis* can manufacture toxins. When allowed to grow to very high numbers on food products, such as rice, they can cause limited food poisoning, resulting in either diarrhea or vomiting.

One *Bacillus* species, *B. cereus,* can cause a rapidly progressing and heavily damaging eye infection, endophthalmitis. *B. cereus* produces several toxins that severely damage the eye's interior, and the organism is motile and able to move around. Rapid diagnosis and antibiotic treatment are critical, as the eye may be lost within 48 hours. The organism usually reaches the eye's interior by trauma, such as debris from industrial machinery. The value of the use of safety goggles cannot be understated.

Bacillus is very good at forming biofilms; sometimes, it gets into a place where it can clog a catheter line. These infections, food poisoning, endophthalmitis, and obstructed catheter lines, are relatively rare. In the big scheme of things, the genus *Bacillus,* despite its ubiquity in nature, is not a very worrisome pathogen for humans. Because many species grow readily on routine laboratory culture media, it is sometimes encountered as a contaminant of specimen collection, and its presence in clinical material is merely an annoyance.

There is one enormous exception to this general statement: *Bacillus anthracis*, the etiologic agent of the disease anthrax. Many eons ago, based on genetic information, *Bacillus anthracis* emerged from *Bacillus cereus*, picked up some genes from other organisms, and turned into a serious pathogen of animals, many of them domestic. It is not a primary infector of humans but of the animals with whom humans often come into contact, such as cattle and sheep. Rare today in developed countries, at one time it would wreak havoc on human populations, more from the slaughtering of vitally necessary farm animals than the direct illness and death of the populace. Mainly a zoonotic infection, anthrax was never a massive killer like bubonic plague, smallpox, or cholera. It is not transmissible from human to human. It is more of a sporadic infection, jumping from animals to humans. It is nonetheless a highly lethal infectious disease.

An ancient disease, anthrax has been a scourge for thousands of years. The species name comes from the Greek word for coal, no doubt because of the black scar characteristic of human skin infections.

At the beginning of the elucidation of the nature of infectious diseases, scientific research on anthrax led to two very important discoveries by two of the greatest investigators of microbes of all time. In the late 1870s, controversy raged over the role of microbes in infectious diseases. The presence of bacteria in ill patients was irrefutable, but the reason for them being there was contentious. Generally, one side claimed their presence was the result of the disease, not the cause of it, while the other maintained they were the reason for the disease. It was not appreciated that there are many different species and strains of bacteria, as they had not been cultured and classified, so the former position seemed tenable. Visualizing unstained bacteria in a specimen may have been the result of putrefaction. Robert Koch's work on anthrax in some farm animals helped settle the matter.

Anthrax was known to affect herds of animals quite differently. Some grazing areas were referred to as "cursed fields" because of their high numbers of infected animals, while other pastures were unscathed. Around the year 1876, Koch, a physician, investigated the death of an excess of 50,000 animals and 500 people over four years in an area that is now part of Poland. At the time, culture media for growing bacteria in the laboratory did not exist. Koch somehow got the idea that he could use a cow's vitreous humor (inside of the eyeball) to cultivate the organisms he had recovered from the bloodstream of infected animals. It worked. The anthrax organisms grew in pure culture, uncontaminated by competing bacterial flora.

Dr. Koch took the anthrax organisms that originated in the dead animals, grew them to high numbers in the cow eyeball, and injected them into some lab animals, inducing the disease. He then injected some of the infected lab animals' blood into other animals, again causing the infection. Over several generations, he continually produced the disease by introducing the organism into healthy animals. Over the following few years, workers in Koch's laboratory perfected the means to grow bacteria in artificial culture, with discoveries such as culture media, agar, and the Petri dish. With more work, Koch could grow different organisms on some media in the laboratory, something that hadn't been done before. He then showed that there are different types of bacteria, and some cause a unique disease. This began the "Golden Age" of microbiology and infectious diseases.

Koch used the anthrax bacillus to establish his theory on the microbial involvement in disease, what was to become known as Koch's postulates: an organism must be isolated in pure culture from a diseased animal; it alone is then shown to induce the disease in a healthy animal; and it must be recovered from that second animal.

Louie Pasteur used anthrax to convincingly demonstrate that altered organisms could induce immunity to the wild type. Koch had shown how to isolate the organism in culture, and Pasteur set about changing it to prevent it from causing disease but still induce immunity. Pasteur had succeeded in this effort with the chicken cholera disease, and his work on anthrax was similarly inspired. Pasteur subjected his cultures to potassium dichromate. They didn't grow all that well, but they did grow, and when he took the viable organisms and put them into lab animals, they didn't develop anthrax. He waited a week and then challenged them with a pathogenic strain. Much to his amazement, the lab animals were not made sick, let alone die.

The laboratory experiment notwithstanding, much controversy existed about microbes, disease, and vaccines. To prove his point to the world, Pasteur announced to the press that he would conduct an experiment on some farm animals in the French town of Pouilly-le-Fort. His experiment was rather dramatic, publicly injecting 25 sheep with his vaccine, leaving 25 unvaccinated. Two weeks later, he gave a second vaccine injection to the 25 previously injected. After a month, he injected all 50 animals with cultures of the live anthrax bacillus. All vaccinated sheep survived, and all unvaccinated perished. The modern era of microbiology and immunology had begun.

While *Bacillus anthracis* hasn't historically killed as many humans as other pathogens, it is arguably the most aggressive and vicious. There are bona fide reports of the staggering numbers of organisms found in the bloodstream of some of its victims: more bacteria than red blood cells. Its initial targets are the cells designed to eliminate it: neutrophils, macrophages, and dendritic cells, the primary line of defense of the innate immune system. As the organisms enter the blood, they are transported to the body's organs, where they continue their wholesale destruction. The mortality rate in untreated patients approaches 100%.

A very good argument could be made that *Bacillus anthracis* is actually a strain of the closely related *Bacillus cereus*. Both share the same genome (as does the insect pathogen *Bacillus thuringiensis*). The difference, and it's a big one, is the presence of two plasmids within *B. anthracis* that code for the formation of the toxins that make the organism such a dynamic killer. (Plasmids are DNA strands, usually circular, distinct from the much larger bacterial chromosome. They replicate independently from the main chromosome and code for specific proteins). One plasmid, pOX1, codes for two toxins that are the primary reason for the organism's extreme virulence: lethal factor and edema factor. The other plasmid, pOX2, is smaller. It codes for the capsule surrounding the vegetative organism, protecting it from phagocyte entrapment. Together, the two toxins and the capsule allow the organism to grow to enormous numbers in the animal host by negating the innate immune response.

All nucleated mammalian cells depend on a vast array of signaling molecules to function properly. Chemical messages received on the surface or within a cell's cytoplasm are often transmitted to the cell's nucleus through a series of chemical reactions that proceed in a cascade-like fashion. Upon receiving the chemical signal, the nucleus is primed to unveil and enable previously sequestered genes to code for and ultimately produce the substances necessary to respond to the stimulus.   An invading bacterium sets in motion many such chemical messages that, if conducted smoothly, will efficiently respond to the threat. One such set of chemical messages is MAPK, or mitogen-activated protein kinase. Several enzyme reactions take part in the MAPK sequence, working in harmony to alert the nucleus to produce the necessary components for the action needed. One of the chain's enzymes is MEK, an essential intermediary. A toxin of *Bacillus anthracis,* the one commonly called lethal toxin, or LT, very effectively attaches to and blocks the action of MEK, completely disrupting the transmission of the MAPK signals from the cell cytoplasm to the nucleus. This significantly delays the cellular immune response. For the first cellular responders of infection, neutrophils, macrophages, and dendritic cells, anthrax LT effectively shuts down their activity, giving the bacterium free rein to grow with impunity. The phagocytic cells are not able to remove the bacteria from the body.

The other toxin, edema factor, or EF, is similar in chemical structure to its neighbor protein lethal factor. The genes for EF also reside on the pOX1 plasmid. EF attacks a different set of chemical signals, protein kinase A, or PKA, resulting in the accumulation of cyclic AMP. Cellular function is severely disrupted, and because of the accumulation of cyclic AMP, fluid loss, with resultant edema, ensues.

Lethal factor and edema factor can't do anything on their own. They must enter the host cell in an active form, and the critical bacterial manager enabling that is a protein called protective antigen, or PA. (The name protective antigen derives from our targeting the bacterial molecule with antibody after vaccination, thus protecting ourselves from anthrax). Protective antigen is produced on the plasmid pOX1, like lethal and edema factors. When made by the organism, protective antigen is a very large, cumbersome molecule. It has two prominent receptor sites on animal cells. Once it attaches to either of those, it is split by a host cell protein. Then, seven or eight slimmed-down versions of PA come together, forming a large tubular molecular structure. After the reaction, lethal and edema factors attach to this active form of protective antigen. The assembled protective antigen then acts as a barge or ferry to get itself and its deadly cargo into the cell. Once attached to the protective antigen, the lethal *factor* and edema *factor* become active. They are now lethal *toxin* and edema *toxin*, ready to do their worst against the cellular enzymes. It's an absolutely remarkable and efficient system.

The activated protective antigen is engulfed by the host cell. Early in the infection, the host cell is a macrophage or a neutrophil. Once the protective antigen, bearing its cargo of lethal toxin and edema toxin enters the cell, it is encased in an endosome, much like an invading virus or bacterium. As the pH of the endosome becomes more acidic, the protective antigen becomes very active, essentially boring a hole in the endosome's membrane, releasing both toxins. The lethal and edema toxins are freed in the cell's cytoplasm.

The deadliest form of anthrax for humans is inhalation, in which the individual breathes spores into the lungs. Two other forms, cutaneous and intestinal, are potentially serious diseases, but the inhalation disease has the highest fatality rate. Despite the entrance of the organism into the lungs, pulmonary disease is not present. When the anthrax spore is inhaled and settles in the lung, it is picked up by a macrophage, which dutifully transports it to the nearest lymph node, most likely in the mediastinal area below the breastbone. Once inside the macrophage, the spore begins to germinate, forming a vegetative cell capable of releasing protective antigen, lethal factor, and edema factor. The "sweet spot" for *Bacillus anthracis* is in the lymph node, where it can invade cells and reproduce at will. The enormous number of vegetative bacteria growing in the lymph node spill out into the bloodstream. Once there, it is only a short matter of time before the bacteria enter other bodily tissues, such as the liver, kidney, and others. Death does not take long to ensue, with edema toxin running rampant and lethal toxin destroying individual cells.

The pulmonary macrophage can take a while to reach the nearby lymph nodes. From the organism's point of view, it must ensure the macrophage remains active to accomplish the transport. The inhaled spore must germinate, and the plasmids must become active to produce the protective antigen, the toxins, and the capsule. To allow all this to happen, the macrophage can't be killed too quickly, lest the organism not reach the lymph node. To ensure the orderly progression of things, the edema toxin acts as an antagonist to the activity of the lethal toxin. Lethal toxin stimulates the host cell to undergo apoptosis and die; edema toxin counteracts it by stimulating anti-apoptotic pathways. While seemingly counterproductive, the process enables the organism to enter the lymph node in a vegetative, active state, fully reproducing and forming toxins. Once the toxin levels rise dramatically, the counteractive effect is overridden.

The first stage of anthrax infection reduces the innate immune response, mainly by attacking neutrophils, macrophages, and dendritic cells. Toxin production, along with the capsule surrounding the organism, ensures the organism's success. Bacteria are multiplying furiously, releasing large amounts of protective antigen and toxins. Most body cells have receptors for the protective antigen, which circulates around the body after the infection has been established. Protective antigen, bearing its toxin cargo, can enter many different tissues, leading to their toxin-mediated destruction. Lethal toxin has a powerful effect on heart tissue and edema toxin on several organs. As the name implies, edema toxin leads to significant fluid loss and swelling throughout the body.

In the natural state, anthrax is a disease of animals, primarily herbivores. An animal in the field eats grass or other vegetation contaminated with spores, then develops gastrointestinal anthrax. *Bacillus anthracis* does not sporulate inside a living animal, but when exposed to air, the genes organizing sporulation kick in. Millions of spores can be produced in a dead, decomposing animal. Some will inevitably make their way to nearby vegetation to be eaten by another animal, thus carrying on the infectious cycle. The spores are incredibly hearty, with credible reports showing them to remain viable for fifty years under the proper conditions. In olden times, the fields where the spores were plentiful were known as "cursed fields." Shepherds would direct their flocks away.

In addition to the inhalation form of the disease, anthrax can be acquired by humans through either the cutaneous or gastrointestinal routes. In the cutaneous infection, spores or vegetative bacteria enter a skin break and a lesion forms after a few days. The wound is painless, and the vesicle is filled with a clear fluid, not pus. If the material in the wound is aspirated with a syringe and examined under a microscope, the examiner typically finds many Gram-positive rods (not spores) and no white blood cells. Presumably, the latter have been destroyed by the action of the toxins. The top of the vesicle is easily removed, and the remaining scar turns black after a week. Untreated cutaneous anthrax has a mortality rate of about 15-20%. If appropriate antibiotics are administered, the death rate is very low.

Gastrointestinal anthrax is the form most animals get as they graze on infected grass. It is the least common form found naturally in humans, who usually acquire it by eating undercooked infected meat. Symptoms are not unique, mainly nausea and diarrhea with intense abdominal pain. Untreated GI anthrax has a mortality rate of about 20-40%.

The treatment of anthrax is usually straightforward and effective. Since the organism's chief means of infectivity is the production of toxins, antibiotics that inhibit protein synthesis in bacteria are the best choice. Ciprofloxacin (Cipro), levofloxacin (Levaquin), and doxycycline have been shown to be effective.

Antitoxins are also available. Raxibacumab (ABthrax) and obiltoxaximab (Anthim) bind to and inhibit the activity of protective antigen. They are both monoclonal antibodies produced in a laboratory. Antitoxins are essential in treating an advanced case, as the toxins are still active in the body even after the organism has been killed. Taking an appropriate oral antibiotic soon after a suspected exposure usually prevents the disease.

Anthrax can kill vast numbers of animals. Whole herds can be wiped out. Historically, when people depended on animals for food, both meat and dairy, animal die-off could be devastating to a community. The disease didn't target humans to anywhere near the extent that human infections like smallpox or plague did, but the repercussions of an anthrax infection of animals were often severe. Thanks to the development of anthrax vaccines, first by Pasteur in the 19th century and then by Max Sterne in 1934, anthrax today is a very rare infection in developed countries. It is by no means extinct, and cases are seen with some regularity in undeveloped areas of the world. Sadly, the organism's extreme mortality rate has made it a high priority for nations intent on developing biological weapons.

Historically, inhalation anthrax affected people who dealt with animal pelts. At one time, it was known as Woolsorters disease. Animal skins contaminated with anthrax spores would be processed in factories, and during the work, the spores would become airborne and inhaled by workers. In the middle 1800s, the area of Bradford, England, became a case study of anthrax's infectivity. Before 1837 Woolsorters disease was not known in the area of Bradford, a major center for processing wool and other hides. But after 1837, animal hides from other countries, most notably mohair (goat fur) from the Middle East and alpaca from South America, were imported into Bradford. It was soon after this that trouble began. Over the years, hundreds of workers in the factories died. The cause wasn't known or even suspected until the work of Robert Koch in the late 1870s describing the organism causing the disease. Eventually, over many decades, appropriate means of handling potentially contaminated hides were adopted, and the disease as an industrial hazard ceased.

Selecting a microorganism to be used as a weapon is a tricky business. Several organisms are known to kill aggressively, but getting them to the target site is problematic. Effective delivery of a biological weapon is critical. The agent that packs the most destructive force and is the simplest to deliver is anthrax's spores. The organism is very easy to grow to large volumes in artificial culture, and the production of spores is also technically not complicated. Creating a dried aerosol requires quite a bit of technical knowledge, as spores tend to clump together and not be in the air for too long. But weapons labs in several countries have developed methods to make massive quantities of spores that repel each other and can stay airborne for several hours, as the lab accident at Sverdlovsk in the 1970s so amply demonstrated. Anthrax as a pathogen for animals and humans is a very rare occurrence in the developed world. But anthrax as a biological weapon is of great concern.

Chapter 30
Under The Influence

From mild to severe,
Uninvited winter guest.
Ever-changing Flu.

Of all the serious infectious diseases afflicting humankind, perhaps the most enigmatic is influenza. It comes to us from animals, but while most of the zoonotic infections that cross over to humans come from mammals, influenza comes to us from birds. Recovery from infection by other viruses, such as smallpox and measles, leads to lifetime immunity. Influenza changes every year. Influenza can greatly harm or kill by itself, but very often it is the presence of another unrelated organism that results in the greatest damage. Some people infected by the influenza virus have what amounts to a common cold, while others are made seriously ill, and some die. The disease influenza shares several symptoms in common with other respiratory viruses, and the term "influenza-like" or "flu-like" is often used to describe an upper respiratory infection (URI). The term flu-like has degenerated among many to simply "flu" so that any URI becomes the flu, confounding the actual disease of influenza with common, much less severe, ailments. Some even use the term "stomach flu," a ridiculous term medically.

The name influenza originated from Latin, by way of Italian. *Influentia* means "influenced by." A long time ago it was believed that the stars influenced illness, and influenza, which usually comes around yearly during the winter, was thought to be the result of celestial events. Since so many viral upper and lower respiratory infections mimic influenza, it's difficult to say with certainty how long it has been infecting humans. Strains of Adenovirus, Enterovirus, and Coronavirus can all cause epidemics that are quite serious. But it is safe to assume that influenza has been around a long time, and because of its unique ability to rapidly mutate and present itself in altered form, it will be around for some time to come.

Three types of Influenza viruses infect humans, designated A, B, and C. Influenza C is something of an outlier, causing the mild symptoms of a common cold. Influenza A is potentially the most serious because of its propensity to mutate and cause pandemics. Influenza B is similar to Influenza A but much less prone to mutation and cause epidemics, but the symptoms it causes can be just as serious as those caused by Influenza A.

Influenza's nucleic acid is RNA. Many RNA viruses infect the upper respiratory tracts of humans, so in that regard, influenza is not unique. But influenza distinguishes itself from other viruses. A significant difference and advantage of the influenza virus is the segmentation of its nucleus. Other RNA viruses have one long, meandering genome. Influenza has the RNA to code for eleven proteins, but the genes are contained in eight individual nuclear segments. They are numbered 1 through 8, with the longest RNA segment assigned the number 1 and the shortest number 8. This segmentation allows for myriad re-configurations of the viral genetic material and the emergence of unique, sometimes serious, progeny.

It is common for two different influenza strains to enter the same host animal simultaneously. The pig is a common target. During viral replication, a genomal segment of one co-infecting strain of the influenza virus can be exchanged for a segment of another. For instance, segment 8 from a duck virus might be substituted for segment 8 of a human virus inside a pig epithelial cell. Just like that, another virus is born. The new virus may not be all that dangerous, and it could very well fade away, but every now and then, a virulent strain of the virus will emerge, bringing with it some dire consequences.

This mixing of nuclear segments between virus strains from different animal species is called antigenic shift. There can also occur relatively minor alterations on the attachment protein, HA, a common phenomenon called antigenic drift. Antigenic drift occurs nearly yearly; the antigenic shift is much less common, but the consequences are potentially far greater.

Of the eleven proteins of the influenza A virus, three are on the surface. The matrix surrounding the virus, holding the whole thing together, is called the M1 protein. Attached to and protruding out from the matrix protein are two attachment proteins. The largest one has a rather unfortunate name, hemagglutination antigen, or HA. (Unfortunate in that the name refers to the ability of the virus to attach to and bring about the agglutination of red blood cells. That's true, but the attachment of the influenza virus to red blood cells has nothing to do with the infection. Influenza does not infect red blood cells. RBCs don't synthesize proteins, and they would be a dead end for the virus). The other surface protein is neuraminidase, NA, the protein the virus uses to break out of the infected cell after viral replication. The two are abbreviated H and N, with numbers attached to indicate their type (H1N1, H3N2, etc.). HA outnumbers NA by a ratio of about 4:1.

Protruding through the matrix covering of the A type is a small channel called the M2 protein, a tiny tube that allows fluid to enter the interior of the virus. The interior of the virus contains eight nuclear segments, each containing different genetic information and each encased by a protein. In addition to the viral matrix covering, each virus is enveloped by a membrane derived from the host cell that has been infected. The shape of the influenza virions is not constant. Sometimes they are round; sometimes, they are elongated.

To infect a cell, the influenza virus must get into the cell. The attachment protein of the virus is hemagglutinin antigen, HA. All our cells have numerous proteins protruding from the membrane into the environment. Many of them are capped by sugar (glycan) molecules, the most prominent of which is a rather odd-looking molecule called sialic acid. Odd in the fact that it has nine carbons, while most active sugar molecules in the body have six. In the cells lining our respiratory tract, the sialic acid topping protein molecules are linked to a six-carbon sugar, galactose. The sialic acid-galactose combination lining our respiratory cells is the point where influenza viruses attach.

The HA of the virus is a long molecule, something like a corn stalk. The part that is farthest from the viral surface is the attachment segment. It is very conserved and doesn't mutate much, if at all. If it did, it couldn't attach to the host cell receptor of sialic acid-galactose. Surrounding the attachment point are four or five (depending on the virus type) protein sites that protect the point of attachment. These hemagglutinin protection areas of the virus change frequently and are immunogenic. To protect ourselves from the virus, we make antibodies to each one. The HA is neutralized when its active site protective proteins are tied up with antibodies, and infection doesn't occur. When one of the viral proteins changes through mutation, though, the antibody to the old variety is no longer effective, and immunity is reduced. If they all change, immunity decreases to zero.

Influenza A is a bird virus, mainly infecting the intestinal tract of wild birds such as ducks. The attachment site for the virus in birds is sialic acid which is bound to galactose by a 2,3-linkage; that is, carbon number 2 on the sialic acid binds to carbon number 3 on the galactose. We don't have the 2,3-linkage on our sialic acid-galactose molecules in our upper respiratory tract; ours is 2,6, with carbon 2 on the sialic acid binding to carbon 6 on the galactose. It doesn't sound like much, but to the virus, it's huge. The HA that binds to the 2,3 of birds cannot bind to the 2,6 of humans. There are 16 different influenza HA molecules capable of infecting birds, but only a few, mostly H1 and H3, have changed over time to bind to the human 2,6 linkage and infect human cells.

Once viral binding to the sialic acid-galactose receptor occurs, several events begin to initiate infection. The HA is made active by being cleaved by an enzyme from the human cell it is invading. After cleavage, the virus combines with the host cell membrane, which encases the virus in an endosome and brings it into the cell's interior. The M2 ion channel on the virus allows the flow of endosomal fluid into the virus, exposing it to a much lower pH. This signals the virus to begin separating and distributing its RNA segments into the cell's interior. HA assists with the endosomal membrane's breakdown, allowing the viral RNA segments to escape. Once released, the viral RNA segments are transcribed to form viral proteins, and more RNA is made to be incorporated into the new virions being manufactured. It is a very efficient process, as the virus uses the host cell's elaborate ribosomal machinery to manufacture its own proteins. In just a day or two, all the viral proteins and RNA are neatly packaged into thousands of new virions, each ready to be released into the surrounding environment to infect more host cells. Neuraminidase, the "N" of the HN type, facilitates the release of the virus from the host cell.

The body's key to defeating invading organisms is the recognition and response to molecules in the microbe that differ from the host cell. Molecular sensors in our cells are ever-present and on guard to detect these pathogen-associated molecular patterns or PAMPs. Once evidence of an invading microbe is detected, our pattern recognition receptors (PRR) become active and trigger other molecules to respond in a cascade fashion. Ultimately, the molecule covering a portion of the genome responsible for the chemical response to microbial invasion is uncovered, and the genes coding for the appropriate chemical responses are activated.

Our cells have RNA, and so do many viruses, but that of the viruses is a little different. Sometimes the end of the viral RNA strand lacks the proper initiation or termination sequences that our RNA has. Also, our RNA doesn't exist in double strands like DNA, but in viruses, the RNA must be replicated and is in a double-stranded form for a while. These RNA differences are detected by our pattern recognition sensors like toll-like receptors (TLR), retinoic-acid inducible gene 1 (RIG-1), and nucleotide-binding domain-like receptor protein 3 (NLRP-3), and an immune response is initiated. To thwart the immune response, a virus must obscure these differences to avoid recognition.

The influenza virus has a very powerful protein that enables it to be a successful pathogen. NS1, or non-structural protein 1, is not very big (its genetic code is carried on the smallest of the influenza segments), but it is essential for the virus's quest to perpetuate. Influenza viruses lacking NS1 are non-pathogenic.

NS1 acts in at least two ways, and it is very efficient. For one, NS1 covers up influenza viral double-stranded RNA by attaching to a part of it. Double-stranded RNA is a dead giveaway that a virus is infecting a cell because our cells don't produce it. The virus' ability to impede the recognition of double-stranded RNA for a time slows the cellular response to the virus. Also, the RNA of influenza lacks the proper chemical cap on one end, called 5', which is crucial in translating the RNA code at the ribosome. The virus must steal the 5' section from the host's cellular RNA for its proteins to be manufactured at the ribosome. NS1 also works to conceal this obvious defect, and the virus can proceed with its multiplication, albeit at a somewhat reduced rate.

Influenza NS1 also mitigates interferon production, the great enemy of viruses. There are three main types of interferon, I, II and III. Type I is divided into alpha and beta forms; type II has only one, gamma; type III is called lambda. Interferon-α, interferon-β, and interferon-λ are employed to counteract the viral attack. (It isn't actually that simple, as there are 13 different types of INF-α, designated by numbers and letters, such as INF-α2a. Differences in activity among the types are rather subtle). Interferons don't directly interfere with viral activity like an antibiotic acts against bacteria. After their release from an infected cell, interferons attach to and alert neighboring cells to put up barriers to viral entry and replication. In a viral infection, the first few host cells are lost, but if interferon production and release occur as planned, the virus encounters a very hostile cellular landscape to continue the infection, and the viral onslaught is halted with minimum damage to the body. Viruses that can interfere with interferon production have an advantage.

The genes to make interferon are always present in the human genome. While interferon benefits our health, there is such a problem as too much of a good thing. Many of the symptoms we experience during a viral infection like influenza don't come directly from the virus itself but from the action of several chemicals and cytokines released because of the virus' presence. This includes interferon, so the genes coding its manufacture and release must be sequestered. Only when an invading virus is an imminent threat are the interferon genes freed to code for their product. All our nucleated cells can make and release interferon, but it is produced in higher quantities in macrophages and dendritic cells. A specialized cell, the plasmacytoid dendritic cell, is particularly adept at interferon production.

All our nucleated cells contain sensory proteins that detect an invading microbe, whether it be a virus, bacteria, parasite, or fungus. Inside our cells is a very important molecule called retinoic-inducible gene-1, or RIG-1. We also have one called NLRP-3. These sensory systems can detect the presence of viruses, including influenza, in the host cell. Each sends chemical signals to the genes in the host cell nucleus to unwrap and transcribe the genes required to produce interferon and other cytokines. There are over 300 such genes, given the collective name of interferon-stimulated genes, or ISGs. The systems are redundant; if they work properly, the influenza virus invading the inside of the host cell is recognized, and interferon is released.

When type I and III interferons are released, they are attracted to interferon receptors on neighboring cells. Ultimately, the receptive cell's nucleus is notified, and the genes that function in the disruption of virus replication are unleashed. There are several, and they effectively interfere with the ability of the invading virus to replicate by using the host cell's ribosomes. Either the viral RNA is negated, or the cell's reproductive machinery is compromised, shutting down the virus with it. In addition to removing the cellular machinery the virus needs to replicate, natural killer lymphocytes are activated, and any cell harboring potential replicating virions is destroyed. As the process moves on, the tools of the adaptive immune system, including B-lymphocytes to make antibodies and killer CD-8 lymphocytes to eliminate infected cells, are activated. It is a very efficient system, and many viruses have been repelled because of it. If a virus is to be successful, it must somehow modulate interferon production or its effects.

Despite our highly developed and exquisite systems of naturally eliminating viruses, some break through and infect us. As our immune system evolved to meet the challenge of viral invasion, so did viruses change through time, with the fittest and most adept surviving. We might think of it as an "arms race," in which a balance between host and tiny predator must be reached. If a virus is too aggressive and deadly, the host animal dies off, and the virus along with it. From the virus' point of view, the immune system needs to be circumvented, not eliminated.

467

Through many thousands of years of infection, viruses have developed several general ways of overcoming, at least temporarily, the host animal's immune system.

In addition to sequestering viral RNA, NS1 disrupts the chemical cascade that sends messages to the nucleus to unblock the genes coding for interferon, especially those sent by the RIG-1 system. Interferon production is mitigated, and viral production continues much faster than it otherwise would. Mutant strains of influenza that lack NS1 are not pathogenic. The person or animal infected by such a virus is not sickened; their interferon is produced in copious amounts and functions properly.

Like any protein produced by an RNA virus, NS1 is subject to mutation. Some versions of it are highly efficient, others not. The viral gene coding for it can mutate in subtle ways, giving a slight change in NS1's activity. There is also the possibility that the entire segment for its coding can be exchanged from one strain of the virus to another (antigenic shift), one of the reasons that now and then influenza epidemics are so forceful. In most years, alterations to the NS1 protein are minor, but sometimes the change in NS1 has a profound effect. The NS1 protein from the H1N1 virus from the infamous 1918-1919 pandemic has been shown in laboratory animals to be a potent force producing drastically reduced interferon levels, with subsequent high mortality.

There is some evidence that NS1 can also interfere with the cellular process of apoptosis, the cell's self-destruct mechanism to prevent viral propagation. The main chemical instigator of apoptosis comes from the mitochondria. NS1 has some ability to significantly slow the process of apoptosis at the mitochondrial level, keeping the host cell alive and able to produce more virus.

Some, but not all, strains of the influenza virus have a second protein that reduces interferon production. Called PB1-F2, it is a small protein with only 90 amino acids. When present, it acts in harmony with NS1 to subdue interferon production by hijacking the chemical messengers being sent to the host cell nucleus. PB1-F2 is most potent when it contains the amino acid serine instead of the usual asparagine at position 66. This unique configuration was present in the horrific influenza virus in 1918-19, as well as the highly virulent "bird flu" H5N1 strains of recent years.

Just as there is genetic variation among strains of a pathogenic virus, there is also considerable variation in the genes of humans. The differences are often subtle, but there can be substantially varied reactions to exposure to viral proteins such as influenza NS1. If one person has a critical section on one of their RIG-1 proteins that has a low affinity for the NS1 protein of a circulating influenza A virus, that individual would most likely produce normal amounts of interferon and have a mild infection. Another person may have a RIG-1 protein that has a high affinity for the NS1 protein and have a near complete shutdown of interferon production and suffer a severe infection. Intermediate reactions could also occur, given the variability of genetic makeup in different people. This is a simplified example, but it is one reason that there can be such different infection severities in members of the infected population.

When the influenza virus infects, it attacks mainly the non-ciliated columnar epithelial cells lining the trachea and the bronchi. Those cells are rich in the sialic acid-galactose combinations bearing the 2,6 linkages. As the epithelial cells are destroyed during influenza invasion, the lining of our airway is left vulnerable to any bacterial species residing nearby that can take advantage. In our noses and mouths, we have many bacteria. Organisms are constantly present, but the species and strains vary over time. We're unaware of it, but there is an ongoing interaction among the bacteria that inhabit our nose and mouth, and organisms come and go regularly. Some of these interlopers are potentially serious pathogens, but our innate immune system and some of our resident microbial flora are up to the task of containing them. Unless, of course, there is a breach in the integrity of the system, thus giving the pathogenic organism an opening. Three bacterial species are especially good at taking advantage of such an opportunity, *Staphylococcus aureus*, *Haemophilus influenzae*, and *Streptococcus pneumoniae*. Many people harbor one or more of these organisms in their upper respiratory tract without ill effects. But trouble may ensue if just the right strain happens to be colonizing a person when the influenza virus infects them.

The bacteria mentioned are all surrounded by a thick, slimy capsule, making it hard for neutrophils patrolling the area to ensnare and destroy them. All can attach to the epithelial lining damaged by the influenza virus and set up an infection. Bronchitis and pneumonia are the most common ailments. All bacteria that may secondarily infect are treatable with antibiotics, but each has shown an ability to resist them. This is especially true of *Staphylococcus aureus*. Pneumonia with a virulent strain of Staph is a serious and sometimes fatal infection.

Such bacterial infections following an attack of influenza are called secondary infections. The three organisms mentioned are the most common and serious, but there can be others. The outcome may be fatal if the infected patient is frail or has a compromising physical condition. Even if the one infected is of robust health, the outcome may be tragic if the infecting bacterial strain is of heightened virulence and/or antibiotic resistance. When one hears of a patient dying of influenza, the virus may have caused it. But quite often, the secondary infection by a virulent bacterium was ultimately responsible.

As mentioned, in humans influenza virus attaches using its hemagglutinin antigen (HA) to surface receptors of sialic acid-galactose with 2,6 linkages. In birds, the natural host of the influenza virus, the attachment is to receptors of sialic acid-galactose with the 2,3 linkages, usually on cells lining their intestinal tract. There are 16 different HAs that can attack birds, but commonly there are only three that can attach to the 2,6 linkage and infect humans. H1 and H3 are the most common, H2 less so. But there are cells surrounding the alveoli in our lungs that have the 2,3 sialic acid-galactose linkage typical of birds, and they are potential targets of bird viruses.

Influenza typically infects wild birds, but it can infect domestic fowl like chickens. In recent years there have been incidents of a bird influenza virus infecting chickens, which then serve as a reservoir for human infections. The hemagglutinin

H5 has been notorious in these severe infections. The infected person doesn't get the virus from another person but from being in the environment of many chickens and their excrement that harbors the virus. Chicken coops can be messy places with lots of airborne material. Exposure to this environment regularly leaves a person vulnerable to any virus that may have been in the birds' intestines. The case fatality rate of these so-called "bird-flu" infections involving strain H5N1 is very high. Because the virus cannot infect the cells lining the trachea in humans, it is not communicable from person to person. But with the virus's ability to mutate, it bears watching.

The symptoms of influenza and their intensity aren't constant from person to person, and any description of them must be generalized. Strain variation, previous recent influenza infection and vaccination history, and an individual's personal immune response capability all come into play. Influenza is a respiratory infection, so the upper respiratory tract is most affected. The symptoms result from our immune system's response to the virus, not anything the virus directly does to us.

The incubation period of influenza is usually about two to three days, the interval from when we get the virus to the display of the first symptoms. Depending on the individual, it may begin as any other upper respiratory infection, with a dry, "scratchy" throat and a gradual general feeling of being unwell. In others, symptoms come on abruptly and forcefully, with sudden profound weakness and muscle aches.

One of our defense mechanisms against viruses is a rise in body temperature. This can be an advantage, as human proteins involved in the immune system are more active at elevated temperatures, while viral proteins are less active. As the body temperature increases, we feel chills until it reaches its set point, usually around 103°F (39.5°C). Fever, and its range, are variable.

The respiratory tract contains mucus to trap microorganisms and other unwanted particles, and during an inflammatory event, the amount of mucus is significantly increased. It must be removed, of course, so the cough reflex is initiated. Coughing and sneezing help rid our body of the virus and decaying dead cells, many of which are neutrophils. Dead neutrophils become pus. The pus in the mucus can lead to a thick, viscous, yellowish sputum.

The release of inflammatory cytokines like TNF-α, IL-1β, and IL-6 can stimulate the digestive system and induce nausea, vomiting, and diarrhea. Swallowing large amounts of mucus can add to the problem. The virus is not a pathogen in the digestive tract of humans (it is in birds), so the symptom of gastroenteritis is the work of the immune system's fight against the virus. Like the expelling of mucus, vomiting and diarrhea are means of expelling a pathogen. Like muscle aches and fever, it is a non-specific reaction because of the body's immune response.

Some influenza patients develop headaches, watery eyes, ear pain, dizziness, and loss of appetite. But the symptoms of influenza are not unique, and all are variable in intensity and duration. Most sickened individuals recover within a week, give or take a couple of days. But some people, primarily those who have an underlying significant medical condition, can become much worse. Sometimes, people who appear to be in an overall healthy condition can develop serious diseases involving severe respiratory failure due to an overabundance of cytokines and chemokines, the so-called "cytokine storm." The more serious conditions are usually due to a secondary bacterial infection, such as *Staphylococcus,* pneumococcus, or *Haemophilus.* It can also be an over-production of cytokines which leads to respiratory failure. Quite often, in the more severe cases of influenza, the disease seems to be progressing normally, with a diminution of symptoms at about day 3-5, but then a more serious disease state sets in as the bacterial infection or cytokine storm advances. Careful intensive medical care is necessary to save these patients' lives.

Antibiotics used to treat bacterial infections don't work against viruses. Most antibiotics suppress the bacterial cell wall or the protein synthesis systems of the microbe, neither of which is present in viruses. Some drugs, though, have shown effectiveness against some strains of influenza. The first one developed was amantadine, used in Germany in the mid-1960s and in the United States a couple of years later. Amantadine blocks the M2 channel of influenza A, preventing the interchange of ions needed to allow the virus to release itself into the cell's interior. Amantadine was never a very good treatment for the disease, but it did have some utility as a prophylactic medication. When one person developed influenza, amantadine could be given to family members and close contacts to prevent them from getting the disease, or at least mitigate the symptoms. Taking amantadine while in the full-blown fury of influenza did little or nothing to end the suffering. Amantadine is no longer an effective treatment for influenza and should not be given. It was vastly overused by Chinese farmers who used it to protect their flocks, and most strains of influenza are now amantadine resistant. It also can cause significant side effects.

A second drug for treating influenza is oseltamivir, introduced in 1999. It interferes with the activity of influenza's neuraminidase, inhibiting the virus' ability to escape from one cell and establish infection in another. Oseltamivir is derived from star anise, a Chinese and Vietnamese spice that grows on an evergreen tree. Star anise is one of the five-spice powder ingredients of traditional Chinese cooking, and it is an important ingredient of Vietnamese pho soup. Oseltamivir is marketed by the trade name Tamiflu. With a drug like oseltamivir, the administration should begin very early in the course of the disease, which is not very easy to do when doctor visits and diagnostic tests usually take a few days. It has no effect against other viruses that cause the common cold that may be confused with influenza, and if one waits for several days before its administration, little or no benefit will be noted. Even when given early in the course of influenza, it is difficult to properly evaluate its effectiveness: would the individual receiving it have had a mild course of the disease, as quite a few do, or did the drug's administration significantly reduce the symptoms? Hard to say. Certainly, oseltamivir is not a magic elixir. There may be some benefit if given early in the disease, but maybe not. Influenza resistance to oseltamivir is common.

It is difficult to develop any anti-viral agent that gives results analogous to those given by antibiotics against bacteria. If one has a urinary tract infection and takes a course of an antibiotic to which the infecting bacteria are susceptible, relief of symptoms takes only a day or two. But in viral infections, many symptoms aren't caused directly by the invading virus but by the immune system's reaction. A drug may effectively kill or significantly retard a virus's growth. Still, the inflammatory cytokines such as interleukin-1β, interleukin-6, and tumor necrosis factor-α are causing the symptoms of the disease, and the anti-viral will not affect that.

One of the great marvels of modern science and industry is the yearly production of the influenza vaccine, usually called a flu shot. Most people take it for granted, which is unfortunate because it is a very complicated and important piece of work. The lives of tremendous numbers of people are saved each year by the simple injection of dead influenza virus into the arm. The work that goes into preparing the influenza vaccine is based on science and depends on dedication to detail, but there is a bit of luck involved as well.

Influenza vaccine must be prepared and administered each year. Sometimes there is little change from the previous year's formulation, but sometimes a great deal. Selection of the most prominent influenza hemagglutination antigen (HA) circulating in the early spring is critical. For influenza A the HA changes constantly. The attachment site on the HA does not change because it must attach to the sialic acid-galactose receptor on the host cell. Without that, nothing happens. But HA contains four or five proteins adjacent to the attachment site. They are all antigenic, and they are subject to variation. Sometimes they vary only slightly from year to year, sometimes a lot. For H1 there are five, designated Sa, Sb, Ca1, Ca2, and Cb, and they can all alter their shapes by substituting one amino acid for another. We make antibodies to all of them, but one or two are usually dominant. If the amino acid substitutions through mutation are minor, then no appreciable change in antibody effectiveness is noticed. But when the change(s) are substantial, the antibody to a previous year's strain is no longer useful, and the virus is not vulnerable. The virus is still of the H1 type, but the antibodies produced to neutralize it from a previous year no longer work. A new set of antibodies must be developed before the new strain of virus attacks.

The manufacture of influenza vaccine is a complex process. Number one on the complication list is that most influenza viruses do not grow well in chicken eggs. Those that do only grow in eggs that are fertilized, and fertilized eggs must be selected in preference to the unembryonated ones. Fortunately, a few strains of the virus grow very well in chicken eggs, and they are used as seed strains. The problem, of course, is that the HA contained in the seed strain is not the same HA as the current strain. The classic seed strain was discovered in Puerto Rico in 1934. A lot has changed since then. Accommodations must be made.

Around late March of each year, scientists worldwide compare notes on the strains of influenza virus they have encountered. Data include the predominant strains, trends in recent weeks and months, and disease severity. A decision is made on which strain of virus is most likely to infect in the winter months six or so months down the road. Clearly, this is a guess, but at least it is an educated one, and it is the most we can ask. Viruses mutate without notice and sometimes rather suddenly, and there is always the chance that a predominant strain in March or April will give way to one that emerges in summer or early fall.

When the decision is made about the strains of influenza virus to be included in the vaccine, viruses containing those HAs are mixed in with the seed strains in fertilized chicken eggs and allowed to grow together. As the viruses multiply within the chick embryos together, they inevitably interchange their nuclear segments (each has eight), with the result being the establishment of the seed strain inheriting a gene segment that contains the proper HAs from the infective strain, giving a virus suitable for vaccine production. Antibodies are administered to the viral culture to eliminate the original seed strain with the wrong HA.

The new virus (the seed strain that grows well in chick embryos endowed with the new HA from the current infective strain) is then harvested and put into freshly fertilized chicken eggs–millions of them. After a suitable time, the vaccine strain is harvested, killed with formalin, and readied for vaccine preparation. The purity of the preparation must be ensured, the titer of the virus carefully measured, and the proper antigen structure firmly established.

Clearly, this is a laborious task and far from perfect. It takes several months to accomplish, and the virus involved, influenza, is notorious for its ability to mutate. Mutations can occur within viral strains within the chick embryos used in vaccine preparation or in the wild, with a new virus strain emerging between the time when the decision was made for strain selection and the final product. There are five antigenic sites on the distal end of the hemagglutinin of the influenza virus. Some may be more immunogenic than others, so in some years the vaccine may be very good at inducing neutralizing antibody production; in other years, not so good.

With all the variables involved with influenza vaccination, it is no wonder the acceptance and compliance rate by the public is variable as well. The vaccine strain may not be a very good match for the strain of influenza circulating in late fall and winter. Some people, especially older people, do not produce a robust antibody response, or they don't produce any response at all. The general populace has a great deal of confusion about the disease influenza, as the "flu" is commonly confused with common colds. Some will say they got a flu shot and they got the flu anyway, not knowing if it was really influenza they got or some other unrelated virus. Some don't get very sick even when they get the influenza virus because they are genetically able to mount a vigorous interferon response. Some people just don't like getting shots.

This is all very unfortunate. Influenza, either directly or through secondary infections, kills many people yearly. In the United States, in a "mild flu" year, there may be around 20,000 who die, while in a "bad flu" season, it may be greater than 50,000. A key point must be stressed: getting a flu shot is not meant only to protect the vaccinee; IT IS MEANT TO PROVIDE FOR PUBLIC HEALTH. If one gets a case of influenza and then passes it to someone who infects someone else, it can eventually find its way to a vulnerable victim. Herd immunity kicks in if the chain is stopped early and the damage is reduced. Much work is being done to produce a long-lasting influenza vaccination that covers all drifts and shifts. If it were easy to do, it would be done by now. With all its shortcomings, the yearly flu shot is the best that can be done, both for the individual and the public.

Chapter 31
Lifelong Companion

Sneaky, invasive,
Lurking serpent; the resident
Persistent menace.

Lots of different viruses can infect us. Mostly they are tiny little critters with a single strand of RNA, a few proteins, and a hard coat to hold it all together and allow it to stick to a cell and invade. We either inhale, ingest, or imbibe them into our body. They infect our cells and make millions of copies of themselves. Our immune system gets engaged to thwart them, and away they go, never to be encountered again. It's one and done, hopefully without too dire a consequence.

But there is one group of viruses that do so much more. They can get into us in any number of ways besides the usual breathing and swallowing, and instead of going away when our immune system reacts to them, they literally become a part of us, establishing their double-stranded DNA in our cells' nuclei. Some can remain in our body for our entire life. They are, of course, the herpes family of viruses, and the old saying "Herpes is forever" is right on the mark.

Compared to other viruses the herpes group is one of the most sophisticated. It's not surprising, as the virus has been around for over a hundred million years. The nucleic acid is double-stranded DNA, just like ours, and there are over seventy proteins produced to protect, escort, and enable it. Most viruses undergo replication and multiplication in the cytoplasm, but the DNA of herpes viruses enters the host cell's nucleus and operates from there. It is transcribed just like our DNA, using the host cell machinery to carry out its work.

The name herpes derives from the Greek word *herpein,* meaning "to creep." The ancient Greeks used the word as a general description for maladies such as cold sores, lupus vulgaris, ringworm, eczema, and other skin conditions. The use of the word herpes as a more definitive diagnosis for the cutaneous disease we know today began in the early 1800s.

The first publication recognizing herpes simplex as a communicable disease was written by French dermatologist

Jean Baptiste Emile Vidal in 1893. Despite the ubiquity and communicability of the disease, it wasn't until the 1940s that the etiologic agent, a very large virus, was identified.

For most people the name herpes makes them think of a skin infection, either around the mouth or the genitalia. But in nature, there are over 100 known herpes viruses, nine of which infect humans with a range of infected sites. In the big picture, they are classified in the Family *Herpesviridae*. For humans, the herpes viruses encompass three groups, or Subfamilies, designated alpha, beta, and gamma. They are all similar in general structure and biology but differ in the diseases they cause.

The alpha herpes includes herpes 1 (mouth), herpes 2 (genitalia), and varicella-zoster, commonly called chickenpox and shingles. The beta Herpes includes the human pathogens cytomegalovirus (CMV), roseola virus, also known as herpesvirus 6A and 6B, and another roseola virus, herpesvirus 7. The gamma group includes the human Epstein Barr virus and Kaposi sarcoma-associated virus. Each group has its own characteristics, and the diseases they cause are unique to each strain.

Each human herpesvirus is assigned a number,
preceded by the letters HHV, for Human Herpes Virus:

HHV-1	Herpes Simplex 1
HHV-2	Herpes Simplex 2
HHV-3	Varicella Zoster
HHV-4	Epstein Barr
HHV-5	Cytomegalovirus
HHV-6A and B	Roseola virus*
HHV-7	Roseola virus
HHV-8	Kaposi's sarcoma-associated virus

*(6A and 6B have been determined to be distinct; hence 9 human Herpes viruses)

The members of the herpes family all have the same general structure. Inside is the DNA. It's a fairly long, linear genome, capable of coding for 70 or more proteins. The genome is immediately surrounded and protected by a tough protein capsule. Made up of 6 different types of proteins, the capsule is very precise in its architecture, and it serves to surround, protect, and escort the DNA inside the host cell like a space capsule protects astronauts. Surrounding the payload of the DNA in its capsule is an amorphous layer known as the tegument. In the tegument are found about 20 proteins that carry out many of the virus' jobs. On top of it all is a membrane not produced by the virus but obtained from the host cell's membrane as the virus escapes. Located in the membrane are around a dozen viral proteins, each associated with a carbohydrate, so they are given the name glycoproteins ("glyco" refers to the carbohydrate portion). They're each designated by a lower-case g and upper-case letter designation, like gB and gD. These glycoproteins protruding through the outer membrane enable the virus to attach to specific receptors on the host cell. A few of them function in evading the immune system.

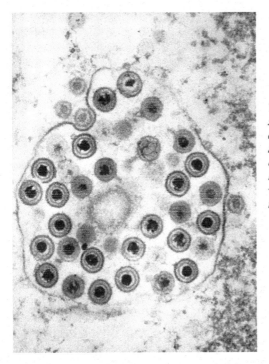

The herpes viruses have double-stranded DNA, surrounded by a complex protein coat. Surrounding that is a tegument of around twenty viral proteins. A host cell-derived membrane with viral attachment proteins encases the virus.

Herpes is a remarkable microbe, millions of years in the making. It infects in two distinct fashions, both beginning with the letter L. **Lysis** is a Greek word meaning to "loosen" or "break apart." The lytic phase of a herpes infection refers to the virus' ability to tear apart the host cell as the newly formed virions escape. **Latent** is from the Latin word *latere*, meaning to "lie hidden," and that's just what the virus does. In the latent phase the virus doesn't produce the seventy-plus proteins needed for a new virus, but just a few to enable the viral DNA to reproduce in synchrony with the host cell and carry out a few other tasks. Since the nucleic acid is double-stranded DNA, just like ours, it rounds up and sits in the cell's nucleus, right near the host cell chromosomes. It can remain there for decades, as anyone who has gone from chicken pox in childhood to shingles late in life can attest.

The first step in the cellular invasion of herpes is the virus's attachment to the host cell's membrane. The virus itself has a membrane that it got from the last cell invaded. Protruding through the surface of the viral membrane are about a dozen proteins, several of which work together to allow the fusion of the viral membrane to the host cell membrane, allowing for the penetration of the viral payload into the host cell.

The viral payload consists of the DNA packaged within its protective protein capsid, accompanied by the viral proteins of the tegument. Early in the host cell invasion stage, the viral DNA is linear, a long string with both ends unattached. The mission for the virus is to get this important bundle to the host cell nucleus. The integrity of the protective protein coat is vital, as DNA isn't supposed to be in the host cell's cytoplasm, only in the nucleus. Molecular sensors are ever-present in the host cell cytoplasm to detect DNA, and if encountered, chemical alarm bells go off, effectively aborting the virus' pursuit. The protein coat prevents this.

Each tegument protein has an important job. For one, a couple of them hook the capsid onto a microtubule in the host cell. Just like a train on a track, the viral DNA package then makes its way up the microtubule directly to the host cell nucleus. A few other tegument proteins allow this to happen.

Once it reaches the nucleus, the host cell's nuclear pore is opened to let the viral DNA in. Again, the accompanying tegument proteins are instrumental. As it enters the host cell nucleus, the capsid proteins are dispersed so the viral DNA enters by itself.

Once inside the host cell nucleus the linear viral DNA rounds up and forms itself into a circle, much like a plasmid in a bacterium. It's considerably larger than a bacterial plasmid but not nearly as large as a human chromosome, so it is given the name episome. The viral DNA is transcribed into messenger RNA for translation into proteins, but not all at once. To do so would result in a sudden release of foreign protein inside the cell and the virus would come to a quick end. By a unique set of circumstances, transcription of viral DNA into RNA goes in stages, called immediate early, early, and late.

The first six proteins produced, those of the immediate early group, are instrumental in directing the activation of the next group of genes, known as the early genes. These earliest genes and their protein products direct the translation of the next group of genes, the so-called late genes, which produce proteins for viral protein production. The final stage is the reproduction of the viral genome. The whole process is carefully structured to allow for the proper amount of time between viral protein production. Making the late proteins too early would result in the misreading of the viral genome and alerting the host cell's immune machinery.

While all this is happening, the virus has proteins that effectively shut down the host cell's metabolism. They are very efficient at it, and the host cell becomes a controlled virus factory. Once the many viral proteins are made and the DNA copied, the virions are assembled and make their way to the edge of the cell, to be released in a process that lyses the host cell. The preferred means of release by the virus is to enter a cell that abuts the original cell, thus avoiding the exterior and the immune defense. This is the lytic phase of the virus, as the host cell from which the virus is escaping breaks apart.

If the lytic phase of the family of herpes viruses were the whole story, we would probably consider them just something of a nuisance. Illness that lasts a few days and then goes away happens all the time, and often we don't know what caused it.

But herpes have perfected a unique feature that makes them a very challenging foe: latency. Being a double-stranded DNA virus that reproduces in the host cell nucleus allows them to remain with us for our whole lives. Usually, they just sit there doing nothing with our not being aware of their presence. But for some people, their long-term presence is potentially catastrophic.

Many of our cells die and are replaced all the time. They live out their usefulness and then are sloughed off or gobbled up by macrophages. It's a normal process. For a virus to infect such a cell is a dead-end; it will die off with the cell. To be a lifelong inhabitant of a cell, the cell it dwells in must itself be lifelong. The herpes family has developed the ability to seek out such cells and infect them in addition to the short-lived cells where it undergoes lytic infection.

Nerve cells aren't turned over. They last our lifetime, so it is no surprise that several herpes viruses can infect nerve cells. The alpha-herpes (simplex 1, simplex 2, and varicella) can all establish a latent infection in nerve cells. Similarly, beta- and gamma- herpes can infect a wide range of cells, inducing them to persist for the life of the infected individual.

The family of herpes viruses is very efficient in cell invasion and propagation. They have been infecting animals for over a hundred million years, and humans for as long as we have existed as a species, so they've had a long time to get it right. A "good" parasite doesn't want to damage its host, at least not very much. The herpes viruses are classic examples of this. Well over half, maybe as many as 90% of humans, are infected by at least one member of the herpes family yet show no symptoms. The most apparent symptoms are displayed by the alpha-herpes group, with simplex 1 and 2 along with varicella displaying pathognomonic signs, but even these are usually short-lived in the initial lytic phase. That's not to say the herpes viruses are entirely benign. Far from it. There is a very broad spectrum of the consequences of infection, from asymptomatic to fatal. The interaction of the virus and the immune system is critical in determining the course of the disease.

One of the first orders of business for the virus after it enters a new host cell is to shut down the cell's protein synthesis. Several enzymes in the viral tegument disable the host cell's RNA before it can be translated into protein at the ribosome. This has the effect of reducing the chances of apoptosis as well as curtailing cytokine production to alert the immune system. The enzymes that shut down host cell mRNA activity are among those produced late in the virus' cycle, so viral mRNA is not impacted nearly as much as the host cell's when the virus traverses the cytoplasm.

One of our most potent immune forces is the ability to display components of an invading virus on a cell's surface. By doing this, T-cells and B-cells can be mustered to attack the virus when encountered. Normally, viral proteins are dismantled, and pieces of them, usually about 5-10 amino acids in length, are put onto an MHC molecule, which displays the peptide on its surface. The peptide-laden MHC molecule is then transported to the cell surface to openly express the little piece of virus. After several steps, the T-cells and B-cells that react with the displayed microbial peptides are activated, and the adaptive immune system is fully engaged to recognize and destroy the virus both inside and outside cells.

The herpes viruses have developed an elaborate system of proteins to greatly subvert this usually efficient system. The host cell has a series of proteins called TAP, which are responsible for attaching the viral peptide to the MHC molecule inside the cell in the endoplasmic reticulum. Herpes proteins interfere with the TAP process, and the MHC molecules never receive their cargo. Viral display on the infected cell's surface is abated, and the adaptive immune response is significantly curtailed.

Our cells can easily recognize double-stranded RNA because our cells do not make it and consider it a foreign substance. At some point in their life cycle inside the cell, RNA viruses create double-stranded RNA, so an immune response to RNA viruses is usually quite vigorous. But the herpes genome is double-stranded DNA, just like ours, so it doesn't look like foreign material. Once the virus becomes latent, it shuts down protein synthesis, so there is no immune response to these foreign proteins. As long as the viral DNA can stay in the host cell nucleus it can remain in the latent state, going unnoticed by the immune system.

But DNA in the cytoplasm, outside the cell's nucleus, is a sign of trouble. Either it means an invading pathogen or a problem with the cell's own metabolism. To detect and react to stray DNA in the cytoplasm cells, human cells have a most elaborate and complex device known as the inflammasome. Diagrams of inflammasomes look something like a spaceship from a science fiction movie, with a large round region on top and long dangling molecules protruding underneath. Inflammasomes don't roam around the cell's cytoplasm, but subordinate components do. When one of them detects the presence of DNA, it becomes active, signaling other molecules that then, in a cascade fashion, form the inflammasome. After all this complicated business, the job of the inflammasome is twofold: to release the inflammatory cytokines interleukin-1 and interleukin-18, and the host cell is instructed to destroy itself along with the invading virus. The host cell's auto-destruction is called pyroptosis. As the words "inflamed" and "pyro" suggest, cell destruction is not an orderly process like apoptosis. It is more traumatic, something of an explosive event. But the host cell dies, taking the invading microbe with it. The system is most used against bacteria since they contain DNA, but the herpes family is the viral exception.

Some herpes viruses have a means of subverting the formation and activity of inflammasomes. A herpes tegument protein, VP22, inhibits an integral part of the inflammasome, a substance called AIM2. Without AIM2, building the inflammasome and its important work is greatly curtailed.

The group of blood proteins known as complement are an important deterrent to invading microbes, including viruses. Complement can work alone against the intruder, or in concert with other members of the immune system such as antibodies and neutrophils. Complement is also vital in giving a chemical alarm about the presence and location of the invader. The family of herpes viruses have developed the means of reducing the effectiveness of complement on initial contact. One of the herpes virus' surface glycoproteins can bind to the critical C3 and C5 complement components, blocking their activity. As a result, the body's initial response to the invading virus is significantly reduced.

A very important group of immune cells working against intracellular pathogens like viruses are the natural killer lymphocytes (NK cells). By chemical sensors on their surface, NK cells can detect a serious problem inside an infected cell and set about the job of destroying it and its pernicious invader. By detecting the presence or absence of key molecules on the surface of cells, the NK lymphocytes can release their appropriate destructive molecular assassins and destroy the infected cell. For herpes viruses, this will not do. Over the eons they have developed the means of counteracting their nemesis NK lymphocytes. One important molecular signal of infected cells is known as MICA, which is displayed on the cell's surface. It is an unequivocal signal to the NK lymphocyte that the cell displaying it needs to be killed. Some herpes viruses have developed molecules to ensure that MICA remains in the cell and the Natural Killer lymphocytes don't encounter it and do their job. The virus, of course, survives. To add insult to injury, some herpes viruses induce the Natural Killer lymphocytes to kill themselves through apoptosis. The result is lots of virus remaining viable within the still-functioning host cell.

One of our most important cells for immunity are the dendritic macrophages, those starfish-looking cells that roam around seeking foreign invaders. They are very good at detecting pathogen associated molecular patterns and internalizing the invading microbe. Once inside the DC cell, the microbe is systematically broken down and carried off to the nearest lymph node for introduction to the appropriate lymphocytes. Dendritic macrophages are especially good at picking up and removing microbes introduced into the skin, like many herpes viruses are. To survive, the viruses must overcome the action of the dendritic macrophages, and herpes is among the best at doing this. The virus can alter the maturation of the dendritic cell phagosome in which it resides, delaying the display of its protein parts on the phagocyte's surface. The virus also interferes with the activity of the important MHC molecules, significantly limiting the recognition of the virus by the rest of the immune system.

All told the family of viruses known as the *Herpesviridae* are extremely efficient and communicable. Most of us have at least one of the nine members, and many have more than one. Just as there is a range of viruses in the family, there is also a wide range of symptoms and sequelae. Just how sick an individual becomes depends as much on the immune reaction to the virus as the invading virus itself.

A brief description of each member of the herpes Family:

Herpes Simplex-1. Technically, herpes simplex-1 (HSV-1) infection is known as herpes labialis, but everyone calls it either a cold sore or a fever blister. More than half the population of the United States has been infected with the herpes simplex-1 virus, but only about one or two in five of those infected develop symptoms. Typically, the signs of a first HSV-1 infection appear before the age of 30, so if you haven't displayed symptoms by then chances are pretty good you never will.

Symptoms occur around the lips and mouth. Before seeing any blisters, the patient feels a bit of tingling and itching for a day or two. When the blisters appear, they are typically red and fluid-filled. There is often quite a bit of swelling and pain. In a couple of days the blisters pop, a yellowish fluid flows, and the skin begins to crust. Usually this is the beginning of the end of the acute phase, and after about a week the patient is right as rain. Healing can progress a little faster if the anti-viral cream acyclovir is methodically applied.

Unfortunately, that's not the end of it. The entire family of herpes viruses have acquired the ability to hold up in some type of human cell. If the virus simply infected epithelial cells it wouldn't last long, as those cells are continually replaced. To survive for a long time in the human host, the virus must enter and quietly inhabit a cell that lasts as long as the infected person. For herpes simplex-1, that cell is a neuron.

Apoptosis is a natural process. Just like leaves dying and falling from a tree, many of our cells die off, either because they are senescent or something inside them has gone wrong. Being infected by a microbe is a good reason for a cell to kill itself if it is easily replaced by an identical cell. One cell type that does not die off, though, is a peripheral nerve cell. Each lasts as long as we do. If one dies it is not replaced, and severe damage occurs. It is into the nerve cells of the face that the herpes simplex-1 virus enters after escaping its primary target, epithelial cells around the mouth.

The trigeminal nerve is just what the "tri" in its name suggests: a three-part nerve. The upper, or ophthalmic, branch innervates the scalp, forehead, and eyes. The middle, or maxillary, branch innervates the nasal cavity, cheeks, and upper lip. The lower, or mandibular, branch communicates with the lower lip and chin. All branches are sensory, relaying touch, taste, smells, and sounds. The mandibular branch is also a motor nerve involved in chewing. The trigeminal nerve is the closest to the lips where Herpes Simplex-1 infects, and it is in this nerve that the virus establishes latency.

Neurons have long branches, called axons, that communicate with their target cell. Axons are equipped with cellular machinery to allow chemicals to travel back to the cell nucleus. The nuclei of peripheral neurons are often found clustered in a group of nerve cell nuclei called a ganglion. Ganglia are a hub of nerve cell nuclei, a central point from which axons branch off to their assigned locations.

After entering a neuron, herpes is able to make its way up the axon to the cell body residing in the ganglion. From there, just as it does in epithelial cells, it enters the nerve cell nucleus, and its DNA is embedded next to the DNA of the neuron. It shuts down most of its DNA transcription and can reside inside the nerve cell indefinitely in what is called the latent phase.

Nerve cells cannot be allowed to die since they cannot be replaced. Apoptosis is not an option. To help keep the nerve cells alive, the cells they innervate continually send them chemical signals to shut down any possibility of apoptosis and the neuron, even if infected, is kept alive. The chemical signals sent are very complicated and come under the general heading of neurotrophins. The neurotrophins are generated by the cells adjacent to the axon and make their way up to the nucleus through the nerve cell's transport system, the same system that the Herpes virus uses.

Neurotrophins are a chemical means by which innervated cells let the attending neuron know everything is OK. But sometimes things are not OK. The cell adjacent to the axon might be infected by a common cold virus, or been overexposed to the UV rays of direct sunlight. Perhaps the affected patient has been undergoing high levels of emotional stress, severely altering the body's cortisol level and immune status. Dramatic shifts in hormone levels, such as those accompanying menstruation and pregnancy, can initiate changes. Whatever the reason, when the cells near the nerve cell axon become stressed, the amount and composition of the neurotrophin they send to the neuron become abnormal. For some yet unexplained reason, this stimulates the herpes simplex DNA to begin lytic transcription—not just a few proteins to enable its own DNA replication, but the whole genome, yielding an entire mature virus. This newly formed virus makes its way down the axon in much the same way the virus traveled to the nucleus. Fortunately for the infected person, the neuron containing them is not lysed as infected epithelial cells are. Neural damage does not occur, but the virus enters the body, not from the outside as it did initially, but from the inside. The result is the production of symptoms identical to those which occurred on initial infection.

Usually, the symptoms produced this second time around (or third or fourth) are milder and more localized than the first episode. Re-infection tends to be on one side of the face and in a restricted location. That of course is not always the case, but much more often than not.

The trigeminal nerve is also called the 5th cranial nerve. It is not that far from the brain, and after being infected it contains viable virus that doesn't go away. In a few cases, the worst happens. The virus makes its way into the brain, causing a deadly serious encephalitis. Usually, the virus travels up the olfactory nerve to the brain. Herpetic encephalitis is a rare disease, with around 2 or 3 cases per million population reported annually in the United States. But it is certainly tragic when it occurs.

Herpes Simplex-2. Closely related to herpes simplex-1 is type 2, which usually infects the genitalia. The two types are very closely related but are clearly distinguishable. Both can infect each other's sites, but HSV-1 is much more efficient around the mouth and HSV-2 is far better at infecting the genital organs. Like HSV-1, HSV-2 can enter nerve cells. In the case of the latter, it is members of the sacral nerve complex, S2-S4, which innervate the pelvic area. Also, like HSV-1, type 2 herpes simplex can become reactivated periodically. In fact, the type 2 variety reactivates twice as commonly as the type 1 type. The two types follow the same pattern of invading the host cell's nucleus and entering both the lytic and latent phases.

With herpes simplex-2 infection, the onset of the first episode of illness is accompanied by systemic signs in addition to localized lesions, with fever, muscle aches, and sometimes headache. The localized lesions' symptoms are mainly itching, discharge, and pain. Quite a few patients with first-time symptoms have pain in the lymph nodes in the groin. Genital herpes infection often lasts longer than oral herpes, sometimes up to three weeks. Also, recurrences are more common with HSV-2.

One great problem of herpes simplex-2 infection is that it leaves an infected person much more vulnerable to infection by human immunodeficiency virus, or HIV. People with herpes simplex-2 become infected with HIV more commonly than those who are herpes simplex-2 negative. No doubt there are several reasons for this, but it is known that herpes infection leads to an influx of CD-4 lymphocytes, the target of HIV, thus increasing the chances of a virus-lymphocyte encounter. Also, laboratory studies have shown that two herpes simplex proteins, ICP0 and ICP4, can increase the rate of reproduction of HIV.

Both types of herpes simplex can be treated with an effective antiviral cream, acyclovir (European spelling aciclovir). It's a prime example of how nature can supply us with effective medications, as it was derived from a shallow water sponge that grows in the warm waters of the Caribbean, (*Cryptotethya crypta*). The sponge has little or no immune

490

system, but it helps keep itself safe by making an enzyme that interferes with viral DNA replication. That's just what is needed to attack herpes simplex, a DNA virus. Acyclovir speeds up recovery by a few days, but unlike bacterial antibiotics, it doesn't remove the virus permanently. Herpes simplex becomes embedded in our nerve cell nuclei, and getting rid of it permanently is a tall order. Most often, the virus persists to re-infect as circumstances allow.

Varicella-Zoster. One of the strangest names of a human disease is chickenpox. Strange in that it has nothing to do with chickens. They don't get sick from the virus, harbor it, or become involved in any way. The most likely explanation for the name is that somewhere, sometime, someone thought the pox marks resembled the result of pecks by a chicken. Be that as it may, the disease has been known to just about every parent for centuries. It has been a very common childhood ailment and, thankfully, usually not too serious in its acute phase. Unfortunately, like other herpes viruses, it does not just go away after the initial illness. It remains with a person for the rest of their life, and for about 30% of us, it can emerge as something much more malevolent: shingles.

The virus has two official names, varicella and zoster, the former referring to the acute "chickenpox" stage, the latter to the shingles stage. In ancient times there was no way of knowing the two were caused by the same virus. In some ways, the childhood ailment resembles a very mild form of smallpox, or variola, hence the "vari" part of the name. The "cella" suffix means diminished or much reduced. *Zoster* is a Greek word for "belt" or "girdle," since the disease shingles often, but not always, attacks the mid-abdomen. The virus is called varicella-zoster virus, usually abbreviated VZV.

Varicella has a typical herpes virus construction but with some unique characteristics. It is a little smaller than its alpha-herpes cousins simplex types 1 and 2, and it attacks by the respiratory route. The incubation period, the time from the first encounter with the organism to the first display of symptoms, is around 14 days, a long time for viruses. Most viral infections incubate just a few days. But just because no symptoms are displayed for two weeks after varicella enters the body doesn't mean nothing is going on. Quite the contrary. The virus becomes very active almost immediately.

After entering the epithelial cells of the upper respiratory tract, it begins multiplying. The virus is best served by getting itself into lymph tissue, either a node or the tonsils. The cells that perform this task for it are the dendritic macrophages, which gobble up free virions and make their way to the lymph tissue. The dendritic cells are designed to digest the virus, display its entrails, and hook up with compatible lymphocytes, which can put an end to the menace. Instead, the dendritic cells serve as chauffeurs to carry the virus around the infected body unmolested. The virus goes from the initial epithelial cells it enters to dendritic macrophages, then to the nearest lymph tissue. It then enters either a lymphocyte or macrophage that carries it to every part of the body, including the macrophages of the reticuloendothelial system. It continues to replicate, making its way into the bloodstream, from whence it is deposited in the cells of the dermis of the skin.

This is quite a journey. From the respiratory epithelial cells to lymph tissue, to various bodily organs by way of the bloodstream, and back into the bloodstream to settle in the tissues of the skin and respiratory cells. All this is accomplished in the face of highly developed immune systems designed to halt such an incursion into the body. But varicella is highly successful in its quest because of its sophisticated armaments.

A major opponent of viral infections is apoptosis, programmed cell death. By killing itself, the cell, which is easily replaced, prevents the virus from using its internal machinery to make more copies of itself; the virus dies with the cell. So to thrive, varicella must be able to prevent apoptosis. On the other hand, after it has replicated and is ready to escape from the host cell, the virus needs to have the cell break apart through apoptosis to release it. Varicella has the capacity to do both in a remarkably sophisticated way. The virus has the proteins that promote the host cell's apoptosis, but only after the virus has had time to replicate and make many copies of itself. This allows the easy release of the virus in an orderly fashion, thus preventing an inflammatory encounter. The virus can then be transported to its next destination. Just like many things in life, the timing of apoptosis is important, and varicella is a master of it.

Another important job of varicella is diminishing the amount of interferon and other cytokines produced by the host cell. Type one interferons signal cells throughout the body about the presence of a virus, and chemical processes are initiated to prevent the spread of the virus. Since varicella infects by going from cell to cell and in and out of the bloodstream, it must quell the amount of interferon produced. It is very good at doing this, with at least three proteins it manufactures designed to substantially halt or slow down both the production of and the response to interferon.

Interferon is powerful in its ability to help us contain invading viruses, but it has a downside: it makes us feel sick with body aches and fever. Interferon must be carefully controlled so that it is released in the proper amount only when necessary. A key protein in controlling the amount of interferon produced is known as suppressor of cytokine signaling 3, or SOCS3. The role of this cytoplasmic protein is to put a brake on excessive interferon production. Varicella has an enzyme that significantly increases the activity of interferon-suppressing SOCS3, thereby using the cell's own chemical to mitigate interferon production.

Human cells infected by varicella should be sitting ducks for natural killer lymphocytes, the blood cell whose job is to destroy their fellow human cells infected by a virus. The signal to the natural killer lymphocytes that everything is all right within the cell it is surveying is the presence of the molecular complex MHC on the cell's surface. Without enough MHC, the natural killer cell detects something is wrong and unleashes several killing molecules to liquidate the infected cell and its viral passenger. But varicella has devised ways to thwart the natural killer cells by modifying the ability of the NK cell to dock onto the surface of the damaged cell. Two stress-induced proteins, ULBP2 and ULBP3, are normally transported to the host cell's surface, where they encounter the surveillance protein NKG2D on the natural killer cell. This enables the killer cell to release its deadly contents and destroy the virus-laden cell. But varicella has several proteins that incapacitate ULBP proteins, not allowing the NK cell to do its job. Instead of killing the cell containing the virus, natural killer lymphocytes can be used by the virus to transport it to other areas of the body. It's kind of like a criminal hijacking a police car to take him to a crime scene.

With the influence varicella has over cell self-destruction and interferon production, it can reproduce and travel around our body with impunity. Ultimately it enters the cells of the dermis of the skin, replicates inside them, then induces the cells to lyse. The result is what we see on the skin's surface, pustules surrounded by a red ring. At first the fluid from the vesicle is clear, but after a short time it becomes thick and milky due to the presence of pus and fibrin. Viable virus is present in the fluid, and when the scabs break by itching or rubbing, the virus can become airborne and remain in the air for some time, allowing it to be transmitted to another individual. Upper respiratory tract cells are also infected, and the virus can be transmitted from there.

Like all herpes viruses, varicella can enter the latent state inside a host cell. The cell type it uses for this purpose is the neuron, which doesn't undergo apoptosis. The virus has several proteins that ensure the infected neuron doesn't destroy itself.

The peripheral nerves from our spinal column come in two major functions, motor and sensory. The motor nerves emanate from the front, or anterior, while the sensory from the back, or dorsal. It is these dorsal sensory nerve cells that varicella inhabits in the latent state. And, like their cousins herpes simplex type 1, they can dwell in the trigeminal nerve of the face. But unlike herpes simplex, which usually inhabits the lower two-thirds of the trigeminal, varicella is mainly found in the upper branch, which enervates the area around the eyes.

Just why varicella in its zoster form breaks out from its nerve cell host is not explained. It most likely has to do with an alteration in the immune status of the infected person, and several things can lead to that, the obvious ones being the aging process and heavy emotional stress.

Not everyone who had chickenpox will get shingles; only about 20-30% do. And not everyone is affected the same. Some cases are rather mild, more of an inconvenience, while others are severe, with a terrible rash, immense pain that doesn't go away, and eye infections that can lead to blindness. Every case is different.

The area served by sensory nerves is called a dermatome. Rather than one specific point, a dermatome covers several centimeters of skin, extending in what looks like a band. It is within this dermatome that the zoster virus is expressed, first as localized pain and irritation, then as an ugly rash. The rash contains viable virus which can be communicated to other people. We don't spread shingles, though; only chickenpox is spread to those who are susceptible.

Shingles near the eye can be devastating. Most times the infection occurs around the orbit of the eye, but sometimes the eye itself can be affected. Blindness sometimes results. Aggressive medical intervention with antiviral agents is vital.

Through the latter half of the 20th century, vaccines were developed for several infectious diseases usually associated with childhood: diphtheria, polio, pertussis, measles, mumps, and rubella can all be prevented by vaccination. Chickenpox was a prevalent childhood disease, but it was presumed by most that it was a mild disease, and a vaccination program wasn't necessary. Since chickenpox is usually a more serious disease when contracted in adulthood, it wasn't uncommon for parents to bring their children to a "chickenpox party," where children would gather in a home afflicted by the disease in the hope that the child would get the disease and get it over with. The very name "chickenpox" suggests a trivial, unimportant malady.

The perception of chickenpox began to change throughout the 1960s and 70s as advances were made in chemotherapy. As steroidal and other chemotherapeutic medications were being used to treat previously untreatable diseases, it was becoming evident that varicella, once considered a benign virus, was, in fact, a killer. Children with leukemia could be treated with a drug that was successful, only to have the child die of varicella. Or a child could contract chickenpox, then visit a grandparent being treated with an agent that suppresses the immune system and unknowingly transmit a deadly disease to them. Vaccinating children for chickenpox would significantly eliminate this threat.

Also in the 1960s and 70s, people were living longer. And the older we get, the more likely we are to contract shingles, and many more cases were being diagnosed and treated. Vaccines for varicella and zoster would also greatly improve public health.

In the 1960s professor Michiaiki Takahashi at Osaka University in Japan obtained specimens from a young boy who had chickenpox. The boy's family name was Oka. In the laboratory, Dr. Takahashi placed the specimen containing the Oka varicella virus on tissue culture cells. Over the next several years the virus was passed to several different cell lines at sub-optimal temperatures. (Most cell cultures are maintained at body temperature, 37°C; Dr. Takahashi did his experiments at 34°C). Different cell lines were used, including human embryonic lung fibroblasts, guinea pig fibroblasts, and other cells from aborted human fetuses, to eventually isolate a strain of varicella that could infect, elicit an immune response, but not make the person sick. In other words, a live attenuated vaccine.

While it was not known then, the vaccine strain had at least eleven mutations in gene number 62, which codes for the viral glycoprotein gE. (The term open reading frame, or OPR, is often used for the term gene. In this case that would be OPR62). Without a properly functioning gE, the immune system easily contains the virus, and the typical chickenpox symptoms are not displayed, or only very slightly, although full immunity is established.

With the introduction of a live varicella virus questions immediately arose. Since it is a live virus, albeit attenuated, is it transmissible to others? Does the vaccine strain enter the latent stage, and if so, can it later re-emerge to cause zoster? If that were to happen, would it cause typical zoster or some abbreviated form? It had been long assumed that immunity to chickenpox was lifelong because people who had the disease as children would be continually exposed to the virus through contact with infected children, thus getting a natural booster of their immunity. If this were true, did the vaccine strain, if not transmissible, give this booster effect?

Because of the long timeframe of infection by varicella answers are not absolute, but it appears some 25 years after the introduction of the vaccine that it does indeed enter the latent stage and persists as the wild-type strain did. There is some evidence that the vaccine strain can emerge as a very mild form of shingles but not anywhere near the severity of the wild-type virus. It is speculation, but the persistence of humoral immunity is likely due to the periodic re-emergence of the virus from the latent stage, prompting an immune response but not yielding any clinical signs. If that is true, then continuous re-exposure to the virus in nature is not needed to keep up immunity. Whether a child immunized for chickenpox will need a vaccine for shingles when they are older is not known.

In the vast number of cases, chickenpox in children is a mild disease. In contrast, shingles in adults is very often a significant ailment. Approximately 30% of adults over the age of 50 develop shingles in their lifetime. Most cases are rather short-lived, a week or two duration, but the symptoms are considerably more troubling than chickenpox. The rash is localized to the affected area and is not particularly problematic, just unsightly and with a small amount of itching. The more serious concern is the pain. The nerves affected are sensory, with pain receptors prominent. Having a mild or no rash with excruciating pain is not unusual. The duration of symptoms varies with the individual, with most over their infection in a couple of weeks. The good news for them is that usually shingles does not recur, and if it does, the second episode is not as severe as the first. The virus remains in the latent stage, but the cellular and humoral immunogenic burst protecting the patient is strong and persistent, preventing or minimizing future episodes.

Some people, though, have a life-altering situation when they develop shingles. When the virus emerges from the trigeminal nerve, it is usually from the upper branch, which enervates the eye region. Eye infections with varicella usually are in the area surrounding the eyes, the orbit. But in some cases, the eye itself is infected with the virus leading to severe medical problems that require a high level of care, with no guarantee of success. Another severe complication of shingles is a condition known as post-herpetic neuralgia, usually called PHN. The nerves in which varicella resides are sensory, which includes pain. Usually, the condition arises a little after the rash subsides, but it can occur without the rash. For some people, and it is impossible to predict just who, the pain is long-term and excruciating. Just a light touch is enough to send debilitating shock waves of pain. The duration of the symptoms is varied, sometimes for a few weeks, sometimes for life.

Just as we now have a vaccine for chickenpox in children, there is a vaccine for shingles in people over 50. In fact, there are two shingles vaccines.

The first shingles vaccine manufactured is the same as the chickenpox vaccine, the live attenuated Oka strain. When given to children, the vaccine is designed to prevent chickenpox in children who have never had the disease. When given to older people, the vaccine is given to people who have presumably had chickenpox as a child and still harbor the latent form of the virus, leaving them potentially vulnerable to an outbreak of shingles. Their immunity to varicella has waned through the years, so giving them the chickenpox vaccine is meant to stimulate their immune response when/if the varicella virus reappears. The live shingles vaccine is given in a much higher dose than that given for chickenpox since the people it is administered to are much larger than children, and their immune response is not as great as that of a child. Recommended in 2006 for use in adults over 60, the live vaccine proved to be pretty good but certainly not perfect. Its effectiveness in preventing shingles was about 66%.

The main difference between the live vaccine strain of varicella and the wild-type is a marked alteration in the surface glycoprotein E. As the technology became available, it was possible to make altered glycoprotein E in the laboratory and administer just that one part of the virus instead of the whole thing. By itself the protein is somewhat immunogenic, but the immune response advances significantly when an adjuvant is administered along with it. The adjuvant ASO1B contains two substances that substantially stimulates the immune response, both in cytokine production and the reaction of CD-4 lymphocytes, the greatest fighter against the cells containing varicella. Approved for use in the United States in 2017, the glycoprotein E plus adjuvant vaccine, known commercially as SHINGRIX, has replaced the live attenuated chickenpox vaccine for the prevention of shingles. While still early in its use, it has been shown to be over 90% effective in preventing shingles. One downside is that two doses are needed 2-6 months apart.

Varicella-zoster virus will always be with us. Vaccines will never eradicate it—they are not 100% effective, the virus is worldwide, and it is very easily spread. While not usually a cause for concern in healthy children, varicella can be devastating in children and older people who are immunocompromised, and shingles in some individuals is often a very serious, life-altering condition. It is a formidable foe.

Epstein-Barr Virus. Epstein-Barr Virus, usually abbreviated EBV, has an unusual history. Even though it infects 95% of the human population, it wasn't discovered until the 1960s. Most viruses are named after the disease they cause, a characteristic of the virus, or the location of their discovery. This one is named for two of the British scientists who first wrote of it in a scientific journal. Given its late discovery and description, one would think it must be non-invasive and benign.

On the contrary, it can be associated with very serious ailments. It causes most cases of infectious mononucleosis (usually just called "mono"), and it can be involved in several types of cancer and autoimmune disorders. The vast majority of people infected with EBV display no symptoms; they don't even know they have the virus. For some, though, the virus is life-altering and highly debilitating.

Epstein-Barr Virus is a member of the herpes virus family, technically designated Human Herpes Virus-4. It is a gamma-herpes, in contrast to herpes simplex and varicella-zoster, members of the alpha group. While structurally the same as its herpes virus cousins, it is larger with about 100 proteins as opposed to the 80-90 of the others. Symptoms like skin eruptions or other observable signs don't accompany the initial infection. After multiplication without symptoms it enters the latent stage. Unlike the alpha herpes viruses that enter nerve cells for their latent stage, EBV enters B-lymphocytes.

Denis Burkitt was a unique researcher. He was a scientist with an unquenching quizzical mind, and a devout evangelical Christian who claimed to have had a vision early in life telling him to serve in remote areas of Africa. Born in Northern Ireland in 1911, he served as a military doctor during World War II. Following the war, he combined his medical knowledge and zeal for his missionary calling to work in Uganda. There he encountered a disease of children that had not been described in medical literature. The children had massively swollen faces along with swollen livers and spleens. It appeared as a type of lymphoma but was markedly different from any yet described. He found it only in children, and it was universally fatal.

In 1958 Dr. Burkitt began a long journey around remote areas of Africa, a trip called the "10,000-mile Safari." He visited many villages and small clinics, treating patients and recording data on several of them, including the lymphoma he had encountered. He found that the lymphoma occurred only in areas of high temperatures and large rainfall, the same regions in which falciparum malaria was found. It seemed possible that a form of cancer was being spread by a microbe, most likely a virus, and that it was perhaps being spread by an insect, the same way malaria was spread.

Dr. Burkitt traveled to England in 1961 to give a series of medical lectures on his experience in Africa. Attending one of his lectures was Dr. Anthony Epstein, who was intrigued by the possibility of cancer being caused by a virus. He and Dr. Burkitt quickly became friends, and it was arranged that biopsy material from the lymphoma patients in Africa be sent to Dr. Epstein's team in London for examination, including observation under an electron microscope. The result of these studies was the first description of what is now known as the Epstein-Barr virus. (There were three authors of the first paper, Anthony Epstein, Burt Achong, and Christine Barr; for some reason, Dr. Achong's name was omitted when the virus was referred to in medical literature, and the virus came to be known as the Epstein-Barr virus).

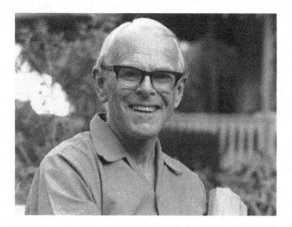

Denis Burkitt was a talented and devoted physician. He spent many years treating the poorest of the poor in remote areas of Africa. After returning to England, he spent the remaining years of his life educating people on the benefits of a high-fiber diet for better health, based on his observations in Africa. (LOC)

The means by which EBV enters the body is saliva. Sharing a drinking cup, glass, water bottle, straw, spoon, kissing, or some similar mechanism is enough to introduce the virus. Once the virus enters the new person, it invades a host cell. There is conflicting data on the type of cell it enters, epithelial or lymphoid; it could be both. No symptoms are displayed during the lytic stage, and as soon as possible the virus enters the latent stage within the nucleus of B-lymphocytes. For the herpes simplex and varicella-zoster viruses, the latent stage is set up in nerve cells, a wise choice since they last the infected person's life. But B-cells have a limited lifespan, so the Epstein-Barr virus must ensure the long-term survival of the infected B-cell. Otherwise, it dies with it. To this end, it has come up with some intriguing mechanisms.

As the rounded-up DNA of the virus sits in the nucleus of the B-cell, it replicates in synchrony with the chromosomes of the host cell, using the host cell's enzymes to attain its purpose. But most of the genes of the viral DNA are not transcribed and turned into proteins. Only about a dozen are. Their job is to ensure two things important to the virus: that the

501

viral DNA replicates while in the latent state, and that the host B-cell stays alive.

One group of viral genes allows the virus to ensure the survival of the B-lymphocytes. The term used is a bit of hyperbole: "immortalization." Clearly, our cells are not immortal. But in the world of immunology and cell biology, a cell that lasts for the infected person's life is as close to "immortal" as it gets. Using a set of gene products in the viral latent stage, the Epstein-Barr virus engages a set of proteins that instruct T-lymphocytes to allow the host B-cell to mature and survive.

The viral genes that work to ensure replication of its DNA are known as Epstein-Barr Nuclear Antigens or EBNA. Several numbered genes work in concert to allow the smooth replication of viral DNA. Two other viral proteins produced during the latent period are known as Latent Infection Membrane Proteins or LMP. There are two of them; their job is to travel out of the B-cell nucleus and make their way to the cell membrane. Through several reactions, they present the infected B-lymphocyte to CD4 T-cells, making the B-cell appear activated and ensuring its survival. It is a highly complex process, but obviously the molecular machinery is very efficient, and the B-lymphocytes perpetuate, taking the included viral DNA along for the ride.

Sometimes the B-lymphocytes infected by Epstein-Barr virus reproduce too rapidly and get out of control. The virus plays a part in this, as the EBNA enzymes operating in the nucleus can transpose a set of pro-growth genes (known as m-myc) from one chromosome to another, where they produce more energy, enabling the B-cells to metabolize and reproduce at an accelerated rate. The most common disease associated with this hyper-reaction of the B-cells is the disease known as infectious mononucleosis, often simply called mono. Normally, CD-8 lymphocytes, often called "killer T-cells," can detect and destroy the viral-infected B-cell. But sometimes, the infected B-cell population has proliferated too rapidly and overwhelms the killer T-cells' ability to maintain it. The activated killer T-cells can be seen in the bloodstream and are referred to as atypical

502

lymphocytes because of their altered morphology. While not specific to infectious mononucleosis, atypical lymphocytes, when observed in the presence of other typical signs, indicate a high probability of the disease.

The classic symptoms of infectious mononucleosis are sore throat, fever, and swollen lymph nodes. The sore throat has been described as "the worst one you've ever had." Sometimes the tonsils are so swollen that they meet in the middle of the mouth. The fever usually isn't too high, but it can persist over several days or weeks. The swollen lymph nodes are usually in the back of the neck and armpits but can also be in other locations. The spleen and liver may also be swollen. Patients often experience extreme fatigue.

Compared with other viral diseases affecting the upper respiratory tract, infectious mono is quite odd. For one, an infected person does not transmit the disease to another, as with influenza or coronavirus. The disease is rare in young children and older people—typically, it occurs in teenagers and early adults. And while the disease is caused mainly by the Epstein-Barr virus, it can also result from several other infectious organisms.

The strangest thing about mononucleosis is the traditional serology test. Historically the disease was known as "glandular fever" since it often involved swollen lymph nodes and tonsils, commonly called glands. In the 1930s, researchers made a very surprising discovery: frequently, infected individuals had in their bloodstream antibodies to the red blood cells of animals like horses, sheep, and cows. How odd. The animals, of course, had nothing to do with the disease, yet here were these antibodies to them. The antibodies were called heterophile ("other loving"). Nobody could fathom why they were there, but the presence of heterophile antibodies was so consistent in cases of mononucleosis that heterophile serology became an established test for the disease. ("Serology" refers to a laboratory test in which the patient's serum is analyzed for antibodies).

We now know that the heterophile antigens don't exist just on certain animals but on various microbes as well. Chances are most humans during their lives encounter some creature that contains the antigen, and since humans don't have it, our immune system considers it foreign and creates an antibody to it. When the Epstein-Barr virus stirs up the B-lymphocyte equilibrium, those primed to generate antibodies to the heterophile antigen ramp up their activity, resulting in detectable amounts. It's an odd happenstance of nature.

It's convenient when the heterophile antibody test (now called the Monospot test) confirms the diagnosis of infectious mononucleosis, but the limitations of the test must be remembered. The antibody is not specific for the Epstein-Barr virus, and even if it was, other organisms can cause mononucleosis. The antibody is only of the IgM type, so it doesn't last long, and if the test is done too early it may read negative. Additionally, some humans don't encounter the heterophile antigen at any time in their life and don't make antibodies to it, giving no chance for a positive test. Also, some other disease conditions induce the production of heterophile antibodies independent of mono. The Monospot can be a helpful aid in establishing a diagnosis of mononucleosis, but a negative test is not definitive.

The age of onset of mono is also interesting. Over 90% of the human population is infected by Epstein-Barr virus, but the vast majority of cases of mono are in patients in their teens or early 20s. The best theory to explain this is that if infected while young our immune system is better equipped to handle the virus, and it is contained in the latent state. If the first encounter with the virus is in teenagers and young adults, it is not as easily contained and more readily causes the rapid proliferation of B-cells, leading to disease. The genetic makeup of the infected person undoubtedly influences disease onset and progression.

With its life cycle of inhabiting a key immune system component (antibody-producing B-lymphocytes), the Epstein-Barr virus can sometimes create havoc. Usually, the virus exists in a tranquil, unobserved latent state, and even when it becomes lytic, no symptoms are observed. But, as clearly seen with Burkitt's lymphoma, circumstances can precipitate dramatic changes in the virus's behavior and the immune system's response to it. Epstein-Barr virus is associated with at least five different forms of cancer. Since the virus has infected most humans for most of their lives, the onset of serious disease appears to be a matter of bad luck. Co-infections with other pathogens and differences in individual immune responses account for most cases. They are, for the most part, unpredictable. With modern drugs, many of the cancers are treatable, assuming the drugs are available. None of the pharmaceuticals directly treat the virus, so it will be with us as long as we live.

Sometimes challenging medical situations arise that have no apparent cause. They are anomalous, sporadic, persistent. The individual suffers greatly from life-altering symptoms, but specific treatments are unavailable. The frustrating aspect of such cases is the lack of physical signs such as a physiologic or laboratory abnormality. Maybe the best example is chronic fatigue syndrome—much of the time, patients are completely exhausted and unable to carry out even simple tasks. It differs from clinical depression and is not amenable to any known treatment in many cases. The frustration is that with the lack of a defining characteristic other than the symptom itself, there can be trouble convincing healthcare providers of the condition's reality.

Any experienced doctor will give plenty of examples of patients with myriad complaints, all highly embellished or figments of the imagination. For attending physicians to distinguish such "symptoms" from a real but non-testable condition is not easy. For the patient suffering from a real, long-term affliction that can mean additional suffering: no one believes you, and it appears like they think you're mentally ill. But the symptoms are real for some, and a latent virus like Epstein-Barr may be somehow involved. But we nearly all have EBV, so just detecting its presence means nothing. So frustrating.

Cytomegalovirus. The largest virus that infects humans is cytomegalovirus, usually just called CMV. Like its herpes virus cousins, it infects most of us. Around 60% of people in developed nations and over 90% in poor countries show antibodies to the virus' antigens. Other herpes viruses have the genes to produce around 80-100 proteins; CMV weighs in at over 200. It is classified as a beta-herpes, as opposed to the alpha and gamma types. In the big scheme of things, CMV is given the name Human Herpesvirus-5.

CMV isn't picky about the type of cell it enters during primary infection. Both epithelial and endothelial cells on different tissues can be infected. Like any virus, CMV induces a vigorous immune system response, both humoral and cellular. To survive, it must substantially mitigate the immune response, and in its millions of years of existence, CMV has acquired the means to produce a wide array of proteins to thwart the immune system:

It shuts down the ability of MHC complexes to pick up little virus parts and transport them to the cell surface to display to compatible T-cells.

It has an array of proteins that interfere with the ability of Natural Killer lymphocytes to recognize and attach to an infected cell.

It significantly curtails the production of interferon.

It makes a protein that functions like the anti-inflammatory cytokine interleukin-10, thereby reducing the amount of inflammation and immune response.

It produces proteins that act as receptors for cytokines, such as tumor necrosis factor-alpha. These act like a cytokine sponge, reducing the inflammatory response.

Despite a wide array of immune-modulating factors, the overall immune response to CMV is very effective, and the virus must enter the latent stage to prevent its elimination. Its preferred cell type for this are those in the bone marrow that give rise to macrophages and neutrophils. It also establishes latency in the cells lining blood vessels, the endothelial cells. These cells don't last forever, so CMV regularly enters the lytic phase, producing virions that can wander about. The body's immune response will destroy most, but some will enter the proper cell where they can re-establish latency. During this latent to lytic cycle, cytokine function is much reduced, so the infected person experiences no symptoms. There is a balance established between virus production and the immune response.

506

Sometimes this balance between the virus and the infected person is upended. The virus remains the same, but changes in the infected person's immune status are the key to opening the door for viral entry. The immune system can become diminished in several important ways, especially as a result of modern technology. There are four main ways in which CMV can cause significant disease:

1) Transplant. CMV sets up house in several organs, especially within the blood vessels of kidneys and lungs. The transplanted organ carries the virus right along with it, and, of course, the receiving patient is administered drugs to diminish transplant rejection. Most transplanted organs, fortunately, don't contain enough virus to cause damage. Still, if the donor has only recently encountered the virus, the amount of virus in their organ is much higher than someone who has carried it at bay for years.

2) Immunosuppression. Patients with a disease such as cancer are often given drugs that knock down their immune system while trying to damage the growing cancer. Those with autoimmune disorders often receive the same general treatment. There are infectious diseases, most notably infection by the human immunosuppression virus (HIV) that can seriously affect the immune response. These immunosuppressive situations enable CMV to gain the upper hand and reproduce in large numbers in the lytic phase.

3) Adult acquisition of virus. When a person is infected by CMV as a young child, their immune system is robust, and the virus is usually easily contained. But when the virus is first encountered as a late teenager or an adult, the virus sometimes gets the upper hand, and symptoms are displayed. It is not unlike the acquisition of the Epstein-Barr virus; teenagers and young adults are the most likely to develop infectious mononucleosis. Such is the case for CMV, which can also cause infectious mono. The symptoms of IM caused by CMV are somewhat different from those caused by Epstein-Barr. CMV rarely causes sore throat, but EBV does in many cases. CMV mono is often accompanied by increased liver enzymes, which is not usually the case with EBV. But infectious mono caused by both viruses displays the hallmark blood counts, with the number of

lymphocytes exceeding the number of neutrophils, with about 10-15% atypical lymphocytes. Fatigue for an extended period is also common to both. Infectious mono caused by Epstein-Barr virus typically affects teenagers and people in their early 20s; that caused by CMV is more likely to be found in people in their early 20s through middle age. CMV does not induce the production of heterophile antigens, so the monospot test will be negative.

4) Babies. Babies' immune systems are immature, so infants depend on the antibodies their mothers produce to protect them. If the mother acquires the virus during pregnancy, her antibody level may be low. This is especially dangerous for babies *in utero*, who sometimes get infected as their mother contracts the virus.

5) Atherosclerosis. The endothelial lining of blood vessels is one known habitat for latent CMV. Atherosclerosis, or "hardening of the arteries," is largely due to the dysfunction of activated lymphocytes that can disrupt the arterial lining, helping to allow the deposition of low-density lipoprotein-carrying cholesterol. It could very well be that latent infection of CMV, with its frequent conversion to the lytic stage, is at least partly responsible for the activity of T-lymphocytes and the subsequent occurrence of atherosclerosis. Other organisms have also been implicated, and cause and effect are speculative, but the involvement of CMV is under active investigation.

Like the other Herpes viruses, cytomegalovirus will always be with us. There are anti-viral drugs available that often work quite well in quelling CMV infections, but establishing a definitive diagnosis is often tricky given the virus' high numbers among the population.

Roseola. The disease of many names. When first described in the early 1900s it was called roseola infantalis, then roseola infantum. Also used commonly is roseola subitem, as well as sixth disease. Each description is apt. The "rose" comes from the color of the rash. "Infantum" and "infantalis" describe the age of the vast majority of patients, infants and toddlers. "Subitum," Latin for "sudden," describes the sudden onset of the rash after cessation of the fever. "Sixth disease" refers to its being one of several childhood diseases involving fever and rash.

Roseola is a disease that is usually uncomplicated in its diagnosis. It overwhelmingly afflicts babies and toddlers six months old to two years, first presenting with fever and usually no other symptoms. The fever is often high, up to 104°F, and can last several days, sometimes a week. But interestingly, there are no accompanying symptoms like runny nose, cough, or sore throat. It's just the fever, and it disappears rather quickly. Just after the fever subsides, the rash appears nearly as suddenly, first on the trunk, then spreading to almost the entire body. The rash lasts a couple of days, and, like the fever, it goes away quickly. Once the disease has run its course it doesn't return. With a high fever, some children experience seizures, but fortunately most of these cases resolve without complications.

This all sounds very simple, but roseola is anything but a simple malady of young children. For one thing, we all have it. Perhaps not all of us, but pretty close. Most of us never have any symptoms like those described, only about 10% of those who acquire the virus as young children do. The virus is of the beta-herpes type, related to cytomegalovirus. It's not as large as CMV, but quite a bit bigger than the other herpes viruses. Biologically it looks and behaves like the other herpes viruses.

For many years since the delineation of the disease in the early 1900s, roseola was considered something of a nuisance, not requiring serious inquiry. The virus itself wasn't described until the 1980s. But recent discoveries have shown that the roseola virus may be involved in a more serious disease than was long thought.

Telomeres are DNA strands fitted on the end of a chromosome. To put it crudely, telomeres help prevent the destruction of the DNA of a chromosome, sort of like a rubber casing placed on the bottom of a chair leg. Over time they wear down, but while active, they aid in the preservation of the integrity of chromosomal DNA.

Like all herpes viruses, roseola enters a latent phase inside the host cell's nucleus. But it does so in a profoundly different way. Other herpes viruses' DNA circles up adjacent next to the chromosomes of the host cell, forming a DNA structure called an episome. It is replicated in synchrony with the DNA of the host cell but independently. The roseola's DNA integrates into the DNA of the host cell's telomeres, thus becoming a part of the host cell's chromosome.

Just how much of an effect this chromosome integration by the virus has on the infected individual is a matter of great scientific interest. Obviously, many variables are in play, such as which cell type is infected, which and how many chromosomes, the immune status of the host, and others. In most cases it is probably a benign situation, but some evidence points to the possibility of more serious consequences.

The axons of many nerve cells are coated by an important substance called myelin. It covers the axon, the extension of the nerve cell that carries the electrical message to the target cell. Axons are so long that they can't create their own myelin sufficiently, so they depend on assistant cells to produce the myelin for them and maintain it. One of the critical myelin-producing cells of the central nervous system is known as the oligodendritic neuron, a cell with many stubby tentacle-like appendages called dendrites, which serve to distribute and maintain myelin on the axon of an adjacent nerve cell. Without the presence and proper function of myelin, neurologic malfunction is inevitable.

Of great interest to researchers is the fact that roseola virus can enter and set up a latent infection in oligodendritic neurons, the cells that produce and maintain myelin on the axons of neurons. After the discovery of the roseola virus in the 1980s, work was done to better characterize the virus, and it was found that there are, in fact, two types of herpes virus 6. They are designated 6A and 6B. Further investigation has shown that the distinction between the two types is not merely a few different proteins but a significant variance in biological activity. Importantly, the 6B type is the one that causes most cases of infant and toddler roseola; the 6A type just a few or perhaps none.

Roseola 6A and 6B have different attachment receptors on the human cells that they prefer. CD43 is a protein that is present on all human cells (except red blood cells). CD43's purpose is to defend the cell against the destructive component of complement, C3, and its presence prevents the cell's inadvertent destruction. Roseola 6A attaches to CD43 for its entry into cells, and since CD43 is present on all our cells, the 6A type has a wide range of human cells to choose from. The 6B type is pickier in its cellular attachment preferences. It has an affinity for the protein CD134, found mainly on activated T-lymphocytes, thus giving it a narrower range of cells it can infect.

When one thinks of myelin and things that can go wrong if it doesn't function properly, one naturally thinks of the autoimmune disease multiple sclerosis, or MS. MS is clearly the result of the immune system's attack on the myelin sheaths surrounding axons. Several factors are involved, including the affected patient's genetics, but the presence of a virus (or viruses) that potentiate the problem has been thought for a long time to play a role. Roseola virus 6A's involvement is an interesting field of study. Perhaps the virus, with its incorporation into the chromosomes of the host cell, somehow alters the chemical structure of the myelin produced by the oligodendritic cells, rendering it immunologically different than native myelin and thus a target for an immune response. Maybe when the virus emerges from the latent into the lytic state, it takes some myelin with it on its surface, thus making the myelin an immune target. There may be some interplay between roseola 6A and Epstein-Barr or some other virus that triggers the immune cascade. Other involvements and interplays are, of course, possible.

Clearly, several factors are involved in the development of MS and other autoimmune disorders. Viral involvement is potentially an important one.

Roseola 7. Human Herpes virus 7 is what might be described as a very successful pathogen. Most of us have it in our bodies, but the disease it causes is thought to be minimal, sometimes causing roseola in young children. The virus wasn't discovered until the 1990s, and even then, it was quite by accident as researchers were looking for roseola 6 virus and stumbled across this one. It is a member of the beta-herpes viruses, resembling the herpes 6 viruses but a little smaller. It seems to produce the same symptoms of roseola, although in a slightly older population of up to six years of age. Of course, as with all herpes viruses, it establishes a life-long residency within the host cells, and the virus's potential to be involved with autoimmune diseases requires further study.

Kaposi's sarcoma virus. The disease we call Kaposi's sarcoma has an interesting history, dating to its initial description in the medical literature by Hungarian dermatologist Moritz Kaposi in 1872. Dr. Kaposi observed and reported on an unusual type of skin cancer in 5 patients. Three of them died in about a year, and it was felt at the time that the cancer was an aggressive one. As time went on, though, Kaposi's sarcoma came to be known as a rare disease, affecting older men from the Mediterranean area with a prolonged progression, taking many years for death to ensue.

In addition to these isolated European cases, the disease was described in sub-Saharan Africa as a not uncommon skin cancer of both children and adults. Males were affected about ten times more than females, usually with a fatal outcome. Given its global distribution, there was some speculation following the description of the disease that a virus caused the cancer, although a virus was not discovered.

Kaposi's sarcoma became a major concern and interest when acquired immune deficiency syndrome (AIDS) burst onto the scene in the early 1980s. Once an obscure malady, Kaposi's sarcoma became one of the defining conditions pointing to an AIDS diagnosis, along with several other diseases usually easily contained by an intact immune system. Losing a large portion of the T-helper cell population in the body dramatically upsets the balance between pathogen and immune system, with a sudden, rapidly expanding cancer resulting.

Kaposi's sarcoma virus was discovered in 1994, and since it was the eighth herpes virus described, it was given the name Human Herpes virus 8. The virus is of the gamma-herpes group, more closely related to Epstein-Barr than the others. Because it causes a type of cancer in humans, it has the further

512

designation oncovirus and is classified as a member of the genus *Rhadinovirus*. Being a herpes virus, its appearance and modus operandi is the same as the other group members: large DNA virus with a protective coating around the DNA, a middle tegument, and an outer membrane bearing several protruding glycoproteins. After entering the host cell, the DNA within its protective coating makes its way into the host cell nucleus, where it takes up residence. The viral DNA rounds up like a plasmid and is loosely attached to the host cell chromosome and, as it enters the latent phase, reproduces in synchrony with it.

Kaposi sarcoma virus contains genes for over a dozen proteins that have no connection to those of other herpes viruses. But they do show a striking resemblance to human genes. Clearly, through the millennia, Kaposi's sarcoma virus has purloined genes from its human host cells and is using them for its own nefarious purposes. Most or all of these interfere with the natural performance of the immune system.

As with all herpes viruses, the assumption of the latent stage greatly assists the virus in evading the body's immune response to it. Instead of producing around 80 proteins, as done in the lytic stage, only a few are produced during the latent stage, making a much narrower target for humoral and cellular initiatives.

Of course, the virus has to ensure that the host cell it resides in during the latent stage continues to live and is not destroyed through apoptosis. There are two main types of cell apoptosis. One is directed by immune cells that detect a problem and instruct the cell to kill itself (extrinsic). The other is directed by chemical mechanisms inside the affected cell (intrinsic). Kaposi's sarcoma virus attacks and disengages both. In extrinsic, a long protein protruding through the cell membrane into the environment is known as FAS (also known as APO-1 and CD95). On the tail end of the molecule inside the cell is what is known as a "death domain," a section of the protein that, when stimulated, can engage the protein caspase 8, which initiates the apoptotic cycle. Kaposi's sarcoma virus produces a protein that blocks the interaction of the FAS death domain with caspase 8, thus preventing apoptosis. On the intrinsic level, a very important protein called p53 controls abnormal cellular proliferation, such as seen in cancer. It also is instrumental in initiating apoptosis when viruses attack. KS virus has several proteins that directly block the activity of p53.

Many questions about Kaposi's sarcoma virus remain unanswered. The first cases described by Moritz Kaposi in the 19th century died after about a one-year illness, whereas most endemic cases of the disease take many years to develop. The virus and the diseases it causes are found much more frequently in sub-Saharan Africa, where it causes a considerable number of deaths. But it is very rare in immunocompetent people in developed countries. The ratio of male to female victims is about 10-1. The virus can modulate the immune system to suit its needs; just what mechanisms and interactions are at play are very complex and need further research. Most cancers involve only one type of cell that goes berserk and continues to reproduce with impunity. Kaposi's sarcoma involves several different cells, mostly endothelial, lymphoid, and monocytes, all multiplying out of control together. The other herpes viruses are found in a large percentage of the population, often over 90%. In developed countries, Kaposi's sarcoma virus is found in only about 10% of people. How they get and transmit it is not entirely known.

The nine members of the herpes virus family are an important part of human health. Nearly all of us have at least one species of the virus within us for most of our lives, and frequently we carry several. Individuals react quite differently to each virus species—some of us develop symptoms of disease, but most don't. Just what interactions occur between the viruses and the immune system in each individual is unpredictable, but it may profoundly affect the person's health, especially with autoimmune diseases and cancer. Getting rid of the virus will not happen. Scientists will have to develop the knowledge and the tools to deal with the myriad consequences of its presence among us.

Chapter 32
Pathogenic Shapeshifter

Ground-to-air attack,
Disruption liberation.
Fungus among us.

In 1891, at the very infancy of understanding the nature of infectious diseases, a medical student in Argentina made a remarkable discovery. A patient named Domingo Ezcurra, a soldier in the military stationed in Buenos Aires, Argentina, presented at clinic with a peculiar-looking purple lesion on his cheek. He also had lesions on his nose, arm, and trunk. First believed to be skin cancer, a biopsy was taken and examined after staining. With careful observation under the microscope, young doctor Alejandro Posadas observed some curious-looking round structures. To the best of his knowledge at the time, the organisms he noticed appeared to be a type of parasite, perhaps one related to the group known as the Coccidia, a large group of parasites that infect a wide range of mammals. The best-known among the human species of Coccidia is *Toxoplasma gondii.* What he actually discovered, though, was the first example of a fungus that infects humans rather commonly in some regions of the world, *Coccidioides immitis.*

This wasn't just any fungus. We're all familiar with fungi that grow as fuzzy white, green, or some other color creature on an orange or slice of bread. That type of fungus is well-characterized and well-studied and usually is of no consequence to human health. But this pathogenic fungus first observed by Dr. Posada is different. It changes its shape and nature depending on where it resides. In the soil, it looks much like other fungi, with mycelial strands forming a matrix of growth. When it enters the body, though, it becomes something very different, with rounded bodies containing multiple spores. Because of this double way of existing, the term dimorphic is applied: *di* meaning "two," *morphic* meaning "shapes."

Since it resembled the Coccidia group of parasites, the genus name *Coccidioides,* or coccidia-like, was applied. In the U.S., much of the early work on the fungus was carried on in the San Joaquin Valley of California. The fungus is resident in the soil in that area, and in the 1930s many immigrants from the Midwest came to the valley to work in agriculture. Being new to the area, they encountered the fungus for the first time, and some became ill. Scientists studying the infection in the San Joaquin Valley were able to provide a great deal of information about the disease.

Because some cases are very serious, the Latin term *immitis*, meaning "not small" or "harsh," was assigned. A similar fungus, the one discovered by Dr. Posadas, is found in parts of South America. It is assigned the name *Coccidioides posadas*, named for its discoverer.

The official disease name for the ailment, coccidioidomycosis, is pretty hard to both pronounce and spell, so the more familiar term "valley fever" is usually used. Workers in the healthcare industry often use the term "cocci."

Coccidioides lives in alkaline, arid soil. This fits the general description of the soil found in the Sonoran Desert, a broad area of the southwestern United States and Baja California, Mexico. It is also found in parts of Central and South America. That sounds simple enough, but in reality, the fungus is very difficult to find just by looking at dirt. A broad swath of land that appears homogeneous might contain very little fungus, which is confined to one small, unique area. It fares better in soils that have elevated levels of minerals such as sodium, sulfates, and magnesium. The organism does not exist on the top of the soil but down about 6-20 inches. How it gets down there is a matter of conjecture, perhaps by rain or hooking a ride on some desert rodent or reptile. There is good evidence to show that the fungus increases in amount in years of elevated rainfall. In endemic areas, this would be during the winter months. It grows primarily as mycelia in the soil during the wet season but forms infectious arthrospores when it dries out in late spring and summer. It contains enzymes that allow it to decompose organic material, so it probably lives where some animal has died or has left some of its food. If it weren't for the fact that it can cause significant human disease, the organism would be of no real importance. But it does indeed cause illness, sometimes very

516

serious, and much has been learned about the fungus' biology and lifestyle.

Since it lives half a foot or more under the soil, it can infect only when the ground has been disrupted, either by natural means like a windstorm, or by extensive digging, such as a construction project. In the soil, the organism exists as mycelia, or strands of long, branching cells. In this regard, it is like many run-of-the-mill fungi. Where it differs significantly is the way it produces spores. Many fungi we are familiar with produce spores on a stalk that project up from the mycelia. A breeze or some other physical event spreads the spores. Think of the fungus you see on an orange, giving off a small cloud of spores when you pick it up. *Coccidioides* lives under the soil, so this type of spore production wouldn't work for it. Instead, it makes what is known as arthrospores, a hardening of the hyphae at regular intervals. The prefix "*arthro*" comes from the Greek, meaning a joint, or combination of two adjoining structures, in this case, two sections of mycelia. The arthrospores are tough and can remain in the ground until the soil is disrupted. Then they fly around like any other fungal spore, blindly trying to find a new place to set up house. If it is on the ground of the desert, it doesn't much matter, but if the arthrospores find their way into the trachea and lungs of a human, trouble begins.

Arthrospores are rectangular shaped, about five microns long. On the outside of them is a hardened coat to protect them from the environment. It doesn't take many arthrospores to set up an infection. Experiments in mice have shown that a single spore is all it takes. Generally, the more spores inhaled, the sooner symptoms will be displayed. Once they enter the lungs, the coat is dissolved away.

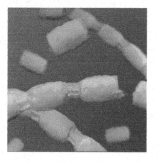 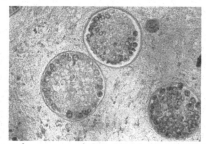

Left, arthrospores of Coccidioides immitis; Right spherules. (PHIL)

The remaining structure rounds up and is known as an endospore. The endospore begins a meticulous and intricate phase when liberated inside the body. It sets up a series of walls, dividing the growing structure into many compartments. Inside each little compartment is a new endospore. When allowed to grow unchecked, the single initial endospore makes a rather large, multi-compartmented structure known as a spherule. Spherules are round, about 30 microns in diameter, and contain about one hundred endospores. Each endospore can create a new spherule, which is what happens. When a spherule gets large enough it ripens, bursts, and releases its many endospores, each capable of initiating another spherule. Clearly, this is not good for the infected person. It doesn't take long for many spherules to infest the lung. They don't invade the lung cells but grow in the spaces between the cells of lung tissue. This crowding eventually restricts the infected person's air space, and shortness of breath ensues. It usually takes 7 to 21 days for symptoms to appear after exposure.

In some cases, endospores and spherules escape the lungs. If uncontrolled by the immune system, the endospores can use the bloodstream or lymphatic channels to traverse the body and end up in remote locations. The skin, especially the area around the nose and lips, is the organ most commonly affected. Coccidioidomycosis can also occur in joints, bones, and the intestinal tract. Meningitis is nearly always fatal if not aggressively treated.

Of course, the immune system cells recognize the danger of the invader and are mobilized. Arthrospores and endospores are small enough to be gobbled up by neutrophils and macrophages, and they bear on their surface a protein that alerts the phagocytes they are foreign material. The fungal protein is called Spherule Outer Wall glycoprotein, or SOWgp. Known as a pathogen-associated molecular pattern, or PAMP, the surface material gives the arthrospores away, and they wouldn't last long if left there. To mask itself, in the early stages of its growth, the organism produces an enzyme called metalloproteinase (Mep-1) to digest the tell-tale SOW and get rid of it. If the

518

fungus successfully removes the PAMP it stands a better chance of evading the phagocytic cells designed to attack it.

Spherules are, of course, much larger than endospores, so neutrophils can't handle them. That leaves it up to CD4 T-helper cells. The immune attack on spherules is similar to that conducted against tuberculosis: wall it off with the formation of a granuloma. The infection can be contained as long as the T-cells are in good working order. If they aren't, it can spell trouble.

Our macrophages and dendritic cells express a group of signaling molecules called Toll-like receptors. Each is designed to react when they encounter a molecule unique to a microbe, sending signals to unleash the molecules of the immune response. In addition to the TLR group, we also have a group of microbe-detecting and signaling molecules called the C-type lectin receptors. An important member of this group is a protein called Dectin-1. Dectin-1 has a specific receptor for a portion of a fungal cell wall, glucans. When they encounter this fungal PAMP, they spring into action, giving a chemical signal to the host genome to unleash appropriate cytokines and other defensive molecules. Two very important immune responses initiated after Dectin-1 becomes active and sends its chemical signals are the Th_{17} subset of CD4 lymphocytes, and interferon-gamma.

The T-helper lymphocytes, which bear the chemical marker CD4, are extremely important in aiding the body's fight against invading microbes. There are several sub-types of the CD4 T-helper lymphocytes. The one known as the Th_{17} variety is activated by the activity of Dectrin-1 after encountering an invading fungus. Among the T-helper Th_{17}'s most important roles are the chemical signals they send to enhance the creation of neutrophils in the bone marrow, and the neutrophils' attraction to and concentration in an infected body site. Neutrophils are very effective attackers of *Coccidioides* endospores, and the more of them at the infected site, the better. The CD4 Th_{17} lymphocytes, stimulated by Dectin-1, are vital in this endeavor.

Macrophages wandering through lung tissue are of two main types, designated M1 and M2. The M1 types are warriors designed to kill invading microbes, mainly by destructive enzymes. The M2 macrophages are tasked with tissue repair. Both are, of course, important. A naïve macrophage gets its signals from cytokines: interferon-gamma stimulates them to turn into M1, and interleukin-4 directs the development of the M2 type. Without the stimulated M1 macrophages, the body's fight against the invading fungus is significantly disadvantaged. Absent the production of interferon-gamma and the attendant recruitment of active M1 macrophages, coccidioidal endospore and spherule production can advance quite rapidly. Dectin-1 and its chemical signals help direct this important mission.

For most people, inhaling *Coccidioides* arthrospores does not result in a serious infection. Neutrophils engulf and digest many of them, and M1 macrophages, activated by interferon-gamma, handle the rest. Neutrophils have many destructive enzymes and any time they are active in an area there is the possibility of local tissue damage, but the M2 macrophages entering the area are very good at cleaning that up. Depending on how many arthrospores are inhaled, the efficiency of the fungus' ability to hide its outer protein, and the number of neutrophils and macrophages in the area, the disease in most people ranges from asymptomatic to a relatively mild flu-like disorder that resolves in a week. In some, it can persist for several weeks or even months, but most cases resolve uneventfully. Many who are infected don't know *Coccidioides* infected them because they are not tested for it; it just seems like a common viral infection.

In some individuals, though, infection by *Coccidioides* is devastating. The fungus progresses at an alarming rate, with the cycle of spherule production, endospore release, and new spherule production progressing at a furious pace. Damage to lung tissue is great, and some of the endospores can escape the lungs, enter the bloodstream or lymphatic channels, and begin to reproduce in other areas of the body. Great systemic damage can ensue.

The attack by neutrophils and macrophages against arthrospores and endospores is part of the innate immune response. The adaptive immune system must be engaged if the infection overwhelms the innate system. The principal mechanism of the adaptive immune response against dimorphic fungi is the activity of CD4 lymphocytes, working in concert with macrophages. Principal among the CD4 cells involved in fighting off *Coccidioides* are the Th_1 and Th_{17} subgroups of cells. Working in concert, they manage the overall coordination of the defense, usually with a good outcome. But in some people, and it is often difficult to predict just whom, the marshaling of the proper CD4 lymphocyte mix is impaired, and the full thrust of the immune system defense is diminished. Certainly, individuals who have human immunodeficiency virus (HIV), and therefore markedly reduced numbers of CD4 lymphocytes, are in great danger of uncontrolled *Coccidioides* infection. That applies as well to someone receiving immunosuppressive therapy. But some people not known to have a suppressed immune system sometimes also develop an overwhelming infection, requiring aggressive, often toxic, anti-fungal therapy. The exact nature of some people's immune system failure to meet the fungal challenge is often elusive. It is probably due to a genetic anomaly giving an imbalance to their adaptive immune response. Members of some racial groups, such as Africans and Filipinos, are at many times greater risk for disseminated infections than whites. Also, pregnant women, especially those in the third trimester, are at higher risk for disseminated infection.

The number of cases of coccidioidomycosis in the southwestern United States, primarily California and Arizona, has been growing in the last couple of decades. Just how much it has grown is subject to speculation. Certainly, population growth in endemic areas directly influences the total number of cases. Better diagnostic testing helps, especially with minimally symptomatic patients. But some serologic tests are subject to false negatives and false positives and may give misleading information, so the answer remains elusive.

Unfortunately, anti-fungal therapy does not kill all invading organisms. It is more likened to bacteriostatic agents against bacteria, which slow down growth without eliminating all organisms. By reducing the number of bugs, we depend on the immune system to clear the remainder. But in disseminated disease that usually doesn't work, and therapy must be maintained for years.

Laboratory workers have known for a long time that *Coccidioides immitis* is a highly infectious organism. It can grow very well on artificial laboratory culture media designed to grow routine bacteria, giving a fuzzy little non-descript creature looking all the world like a contaminant. It's a noteworthy hazard of the occupation. But because it is so easy to grow on lab media and so few arthrospores are needed to start an infection, the fungus has been classified as a potential bioweapons threat. It wouldn't be able to kill millions, but it can sicken many, and its widespread use would certainly sow panic.

There is currently no vaccine for coccidioidomycosis. Treatment with anti-fungal medications has not been shown to be effective for mild cases, but for serious cases, drugs such as amphotericin and fluconazole can manage the disease, but unfortunately, they usually don't eliminate it.

Chapter 33
Budding Trouble

With us since our birth,
Fungal companion bides time.
Equivocal germ.

The words infectious and contagious are not synonymous. "Infectious disease" conjures an image of a microbe we pick up by eating, drinking, breathing, having sexual relations, or being exposed to an insect. But there are some infectious diseases that we get from ourselves–the organism responsible is part of our internal microbiota. The term for that is endogenous or "generated from within." Such infections are nearly always the result of some failure or shortcoming of our immune system, whether our integument, resident microbiota, or our innate and/or adaptive cells and molecules.

All or most of us have somewhere on or in our body organisms like *E. coli, Staphylococcus aureus, Streptococcus agalactiae, Klebsiella, Clostridium difficile,* and one or more species of *Candida.* All of these, and many others, are capable of causing serious infections, but usually they are a non-descript part of our normal microbes. For one of them to break through and infect us, some event that disrupts our balance of health must occur.

One organism that is particularly good at causing endogenous infections is the yeast, *Candida.* The species we often encounter is *Candida albicans,* but there are several others. It has been estimated that *Candida* benignly colonizes about 60% of the human population, but when the right circumstance arises, the road from normal flora to an infectious agent can be a short one.

Candida albicans is easy to grow on simple laboratory media, giving a round white to off-white colony. The color of the colony provides the organism with its name, from the Latin *candidus,* meaning "bright" or "light," and *albus,* meaning "white." On laboratory media, it grows as a yeast that divides by binary fission; one organism divides into two by budding. The two daughter cells tend to stick together, and it's not unusual to see a clump of several organisms under the microscope.

Technically, the yeast cell is called a blastospore; the term "blast" comes from the Greek word *blastos,* meaning a sprout or bud. It is asexual reproduction. *Candida albicans* also assumes another form, filamentous hyphae. In the presence of serum, elevated carbon dioxide concentrations, and slightly alkaline pH, like the conditions found in some areas of the body, the organism goes from the yeast form to the filamentous hyphal one. This is significant because the hyphal form is the more invasive.

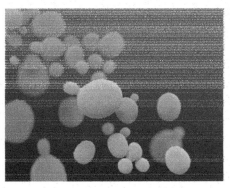

Candida as budding yeast. (PHIL)

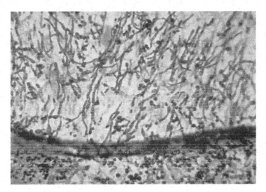

Candida as pseudohyphae. (PHIL)

Candida albicans has a lot of virulence tools in its arsenal. One is the ability to stick to just about anything. They can adhere to bacteria, human cells, non-biologic materials like plastic and metal, and each other. This adhesion property serves the organism well when it gets an opportunity to set up an infection, as clumps of organisms are harder for phagocytic cells like neutrophils and macrophages to digest.

A remarkable feature of the yeast is that it can enter human cells through two different mechanisms. One is the common method of adhering to a receptor on the host cell surface and inducing the cell to bring it inside by endocytosis, forming a yeast-containing vacuole. The other method is direct invasion, or active penetration, whereby the organism powers its way into the host cell. The former is employed by yeast-phase cells, the latter by hyphae.

Given the adhesive properties of *Candida,* it's no surprise that it is adept at forming biofilms. Once they gain a foothold and are supplied with proper nutrients, the film formed is a hard, tenacious mass of cells and extracellular material that is very difficult to eliminate, both by our immune system and anti-fungal drugs. The first yeast cells that attach to a surface lay down a matted floor of organisms. Once bound, they transform into hyphae. On top of this comes more hyphal cells. As the biofilm matures, a hard, crusty material is incorporated. More yeast cells form on top. The upper cells are loosely attached and can be dispersed to set up an infection elsewhere. It is not unusual for patients with Candida-occluded catheter lines to have the yeast enter their bloodstream, causing a serious infection.

Candida albicans secretes a large number of enzymes, many of which assist it in establishing an infection. There are two main types, some attacking proteins and others lipids. Working alone or in concert, these yeast enzymes assist the organism in penetrating human cells. Some strains of the organism are more aggressive than others because of the amounts and kinds of enzymes they excrete.

The human body has a wide range of acid-base environments. Blood and tissues are slightly alkaline, with a pH of about 7.4. The intestinal tract is varied, with some very acidic areas with a pH of around 2.0 and others with an alkaline pH. The vagina has a pH of about 4.0. *Candida albicans* can colonize and grow in all these environments. The organism possesses several molecules that can sense the external pH. One called PHR1 is activated at neutral to slightly alkaline pH, and one called PHR2 becomes active in acidic environments. After becoming stimulated, the respective pH sensor sends a chemical messenger to the nucleus to unlock the genes that will produce the most appropriate proteins for the situation. In slightly alkaline pH, *Candida* assumes the hyphal type; in acidic environments, the yeast form predominates. *Candida* can also affect the local environment by metabolizing amino acids, converting the end-product to ammonia, and exporting it to raise the pH of an acidic environment.

With its impressive array of virulence factors, *Candida albicans* is a formidable foe. While oversimplified, it is convenient to divide the infections it causes into two major categories: skin and mucosal layers, and deep-tissue invasion. The former are quite common and, for the most part, more of a nuisance than a threat to life. The deep-tissue infections are far more dangerous and potentially fatal.

Skin and mucosal yeast infections are most commonly diaper rash, vaginal infection, and mouth infection, sometimes called thrush. *Candida* is a part of the normal residential flora of each of these areas, the stool, the vagina, and the mouth, usually without any untoward events. But sometimes the status quo is upset; the microbiome becomes unbalanced, the little yeast grows excessively, and infection results. Our primary defense against the invading yeast is our neutrophils.

Diaper rash is a very good example of how *Candida albicans* establishes an infection. The term "diaper rash" is broad, meaning just what it says. Stool and urine irritate a baby's tender skin, and a mild rash often develops with some friction from the diaper. It is usually easily remedied with gentle washing and a commercial cream. But when the baby has *Candida albicans* in the bowel, it can take advantage of the damaged tissue and colonize the skin. Especially vulnerable are the folds and crevices.

The immune reaction to this infection is the influx of neutrophils, a very effective response for getting rid of the yeast. Unfortunately, neutrophils are equipped with very powerful toxic granules that release several chemicals like myeloperoxidase that damage the skin and add to the inflammatory reaction. The result is a very reddened, painful rash. Simple washing and creams are usually insufficient to clear up a case of diaper rash due to *Candida;* an anti-fungal treatment is often necessary.

Yeast vaginitis is a common ailment most women experience at least once in their lives, some a whole lot more. The vagina is acidic, with a pH of about 4.0, so *Candida* exists there in the yeast rather than hyphal form. The yeast must compete with bacteria in the area for nutrients, and some bacteria produce enzymes detrimental to yeast growth, keeping their numbers down. *Candida* can rapidly multiply when something disrupts this yeast-bacterial balance, resulting in a yeast infection. Administration of an antibiotic that kills the competing resident bacterial flora, oral and local contraceptives, and sexual activity can precipitate a yeast infection. Like in diaper rash, the immune response is an influx of neutrophils, resulting in inflammation and tissue damage. Under the microscope, smears taken from the vagina reveal many yeast and white blood cells.

In the case of diaper rash and vaginitis, most of the symptoms experienced are not directly from the yeast but in the immune response to it, namely neutrophils in very high numbers. The epithelial cells are not equipped to fight off the yeast but do a good job detecting the organism's presence. They contain two main detection molecules, a Toll-like receptor and a C-type lectin receptor, each recognizing a unique molecular pattern on the yeast. Activation of these sensors eventually leads to the release of several chemical signals. One signals the nearby blood vessels to extend an integrin to capture neutrophils as they tumble through the bloodstream. Another is the neutrophil-attracting chemokine interleukin-8. The result is large numbers of neutrophils infiltrating the area. Macrophages are involved too. These phagocytes are very good at attaching to, engulfing, and killing the yeast, but the resultant inflammatory reaction is responsible for most of the symptoms.

Candida albicans is found with no ill effects in many people's mouths. Present in low numbers, the organism is readily contained by the resident bacterial flora and a valuable substance found in saliva, histatin. Histatin is not a single but multiple substances, each of which works in unique ways, but a couple of them attach to the cell membranes of yeast, disrupting them and helping to control their growth. Also of great value in keeping the numbers of *Candida albicans* in the mouth to a minimum are CD4 lymphocytes, also known as T-helper cells. The mouth is usually slightly alkaline or slightly acidic, encouraging the development of the hyphal rather than the yeast form of *Candida*. The hyphal forms of fungi are monitored and dealt with by lymphocytes, particularly the CD4 helper cells. They interact with other cells and systems to contain the pathogen.

The CD4 cells are subdivided into groups depending on their specialty. Early in the discovery of lymphocyte cell types, the terms Th_1 and Th_2 were applied, the T-helper-1 types involved in controlling intracellular bacteria such as tuberculosis, and the T-helper-2 types assist in ridding us of extracellular organisms such as parasites. As research evolved, it was found that there were other T-helper cells in addition to the Th_1 and Th_2 types. One that is very important was found to assist with bacteria and fungi that persist outside the cell. One might think the logical designation for these T-helper lymphocytes would be Th_3, but as fate would have it, another label was assigned. The principal cytokine these cells emit is interleukin-17 or IL-17, so the cells became known as Th_{17}. Whatever we call them, they function as CD4 T-helper lymphocytes, and the control of *Candida* in the mouth is one thing they do very well.

Because *Candida* colonizes the mouths of most people, it's no surprise that oral infections occur. Sometimes they begin very early in life. Oral candidiasis, commonly known as thrush (from an old Nordic word for throat), is seen in infants. It presents as discreet white patches on the tongue, cheeks, and/or gums. Babies no doubt acquire the organism from their mothers, probably during birth. Why some babies develop thrush is unknown, but it may be due to their Th_{17} lymphocytes not being sufficiently active. Sometimes the oral *Candida* is swallowed, enters the intestinal tract, transforms into the yeast phase, then causes diaper rash. With all that yeast around, the mother's nipples may also be infected. Oral candidiasis in babies is usually relatively easily treated with a topical anti-fungal agent

528

on a sponge or swab. As the child matures, so does the activity of its CD4 lymphocytes, and the disease is rarely a problem.

Clearly, the CD4 lymphocytes, especially those of the Th$_{17}$ type, are critical in containing fungi, including *Candida*. Whenever there is a suppression of their numbers, oral candidiasis can emerge. It is not uncommon in people with immunosuppressive therapy for cancer, and it is one of the hallmark conditions in individuals with untreated human immunodeficiency virus, HIV. Some people who take an antibiotic for an unrelated condition can sometimes also develop the disease, as the competing microflora of the mouth is compromised.

Another oral problem caused by *Candida* is the contamination of dentures. The organism readily adheres to just about any type of surface, denture material included. Here it forms a biofilm with a very firm attachment. Once it sets up shop, it isn't easy to get rid of. A result is a large number of yeast being produced in the mouth continually, with tissue damage resulting from the organisms' enzymes and the infiltration of neutrophils. A mature biofilm is extremely difficult for the immune system to attack, as the mineral material incorporated in the film reduces the entrance and activity of neutrophils and lymphocytes.

Besides oral, diaper, and vaginal candidiasis, *Candida* can initiate a far more severe and life-threatening form of the disease, invasive infection. Normally neutrophils and macrophages, working in concert with other members of the immune system, prevent the organism from getting out of control and entering our deep tissues. If it infects at all, it's on the skin, vagina, or mouth. But there are times when the immune system is compromised, or invasive medical procedures are undertaken, and the yeast invades the blood and spreads to one or more organs. Once established, an invasive *Candida* infection can be very difficult to eliminate.

Many people have *Candida albicans* residing inconsequentially in their bowels. It is kept in check by patrolling neutrophils and by competitive bacterial flora. We also have some anaerobic bacteria in our gut that secrete substances that induce the cells lining the intestine to produce anti-fungal molecules, limiting the number of *Candida* present. Problems arise whenever one or both of these protective factors are altered. The neutrophil count can be drastically reduced by several types of chemotherapy to treat cancer, and the gut microbial flora impacted by large doses of broad-spectrum antibiotics. These measures, of course, are not taken lightly but are often necessary to help combat serious life-threatening ailments. The emergence of *Candida* is, unfortunately, collateral damage.

Candida albicans excretes enzymes that can damage the membranes of many of our cells. The good news is that normally the numbers of organisms present are kept low by the immune system and other factors, so the destructive power of the enzymes is not realized. Trouble arises when the number of yeast increases prodigiously. When in the bowel in large numbers, they can cross the intestinal membranes and enter the bloodstream. From there, they can travel to many locations, adhere to the organ linings, and produce damage. If the neutrophil response is subdued, the infection can continue with potent force, and tissue damage ensues. The result is sometimes organ failure and death.

Candida's ability to adhere to non-biologic material gives it another avenue to create an invasive infection. Catheters and indwelling prosthetic devices can become colonized with the organism, which then creates a biofilm. Biofilms are very difficult to clear, short of removing the device. Even then, the organism may have spread to other organs and set up localized infections, which may seed the blood and other devices inserted later. When those devices are necessary to sustain life, the resurgent yeast infection is very frustrating.

There has been a direct parallel between the advancement of medical procedures in hospitals and the number of severe *Candida* infections. Antibiotic use, vascular and urinary catheters, drainage tubes, and other technical marvels are very important in saving many people's lives. But by themselves or in various combinations, they sometimes allow for yeast infections that can become serious. Candidal infections tend to be relatively silent and under the radar compared to infectious diseases caused by bacteria. The Gram-negative rods stimulate a rapid, profound immune response of cytokines triggering high fever, muscle aches, and other symptoms of septic shock. Serious infections caused by Gram-positive organisms such as *Staphylococcus* also are accompanied by unmistakable symptoms. But invasive yeast infections are less obvious. The test most used to detect it is the blood culture, in which about 10 milliliters of blood are placed in culture broth and incubated. Typically, two bottles are inoculated, one containing air and the other anaerobic, to allow for strictly anaerobic bacteria. Yeast are aerobic organisms and don't usually grow in the anaerobic blood culture bottle. Also, yeast tends to stick together and not occur in high numbers of the blood. So blood cultures for yeast are often false-negative despite a significant infection, and the infection can proceed untreated for a considerable time.

Several classes of anti-fungal drugs are usually quite effective in treating invasive *Candida* infections. Azoles and echinocandins are the most used. But anti-fungal drugs aren't as effective at killing yeast as antibiotics are at killing bacteria. They only kill about 80% of the organisms present. The effectiveness is even less if the yeast is present as a biofilm and/or the patient has a very low neutrophil count. In addition, resistance to anti-fungal drugs is rising. These facts and the often-delayed administration of a proper drug make for a very difficult disease to treat.

There are over a dozen species of *Candida*. Besides *albicans,* the more commonly seen species are *tropicalis, glabrata, krusei,* and *parapsilosis.* All can initiate an invasive infection in hospitalized patients. Laboratory methods for isolating and identifying the organisms are not difficult, but successful treatment and eradication are another matter.

A species of *Candida* that was first described in 2009 is troubling. It was first isolated from a patient's ear, so it was assigned the name *Candida auris* (auris is the Latin word for ear). *C. auris* can cause the same serious invasive yeast infections as *Candida albicans*. What is of deep concern is the yeast's resistance to anti-fungal drugs. It is resistant to most available drugs. Some strains have been resistant to all of them (pan-resistant). Like *Candida albicans*, *C. auris* needs an opportunity to infect. It has been found almost exclusively in patients hospitalized for serious conditions for a long period of time. The organism has been found worldwide, and its incidence is growing.

Candida albicans is a well-adapted organism; its only known reservoir is human beings. It usually lives in concert with its host and neighboring commensal organisms, but infection can ensue when circumstances allow it to grow to disproportionate numbers. The more superficial infections like diaper rash, vaginitis, and thrush are usually relatively easily managed, but when it enters the blood and spreads throughout the body, it can be a deadly pathogen.

Chapter 34
Split Personality

Deadly passenger.
Lurking, plotting, seeking a
Means to overrun.

One of the more descriptive words in medical parlance is "fulminant." It comes from the Latin *fulminare*, meaning "to throw bolts of lightning." A fulminant disorder is rapid, intense, and catastrophic. Another word coming from the same root is fulminate, a description of explosives.

An infectious disease that certainly deserves the description fulminant is Neisserial meningitis. A person can go to bed at night entirely well, wake up the following day feeling a little rough with maybe a slight fever and scratchy throat, and be dead by evening. Tragically, it strikes the young much more than the old, with children and teenagers its primary victims. Not all cases proceed as rapidly as described, but the condition is often life-altering or fatal without immediate and vigorous medical attention.

Nature has gone to great lengths to protect our central nervous system. The skull encases the brain, and the vertebral column covers the spinal cord. While not especially thick, about 7 millimeters, the skull is very strong because of its shape, somewhat like an egg. The vertebral column effectively shelters the nerves it contains while allowing movement. These bone coverings give solid protection, but the central nervous system is further fortified by its own specialized covering, the meninges. The term derives from the Greek word for membrane, *meninx*. The membrane has three distinct layers, so it is pleural. Each of the three layers has its own name, but each bears the designation "mater," the Latin word for mother. Presumably, the covering shelters and protects us as a mother does her child.

The outer layer of the meninges is the **dura** mater, "dura" meaning hard or tough, as in durable. It is the layer that lays closest to the skin. The word mater is omitted in much medical terminology, and only dura is used, as in epi-dural or sub-dural.

In contrast to the tough outer dural layer, the inner lining of the meninges is called the **pia** mater, "pia" meaning soft or gentle. It is very thin and pliable, like moist tissue paper. It has to be because it lies in very close proximity to the brain and spinal cord and must accommodate the underlying tissues' peaks, valleys, and undulations.

Between the dura and pia mater lies an area that resembles a spider web, so it is assigned the name **arachnoid** mater. The arachnoid has many extensions, called trabeculae, which run from the top part of the layer near the dura mater to the pia mater, where they connect, hence the name "spider web." The area filled with the trabeculae contains a clear fluid, the cerebrospinal fluid, CSF. It circulates around the central nervous system, cushioning the organs and carrying nutrients and waste products.

These physical barriers are extremely helpful in protecting our precious central nervous system, but the shield doesn't stop there. Circulating blood can contain noxious materials or microorganisms. Much of this can be cleared by special organs such as the liver, spleen, and kidneys, but if the material were to enter the central nervous system before it is removed, it could cause irreparable harm. To prevent the migration of these undesirable elements into the cerebrospinal fluid and eventually into the brain, the cells of the endothelial lining of the blood vessels in the area are specialized. All our blood vessels are lined by cells that prevent the leakage of fluids and nutrients, but they are designed to allow the contents of the bloodstream to communicate with the tissues nearby easily. Nutrients, white blood cells, and other materials, when necessary, can traverse the endothelial lining of blood vessels and make their way outside.

The situation is different in the endothelial cells lining the central nervous system. The junctions between adjoining cells are very tight, as opposed to just plain tight in the rest of the body. A crude example would be a bolt that in some cases can be "finger tightened," while a firm wrench turn is required in others. The brain and spinal cord junctions are so tight that

534

only very small molecules, like oxygen and water, can pass through. Other materials, such as glucose, must be actively transported in. It makes for a formidable impediment to any would-be invader. It is rightly called the blood-brain barrier, BBB.

Not many microorganisms can penetrate the blood-brain barrier of the meninges, but a few do. The most common one in the developed world is *Streptococcus pneumoniae*, which, as its name suggests, is more known for causing pneumonia. Still, under the right circumstances, it can enter the bloodstream, localize in the central nervous system, and set up an infection known as meningitis. *Haemophilus influenzae* and *Listeria monocytogenes* can also cause meningitis, the former more commonly in young children and the latter in people whose immune systems are compromised. *Streptococcus agalactiae,* commonly known as Group B Strep, sometimes causes sepsis and meningitis in newborn babies. Other bacteria and viruses, as well as some fungi and even amoeba, can rarely cause meningitis. But the most serious pathogen involved in the disease is *Neisseria meningitidis,* more commonly referred to simply as meningococcus.

We all have bacteria belonging to the genus *Neisseria* in our mouths. They are part of a mixture of bacteria that colonize the oral cavity and don't harm us. There are about twenty different recognized species of *Neisseria,* and around a dozen of them can colonize the oral cavity of humans. All of them are non-pathogenic.

All but for one notable exception, *Neisseria meningitidis.* Actually, *N. meningitidis* is usually non-pathogenic when it colonizes our mouths. About ten percent of the population harbors it without ill effects. Usually, the organism comes and goes unnoticed, competing with the resident bacterial population of the upper respiratory tract for nutrients. Some strains, though, have the genetic means to make them hyper-invasive when the right circumstances present. Even these virulent strains are not necessarily deadly, but if the host has an immune system deficiency, the organism can take advantage and cause great damage.

On the surface, all strains of *Neisseria meningitidis* look alike. On a Gram-stained preparation under the microscope, they appear pink and round, Gram-negative cocci. Two organisms don't break away from each other but share a common side, a form called diplococcus. It is a very distinctive morphology, and if one gets a specimen of spinal fluid, does a Gram-stain, and sees Gram-negative diplococci, it is diagnostic of Neisserial meningitis. Nearly always, when the organism is seen on smears from spinal fluid, the organisms are noted to be inside neutrophils. The laboratory report is "intracellular Gram-negative diplococci," a very strong indication that the meningitis is meningococcal. On common laboratory culture plates like blood agar and chocolate agar meningococcus takes about 24 hours to develop colonies. The organism grows as flat, gray colonies with varying degrees of a glistening mucoid look. Most colonies are sticky when picked up off the culture plate with a bacteriologic loop.

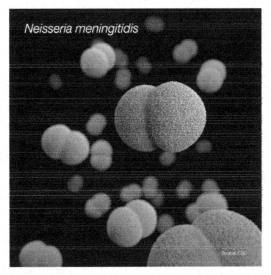

Neisseria meningitidis is a Gram-negative diplococcus (PHIL)

But superficial appearances don't tell the whole story of the potential virulence of the organism. Some strains of Neisseria meningitidis are quite benign, no more invasive than the typical non-pathogenic species we all harbor in our mouths.

Others, though, are endowed with the genes to manufacture several virulence products that can make the organism deadly. These hyper-invasive strains do not always cause a fulminant infection, but they can wreak havoc when the right circumstances arise.

The highly pathogenic strains of *Neisseria meningitidis* possess pili, short hair-like projections extending from the bacteria's surface. There are several proteins on our cells to which the pili can attach, especially on the epithelial cells in our mouths and the cells lining the meninges. Once attached to a human cell, meningococcus can do something unique: form micro-colonies on top of the cell. Micro-colonies are not biofilms; they are just a collection of dozens of microbes all attached to the same host cell. Some of the bacteria of the colony break away to attach to other cells; some stay right where they are and metabolize and replicate. But the invasive strains of *Neisseria meningitidis* have a unique ability. They can directly penetrate the host cell to which they are attached and travel right through it to emerge on the other side. Once through, they begin the micro-colony formation on the next layer of cells. They keep going until they reach the bloodstream. Once there, the organism causes extensive damage, including sepsis and meningitis. If not treated appropriately and immediately, death is likely.

The immune system, if functioning correctly, doesn't just stand by and let this happen. Two well-established innate immune system components are immediately engaged once an organism penetrates cells: complement and neutrophils. They can act in concert or alone, but they represent a most efficient defense against invading bacteria that are outside human cells. Neutrophils engulf and digest the invader. Complement, activated by the engagement of antibodies or responding directly to the organism's molecular pattern, can destroy the invader or assist the neutrophils in their endeavors. Both methods are highly efficient, and bacteria that enter and penetrate our epithelial lining are normally eliminated in short order, usually without any residual evidence that they were there.

Strains of *Neisseria meningitidis* that are successful pathogens have developed methods to counteract the effect of neutrophils and complement. For one, they are surrounded by a slimy capsule, making the job of the neutrophil more difficult. They just bounce off like a wet bar of soap. So, much of the burden of encountering and destroying the invading organism falls to the complement system, an elaborate, complicated cascade of around 30 proteins designed to work either alone or in concert with antibodies and neutrophils to quell the encroaching foe. The complement cascade can be initiated in three ways: (1) attaching to and working with antibody that has already bound to the incoming microbe (classic pathway); (2) mannose-binding lectin pathway, or MLB, whereby a portion of complement attaches to a mannose-bearing molecule on the microbe's surface, initiating the complement cascade; (3) the alternative pathway, which is the most primitive. (See Chapter 8). In the latter, a major part of the complement system, C3, spontaneously binds a water molecule forming $C3_{H2O}$. This highly destructive and volatile molecule lasts only a few milliseconds before breaking down, but if three serum factors are immediately present, the C3 can actively pursue an attacking microbe. Factors B and D, along with properdin, are normally present in the serum but in greater numbers when an infection arises. They stabilize the activated C3 and enable it to do its work.

Human cells are vulnerable to activated C3, but we have safeguards. One of these is human Factor H, which is present both in serum and attached to our cells. Factor H mitigates the activity of C3 and renders it harmless to our cells; microbes lack it and are fair game. The alternative pathway is very effective, although non-specific.

Hyper-invasive strains of *Neisseria meningitidis* have developed a novel means of reducing the effects of complement, to which it is highly susceptible. The organism produces a protein that binds human Factor H, preventing it from stopping the activation of complement. From the organism's perspective, this seems like a strange thing to do, making more of the substance that can destroy you, but the result is the activation of lots of complement throughout the body. There are only so many complement molecules available, and if they are activated and tied up due to the lack of Factor H, then complement won't

538

be available for the other two complement pathways, classic and MLB. It takes a while for the liver to manufacture a re-supply of complement factors; by that time, the organism may have gained a foothold.

There are 13 known capsule types of *Neisseria meningitidis,* but five predominate in clinical infections–A, B, C, Y, and W-135. The organism normally colonizes our mouths, and when they produce a capsule, we naturally make antibodies against it. Some other, unrelated organisms can contain antigens that mimic the antigens of *Neisseria meningitidis,* and if we make antibodies to them, that antibody will cross-react and attack the *Neisseria.* The older we get, the more likely we will be exposed to *Neisseria meningitidis* or some other bacteria that mimics it. Eventually, we have plenty of antibodies on board to counteract the invading microbe. If our complement system is working well, the antibody hooks up with complement, which helps attach it to a neutrophil, and the organism's invasion is short-lived.

Two things can interfere with this happy outcome. Young people haven't had enough exposure to the various forms of the organism or other organisms that chemically mimic it, so antibody is not formed. That's a major reason Neisserial meningitis is a disease primarily of the young (those under 25) and not older. Also, a defect in one or more of an individual's complement components can hinder the immune response and render the person more susceptible to deep infection. Studies have shown that many people who get Neisserial meningitis have a defect in one of their complement components, usually C5 through C8. In addition to the organisms' ability to reduce the complement components in the bloodstream, such a complement defect can give the microbe an advantage in establishing an infection.

Neisseria meningitidis is Gram-negative, containing the highly toxic Lipid A in its cell wall. Other gram-negative organisms have lipo-***poly***-saccharide, but *Neisseria* has lipo-***oligo***-saccharide, meaning the carbohydrate associated with Lipid A is of shorter length. This presumably makes it a lesser target for the immune system, especially B-lymphocytes that make antibodies.

All pathogenic bacteria require iron. Our bodies have a lot of iron, but it is tied up in various forms, like ferritin, transferrin, lactoferrin, and hemoglobin in red blood cells. Pathogenic strains of *Neisseria* possess several enzymes that allow the organism to steal iron from the body, enabling its proliferation at a very rapid rate.

Pili, capsule formation, human Factor H binding, and iron sequestration, the four pathogenic factors of *Neisseria meningitidis,* allow the strains that possess them to be one of the most virulent pathogens of humans. Once the organism passes through the lining of the oral cavity and enters the underlying blood vessels, it can establish an overwhelming infection in susceptible individuals.

After entering the bloodstream, the organisms still make micro-colonies, only now it is on the endothelial lining of small blood vessels. These can occlude the tiny vessel, and their ability to conduct blood containing oxygen to nearby tissues is significantly compromised. Added to this is that they are Gram-negative and therefore contain endotoxin. All that endotoxin circulating around the body induces the monocytes of the blood to produce copious amounts of inflammatory cytokines such as interleukin-1β, interleukin-6, and tumor necrosis factor-α, with resulting septic shock and the onset of intravascular coagulation. One of the hallmark symptoms of Neisserial meningitis and sepsis is the appearance of purplish blotches on the skin, known as petechiae (pronounced 'pet-teek-ee-eye'). Along with septic shock is the lack of blood supply to the extremities, often resulting in the need for amputation to save the patient's life.

Not all circulatory *Neisseria meningitidis* enter the central nervous system, but it often occurs. The organism can attach its pili to the endothelial cells of the meninges, thereby altering the host cell's ability to maintain the tight junctions of the blood-brain barrier. The organism can then move right into the arachnoid mater. Once there, the body's inflammatory response is in full gear, with enormous numbers of neutrophils entering the space. Ordinarily, one cubic milliliter of spinal fluid

540

contains 0-1 neutrophils. In full-blown Neisserial meningitis, there may be upwards of 50,000. Rather than clear like water, the CSF has a turbid white appearance.

Meningitis caused by *Neisseria meningitidis* is a medical emergency. Minutes count because the disease progresses so rapidly. When a lumbar puncture is performed, the spinal fluid has a cloudy appearance. On examination in the clinical laboratory, the fluid under the microscope is noteworthy because of the large number of neutrophils. On Gram stain for bacteria, some of the neutrophils are seen to encase Gram-negative diplococci, a dead giveaway for *Neisseria meningitidis.* The lab comment denoting the observation is "intracellular Gram-negative diplococci." Appropriate antibiotics must be administered immediately to save the patient's life.

Not all antibiotics can enter the meninges. The blood-brain barrier does a great job of prohibiting the entry of many substances into the central nervous system, including antibiotics. Penicillin can enter, but only if there is inflammation. An antibiotic that can cross the blood-brain barrier and kill the pathogen is the best choice, and third-generation cephalosporins, like ceftriaxone, fill the bill. If given early enough the treatment usually is effective, and the patient's life may be spared.

Neisserial meningitis is not a common disease in developed areas of the world. Typically, it occurs spontaneously in a single individual, often a teenager or someone in their early twenties. It is not usually a disease that spreads easily from an infected person to a non-infected one. The organism may indeed spread and colonize contacts of the index case, but the immune response of the newly colonized person is usually enough to thwart the infection.

There are a few notable exceptions to this generalized rule. A patient showing severe symptoms from the disease often harbors large numbers of organisms in their mouth and throat. The bug can spread to others when very large numbers of organisms are present, and immediate contacts may get such a sizeable infective dose that it can overwhelm their immune system. Family members and healthcare workers in very close contact with the victim should be given an antibiotic as soon as the diagnosis is known to prevent their heavy colonization. Ciprofloxacin is often used and is very effective.

Historically, Neisserial meningitis has stricken those who have traveled and entered a social setting of many other travelers. Military recruit bases and college dormitories are classic, but there are others. Young people enter these settings, and if a person from another area of the country or world should harbor a hyper-invasive strain of *Neisseria meningitidis*, it can be easily transferred throughout the immediate population and enter a susceptible person. Stressful emotional and physical activities can add to a person's vulnerability. Individuals in such circumstances often develop relatively mild upper respiratory infections caused by many different organisms, primarily viruses. But a hyper-invasive strain of *Neisseria meningitidis* clearly takes things to a much higher and more dangerous level.

To prevent a potentially catastrophic occurrence in environments like military recruit stations and college dormitories, pre-existing antibody levels to the most common serotypes of the organism are obviously desirable. Unfortunately, there is no easy way of knowing which individuals have naturally acquired appropriate antibodies. A multi-valent vaccine containing the capsular material of the most common strains of infectious *Neisseria meningitidis* ensures that an individual exposed to a pathogenic strain of the organism for the first time can mount an effective immune response.

Neisseria meningitidis contains several unique surface antigens, but the capsule is the most obvious target for antibodies. Without it, the organism is easy prey for neutrophils and complement. All the capsules of the organism are chemically well characterized and relatively easy to prepare in relatively pure form. Unfortunately, they are all polysaccharides, mostly resembling sialic acid. All induce an immune response in the form of antibody, but the antibody is of the IgM type, which doesn't last very long. Also, the response involves only B-lymphocytes, not T-cells, so there is little or no immunologic memory. After a couple of years, the humoral immune response and immune memory disappear.

The answer to this dilemma is to attach the polysaccharide capsular antigen to a protein. Doing so gives both a T-cell response and immune memory, and longer-lasting antibodies of the IgG class are produced. The best protein carrier is a neutralized diphtheria toxoid, which binds to the capsular material. As in the diphtheria vaccine, the toxin is denatured by formalin, leaving it immunogenic but non-toxic. A non-virulent derivative of the diphtheria toxin, CRM-197, is used. It is a well-known diphtheria toxin with a mutation at position 197, making it non-toxic, even before formalin denaturation. In most individuals, the immune response to the combination of Neisserial capsule material and diphtheria toxoid is vigorous and presumably protective.

The vaccine has been shown to be safe and effective for four of the five most serious and common types, the so-called ACWY preparation. Notable by its absence, however, is type B. The reason is that the chemical structure of the B polysaccharide very closely mimics the structure of human sialic acid. Hence, the immune system recognizes it as self, and antibodies are not produced. Fortunately, the surface of *Neisseria meningitidis* has other antigens besides the capsule, and they can be used as antigens in the vaccine. One vaccine preparation uses two variations of the organism's factor H binding protein. Another one uses that protein and adds the bacterial proteins Neisserial adhesin protein A, Neisserial heparin binding protein, and one called PorA. None of these are unique for the type B serotype, so they can most likely protect against the ACWY types.

Neisserial meningitis is a devastating disease, but it is not common in developed countries. Before the introduction of antibiotics, outbreaks of the disease were sometimes seen, with several people in a community presenting with symptoms. It didn't spread through the population like influenza or coronavirus, but a strain of *Neisseria meningitidis*, usually type A, would show up and sicken dozens of people every few years. In the pre-antibiotic era, the only treatment available was the serum of patients who had had the disease and recovered. The antibodies it contained were effective against the invading strain. This passive immunity was often effective, and quite a few lives were saved. After the 1940s, antibiotics became the treatment of choice, usually a derivative of penicillin or a cephalosporin.

Epidemics of meningococcal disease still strike part of the lesser developed world. Most notable is the "meningitis belt" of sub-Saharan Africa, which stretches from the Atlantic coast to the Indian Ocean. Every few years, as immunity wanes, strains of *Neisseria meningitidis*, usually type A, infect and kill many, usually children.

Outbreaks of Neisserial meningitis used to be characterized by identifying the capsular type involved, A, B, C, Y, and W. With the laboratory tools available today, the offending strain can be much further characterized according to proteins other than the capsule. Genotyping is very helpful in identifying infecting strains, and designations such as ST-5 and ST-11 go a long way in establishing the presence of especially virulent strains and the damage they do.

With the introduction of effective vaccines, the number of cases of Neisserial meningitis has substantially decreased. But the organism is far from extinct. Extreme diligence is essential. The consequences are much too dire.

Chapter 35
The Crown of Thorns

Worldwide traveler
Pounces unexpectedly.
The spiked intruder.

Coronaviruses infect many species of animals. Humans are no exception. Historically, four main types of the virus routinely infected humans. They have the forgettable names HCoV-229E, HCoV-OC43, HCoV-NL63, and HCoV-HKU1. Infection by each of them results in what is usually referred to as the common cold. Like many viruses, they circulate freely throughout a population for a season, then are absent for a few years. Since immunity to one does not give immunity to the others, they take turns infecting seasonally.

The illness that traditional coronaviruses cause is often called a common cold. There is often a sore or scratchy throat, and a runny nose. The chief symptom is the production of mucus and phlegm, which induces a cough. Other common cold symptoms can be present, such as fever, muscle aches, and listlessness. All of these vary from person to person. It is not uncommon for a person to become infected, shed the virus, but display no symptoms.

All viruses home in on a specific receptor on the human cells, and the one that is targeted by traditional coronaviruses sits on cells that bear cilia. Cilia are the moving hairs atop the cell that project into the airway. They beat rhythmically to expel mucus. But when the virus attaches to a ciliated epithelial cell and enters it, the cell is killed, and so is the movement of the cilia. The mucus just pools there. The only way to expel the mucus is to cough, which, of course, enables the virus to spread to other individuals, perpetuating itself. Coronavirus is not what one would call a "super-spreader," as one patient may infect only a few others. But that's all it takes to move the virus around the community quickly.

The typical incubation time for a coronavirus common cold is about 2-3 days. Sometimes it can take a week, and rarely, it can take up to 14 days. The infection with traditional human coronavirus lasts several days, and most patients resume normal activities about a week after showing their first symptoms. The traditional coronavirus strains have adapted themselves very well to humans, making us sick for just a few days before we return to normal health. A "good" pathogen doesn't kill its host because it just dies with it. Through eons of interaction, humans have adapted to the virus, and the virus has adapted to us.

In November 2002, a new chapter in the coronavirus story began. In Guangdong Province, China, a novel strain of coronavirus emerged. Used in this context, the word "novel" refers to a microbe that had formerly infected an animal but can now infect humans. The new strain produced the usual symptoms of traditional human coronavirus, but the virus sometimes entered and severely affected the lungs. The mortality rate exploded, and extreme measures had to be taken to contain the virus. The disease it caused was named Severe Acute Respiratory Syndrome, SARS for short. Fortunately, those containment measures were successful, and the virus did not spread very far, and it has not become endemic.

Another novel coronavirus emerged in 2012 in a most unusual place, the desert of Saudi Arabia. Because of its first detection location, it was called Middle Eastern Respiratory Syndrome Coronavirus, abbreviated MERS-CoV. The virus most likely spread from bats to camels, then from camels to humans. Human-to-human spread has occurred, but usually in settings like hospitals where very close, prolonged contact is common. The MERS virus attaches to a receptor on the host cell that differs from that used by the SARS virus (dipeptidyl peptidase 4 for MERS versus angiotensin-converting enzyme 2 for SARS).

In late 2019, another novel coronavirus arose from China in the Hubei Province, city of Wuhan. This newer strain spreads at the same rate as the traditional coronaviruses but is more deadly than the usual human strains. The name assigned to the new strain is SARS-CoV-2. The disease it causes has the more common designation COVID-19, an acronym for COronaVIrusDisease, 2019.

Coronavirus derives its name from its appearance, that of a crown or corona. The spikes from the virus's core are the attachment vehicles, which the virus uses to hook onto a ciliated cell in the respiratory tract. Like all viruses, the molecular composition of these spikes can change due to genetic mutation. These changes may mean that a different receptor on the host cell is sought, and entrance may be more vigorous. The major change in coronavirus virulence came from the alteration in the spike protein and the human cells the virus could enter. OC43, 229E, and HKU1 all attach to host cell receptors located only on upper respiratory epithelial cells. The more virulent SARS strains bind to the receptor angiotensin-converting enzyme 2 (ACE2). ACE2 is abundant on the upper airway epithelial cells, but it is also prominent on many other cells in the body, especially the lungs, and therein lies the problem. (Interestingly, the traditional coronavirus NL63 also attaches to ACE2, but it uses a different, less efficient enzyme to initiate cell penetration). Because of the expanded range of cells bearing its receptor, the early symptoms of the SARS viruses are similar to those of other respiratory viruses, namely scratchy throat, runny nose, and muscle aches. There is also cough with significant amounts of phlegm.

Coronavirus is very large compared to other viruses that cause respiratory infections. Influenza has eight genes that code for eleven proteins. RSV has ten genes and eleven proteins. Human coronaviruses contain twenty-six proteins. Four are structural, sixteen are non-structural, and six are accessory. The structural proteins hold the virus together and facilitate its entry into and exit from the host cell. The nonstructural and accessory proteins assist the virus with its replication and formation of new virions. They also work to reduce the immune response of the host.

The receptor for the SARS strains of human coronavirus is a protein extending out from the host cell surface called angiotensin-converting enzyme 2 (ACE2). ACE2's reason for being is to ensure a steady state in blood vessels, helping to regulate vital functions like blood pressure, coagulation, and blood vessel permeability, among others. ACE2 is abundant in different tissues and is especially prominent in the lungs.

The spike proteins of both SARS-CoV-1 and SARS-CoV-2 attach to the ACE2 projecting from human cells. The attachment of SARS-CoV-2 to ACE2 is 10-20 times stronger than SARS-CoV-1. The spike protein of SARS-CoV-2 is divided into two sections. The outer one, S1, attaches to the human ACE2 receptor. The lower section of the spike protein, S2, is connected to the outer S1 section by a short amino acid bridge. The short amino acid bridge is key to making SARS-CoV-2 an effective pathogen.

We have lots of enzymes that exist in an inactive form. To become active, they must be cleaved by another enzyme. The enzyme that does the cleaving doesn't participate in the target enzyme's activity; it merely activates it. An important cleaving enzyme is furin. It is found in the membranes of many of the body's cells, and it works to activate many different human enzymes. SARS-CoV-2 somehow developed a short amino acid bridge between its S1 and S2 sections of the spike protein that is readily cleaved by the human enzyme furin.

Immediately after furin cleaves the amino acid bridge between the S1 and S2 sections, the S1 section becomes more firmly attached to the ACE2 receptor. This makes the S2 section start to wiggle and shake, leaving it open to the activity of two other human enzymes. One is Transmembrane Serine Protease, TMPRSS2. The other is Cathepsin L, an enzyme that spends most of its time in lysosomes inside the cell. But some of it is released to the outside of the cell. Whichever of these two enzymes is used by the virus, the lower half of the viral spike protein, S2, is activated and fuses with the host cell membrane. The virus, now inside its host cell-derived membrane, is taken into the host cell where it can do its mischief.

All coronaviruses have positive-sense RNA, so as soon as the virus breaks free in the host cell cytoplasm the RNA gets right to work, migrating to the cell's ribosomes to be copied. Several of the viral non-structural proteins assist with the process.

548

All our nucleated cells can detect foreign RNA. Our cells don't create double-stranded RNA, but viruses do, and our cells have the means of detecting it. Also, the RNA of coronavirus has a cap on one end that is different from that on our RNA, another sign to the host cell that a viral invader is present. Two important chemical sensors our cells have for detecting the presence of a virus in the cell are known as RIG-1 and MDA5. RIG-1 detects the virus' unique chemical arrangement on one end of its RNA strand, and MDA5 recognizes double-stranded RNA. We also have Toll-like receptors that do a similar job. It's a redundant system.

Interferons are the most potent weapons we have to shut down the effects of an invading virus in the early stages of an infection. Interferons don't kill the virus directly like an antibiotic, but the infected cell sends these chemical messengers to neighboring uninfected cells, alerting them to gear up to the impending danger. Most of our cells have receptors on their surface to allow interferon to attach and enter them. Once inside, interferon can direct the uninfected cell to do several things. Interferon can induce the cell to manufacture substances that degrade viral RNA. It can shut down the enzymes the virus needs to replicate in the host cell ribosomes. Interferons can also stimulate the activity of dendritic cells, helping to give a more robust acquired immune response. Finally, because of the action of interferons, lymphocytes and macrophages can increase the formation of MHC class I molecules, also enabling a more vigorous immune response.

There are three types of interferon, conveniently called Types I, II, and III. Type I interferons are subclassified into alpha and beta. The alpha types are subclassified into over a dozen subtypes. Beta interferon has just two. All nucleated cells of our body can create interferons alpha and beta when invaded by a virus, but some cells are much more efficient at it. Type II interferon is interferon-gamma, a very important one, but it doesn't play an important role early in acute viral infections. Type III interferon is known as interferon lambda. There are four subtypes. It doesn't get much attention compared with the others, but it is still important in upper respiratory infections. It is secreted only by cells of the upper respiratory and intestinal tracts and only protects those cells, but that is very important in infections like those caused by viruses like coronavirus and Influenza.

The cell that is the grand champion at interferon production is the plasmacytoid dendritic cell, pDC. Plasmacytoid dendritic cells constitute a small fraction of our dendritic cells but are a major player in defending us against viruses. pDCs start in the bone marrow, then travel mostly to lymph nodes. They become activated if they come into contact with a substance found exclusively in viruses, like double-stranded RNA. pDCs can crank out as much as a thousand times the interferon that other cells do. pDCs are a bridge between the innate and acquired immune response. Their action slows down the invading virus' activity, so cells responsible for antibody production and cellular responses can become active.

Natural killer lymphocytes also play a crucial role early in a coronavirus infection. Cells that are in trouble send chemical signals to their surface. The NK cells interact with the infected cell, injecting enzymes that cause its death (Chapter 11). The virus dies with the cell, and parts of the virus are then displayed on antigen-presenting cells, initiating acquired immunity. Interferon production and NK lymphocyte activity are vital parts of early innate immunity. When all goes well, an invading virus is eliminated in short order. Successful viruses have the means to curtail both interferon production and NK cell activity.

Coronavirus is equipped with several factors that help it drastically reduce the activity of interferons and natural killer cells. As soon as the virus begins replicating, it induces the formation of a double membrane vesicle to surround its RNA. This is a clever way of concealing the unique viral RNA from the host cell's chemical sensors, slowing down interferon production.

Without the presence of a virus, the DNA sections on our chromosomes responsible for coding for interferon are sequestered, lest interferon be produced for no good reason. Interferon is technically a cytokine, and many cytokines make us feel sick. Interferon is no exception, so it is kept under wraps until needed. Each sentinel system designed to alert the host cell's chromosomes to unlock the interferon genes employs a pathway of chemical reactions. Typically, chemical sensors like RIG-1, MDA5, and the Toll-like receptors detect the presence of viral products, and latch onto the unique viral piece. This alters the sentinel molecule's shape. This gets the chemical reactions going, step by step, ultimately sending a chemical messenger to the host cell nucleus instructing it to begin coding the interferon genes. This translates into messenger RNA, which then migrates to the ribosomes to produce interferon. The system is redundant, so if one part doesn't fire, others will take its place.

Coronavirus is a master at disrupting these systems. It is large compared to other viruses that cause upper respiratory infections, containing over three times the number of genes and proteins. Many of these coronavirus proteins have the job of disrupting the production and release of interferon. Besides encasing its tell-tale viral RNA in a vesicular bubble, it has enzymes that can blunt host cell interferon signaling reactions. These include the recognition of the virus, subduing chemical reactions along the chemical pathway to produce the chemical messenger to the nucleus, and interfering with the transport of host messenger RNA to the ribosomes, including the genes coding for interferons.

Another vital part of the early battle against invading viruses is the activity of Natural Killer lymphocytes (NK cells). Cells that have gone awry alert the NK cells that all is not well. The NK cell then organizes the cell's destruction through apoptosis, and the virus is liquidated with it. It's not known precisely how the virus does it, but the number of circulating NK cells is reduced in the early stages of a SARS-CoV-2 infection. The cell in which the virus is replicating is allowed to proceed, cranking out more virus.

SARS-CoV-2 infections can be divided into three stages. First, there is the invasion of the virus and its early stages of replication. Late in this phase the infected person may not feel symptoms but can still shed the virus. Next is the appearance of symptoms, those usually associated with a common cold. If interferon, Natural Killer lymphocytes, and the other members of the innate system function normally, the infection stops there. The infection will run a course of about 3-5 days. While the virus can subdue the production of interferon and the activity of Natural Killer cells, it doesn't shut them down entirely. People differ in their reactions, probably due to differences in their genetic makeup and their immune system status. Some folks have a rather robust interferon and NK Cell response, while others are less so.

Meanwhile, the acquired immune system with long-term immunity is being assembled. With most traditional coronaviruses, such as 229E and OC 43, the story is a short one. The infection is halted, and long-term acquired immunity is assembled.

Most infections caused by SARS-CoV-2 follow this pattern. But in some people, there are complications. This is especially true in older people and those with a pre-existing medical condition, often called a comorbidity. The disease in these patients can proceed to the third stage, lung infection.

A major reason for the sometimes catastrophic complications of SARS-CoV-2 is the location of its receptor, ACE2. The receptors for other viruses that infect the upper respiratory tract are located there exclusively, usually on the epithelial cells lining the upper airway. But ACE2, the receptor for SARS-2, is situated on a wide range of cells, including the inner lining of blood vessels and cells in the lungs. Therein lies the problem.

For most people, the initial infection is effectively ended by the activity of the innate immune system, primarily the actions of interferon and NK cells. While the virus can mitigate their activity, it doesn't eliminate it. Especially important is the activity of the plasmacytoid Dendritic Cells. They can pick up enough viral material, including viral RNA, to initiate the production of significant amounts of interferon. But some older people and those with comorbidities don't have as many pDCs as younger people. Also, the number of active NK cells is lessened in older people. For a person with a condition that causes chronic inflammation, the immune system is given chemical signals to reduce its activity so that the inflammatory

552

condition won't get out of control. It amounts to being slightly immunocompromised. The result is reduced activity of cells like pDCs and NKs.

If the initial battle between the virus and the innate immune system results in something of a standoff, with some of the virus surviving the first few days, the situation can turn dangerous. Most virus is contained in the upper airway, but if it hangs around long enough, it can relocate to the lungs, where there is an ample amount of its favored ACE2 receptor. In the lungs, the virus begins another frontal attack, and the immune response can spin out of control. In addition to damaging lung tissue, the virus can injure the endothelial lining of the blood vessels. All this damage is inflammatory, and immune cells and chemicals storm into the area. Neutrophils are prominent, even though they aren't helpful against a virus. The condition has been described as a cytokine storm, with the lung tissue and blood vessels damaged. Heroic means are needed to save the patient's life.

Developing a vaccine was critical when the COVID pandemic furiously struck the world in early 2020. Until then, the vaccines available for preventing viral infections were of two types. One used virus grown in laboratories in tissue culture. After growing to large numbers the virus is denatured. The dead virus is then injected into the patient. Vaccines for polio and influenza are the most common examples. The other type uses live viruses that are attenuated. SARS-CoV-2 presented problems for both. It doesn't grow well on laboratory tissue culture media, so there isn't enough virus to harvest for massive numbers of vaccines. Also, it takes years to generate an attenuated virus, with hundreds of passages through tissue culture or animals. The urgency of the COVID pandemic required an accelerated and innovative approach.

Many laboratories worked on vaccine development using different approaches. Two types of vaccine production emerged. One was to take a small piece of the virus and insert it into an unrelated virus that can be grown easily in the laboratory. That virus, bearing the antigens of the coronavirus, could be harvested and inoculated into the person being vaccinated. That approach had been used successfully before, notably in developing vaccines for Ebola and malaria.

The other approach was innovative and remarkable in its complexity. In essence, scientists began from scratch and constructed what amounted to a novel virus in the laboratory. Single-stranded RNA that could function in human ribosomes was used for nuclear material. The RNA carried the genetic code for the entire spike protein of SARS-CoV-2, all 1273 amino acids. (There are 672 amino acids in the S1 subunit and 588 in the S2. A few extra ones help stabilize it). The mRNA is wrapped in a coat of lipid nanoparticles to allow it to be protected and incorporated into the host cell. Without the lipid nanoparticles, the mRNA would be useless. It couldn't get into the human cell, nor could it travel to the ribosome to be transcribed. There are four types of nanoparticles. One binds the stuff to the RNA, and another helps stabilize the group. Two others, phospholipids and cholesterol, help protect the whole thing from enzyme destruction and assist the incorporation of the particle into the human cell.

The vaccine acts just like a virus, entering the cell and allowing its payload of RNA to be transcribed into a protein. The protein produced is the entire spike protein of SARS-CoV-2. Only in this case the additional proteins that inhibit the production of interferon are not produced. The immune system recognizes the spike protein produced as foreign material, even though it was manufactured by a human cell. Antibodies are produced to neutralize it, enhancing immunity.

The COVID pandemic of the early 2020s brought to light many of the interesting features of infectious disease epidemics. Most notably, people react differently. Some were infected but displayed no symptoms, others suffered terribly, and millions died. People also varied significantly in their emotional responses. The pandemic produced a wide array of social and political reactions.

SARS-CoV-2 has become endemic. Most people worldwide have some level of immunity to it, either by vaccination or natural infection. The virus, though, is notorious for its mutation rate. How the virus mutates and re-combines its genetic material is key to the future of the disease.

Chapter 36
Pyogens

Thin liquor puris:
Symptom of hope? Sign of doom?
The suppuration.

Bacteria are everywhere. That includes on and in our bodies, by the billions. Most of the time, they are controlled by our immune system, including our skin, mucus membranes, and other barriers to their entry into our soft tissues. We also have specialized members of our innate immune system always at the ready to engage and destroy potential invaders. Complement, neutrophils, and macrophages are programmed to hook up to and disable any bug displaying surface molecules peculiar to them and not us, the so-called pathogen-associated molecular pattern, commonly called PAMP. It is a very efficient protection system, especially when you consider how many bacteria regularly colonize us.

A major type of organism that benignly colonizes our bodies are the Gram-positive cocci. The word coccus is from the Greek *kokkos*, for "berry." Two genera predominate, *Staphylococcus* and *Streptococcus, staphylo* meaning a "bunch of grapes," and *strepto*, meaning "a twisted chain." The terms refer to the organisms' microscopic appearance on a Gram stain; *Staphylococcus* divides into three planes, so it does indeed look like a bunch of grapes (they stain purple on Gram stain), and *Streptococcus* divides only end-to-end, giving either pairs or chains. The organisms are quite different biologically, but they both have found a way to colonize our bodies with impunity. *Staphylococcus* is usually referred to simply as Staph, and *Streptococcus* as Strep.

Staph prefers our skin, where over a dozen species can be found. Strep prefers the mouth and other mucus membranes like the bowel and the vagina, where multiple species are prevalent. Most of the species of Gram-positive cocci that colonize us are beneficial, mainly by keeping away other types of bacteria that might harm us. Some bacteria produce substances known as bacteriocins, proteins that can kill other organisms and keep them away. They are natural antibiotics produced by our bacterial flora that help protect us. Other interactions among our resident bacterial flora similarly protect us from more invasive creatures.

But sometimes, even harmless or beneficial bacteria can do us damage if they end up in the wrong place. If there is a breach in our immune defenses and damage to one or more of our tissues, normally benign bacteria can take the opportunity to set up an infection. One of the most notorious of these situations is a disease called endocarditis.

The heart valves are made up of the inner lining of the heart, the endocardium. When a valve becomes damaged, either by an autoimmune reaction or a foreign substance like injected narcotics, the body's response is to repair the damage by establishing a fibrin layer, forming a hardened mesh over the damaged heart valve. (Fibrin is a hard stringy protein that makes a blood clot tough). Over time, these small fibrin layers grow to a formidable size, which can then become a nesting area for bacteria from our mouth, bowel, or skin. We sometimes have minor tears in our mouth or skin that allow the introduction of a few bacteria into the bloodstream. Usually, they are dealt with in short order by the innate immune system, but if a heart valve is damaged, the bacteria can enter the valve's fibrin growth and begin to multiply. The result is many bacteria growing in a shield of fibrin, known as a vegetation. Little pieces of this large vegetation, carrying bacteria, can break off and end up in the arterioles of other organs, such as the brain, lungs, or kidneys, resulting in harmful clots. Of course, the infected heart valve is damaged, and cardiac disease results.

Before the availability of antibiotics, endocarditis was a universally fatal disease. Rheumatic fever, which results from a streptococcal infection, is well known to damage heart valves. In the 1930s, 40s, and 50s, rheumatic fever was a highly significant disease, mostly in children. The damage to heart valves often precipitated the disease endocarditis, sometimes much later in life. Today in the developed world, rheumatic fever is rarely seen. But other conditions may also injure heart valves, making them vulnerable to endocarditis.

Fortunately, antibiotic therapy and, if needed, heart valve replacement surgery, have greatly reduced the mortality rate of endocarditis. Many organisms can be involved in endocarditis, but the most common is the usually benign Strep from the oral cavity, traditionally called the viridans Strep. Viridans comes from the Latin *viridis* meaning "green," and is used because there is often a green halo around colonies of bacteria on common laboratory culture media. Viridans Strep are usually harmless, but in the setting of endocarditis, they may cause a fatal infection.

Another place where ordinarily harmless bacteria can cause serious infections is implanted medical devices. The usually harmless *Staphylococcus epidermidis* and related bacteria can attach themselves to the device, whether plastic or metal, and form a biofilm that can be extremely hard to dislodge. As in endocarditis, little pieces of the growth can peel off, enter the bloodstream, and lodge themselves in an arteriole, resulting in reduced blood flow to a vital area, a dangerous situation. Sometimes the medical device must be removed and replaced, if possible.

Endocarditis and medical device infection are two ways our harmless bacterial colonizers can cause a serious infection. Normally the bacteria are not a threat, but if the body is compromised in some way and bacteria gain access to the bloodstream for a short time, illness may result. They are the ultimate opportunistic pathogens.

While most of the streptococci that inhabit our mouth are harmless in that environment, one that can cause local damage is *Streptococcus mutans*. It has some unique abilities. For one, it has strong attachment proteins allowing it to adhere to the surface of teeth. It can also form biofilms, engaging with other species of bacteria to form what can become dental plaques. When *Strep. mutans* metabolizes sugar, mainly sucrose found in sugary beverages and foods, the result is lactic acid. Acid on tooth enamel is not good, especially when it is trapped in place by dental plaque. Tooth decay, also called dental caries, can result. There is currently no therapy specific for *Streptococcus mutans*. Vaccine trials to date have not been successful. Sugar avoidance and assiduous dental hygiene are the best means to prevent tooth decay.

Another genus of bacteria that normally inhabits us without incident is *Enterococcus*. It looks just like *Streptococcus*, and it was included in that genus at one time. As the genus name suggests, the enterococci are part of the resident bacterial flora of our bowel. Just like their viridans streptococcal cousins in our oral cavity, they typically exist there with no harm to us. But they possess two characteristics that enable them to set up an infection: the ability to form biofilms and a propensity to develop resistance to antibiotics.

As with the viridans Streps, *Enterococcus* can cause endocarditis, most of which arises in the community. But the vast majority of *Enterococcus* infections are nosocomial, that is, acquired while the patient is in the hospital or healthcare setting. The most common infection is urinary tract infection (UTI), mainly after the insertion of a bladder catheter. Also seen are infected wounds of damaged tissue. The organisms are very hardy and able to survive on environmental surfaces for extended periods. A person can easily acquire them during hospitalization, and if the patient is vulnerable to infection, potentially serious consequences may follow.

Enterococcus's innate and acquired resistance to commonly used antibiotics is a very troubling characteristic. Antibiotics are frequently used in hospitals, and the organisms that are resistant to them survive. When an opportunistic situation arises, they can set up an infection. An antibiotic often used to combat enterococcal infections is vancomycin, which has also been used to battle Staph infections. Unfortunately, vancomycin-resistant enterococci, or VRE, are now commonly encountered in the hospital environment and can be extremely difficult to treat.

There are two species of Gram-positive cocci, one a Strep and the other a Staph, which have attained the role of aggressive pathogens. *Streptococcus pyogenes,* often called Group A Strep, and *Staphylococcus aureus,* can and often do cause serious infections. Most of humanity will get infected by both of these organisms. Another species of Strep, *Streptococcus pneumoniae*, is also capable of causing serious disease, but most strains behave more like the viridans Strep and are benign. Our innate immune system is vital in protecting us from these potentially severe pyogenic pathogens.

The word pyogenic means pus-forming. The prefix "pyo" is from the Greek word for pus *pyon*; "genic" is also from the Greek word *genes*, meaning "born or producing." The technical name for it is liquor puris. Pus, of course, is made up mainly of dead neutrophils because it is the neutrophils that respond quickly and in large numbers to the invasion of pyogenic organisms like *Streptococcus pyogenes* and *Staphylococcus aureus*. Other debris from damaged tissue is also present.

***Streptococcus pyogenes* (Group A Strep).** Since the early days of clinical microbiology, it has been known that when some species of *Streptococcus* are grown on culture media containing whole blood, the red blood cells on the culture plate are destroyed (lysed). There is a clearing around the colony of growing bacteria, a phenomenon called hemolysis. It was also well known that most strains of Strep isolated from serious infectious diseases are hemolytic. But there are also species of Strep that are hemolytic that do not produce serious disease. In the 1930s, a scientist named Rebecca Lancefield of the Rockefeller Institute in New York sought to differentiate the virulent from the benign. Using antibodies to various cell wall carbohydrates, she found that the hemolytic Strep could be divided into well-defined groups, which she labeled with capital letters, starting with A. Such strains were found throughout nature, ranging from Groups A to M, but those most associated with humans at the time were A, C, and G. Of these, by far the most pathogenic for humans was Group A, also known as *Streptococcus pyogenes*. (In the 1930s, the hemolytic strain associated with cows was Group B, for bovine; at that time, it was not found in humans).

The first responders to an invasion by Group A Strep are complement, neutrophils, and macrophages. Their job is twofold: attack and destroy the invading organism and signal other components of the innate immune system of the invader's presence.

Complement, as described in Chapter 8, can recognize the organism either by antibody assistance to the bug or by two alternative pathways. Once engaged, the C3 portion of complement splits into two sections, the larger 3b and the smaller 3a. The C3b portion has two roles. One is to attack the outer membrane of the invading microbe directly. The other is to enable the activation of C5, triggering the rest of the complement cascade. The smaller C3a portion is tasked with traveling to areas outside the infected site to attract a variety of immune responders, including macrophages and neutrophils. One of the co-products of C5 induction is C5a, which has a similar job.

Neutrophils are killing machines. They detect invading bacteria, surround them with a pseudopod and engulf them, then destroy them with numerous granules within their cytoplasm. The neutrophil also dies; their collection makes most of the pus in an infection site. Often the neutrophils are assisted in their mission by complement, which can bind the microbe to the neutrophil in a process called opsonization. In some cases, antibody is also involved.

Neutrophils are formed in the bone marrow. Some remain in the bloodstream after they mature; others enter the tissues to act as sentinels and guardians. As discussed in Chapter 7, elegant mechanisms are in place to attract copious numbers of neutrophils to the site of infection, resulting in inflammation. Some symptoms we experience, such as swelling, redness, and pain, result from this inflammatory response. Macrophages are also intimately involved in the early response.

The combination of macrophages, neutrophils, and complement is a powerful force to engage the invading Group A Strep. For most bacteria, it is insurmountable, and they are summarily eliminated. But the crafty Strep has some defensive munitions of its own, and therein lies a great problem for us.

Our bodies are awash in a substance called hyaluronic acid. It's a gooey material that acts like a lubricant, coating cells and the matrix that envelope them. Without hyaluronic acid, our life wouldn't be very good, all stiff and unbending. Somewhere along the natural history of Group A Strep, it acquired the genetic material to manufacture hyaluronic acid in the exact same chemical composition as the human type. The organism expresses it as a capsule surrounding itself, thus impeding potential phagocytizing neutrophils. Since bacterial hyaluronic acid is the same as the typical human type, we don't make antibodies to it. That means the classic mode of complement action, opsonization with antibody, doesn't work very well for Group A Strep.

Unfortunately, the other two complement pathways, known as alternative and lectin, are diminished in their effectiveness by a malevolent force on the organism's surface, the M protein complex.

The M protein is a long, coiled structure anchored in the bacterial cell wall. It has three general sections, the anchor, the stalk, and the outer part that extends out the furthest from the bacterial cell surface. The section closest to the bacterial surface is very similar between different strains, while the end extending into the environment varies with the strain of bacteria. Around a hundred different M proteins are known, but some are involved in Group A Strep disease more commonly than others. In fact, some M-types are associated with specific diseases, like Strep throat or puerperal sepsis.

Two major functions of the M protein are the disabling of complement and the activation of coagulation. M protein can bind to some complement components, rendering them inactive and interrupting the cascade, giving the organism a better chance of surviving the attack by macrophages and neutrophils. M protein also activates coagulation early in the infection. The deposition of fibrin and other clotting components slows down the immune response, much like the deposition of a clot in the case of endocarditis helps a much less pathogenic strain of Strep become infectious. The M protein, along with the hyaluronic acid capsule, gives the organism a significant advantage in its early advances, enabling it to thwart the protective efforts of complement and neutrophils.

While bacterial hyaluronic acid is not antigenic because it resembles our own, the M protein is unique and induces antibody production. However, there are many different M proteins, and immunity to one type does not confer immunity to the others. That's why we don't have an effective vaccine for Strep throat; if we get infected by one strain and develop antibodies to it, other strains with different M proteins can still infect.

Some pathogenic bacteria penetrate and invade a human cell, setting up the infection intracellularly. Group A Strep does not enter the human cell but sets up the infectious process outside. To do this, they must adhere to the cell's surface, or the matrix surrounding the cell, while at the same time evading the immune defense forces. The M protein is important in this endeavor, but over a dozen other bacterial surface proteins also play a role. Of great importance here is lipoteichoic acid or LTA. LTA is most likely the first bacterial adhesin to attach to the human cell surface, enabling the other factors, including the M protein, to enhance the binding. Interestingly, some bacterial adhesins other than LTA and M protein are active in high oxygen concentrations, thus important in skin infections. In contrast, others are active in high concentrations of carbon dioxide and are important in infections in the soft tissues.

The critical component of LTA is the "L" part, lipo. Being a lipid, it can integrate with many different human cell surfaces so the organism can set up an infection in many different areas. Another vital attribute of LTA is its ability to bind fibrinogen. That is the substance that helps form a matrix web around the cells of a tissue, helping to bind them all together. Binding fibrinogen in the extracellular matrix gives the organism another solid binding site and a place to set up an infection.

Once they gain their way into a human tissue and begin to set up an infection, some strains of Group A Strep can manufacture toxins, which are released in a timely fashion to meet the organism's need for nutrients. Not all strains of Group A Strep are the same; there is a wide variance in different strains' ability to create and excrete toxins. Just which toxins are produced and released goes a long way in determining which strain is highly virulent, even deadly, and which are much less so.

Most strains of Group A Strep produce two substances known as hemolysins (pronounced he-MOL-asins). First noticed by their ability to break apart red blood cells in the culture medium, hemolysins are an integral part of streptococcal virulence. There are two hemolysins, denoted O and S. The designation O for oxygen is somewhat confusing in that it is not produced in the presence of oxygen but only in its absence. The S stands for serum, as the substance is only produced when serum is present, as it is in blood. While chemically different, the two hemolysins are both very important in the organism's assault on the host.

Breaking up red blood cells on culture media is how we notice the hemolysins' activity, but that is of little importance in their attack. What really matters is the ability of these two toxins to disrupt the cell membranes of several types of human cells, including neutrophils, epithelial cells, and platelets. They work in concert with the attachment organelles of the organism to initiate an infection while disrupting the immune response designed to halt it. As neutrophils and macrophages approach the bacteria with the intent of gobbling them up and killing them, the opposite occurs, with the bacteria destroying the phagocytes. The result is the formation of pus, along with significant inflammation.

With many neutrophils killed off in such a rapid manner, their nucleic acids, mainly DNA, tend to aggregate in the surrounding milieu, forming what is known as Neutrophil Extracellular Traps, or, appropriately, NETs. This mesh of nucleic acids acts to trap bacteria, giving other living phagocytic cells a better shot at destroying them. To free themselves from this web-like confinement, many strains of Group A Strep excrete an enzyme known as DNase, which is effective at breaking down the DNA strands, thus freeing the organism.

With its armament of a capsule, M proteins, hemolysins, and DNase, Group A Strep is a powerful invader once it gains a foothold. While not eliminated, the usual members of the innate immune response, complement, macrophages, and neutrophils, are significantly diminished in their activity, giving the invading

564

organism an advantage as it sets up an infectious process. But some strains of the organism do more. Some are endowed with the genes to make toxins that can inflict damage not just near the initial infection but in remote areas throughout the body as well.

Many of the toxins Group A Strep produces are known as "super-antigens." Routinely, foreign proteins, including toxins, are processed inside a human cell, most often a macrophage or dendritic cell. Through a complicated process, the foreign protein, or a part of it, is mounted onto a scaffold-like appendage of a Major Histocompatibility Complex, or MHC. There are two MHCs, and most toxins are handled by those designated MHC class II. The foreign protein, an antigen, is snugly fitted into a notch in the MHC, and the whole complex is transported to the cell's surface. The antigen, while still attached to the MHC, is then displayed on the cell's exterior surface, now known as the antigen-presenting cell (APC). There it waits for the arrival of a T-cell or B-cell with a protein on its surface that precisely matches the antigen presented. When matched, the T or B-cell begins to reproduce, and the acquired immune response is initiated, with either activated T-cells or antibodies produced by the B-cell line. There aren't that many T or B cells in the body to hook up with the presented antigen, just one in millions of lymphocytes.

Superantigens do it differently. Instead of fitting snugly into the presenting groove of the MHC, they are chemically arranged to fit outside it. The superantigen is transported along with the MHC to the cell surface, but in this askew position. That doesn't sound like much, but the result is a massive activation of T-cells, triggering a tremendous cytokine release. Instead of just the rare compatible T or B cell coming along to hook up, as many as 20% of those encountered become activated because of the odd arrangement of the toxin on the MHC, which is chemically determined by the molecular structure of the toxin. Much of the toxicity of Group A Strep infections is due to this superantigen phenomenon and the resultant intense systemic cytokine release.

Group A Strep can attack just about any organ in the body, but most of the diseases it causes are fairly well-defined. A list of the most common:

Strep throat. The disease streptococcal pharyngitis, commonly called strep throat, is one of the most common infections afflicting the human race. It strikes all ages, ethnicities, and geographic locations. Individuals can be infected multiple times, albeit with different bacterial strains. It occurs so commonly that the term "Strep Throat" is often used to describe any "Sore Throat," whether Group A Strep causes it or not. Of course, proper testing must be done to determine the presence of Group A Streptococcus to be sure that it is really the culprit. Sore throats caused by other organisms can and often do mimic those caused by Group A Strep.

Strep throat is spread like many respiratory tract organisms by oral passage from person to person. The classic signs of Strep throat are sudden onset of sore throat, fever, muscle aches, and often discreet white patches on the tonsils with distinct reddening of the throat. The tonsils are often enlarged, so much so that they can almost meet in the middle of the mouth. The onset of the disease is usually quite sudden, with a person going from feeling fine to being overwhelmed in just a few hours. Younger children often get diarrhea and vomiting, but these signs are usually not seen in older children or adults. The fever is about 101, and the white cell count in the blood is about 12,000, somewhat elevated. If treated with penicillin or another appropriate antibiotic soon after symptoms present, the disease usually diminishes in a few days. If diagnosis and treatment are delayed a few days, the illness may last a week to ten days.

Antibody forms to several Group A Strep antigens, including the M protein and Streptolysin O. The antibodies persist, but, unfortunately, they do not protect against other M-types, and subsequent infections can, and often do, occur. That's a big reason we don't have a vaccine for Group A Strep—too many M-type strains. (Originally, Strep typing was done using antibodies specific for each M type, serologic typing. Genetic technology is used today, and the gene set for M proteins is designated *emm*. Serologic and genetic testing correlate very well, and the proper designation now is, for instance, *emm*1 for the gene set instead of the previous designation M1 for the antigen).

Not all cases of Strep throat present in the classic pattern. Some are more subtle, with just a few symptoms, none distinct. Proper laboratory testing is required to establish the diagnosis. The standard test for determining Strep throat is a throat culture, in which the tonsils and back of the throat are swabbed, and the material is placed on blood agar culture plates in the laboratory and incubated overnight. On the Petri dish the next day, the tell-tale clear zone around the colony where bacterial toxins have destroyed the blood gives the lab worker a significant clue suggesting the presence of Group A Strep. It is an indication to perform further tests to rule it in or out. Another test uses the same sample with results available in less than an hour rather than the full day required for culture. The rapid test detects an antigen unique to Group A Strep. While more convenient in terms of time, it is less sensitive than the throat culture, and negative tests should be confirmed with the overnight test.

Many bacteria have developed resistance to the penicillin class of antibiotics through the years, but not Group A Strep. Some Group A Strep strains show resistance to other antibiotics, but not the penicillins. If a patient is not allergic to penicillin, that drug, or a derivative of it, such as amoxicillin, is the drug of choice. There has been much discussion in medical circles on the need to treat Strep throat, with the possible induction of bacterial resistance to antibiotics being a major concern. Some maintain that the use of antibiotics does not much alter the progression of the disease, and the development of antibiotic resistance by other bacteria wouldn't occur as frequently. Others maintain that antibiotic use reduces the spread of the disease and can prevent other sequelae from occurring. Most physicians treat with an antibiotic.

Scarlet fever. Most people have heard of scarlet fever, but few have had the disease themselves, nor know anyone who had it. Before the 1930s, and presumably throughout all human history, it was a widespread infection, considered one of the common

567

infectious diseases of childhood, along with chicken pox, measles, and mumps. Then it gradually began to almost disappear, with very few cases diagnosed in the developed world in the latter 20th and early 21st centuries. It has recently made a comeback, with its future still up in the air.

Scarlet fever is an odd one, with some unexpected facts. The characteristic rash results from a toxin released by the bacterium, but *Streptococcus pyogenes* does not have the genes to make it. The toxin is produced by a virus that infects the bacterium. (It is similar to what occurs in the disease diphtheria, in which a virus infects the bacterium and produces the toxin). Since it is a toxin that is produced, it is fair to assume that the toxin is directly responsible for the skin rash. But the toxin, a superantigen, stimulates the cells of the immune system, T and B lymphocytes, and their reaction causes the rash. Think of it as an allergic reaction. Also, one cannot show the signs of scarlet fever unless they have previously had a Group A Strep infection. Usually, the previous infection was strep throat, but it could also have been a skin infection.

Several toxins can be involved, but the most important is Streptococcal Pyogenic exoenzyme C or SPeC. It is a superantigen in that it becomes attached to the outer part of the MHC-2 molecule and therefore incites many T and B cells to become active, whether they have a receptor for SPeC or not. The activity of all these T and B cells results in an allergic reaction in the skin. A good question is just why it benefits *Streptococcus pyogenes* to make the adaptive immune system cells behave in such a remarkably unproductive way. One theory holds that many reactive lymphocytes are B-cells, potential antibody producers. If induced to pursue this highly aberrant activation folly, B-cells die by apoptosis. In that case, they can't do the job they were designed to do, making antibodies to the invading *Streptococcus*. The fewer antibodies, the greater the chance the organism has to go on reproducing. It's only a theory, but it makes sense.

Most cases of scarlet fever are self-limited, with the rash going away at about the same time the primary infection does. But occasionally, the invading Strep strain has more than just the single SPeC exotoxin. It can also contain a more virulent toxin, a superantigen that induces septic shock with potentially dire consequences.

Rheumatic fever. Like scarlet fever, rheumatic fever was much more prevalent over sixty years ago than it is today. It is probably the best studied of the autoimmune disorders, in which the body's immune system, after the invasion of a pathogen, directs its full force against the patient's own organs, causing significant and, in some cases, irreparable harm. Just why the disease has decreased in incidence in developed countries is open to speculation. It seemed to coincide with the introduction of antibiotics, so that must play a role, but other factors may be at play.

Most of the epidemiologic data come from a time when rheumatic fever was much more prevalent than today. In the early 1900s, about 3% of children with strep throat developed rheumatic fever. The incidence today is much less. It is no longer a reportable disease to Public Health centers, but some studies put its incidence at around 0.3% in some areas. Interestingly, it is more common in poorer areas with more crowding and less sanitation. Worldwide, there are about 500,000 yearly cases of rheumatic fever today. About 30 million people have a heart problem from having had rheumatic fever as a child. The most common age affected by far are children ages 5-15.

Group A Strep has lots of antigens, and it is difficult to discern just which one(s) are responsible for initiating rheumatic fever. Most likely, it is some part of an M-protein, probably the variable part on the distal end, but it could be one found on the M-protein stalk. The type-specific carbohydrate in the bacterial cell wall is antigenic and could also be involved.

Whichever bacterial antigen it is, the immune antibody and T-cell response to the *Streptococcus* cross-react with a protein in one of the patient's tissues. The four organs involved are the large joints, heart, skin, and brain. Not every patient has the same organ involvement, suggesting multiple antigens and antibodies are in play. It can be a very painful, debilitating disease, with some patients confined to their beds for long periods. Even when the patient passes the acute phase of the disease, some problems persist for years.

Joints. Vimentin is a protein found in several tissues and is especially prominent in joint tissue. In some individuals, the molecular structure of their vimentin closely resembles that of one of the antigens of Group A Strep, and antibodies directed against the Strep also are active against vimentin in the joint. T-helper lymphocytes are also activated and enter the active area of the joint, leading to marked inflammation. Joint pain and fever are often the first signs of rheumatic fever. Usually, the joints affected are large ones, like the hip and shoulder. Inflammation and pain often travel from one joint to another. About 75% of patients with rheumatic fever have joint pain.

Heart. The heart has several proteins that can cross-react with the antibodies formed against Group A Strep, including myosin, laminin, tropomyosin, troponin, and actin. These are found in all three layers of the heart, and, depending upon which one mimics the Strep antigen, that area can be attacked by antibodies and immune cells, giving distinct symptoms. When the heart valves are involved, vegetations grow, forming a seedbed for organisms that have entered the bloodstream, resulting in the potential to develop endocarditis. Around 50% of patients with rheumatic fever have a heart condition.

Skin. Keratin is the skin protein thought to cross-react with antibodies formed against a component of invading Group A Strep. In rheumatic fever, the classic appearance of the skin is known as erythema marginatum, a distinctive skin lesion of red edges, round margins, and a clear center. Sometimes they resemble a bullseye and are found mainly on the trunk and upper arms. While only about 5% of patients with rheumatic fever display skin lesions, they are a very helpful diagnostic aid.

Central nervous system. The brain, specifically the ganglioside nuclei, is a less common but very important 4th organ system that can be affected by cross-reacting antibodies to Group A strep in some people. The area of the brain which controls movement and some cognition contains many of these proteins. When impacted by antibodies and invasive T-cells and the inflammation that goes with it, the result is a condition known as Sydenham's Chorea, characterized by rapid uncontrolled movements, especially around the face and the arms. Less than 5% of patients with rheumatic fever get this disorder, but it can be quite debilitating.

The word mimic is fitting in talking about rheumatic fever, as the antigens of the Streptococcus strongly resemble those of the human host. Also, the symptoms of the disease can mimic those of other ailments: fever, arthritis, heart disease, and others are not unique. The criteria for diagnosis is to have at least two major symptoms, such as those of the joints, heart, nervous system, and skin, OR one major symptom plus two minor ones, the so-called Jones criteria. There must also be a history of Group A Strep infection, demonstrated by culture, antigen detection, or serology (ASO titer), to confirm the diagnosis.

Other sequelae to Group A Strep infection don't come under the heading of rheumatic fever but are an autoimmune reaction due to cross-reacting antibodies. Glomerulonephritis (inflammation of the kidney resulting in blood and protein in the urine), and post-streptococcal reactive arthritis, PSRA (generalized arthritis lasting a few weeks or months after infection), are such ailments. A neurologic disorder of children called PANDAS, an acronym for pediatric autoimmune neuropsychiatric disorders associated with Strep infections, is attributed by some researchers to post-Strep infection. Its cause is considered speculative, but there will always be the question of this and other diseases being due at least in part to a cross-reactive autoimmune reaction to a Group A Strep infection.

Rheumatic fever is not a malady of a bygone age. It's still with us today, albeit in much lower numbers in the developed world than over a century ago. When one gets Strep throat, is diagnosed, and prescribed appropriate antibiotic treatment which is taken assiduously, the chances of developing rheumatic fever are nearly zero. But the medication must be taken as prescribed for the duration of treatment. Children are the victims of the ailment, and, as we all know, getting kids to take their medicine is not the easiest job. There are no simple means of predicting who will get rheumatic fever after a Group

A Strep infection, so it is best to proceed as if it were possible. At the very least, proper dosing of antibiotics reduces the chance of spreading it to others.

Impetigo. A large variety of bacteria colonize our skin, most of them Gram-positive. This is because the Gram-positives, as opposed to the Gram-negatives, are rich in teichoic acid, which allows the organism to bind to the skin. Many of these adhering bacteria produce substances called bacteriocins that kill and prevent other harmful bacteria from colonizing. Intact skin presents a formidable barrier to microorganisms, and we usually reach a steady state of resident bacterial flora living on our skin's surface which helps keep away the harmful ones. But occasionally, especially in young children ages 2-5, a pathogenic interloper takes its place among the skin flora, and trouble ensues.

Group A Strep, along with the other prominent pyogen *Staph. aureus,* can colonize the skin transiently. If there is some disruption to the skin's integrity during this encounter, like a scraping or an insect bite, the pathogen takes advantage. It infects, causing a condition known as impetigo. The term impetigo comes from the Latin word *impetere*, meaning "assault" or "incursion." The chief attachment organelle for Group A Strep is the M-protein, which can attach to the fibronectin surrounding the cells of the dermal layer. Once attached, the infection proceeds similarly to what occurs in the pharynx, with pus and serous fluid forming. This scabs over, with resulting lesions on the skin.

The streptococcal M-types responsible for impetigo differ from those which cause Strep throat. They have a greater predilection for the cells of the skin than those of the throat. Their different antigenic structure is also displayed by the fact that the more common sequela of skin infection is glomerulonephritis (kidney inflammation), while that of strep throat is rheumatic fever.

Group A Strep can also cause dermal infections in older people. Erysipelas is characterized by large red swollen areas of the skin that are clearly demarcated from the surrounding skin. Cellulitis is a tender swelling usually following mild trauma.

Occasionally the organism can invade the deeper tissues, and prompt effective antibiotic therapy is necessary.

Puerperal sepsis. In reading books of history, either novels or non-fiction, it is not unusual to come across the statement, "She died in childbirth." While much less common today in the developed world, severe complications and death happened with some regularity in times gone by. While there are many reasons for complicated births, a particularly vile one is an infectious disease that attacks the uterus at the time of or shortly after birth, puerperal sepsis. The term puerperal is from the Latin *puerperalis,* meaning "related to childbirth." Following a vaginal birth, the woman's tissues are vulnerable to infection, and several organisms may play a role. The worst one to get is *Streptococcus pyogenes* because of its highly virulent abilities. Group A Strep is not normally found as part of the vaginal flora. But if it is introduced during or shortly after birth, it can cause the very rapid and deadly infection of puerperal sepsis (sometimes called puerperal fever).

Puerperal sepsis has an important historical place in the discovery of infectious diseases. In the 1840s, most women had midwives to assist them in birth; physicians usually shunned the procedure as beneath them. But financially well-off women could afford to hire a personal physician and often did for childbirth. At the General Hospital in Vienna, there were two obstetrics wards: one for wealthy women and their physicians and one for poor women and their midwives. Amazingly, the rate of puerperal sepsis in the upper-class ward was about ten times greater than that of the other. In the 1840s, such infections were attributed to "miasma," or "bad air." That made no sense since the two groups were in the same building.

A young obstetrician named Ignaz Semmelweis noticed one day that a cut on his finger he incurred while doing an autopsy had become infected. He hypothesized that the source of his infection might be the same as that causing the high number of cases of puerperal sepsis in the affluent OB ward. (At the time, the ailment was referred to as "childbirth fever"). It was not unusual for a doctor to examine a patient after coming from the autopsy room or another patient without washing his hands. Microorganisms were unknown, so the only reason to rinse one's hands would be to get the gross material off them. Soap was rarely used, only water. Semmelweis argued that some "particle" of the corpse or patient might be spread by way of the doctor's hands. When he became director of the unit, Dr. Semmelweis insisted that all physicians scrub their hands in dilute phenol (carbolic acid), a rather noxious substance that when used regularly imparts drying and roughness to the skin. The number of cases of childbirth fever dropped dramatically. Despite being an effective procedure, this command did not go over very well with the medical staff. Semmelweis was severely criticized, forced out, and lived a wretched life in disgrace. But with its dramatic success, the incident went down in history as one of the first examples of sanitation saving lives and misery.

Because puerperal sepsis is so rare in developed countries today, it is difficult to know what Streptococcal strain(s) are chiefly responsible. It most likely produces streptococcal pyogenic exotoxins that destroy local tissue and allow the rapid spread of the organism, resulting in toxic consequences. The strains most implicated are M-1 and M-28, but which were involved a hundred years ago is anyone's guess. Antibiotics, first sulfa drugs, then penicillin, dramatically reduced the number of women infected. Thankfully, puerperal sepsis, the scourge of women throughout the ages, is an extremely rare possibility today in the developed world with aseptic technique and antibiotics. Sadly, however, it persists in impoverished countries.

Necrotizing fasciitis. A scene sometimes used in movies involves a physician giving a diagnosis to a patient using sophisticated medical terminology. The patient then responds something like, "Can I have that in English, please?" The response that one very much does not want to hear from the doctor is "flesh-eating bacteria." Somewhere in the journalistic lexicon, this unfortunate phrase took form. "Flesh-eating bacteria" suggests the most horrific, god-awful affliction that can befall a human being. Better to just use the scientific term necrotizing fasciitis or its medical jargon term, "nec fash."

The medical terminology describes the disease very well. Necrotizing refers to tissue death; fascia is a thin covering of tissues, including muscle. That's how the disease starts. Our muscles have a very thin covering overlaying them, the fascia, that looks and feels something like delicate cellophane. When the organism, Group A Strep, gets inside the fascia but outside the muscle, it can metabolize and reproduce with impunity. The immune system has little effect on its progress. If the strain of Strep infecting has the proper array of toxins, such as Strep Pyogenic Exotoxin B (SpeB), all hell breaks loose. The muscle tissue and the fascia surrounding it are rapidly degraded, and the resulting reaction affects the entire body—septic shock.

Treatment of necrotizing fasciitis is draconian. A skilled surgeon must debride a large part of the muscle tissue; often, amputation is the only recourse. Even with that, patients often don't make it.

Group A Strep is not the only organism that can cause the disease but it is the most aggressive. With the production of toxin, the surrounding tissue is rapidly destroyed, or necrotized, and it spreads rapidly. While the infecting organism is very susceptible to the antibiotic penicillin, getting the drug to the site of infection is much reduced because of its location and the accumulation of dead tissue, and the bug replicates unabated. In addition, when the organisms reach a very high number, they have a chemical signal between them that shuts down their reproductive activity, leaving them in a state of reduced metabolism, the stationary phase. Penicillin, even if readily available, is less effective than it usually is during this reduced growth state of the bacteria. But the organism is still pumping out the toxin, the production of which is not affected by penicillin, which only affects the cell wall. A second antibiotic that can inhibit protein synthesis (and thus toxin) must be added to the regimen. Clindamycin fits the bill. This phenomenon of reduced bacterial cell wall synthesis and robust toxin production is known as the "Eagle Effect," named for Dr. Harry Eagle, a British pathologist who first described it.

How Group A Strep gets into the muscle fascia is a question not easily answered. Sometimes it seems like a sharp object causing a puncture wound picks up the organism residing on the skin and deposits it adjacent to the muscle. In many cases, the disease is preceded by a jolting, non-penetrating injury that damages the tissue enough for the bug to take advantage and invade. But most times, the source of the infection escapes detection.

Streptococcus pyogenes can bring great harm to humans, its only natural host, causing several serious types of infections, even more than those mentioned above. It can attach to the cells of all human tissue and, depending on the strain, manufactures and releases several potent toxins. We will never rid ourselves of it. No vaccine is available, and with the number of different M-protein strains, there will always be the chance of re-infection. Good hygiene has been shown to reduce, but not eliminate, the chances of infection. Fortunately, the organism has never achieved the means to resist penicillin, which is very effective against it. Other antibiotics are also effective. Early detection and prompt antibiotic therapy are the best means of reducing this virulent pathogen's damage.

Streptococcus pneumoniae has caused enormous suffering and death by the means its name suggests, pneumonia. It also causes other infections. Under the microscope, it has a unique appearance, nearly always two cells bound together. The joint between the cells a straight, flat line, and the opposite ends somewhat pointed. The descriptive term "lancet-shaped diplococcus" is applicable. At one time, the organism was known as "*Diplococcus pneumoniae.*"

We have many species of *Streptococcus* in our mouths and throats that are supposed to be there. They don't normally harm us, and they exist to our benefit in several subtle ways. Some of these oral Strep produce a substance that can metabolize hemoglobin. When grown on solid laboratory media containing blood, they reduce the hemoglobin to methemoglobin, which has a green color. When the organism is grown on a culture plate it produces a gray colony surrounded by a green halo, commonly called alpha-hemolysis. The species that produce the green-haloed colonies are collectively known as Strep viridans. It is not a valid species but a general description of the organism's appearance on blood agar plates. The term alpha-Strep is often used as well.

Long ago, one of the members of this viridans group began to acquire genes that enabled it to transform itself from the state of a benign colonizer into a virulent pathogen. We now call this species *Streptococcus pneumoniae.* While it still has the green halo around its colony when grown on blood agar plates, it differs considerably from the other oral Strep.

The most apparent laboratory difference between *Streptococcus pneumoniae* (usually just called pneumococcus) and garden variety alpha-Strep is the presence on the former of a carbohydrate capsule surrounding the bacterial cell. The carbohydrate is a thick, gelatinous material. When a colony of the organism growing on an agar plate is touched with a wire loop, the capsule gives the colony the texture of slimy goo. Another feature of the colony of pneumococcus is the suppressed center of the colony, looking volcano-like. In a mature bacterial colony, the older cells in the middle of the colony break apart in an act known as autolysis, wherein they kill themselves, similar to apoptosis in human cells. With the death of these older cells, the middle of the colony collapses, giving the appearance of a crater in the middle. These two features, a slimy colony with a crater in the middle, give the lab worker a high suspicion of pneumococcus.

The capsule gives the pneumococcus a big advantage when confronted by a neutrophil attempting to engulf it. It just bounces off and skips away. If antibodies to the capsule and complement are present, the neutrophil becomes much more efficient, and the organism has less chance. But in the early stages of infection, the bug has the upper hand, and infection may result.

Another potent weapon pneumococcus has acquired is a protein called pneumolysin. It's a force. Just where the pneumococcus acquired it in the distant past is a matter of conjecture, but a similar molecule is found in *Clostridium perfringens,* an anaerobic Gram-positive rod that can cause gangrene. Just how the genetic material was passed from one organism to another is hard to say, but by having pneumolysin, the pneumococcus, once probably just another benign member of the oral flora, became a potentially serious pathogen.

Pneumolysin is a complex toxin made up of four distinct sections. One of those sections allows the molecule, and therefore the entire organism, to bind to cholesterol. Cholesterol is a component of our cell membranes, so the pneumolysin-cholesterol binding enables the adhesion of the bug to our cells. Like the other streptococci, *Streptococcus pneumoniae* does not penetrate and reside inside the human cell. It remains outside. But with pneumolysin, pores (holes) are bored into the human cell membrane with resultant fluid and electrolyte leakage. The mitochondria are damaged, and they send out their signal for apoptosis, self-destruction. The infected area then becomes a red-hot mess of dead cells and a strong attractant for neutrophils, which also can damage tissue. Fluid seeps into the area, and if the tissue infected is the lungs, pneumonia is the result.

In some cases, the organism enters the bloodstream. Sometimes that's the end of it, but pneumococcus can potentially attach itself to the lining of the central nervous system, the meninges, and using its powerful weapon pneumolysin, enter the area. The result is meningitis.

Another body site pneumococcus frequently infects is the middle ear. Most children will get a middle ear infection. Some will get more than one. Several organisms, both bacteria and viruses, can be the cause, but *Streptococcus pneumoniae* is the one most encountered. The organism commonly colonizes the throat, and when conditions are right, it ascends the Eustachian tube, going from the mouth to the middle ear. There it establishes an infection with the assistance of pneumolysin.

Streptococcus pneumoniae is a serious pathogen, a major cause of pneumonia, meningitis, and middle ear infection (otitis media). But unlike many other pathogenic organisms, it isn't something we suddenly catch and then become ill. We don't directly get any of the infections it causes by coming into close contact with a person with that disease like we would Strep throat or influenza. We get the organisms from other individuals, but usually the bug resides in our pharynx quite harmlessly, along with hundreds of other species. Periodically, we gain one strain of the creature, harbor it for a while, then it goes away only to be replaced by another. It goes on this way for our whole life. What turns the organism into a holy terror is a precipitating event that upsets the dynamic of peaceful colonization. Usually, that precipitating event is a viral infection.

When a virus infects, the ordinarily stable environment of our upper respiratory tract is thrown into chaos. The human cells involved send out chemical signals in the form of cytokines. They also alter their surface molecules. Inflammation results, and normal host defense mechanisms can be compromised. It is into this type of disrupted situation that pneumococcus can pounce. Whether it is into the lungs to cause pneumonia, up the Eustachian tube to the ear, into the bloodstream to eventually colonize and infect the meninges, or into the sinuses to infect one or more of them, it is a formidable foe.

There are many strains of *Streptococcus pneumoniae*. Some are much more virulent than others, depending on their capsule type. Since different strains are constantly cycling through our upper respiratory tract, it becomes a matter of luck as to which strain we have and the amount of damage done by the precipitating event, like a viral infection.

The carbohydrate capsules of pneumococcus are antigenic, and we make antibodies to them. But carbohydrates are poorer antigens than proteins, and the plasmacytes producing antibodies to a complex carbohydrate cease to function after a few years. Also, babies and very young children make few antibodies to carbohydrates, if at all. That, of course, leaves them more vulnerable to infection by pneumococcus. The same holds for older people.

There are around 90 different types of pneumococci based on carbohydrate capsule content. To make a vaccine against all these different types would be impossible, but some capsular types are associated with more virulent diseases than others. Pharmaceutical companies have prepared vaccines to include the most common and virulent types of pneumococci. They are not designed to be administered to everyone but only to those most vulnerable: the very young, the old, and people with compromising medical conditions. There are two formulations.

Since babies and young children do not make antibodies to carbohydrates very well, the capsule materials of the vaccine strains are attached to a protein, then injected. With this protein-carbohydrate conjugate, the immune system cells make a vigorous antibody response. The protein carrier is a non-toxic form of diphtheria toxin called CRM_{197}, which is widely used as a carrier for carbohydrates used in vaccine production, including *Haemophilus* and meningococcus. With the dual induction of antibodies, T-cells are activated along with the B-cells, and the vaccine is much more effective and lasts longer.

Several formulations of pneumococcus vaccines have been used, but two predominate. The one for young children, conjugated with CRM_{197}, is called PCV for Pneumococcus Conjugated Vaccine. The number attached gives the number of strains of pneumococcus capsular types included. An example is PCV13, indicating that carbohydrates from 13 pneumococcal capsules are included.

The other vaccine does not contain the CRM_{197} component and is a carbohydrate, or polysaccharide, only. The abbreviation here is PPSV, for Pneumococcus PolySaccharide Vaccine. Like the PCV, it is followed by a number of capsular types included, such as PPSV15 or PPSV23.

The health departments of most countries recommend that pneumococcal vaccine be given to children, people over age 65, and any others with potentially serious health problems. The vaccines do not prevent all pneumococcal diseases. Strains of other capsular types can still infect. Also, other organisms can cause the same infections as pneumococci, such as pneumonia, sepsis, meningitis, sinusitis, and middle ear infection. But pneumococcal vaccines reduce the number and severity of infections in the general population.

Group B Streptococcus. At one time, Group B Streptococcus only rarely colonized and infected humans. It was chiefly a pathogen of cows, infecting their udders, giving a disease known as mastitis. The species name of the organism is *Streptococcus agalactiae,* which means roughly "no milk." When Rebecca

Lancefield did her classic work on streptococcal classification in the 1930s, no thought for human disease was given to Group B, which was assumed to be of veterinary interest only, and the letter B was assigned to the group for bovine.

That changed in a big way in the 1970s. The first sign that Group B Strep was evolving into a serious human pathogen was the sudden occurrence of newborn babies suffering from sepsis and meningitis. An organism isolated from the babies' blood and spinal fluid specimens was a *Streptococcus*, but it was different from those usually seen at the time. They were hemolytic on blood agar, but the clearing around the colony was smaller and with a hazier appearance than that shown by Groups A, C, and G Strep. The typing kits used to identify hemolytic Strep at the time didn't include antisera for Group B; lab workers had to refer to veterinary texts to find tests to conclusively identify the organism.

It became apparent through the 1970s and 80s that Group B Strep had undergone a profound alteration in its affinity for human cells and had become an established colonizer. It was found that a large percentage of women had Group B Strep as a member of their vaginal flora, and many people had the organism in their stool specimens because it colonized their bowel. In the vast majority of cases, the organism was simply a harmless colonizer, just another member of the normal bacterial flora. But it had gone from non-existent to common in just a decade.

How this transformation occurred is a matter of conjecture. But certainly, it was due to the organism's acquisition of genetic material from other bacteria, most likely other species of streptococci. Bacteria exchange DNA all the time, and Group B Strep picked up a packet of genes from other organisms, which allowed it to harmlessly colonize human epithelial cells. Occurring at the time was women's use of oral contraceptives. Some have argued that their use hormonally altered the surface proteins of women's cells, perhaps enabling Group B Strep to attach more firmly. Whether this had anything to do with the organism's ability to adhere to human cells and begin a new environmental regimen is anyone's guess, but today the organism is firmly entrenched as a regular member of human microbial flora.

As more information about Group B Strep became available through scientific research, it is not surprising that the bug could jump from cows to people. On the organism's surface, there is an array of different attachment proteins, enabling it to hook onto many different cells and proteins of the matrix surrounding them. The genes of these attachment proteins are very adaptable; the bacterium can turn them on or off as the situation dictates. If the organism finds itself in an environment where it needs more of one adhesin molecule and less of another, chemical signals sent to the bacterial chromosome suppress one set of genes and enliven the ones needed. The organism is also adept at forming biofilms, enabling it to keep a low profile and thus avoid the immune system's weapons. It is an elegant system; Group B Strep can be found in many locations throughout the body.

Usually, this is inconsequential to us. We don't get sick from Group B Strep as we do from Group A. It usually just sits there harmlessly, unnoticed. But, when the proper situation arises, Group B Strep can become a serious pathogen, sometimes deadly. Interestingly, Group B Strep colonizes the vagina and intestinal tract, but it doesn't cause vaginitis or gastroenteritis. The infections it causes are in different areas, most notably newborn babies, and in wounds, especially in diabetics.

At birth, the intestinal tract of babies is sterile. During vaginal delivery, the baby normally swallows material in the birth canal, and these organisms begin to colonize the baby's gut. This is a normal, healthy event. But trouble may ensue if one of the organisms present is Group B Strep. Group B Strep has several factors that enable it to colonize the intestinal tract, pass through the gut lining, and enter the bloodstream. This happens more readily in a newborn's gut because the tight junctions between cells are not fully formed. Also, the newborn's immune system is not well enough developed to thwart the invading organism. From the blood, the organism can then attach to and infect the meninges, resulting in meningitis.

582

Such an event requires intensive medical care to save the infant's life.

There is no vaccine for Group B Strep, but in the late 1990s a medical procedure was introduced that substantially reduced the number of cases of Group B Strep sepsis in infants. About three weeks before the expected delivery (due date) the mother's vagina is swabbed, and the material cultured for Group B Strep in the clinical laboratory. If she harbors the organism, an antibiotic such as ampicillin is administered intravenously at the time of delivery. This is not to clear the organism from her vagina. The antibiotic enters the baby's circulation, so if the infant is exposed to Group B Strep during birth, there is a good chance the invading bacteria will be eliminated before the infection begins. Following the introduction of the procedure, the number of cases of Group B Strep sepsis and meningitis in newborns dropped dramatically.

Group B Strep is also very good at attaching to damaged tissue. If the tissue does not readily heal, such as that seen in a wound of a person with diabetes, the organism forms a biofilm over the area and the wound festers. In some cases, the infected wound is refractory to treatment, and chronic infection results.

Like Group A Strep, Group B comes in many strains. Mostly they are distinguished by which adhesin appendages they carry, but a few strains can make an exotoxin that can act as a superantigen. Sometimes toxic shock syndrome is the result.

Staphylococcus aureus. Most of us will get a Staph infection sometime in our life. Usually, it is relatively minor, like an infected cut or the red, tender swelling we can get around a finger or toe. But the organism's potential is anything but minor, and given the right circumstances, the infections caused by this common organism can be severe, even deadly.

The species name "aureus" comes from the Latin word for gold, *aurum*. When grown on laboratory culture media, the colonies that develop have a golden color due to a pigment it produces.

Staph aureus can make us ill in three general ways: toxins produced while growing on food we eat, toxins produced while the organism grows inside our body, and direct infection of tissues. There are many strains of Staph, and which one(s) we encounter will make a big difference in how ill we become.

Staph aureus is one of the leading causes of food poisoning. It can grow on many different types of food, but we usually get sick from consuming meats or cheeses that have been processed, then contaminated by a toxin-producing of Staph. The source of the organism is usually the food handler, who has the organism colonizing some body part, and it gets onto their hands. Two conditions are necessary for Staph food poisoning. One is that the food must sit at room temperature for some time, allowing the organism to grow. The other is that organisms other than Staph have been removed by cooking. Staph doesn't compete well with other organisms, so to produce a large amount of toxin, it needs to be able to grow without many competitive bacteria.

While growing on food products, some strains of Staph can produce very high amounts of enterotoxins. They are technically known as Staphylococcal Enterotoxins, abbreviated SE. There are around 20 known toxins, each abbreviated by a letter: SEA, SEB, etc. The toxins are not destroyed when the food is cooked, but the organism is. A key factor is the amount of time the organism has to grow on the food product; the longer the growth time, the more toxin produced.

Staph enterotoxins are superantigens, but fortunately, they are not absorbed into the bloodstream. They stay in the intestinal tract. They do, however, stimulate the vagus nerve, which is responsible for vomiting and nausea. Our body does not want these toxins to stick around. So, just like the procedure in the ER for a drug overdose, the vagus nerve induces a natural "stomach pump," with vomiting removing most of the toxin. Typically, the symptoms occur six to eight hours after eating, and nausea and vomiting resolve without complications in about twenty-four hours. Staph food poisoning is not transmissible from one person to another, but when multiple people consume the same contaminated food, they will all get sick.

When consumed in food, the enterotoxin of *Staph aureus* doesn't enter the bloodstream. But if the organism is growing unabated in an area of the body, sometimes called a "pus pocket," the toxin can enter the bloodstream. The toxin is a superantigen, and when a high level of it is present in the body, a severe reaction ensues. The prime example is toxic shock syndrome. To get toxic shock syndrome, the correct strain of Staph must be involved, one capable of producing the toxin. It must grow unfettered in a walled-off area of the body, with toxins freely able to enter the circulation. It is a rare event, but when it strikes, it is devastating.

Staph aureus has a wide array of virulence factors in its arsenal. One group of them, the adhesins, allow the organism to stick to many different receptors in our bodies. Depending on which tissue Staph enters, the correct adhesin can be produced in short order to facilitate attachment. The bug is very adept at adhering to the extracellular matrix.

Our tissues contain millions of cells that have attachment molecules for each other. Tight junctions are formed between cells, giving stability to the tissue. Besides that, our cells are encased in an elaborate web of proteins outside the cells called the extracellular matrix (ECM). The ECM is necessary for the tissue's structural integrity and is extremely important in cell communication and signaling. There are many components of the ECM. Integrin originates within each cell and extends out into the environment, where it attaches to fibrinogen. Fibrinogen binds to collagen, the most abundant protein in our body.

Staph aureus has many adhesins extending out from its cell wall, enabling it to attach to each of the ECM components, as well as the membranes of cells. It is particularly adept at attaching to fibrinogen. When it binds to a receptor, Staph is either attached to a human cell or situated in the ECM, a very short distance from the membrane of the nearest cell. If it finds its way here and gets established, trouble starts.

Being stuck to a receptor outside the cell is not a great place to be if you're a bacterium. There aren't many nutrients there, and the bug is vulnerable to the activity of several immune system components. To overcome this situation, *Staph aureus* has several factors it employs to its advantage.

Staph aureus is notorious for the many toxins it produces and releases. Four of the best known are called hemolysins because they easily disrupt (lyse) red blood cells. This phenomenon is easily seen in the microbiology laboratory when the organism is grown on culture media containing blood. A colorless halo immediately surrounds the bacterial colony of Staph growing on culture media containing blood because the bacterial toxin lyses the blood in the media. The hemolysins are designated alpha, beta, gamma, and delta. While the action of these toxins is easily noticed because they disrupt red blood cells, that isn't the most important advantage for the organism. The hemolysins destroy the cells of human tissue as well. This tissue destruction releases nutrients the organism uses to its advantage, and it can grow apace. This rapid growth of the bacteria and the destruction of surrounding tissue attracts myriad neutrophils and macrophages. As the neutrophils engage and die off, pus is left in their wake. Sometimes it is present in copious amounts.

Staph must protect itself against the action of the immune system, which is vigorous. A major factor in the virulence of Staph aureus is its ability to cause the coagulation of plasma. It makes two enzymes called coagulase, one of which remains bound to the bacterial cell wall, and the other is released into the surrounding environment. By binding coagulated plasma to itself, the organism forms a type of capsule, making it more difficult for neutrophils and macrophages to engulf it. It also produces its own carbohydrate capsule to accomplish the same thing.

The coagulation of plasma in the surrounding tissues makes it more difficult for anti-bacterial cells and molecules to enter the area of infection. The enzyme the organism produces that causes the clotting is called "free coagulase" because it does not remain attached to the bacterium.

The production of coagulase sets Staph aureus apart from other staphylococci. When the lab test for coagulase is positive, the organism is identified as Staphylococcus aureus. When it is negative, the report goes out as "coagulase-negative Staphylococcus," usually called "coag-negative Staph." Coag-negative Staph are usually contaminants from the specimen collection, so their exact species designation is unnecessary. Occasionally, though, they cause disease, and the organism must be fully identified. There are over a dozen species of coag-negative Staph seen clinically.

A very important factor in infections caused by *Staph aureus* is Protein A. Antibodies are long molecules that look something like the letter "Y." The "Y" end is variable, specific to the antigen it is designed to hook onto and incapacitate. The other end is constant and is the same in all antibodies of the class, regardless of the antigen. It is designated Fc. The Protein A produced by *Staph aureus* binds to the constant or Fc portion of the antibody molecule rendering it ineffective. This reduces the effectiveness of complement and neutrophils as well.

The presence of a carbohydrate capsule, the coagulation of plasma, and the activity of Protein A mitigating the activity of antibodies, complement, and neutrophils, all make *Staph aureus* a formidable foe. Once it gets established in a tissue, infection often proceeds rapidly.

Unlike Group A Strep, *Staph aureus* can enter the infected cell. Some human cells are more accommodating to Staph invasions, such as skin, bone, and kidneys. By entering the cell and metabolizing inside it, the organism is less of a target for the immune system. Cellular invasion is one reason some people get recurrent Staph infections.

Staph aureus differs markedly from Streptococci in a very important way, its ability to resist antibiotics of the penicillin class, known as the beta-lactam group of antibiotics. The lactam ring of penicillin contains four carbons. In a diagram, they are arranged in a square. This beta-lactam ring is the center of the penicillin class of antibiotics.

Early in the development of penicillin in the 1940s, it was noted that most infections caused by Staph responded to the therapy, but a few didn't. It was discovered that resistant strains produced an enzyme, first called penicillinase but now more appropriately called beta-lactamase, which destroys the beta-lactam ring, rendering the antibiotic useless. In those cases, treatment with an alternative antibiotic was required. As time passed, more strains of Staph were resistant to penicillin. Today, most strains are resistant.

An ingenious means of countering the organism's beta-lactam-destroying enzyme came from a drug called methicillin, developed in the early 1960s. Adding methyl groups around the beta-lactam ring effectively "hid" the ring from the organism's beta-lactamase enzyme. The bacterial enzyme couldn't access the ring and inactivate it. The drug was called methicillin, and it served the great purpose of allowing a penicillin drug to treat Staph infections. Similar drugs followed, each with the same mission of hiding the beta-lactam ring from the bacterial beta-lactamase.

Like all bacteria, staphylococci must continually make cell walls. An important cell wall structure is peptidoglycan, which is stitched together by enzymes. One critical enzyme in the cell wall construction process mistakes penicillin for the chemical needed to be inserted into the growing wall. The whole thing falls apart with penicillin inserted, and the bacterium leaks and dies.

Staphylococci produce an enzyme that inactivates penicillin, beta-lactamase, allowing the cell wall to grow as needed. Methicillin and drugs like it overcame the effects of beta-lactamase, and for a while, Staph infections could be treated with such medications. But not long after these were put in use, pathogenic staphylococci acquired an enzyme that didn't recognize the penicillin drugs and mistakenly insert them into the growing cell wall. Penicillin drugs weren't just inactivated; they weren't incorporated into the growing cell wall. The bacteria could grow despite the antibiotic's presence. Since methicillin was the first such drug used, the strains of Staph that grew despite the antibiotic were called Methicillin-resistant *Staphylococcus aureus*, abbreviated MRSA.

"Methicillin-resistant" is a most unfortunate term. For one thing, methicillin isn't used anymore, so on the surface, an organism's resistance to it shouldn't matter. But the bacterial mechanism that allows the organism to develop methicillin resistance enables it to resist all antibiotics having a beta-lactam ring. That would be all drugs of the penicillin and cephalosporin classes. These antibiotics work best against a Staph infection,

588

but alternatives must be used if the bug is resistant to them. A better name for the resistance by the organism would be "beta-lactam resistant *Staphylococcus aureus*," but the term methicillin-resistant came first and is in common usage, so MRSA it is.

After its emergence in the early 1960s, nearly all cases of MRSA were acquired in the hospital setting. Staph can persist on environmental surfaces for an extended time, and patients undergoing treatment in a hospital are often vulnerable to MRSA persisting in their vicinity. It is not unusual for a person to enter a hospital for one disorder only to develop another, namely an MRSA infection. Sometimes these hospital-acquired infections are serious, even fatal. Hospital workers are very aware of the danger and go to great lengths to prevent MRSA and other hospital-acquired infections. But sadly, they do occur.

Around the year 1999, another strain of MRSA emerged. Instead of originating in a healthcare setting, these bugs were acquired in the community. The worldwide outbreak began slowly, and there was some initial confusion about the cause of the infections. Staph is known to cause skin infections, primarily boils (furuncles) and carbuncles (a collection of boils). These primarily affect hair follicles, where pus collects. The newer community-acquired (CA) MRSA strains first seen in the late 1990s caused small discreet skin eruptions that then spread to produce larger lesions, not the classic boil. Many patients presented for healthcare with the initial complaint of "spider bite," even though the alleged spider was never seen, and spiders are not known to give such a reaction. It soon became apparent that this rapidly erupting disease was caused by a newly developed strain of *Staph aureus* resistant to beta-lactam antibiotics and mainly acquired in the community (CA-MRSA).

An important factor in the elevated virulence of CA-MRSA is their production of a toxin known as Panton-Valentine Leukocidin (PVL). PVL is not produced directly by Staph bacteria but by a virus that has invaded it. The toxin consists of two large proteins that join together in the membranes of neutrophils and macrophages, essentially forming a hole in the phagocytes' membranes leading to their death. Thus, the

589

primary weapons of the innate immune system in the battle against the invading Staph, neutrophils and macrophages, are severely compromised. Without immediate therapy, an infection by CA-MRSA can quickly become a very serious disease.

Staphylococcus aureus has an exceptional ability to absorb the DNA and genes of other bacteria, even those of other genera. Analysis of *Staph aureus'* genome shows it is most likely related to the harmless soil bacterium *Bacillus subtilis*. But through the eons, *Staph's* ability to utilize the genetic information it appropriates from its fellow bacteria has turned it into an inhabitant and sometimes pathogen of humans. About 30% of people harbor *Staph aureus* on their body, usually in the anterior of their nose, sometimes in areas of elevated moisture. Staph colonization is not a problem, but the organism is set to pounce if there is a breach in our immune defenses. Because of the organism's ability to incorporate the DNA of many other microorganisms into its own genome, there are a vast number of strains of Staph. Some are highly virulent. Others are less virulent but, given the right circumstances, can still cause serious infections. Sometimes, the patient's status is as important as the virulence of the infecting pathogen.

Chapter 37
Imperiled Infants

Beautiful baby,
Source of joy, aspirations.
So vulnerable.

Humans have an innate and admirable instinct to protect and look out for our most defenseless. Not so the microbes that cause infectious diseases. They are programmed by nature to take advantage of whatever opportunity presents. Sadly, that includes our most vulnerable at the extremes of life, the very young and the very old. The immune system of newborns is not fully developed, and in the elderly, it is past its prime. That's not to say it is non-functional, but it's not at its optimum level of performance.

With infants, some microbes and their virulence capacities have a distinct advantage. As discussed in Chapter 36, Group B Strep is aggressive against newborns. *Listeria monocytogenes*, a bacterium usually contracted from dairy products, can seriously infect both mother and child (Chapter 16). Many babies are infected by the yeast *Candida albicans*, either as an oral infection or diaper rash, often both (Chapter 33). Cytomegalovirus, CMV, can sometimes infect infants, especially *in utero* (Chapter 31). *Bordetella pertussis* (whooping cough) can infect people of all ages, but it is especially dangerous when it attacks the very young (Chapter 17). The parasite *Toxoplasma gondii* is potentially harmful when the baby's mother is infected by it during her first six months of pregnancy (Chapter 26). Zika virus, spread by mosquitoes, can be devastating to the infant when it infects a pregnant woman (Chapter 23). Of course, many other microbial pathogens can infect infants just as they can infect the rest of the population. Three that can be merciless with infants deserve special attention: respiratory syncytial virus (RSV), rubella, and *Cronobacter sakazakii*.

The word syncytial (pronounced sin-SISH-el) comes from two Greek words, *syn*, meaning "together," and *cyto*, meaning "cell." Combining two or several human cells into one, with multiple nuclei and other cellular organelles, is not normal or desirable. Such an event is invariably the result of the activity of a microbe, usually a virus. As its name suggests, respiratory syncytial virus, often referred to as RSV, accomplishes this combination of cells very well.

RSV is an enigma. It is not a big virus, just ten genes and eleven proteins. Its genome is single-stranded RNA. When it reproduces inside a cell lining our respiratory tract, it doesn't make many copies of itself. The cells lining our respiratory tract are the only ones in our body to which it can attach and penetrate. That sounds non-descript, like many other viruses that cause upper respiratory tract infections (URI), usually called a common cold.

But RSV has several factors that distinguish it from other viruses causing respiratory tract infections. It can be a formidable pathogen, especially in the very young and people with compromised immune systems.

In medicine, one never says never or always; there are always exceptions. But with RSV, we are not too wrong in saying that all of us will contract the virus. Many of us get it twice or more. It spreads very easily. RSV is spread from person to person when they are close together, less than three feet apart. But it is a very hardy virus that can survive on environmental surfaces like furniture and clothing for several hours. Also, it can infect not only through the mouth but the nose and eyes. When one person has the virus, it spreads easily to all other household members.

Many viruses have one molecule on their surface which allows them to attach to the host cell's membrane and initiate penetration and replication. RSV has three such attachment molecules, the F, G, and SH proteins. The largest of these is the G, which is responsible for binding the virus to the outside of the ciliated columnar epithelial cells lining the trachea, the first step in infection after the virus enters the body. With some assistance from G, the F and SH proteins are responsible for the fusion of host cells, leading to syncytia formation. It is this cell fusion characteristic that makes RSV unique and potentially dangerous.

Unlike the adhesions of many other viruses, the F and G molecules are not just proteins. They are glycoproteins, the "glyco" referring to a carbohydrate moiety attached to the protein. We can produce antibodies to carbohydrates, but they tend to disappear after a few years with no immune memory. That means we become vulnerable to re-infection after our first episode. Babies' immune response to carbohydrates is very poor, and they may make few antibodies to the viral attachment glycoproteins or none at all. For the first six months of life, babies depend a great deal on the antibodies acquired from their mothers while in the womb for protection against RSV.

Other respiratory viruses exit the host cell after replication, with many newly formed virions wandering about seeking other cells to infect. RSV does that too, but it also moves from cell to cell by forcing their fusion, then simply migrating from one cell to another to continue replicating. Doing it this way, the virions are not exposed to the external environment, and the immune cells present there, thus protecting themselves. While the infection starts in the upper respiratory area, through syncytia formation and its hidden replication, the virus can work its way down to the lower respiratory system, namely the bronchioles and the alveoli. It is here that serious repercussions ensue.

RSV has a non-structural protein, NS2, which causes the cell the virus is infecting to round up, die, and slough off. RSV infection also stimulates the cells underlying the epithelial cells, those of the basal layer, to turn themselves into goblet cells. Goblet cells produce mucus, and with the increase in their number, more mucus is excreted into the airway. The result is inflammation with the accumulation of pus and mucus, potentially obstructing the airway.

As the virus works its way into the lungs and the inflammation increases, neutrophils and macrophages are attracted to the area. As they die off, their nucleic acids, primarily DNA, accumulate to form a matrix of sticky material, the so-called Nuclear Extracellular Traps (NETS). This material is very useful when dealing with bacteria, holding the microbe in place so other neutrophils can attack it. But when formed in the bronchioles and alveoli of the lungs during a viral infection, it only serves to hold the accumulated debris in place, exacerbating the situation.

This is especially worrisome in babies, as they don't have the strength to cough out the perilous material, and their breathing is compromised. Medical assistance is often essential to keep the young ones alive.

The action of our immune system, both innate and acquired, helps us counter the RSV attack. For most of us, RSV is a nasty cold that induces a productive cough that lasts about a week and then goes away. But the immaturity of the immune system of infants makes them more vulnerable.

The newborn relies heavily on the antibodies its mother produces, which are passed on to the baby in utero. If the mother does not have many or any antibodies to RSV, the infant is on its own to produce them, and at its young age, that can be a problem. Most of the mother's antibodies of all types are passed on to the baby in utero during weeks 35-40 of the pregnancy. If the baby is premature, a full amount and range of antibodies are not passed along, leaving preemies more vulnerable.

An essential part of our immune response to a viral invasion is the activity of cells known as plasmacytoid dendritic cells, abbreviated pDC. The pDCs recognize the presence of viruses by their unique viral molecular patterns. Unlike their dendritic macrophage cousins, the pDC don't act as antigen-presenting cells but serve to excrete type I and III interferons, alerting neighboring cells to the virus' presence. Alerted by interferon, these cells alter their receptors and metabolism, making it much more difficult for the virus to infect them. Unfortunately, the plasmacytoid dendritic cells are not well developed in infants, so their interferon levels and cellular resistance to RSV are not robust.

Besides antibodies, a critical component in controlling RSV infections are the killer lymphocytes, the CD8 cells. Matured in the thymus gland, the CD8 cells are primed to destroy any human cell harboring the virus, killing the virus along with it. In babies, the thymus gland is not mature, so the CD8 lymphocytes aren't yet up to the task. As we mature, our T-cell population becomes more efficient, so infections like those caused by RSV are more manageable. But as we grow into our older years, into our 70s and beyond, the effectiveness of our T-cells, including the CD8 variety, begins to wane, leading to greater vulnerability to RSV infections. It is estimated that over 10,000 older adults in the U.S. every year succumb to RSV infections.

Like most respiratory viruses, RSV infections are seasonal, with a rise in cases seen in late September and cases peaking in December through February. Numbers vary by year, but in the United States, annually, around two million children under the age of five are taken to a hospital emergency room because of RSV infection. About 60,000 to 80,000 need to be hospitalized, and several hundred die.

An effective vaccine could significantly reduce these dire numbers, but RSV presents a complex set of circumstances. Infants are most at risk, but their immune system is not advanced enough to handle a vaccine. A vaccine to protect them would have to be given to the mother, who would then pass her anti-RSV antibodies to her baby in the womb. The level of protection for the baby would be difficult to measure, especially in cases of premature birth.

The history of attempts to vaccinate babies against RSV infection is a tragic one. In the early 1960s, with the success of the polio vaccine as a model, it was felt that the RSV virus could be grown in tissue culture in the lab, de-natured with formalin, then injected as a vaccine. A trial was done. The result was catastrophic. Forty children were not given the vaccine and served as controls. Twenty-one of the forty in the control group went on to be diagnosed with RSV, and only one required hospitalization. Thirty children were given the trial vaccine. Twenty of the thirty went on to develop RSV, a higher rate than the control group. The most remarkable difference was the number of vaccinated children who required hospitalization, sixteen, who acquired the virus after vaccination. Two of the sixteen died of respiratory failure. Clearly, the trial vaccine against RSV had the opposite result of the one expected: not only did it not prevent the acquisition of the virus, but it also made the vaccine recipient more seriously ill when they did contract the virus. This tragic setback put a huge damper on RSV vaccine development for decades.

The apparent reason for the failure of the first RSV vaccine attempt was that the antibody developed by the babies had a poor avidity for the surface glycoproteins of the virus. The deactivated virus of the vaccine was loosely attached to an antibody but not inactivated. This led to the increased activity of T-cells, damaging the lung tissue when wild-type RSV was naturally acquired.

Today we have many more techniques available to produce vaccines. Administering the vaccine to the mother and allowing her to pass the antibodies to her infant in the womb is the method of choice.

The U.S. Food and Drug Administration has approved two vaccines protective against RSV for people over 65. There are two strains of RSV, A and B, with subtle genetic differences between them. The vaccines cover both strains. The vaccines are recommended for older people with potentially severe underlying health problems.

A commonly used monoclonal antibody is available to treat or prevent RSV. Palivizumab is a monoclonal antibody directed against the F protein of the virus. It can be administered to high-risk infants during the RSV season. It serves the same role as the mother's antibodies protecting the baby for the first six months after birth.

Respiratory Syncytial Virus is a ubiquitous pathogen uniquely equipped to infect billions of people. Most of us suffer a mild to moderate respiratory infection for a week or two. But it can be a life-endangering scourge to the most vulnerable of our population.

Rubella. The Latin word for "red" is *rubrum*. The technical term for measles is rubeola, owing no doubt to the red rash. At one time, it was felt that the disease we now call rubella was a minor variation of measles, and it was given the name rubella, meaning "little red." But the viruses aren't related. German researchers distinguished the two diseases in the early 19th century. Most of the information about the subject was published in German literature, so rubella, for a long time, was called "German measles." Of course, rubella isn't measles at all.

For many years rubella was considered a common, relatively minor childhood disease. Most children between the ages of two and seven got the disease, which persisted for just a few days with a mild fever, slightly swollen lymph nodes around the neck, and a mild rash. Recovery rendered one immune for life, and complications were rare. Other infectious diseases of childhood present in a similar fashion, including hand, foot, and mouth disease (caused by a Coxsackie virus, a type of Enterovirus), roseola (caused by herpes viruses 6 and 7), and fifth disease (caused by parvovirus B19). These viruses are unrelated, but the symptoms are similar when they infect. Usually, they are thought to be mild, nuisance-type diseases in young children. (The technical term for rash is exanthem).

The great significance of rubella came to the medical world's attention in 1941 when Australian physician Norman Gregg, an ophthalmologist, treated a very high number of infants with severe cataracts. In his own practice he saw 13 cases, an unusually high number. In consultation with colleagues, 65 more cases were encountered, a total of 78. A diligent investigator, Dr. Gregg took it upon himself to investigate this most unusual occurrence.

In 1940 there was a widespread outbreak of rubella throughout Australia. When the mothers of the affected babies were interviewed, 68 reported they had contracted German measles during their pregnancy, most of them in the first trimester. Further examination of the children revealed other problems, such as heart defects and deafness. Dr. Gregg wrote an eloquent description of his findings in a medical journal.

At the time, it was assumed that all congenital malformations were inherited due to genetic defects. Infectious agents were not considered. Dr. Gregg's work was groundbreaking. Initially, there was great reluctance to accept it outside of Australia, but eventually, the magnitude of the discovery was realized. The rubella virus was responsible for causing serious permanent damage to babies in utero. (Dr. Gregg was a gifted individual, excelling in athletics and academia. Colleagues described him as being affable, quick-witted, and having an easy smile. He was knighted for his work by Queen Elizabeth II in 1953; he is formally known as Sir Norman Gregg).

The extent of the damage done to the developing baby depends upon at what stage of the pregnancy the mother is infected with the virus. If she becomes ill during the first two months of pregnancy, there is about a 70-85% chance that the baby will be affected. If infection occurs during the third month, the chances are about 30%; during the fourth month, it is about 10%. The chances of the infant being affected if the mother is infected during the third trimester are rare. Also, babies affected early in the pregnancy more commonly develop a greater number of more severe abnormalities.

Many scientific and medical terms come from Latin, and the classification of rubella virus is one of the best uses of the language. The viral family is *Togaviridiae,* with "toga" referring to its prominent outer coat. Rubella, or *Rubivirus rubellae,* is unique in that it is related to viruses that infect through a mosquito bite, the alphaviruses. But rubella only infects by the respiratory route. Also, it only infects humans. It's something of an outlier, with no other viruses infecting humans closely related to it. Rubella is a small virus with only five proteins. Two of its proteins, E1 and E2, extend out from the virus' surface and are responsible for binding and entry into host cells. The RNA is single-stranded. It is positive sense, so it is transcribed soon after being introduced into the host cell. The combination of E1 and E2 is responsible for releasing the virus from the cell into the environment or an adjacent cell.

Infection by the rubella virus is not complicated. We breathe it in from an infected person, and it enters the upper respiratory tract cells and begins to reproduce. It then enters the cells of nearby lymph nodes, causing them to swell. Following that, the virus enters the bloodstream, a condition known as viremia (virus in the blood), and a mild fever usually accompanies that. By this time the immune system is fully activated, and immunity is quickly established. Adaptive immunity, both of the B-cell and T-cell variety, lead to a lifelong immunity to rubella. Get it as a kid, and you never have to worry about it again.

The major impact of rubella is its effect on babies early in gestation. Having the virus in the mother's bloodstream is critical, as the virus has a strong attachment to some of the cells of the placenta. After replicating in the placenta, the virus enters the developing fetus, which has little or no immune defenses during the early stages of development. In the latter stages of gestation, especially in the third trimester, the mother's antibodies enter the baby's bloodstream, enhancing the baby's immunity. But early in the pregnancy, maternal antibody in the baby is meager or nonexistent. The virus can replicate with impunity.

In the early descriptions of the congenital damage caused by prenatal infection by rubella, four conditions predominated: severe eye cataracts and glaucoma, deafness, heart problems, and mental retardation. It was later found that many more organ systems could also be affected. Fetal death is not uncommon.

The E1 and E2 attachment proteins can adhere to several receptors on human cells. Most are not known, but one that has been studied is myelin oligodendrocyte glycoprotein, MOG. Oligodendrocytes manufacture myelin, which covers nerve cells. By infecting these cells, rubella can wreak havoc on the baby's developing cells.

Rubella used to come around every four or five years. Some years were worse than others, and 1964-65 were particularly bad. In the U.S., there were over twelve million cases of the disease, with around 20,000 cases of congenital rubella reported. During the epidemic, a group of pediatricians at the University of Pennsylvania headed by Dr. Stanley Plotkin set about developing a vaccine for rubella. The researchers found that the virus changed over time by passing the rubella virus (a strain labeled RA27/3) on cells derived from a human fetus (cell line WI-38, for Wistar Institute) at reduced temperatures. The vaccine strain could infect cells weakly but produced no symptoms and was not spread from person to person. After clinical trials, the live attenuated rubella vaccine was widely available by the late 1960s. In 1971 it was incorporated with two other live attenuated vaccines, one for measles and the other for mumps, yielding what has come to be known as the MMR vaccine.

The reduction in the number of cases of rubella following the introduction of the vaccine has been astounding. What had been a common childhood ailment with over 90% of children infected came to be a rare, nearly extinct condition in the developed world. Unfortunately, that cannot be said for the underdeveloped areas of the world, where over 100,000 babies are born yearly with rubella-caused congenital abnormalities.

Cronobacter sakazakii. Most virulent microbial pathogens are well known. *Neisseria meningitis* causes meningitis, *Salmonella typhi* causes typhoid fever, and *Mycobacterium tuberculosis* causes tuberculosis. There are many other examples. They are widespread and found in millions of people. But a few organisms that can cause a devastating infectious disease are rare and attack only under a unique set of circumstances. Such an organism is *Cronobacter sakazakii*, whose primary victims are young infants, especially those who are bottle-fed with infant formula.

Cronobacter is a member of the bacterial family *Enterobacteriaceae* and is therefore related to *E. coli* and others commonly found inhabiting humans. But *Cronobacter* is not part of normal human flora. It is found in the environment and is mainly associated with plants. Older children and adults are not affected by the organism except under very rare circumstances. But young babies can be ravaged by it when exposed to a virulent strain.

When seen on common clinical laboratory culture media, the organism produces a dry, wrinkled colony that is very tough when touched by a wire loop. These characteristics distinguish the organism from other members of the *Enterobacteriaceae*. It was initially called *Enterobacter sakazakii*, but it was later determined that since it differed enough from the genus *Enterobacter*, it should be placed in another genus. Given the organism's propensity to seriously infect young babies, the name *Cronobacter* was selected. The name comes from the Greek god Cronos, who, in mythology, swallowed his own children out of fear that one of them would one day overthrow him. The species name sakazakii was assigned by researcher John Farmer in honor of Japanese bacteriologist Riichi Sakazakii in the 1980s.

Cronobacter sakazakii has several properties that allow it to cause disease. It tends to aggregate. Most bacteria are found in nature as single or a few organisms or in small clumps like Staph or chains of Strep. *Cronobacter* often aggregates into large clumps, thus allowing for the formation of a biofilm. It contains two outer membrane proteins that enable it to attach to epithelial cells, especially those of the intestinal wall. It also has surface proteins that allow the bug to bind to fibronectin, the "glue" that helps hold groups of human cells together. By an unknown mechanism, the organism can survive inside a macrophage and use it to carry it around the body. And, most unfortunately, *Cronobacter* can attach itself to the cells of the blood-brain barrier and gain entrance to the meninges and brain tissues.

One thing *Cronobacter* can't do very well is compete with other bacteria. The human gut is replete with billions of organisms, and *Cronobacter* has no chance of out-competing them for a place in the human gut. Except for babies. The microbiome of babies is not complete and is still assembling, giving *Cronobacter* an advantage. Also, the junctions between the intestinal cells of babies are not as tight as those of adults, and fibronectin, an attachment site for the organism, is readily available. So, in young babies, *Cronobacter sakazakii* finds the perfect opportunity: little competing bacterial flora, loose junctions between intestinal cells, lots of fibronectin, and macrophages that give them safe passage. After entering the bloodstream, the meninges present an attractive target, and crossing the blood-brain barrier is not difficult. Meningitis results. The result for the little baby is sepsis, meningitis, and possibly death. Sometimes the cells lining the baby's colon are killed and disrupted, leading to necrotizing enterocolitis, a severe condition of the intestinal tract.

Another feature of *Cronobacter* is its ability to survive in the wild. It resists drying, temperature extremes, and acid-base variations. It's a hardy little creature, and getting rid of it in the preparation of infant formula is not easy. Dry powder can't be boiled or pasteurized. *Cronobacter* grows on plant material and sometimes can find its way into the preparation. It resists drying and can hang around for a long time. If the manufacturer tests for its presence by culture, two problems present. Not all strains of *Cronobacter* are pathogenic, so isolating the organism while testing baby formula in the lab may be misleading. Also, the organism can enter a quiescent stage where it cannot be cultured but is still viable. Getting *Cronobacter sakazakii* out of baby formula is easier said than done.

Cronobacter grows on plant material, including fruits and vegetables. It's possible the organism can get onto the hands of a person working with produce and find its way into a baby bottle, one filled with either infant formula or expressed breast milk. Often the source of the organism in an infection is not apparent.

As pathogenic bacteria go, *Cronobacter sakazakii* is a crude outlier. It does not inhabit humans and isn't transmitted from person to person. While several factors allow it to invade the human body, older children and adults are not bothered by it. Only the very young are affected, and even there, only very rarely. But when it does attack, the result can be devastating.

Other organisms besides those mentioned here can infect babies. The sexually transmitted organisms *Neisseria gonorrhoeae* and *Chlamydia trachomatis* can cause disease in newborns if they acquire the organism from their mother. Eye infections are especially problematic. Organisms that typically infect the bloodstream, like syphilis, malaria, HIV, and others, can enter the baby *in utero* and cause a congenital infection. Good prenatal care of the mother is indispensable for a healthy infant.

Of course, the mother's health while carrying her baby is critical. The mother's T-helper lymphocyte population changes during pregnancy, shifting from a preponderance of the Th_1 variety to Th_2. The former are equipped for intracellular pathogens, while the latter are more involved in the humoral response to extracellular organisms. Sometimes this change in

T-cell organization can leave the mother more vulnerable to infections. The baby shares in that vulnerability.

Chapter 38
Peptic Predator

Stomach disrupter
Slithers under the surface.
Run silent, run deep.

Common knowledge. Conventional wisdom. Scientific consensus. Dominant ideology. Shared beliefs. Take it for granted. Some things in life, and medicine, are just accepted, probably because that's how it's always been, and no reasonable alternative exists. Some beliefs are held sacrosanct despite no compelling scientific evidence for support. Sometimes "facts" become so entrenched that their challenges are met with derision and ridicule.

It doesn't happen often, but a commonly held belief is sometimes proven wrong. Achieving widespread acceptance of the new theory is frequently fraught with years of frustration, squabbling, and often acrimony. Fortunately, scientific evidence is the foundation for medical opinion, and eventually, the truth will prevail. Such was the case for a common human ailment, peptic ulcers.

Ulcers were once common. They were mainly life-inhibiting, with bouts of intense stomach pain that could last several days. Often there was nausea, bloating, and loss of appetite. These episodes would come periodically and were usually treated with antacids and a "bland" diet.

Some ulcers were more serious. They were marked by intense, unremitting pain and hemorrhage. Surgery was sometimes necessary to stop the bleeding. A peptic ulcer could be fatal if medical intervention was unavailable or unsuccessful. Rarely, a patient with a peptic ulcer developed stomach cancer. Many suffered.

Such a common, painful, and often severe medical condition required an explanation. For many years the one widely accepted was the production of excess acid in the stomach. Stomach fluids are acidic under normal conditions, but it was supposed that the contents were more acidic than typical in some people. This excess acid was held responsible for the erosion of the stomach and duodenum lining, leading to ulcer formation. The reason for the extra acid formation was often attributed to the nervous state of the patient: some people, because of the stress in their life, produce more stomach acid and, as a result, suffer more from ulcers. The common term "case of nerves" was often used.

Proving such a hypothesis is obviously tricky, but some tried. In one experiment, mice were outfitted in little mouse straitjackets and lowered into near-freezing water, clearly a stressful situation. Their stomach contents were then measured for acidity, and, sure enough, it could be concluded that stress resulted in the formation of excess stomach acid.

With such a straightforward explanation for the malady, the remedy seemed clear. Consume antacids, cut down on stress, and eat bland, non-spicey foods to reduce the acidity of the stomach contents. The stress reduction part was the least medically controllable. It was not uncommon for ulcer sufferers to have their stress levels enhanced by thoughtless people essentially blaming them for their own trouble. "Calm down, you'll aggravate your ulcer!" "Your ulcer's all in your head!" Needless to say, this didn't help.

Barry Marshall was the ultimate "free-range" kid. He was born in 1951 in Kalgoorlie, a gold mining town 400 miles east of Perth, Australia. His father worked as a mechanic, and his mother was a nurse. They often moved around from job to job, and little Barry was never at a loss for adventure. He was a clever boy and had an insatiable need to find out how things worked. His father often accommodated him, showing Barry the inner workings of the machinery he worked on. Young Barry also had a great interest in his mother's medical books. After graduating from college, he chose to enter medical school. Internal medicine with an interest in research was his career goal.

Dr. Marshall spent the third year of his medical rotation at Perth Hospital in gastroenterology. Third-year doctors were required to do an investigative study, and around that time he met Dr. Robin Warren, a pathologist. The two struck up a friendship and often met in Dr. Warren's office in the hospital basement. During their conversations, Dr. Warren mentioned that he frequently observed some unusual, curved bacteria on biopsy specimens of stomach tissue submitted because of possible stomach cancer. At the time, the stomach was believed to be free of infection by bacteria because of the level of acidity present and the inhospitable environment it presented. By the early 1980s, with a hundred years of investigation into the causes of infectious diseases, no one had proposed that bacteria could cause a stomach infection. Coincidentally, a few years before, another small, curved bacteria, *Campylobacter*, had been proven to cause gastroenteritis, a disease similar to that caused by *Salmonella*. No one had seen that one coming either. Dr. Marshall was intrigued and got a list of patients with the mysterious stomach bacteria from Dr. Warren.

After doing a good deal of investigating, Dr. Marshall concluded that there likely was an association between these curved stomach bacteria and peptic ulcers. But there was trouble in proving it. The first step in demonstrating an organism's association with disease is the isolation and characterization of the bug. For bacteria, this usually means growing it in pure culture (the term "pure" means by itself, independent of other organisms). In 1982, the mysterious organism was only seen under the microscope in a pathology lab, so more work was needed. Dr. Marshall worked with members of the microbiology lab to try to grow the organism like other pathogenic bacteria they commonly worked with. Clinical specimens from biopsies and gastric washings were inoculated to solid culture media and placed in an incubator. After one and two-day incubations, the cultures were examined for bacterial growth. A simple, routine bacterial culture, but since the organism had never been described, it was hit-and-miss. The first attempts were unproductive.

Sometimes the culture plates were overgrown by non-pathogenic bacteria. Common bacteria can't survive long or multiply in stomach acid, but they can survive transiently. Bacteria on recently consumed food or resident flora of the mouth that is swallowed can easily gum up a culture of stomach material by growing rapidly and abundantly, overwhelming the culture media. Typically, culture plates are held in the incubator for 48 hours, and if no growth on the plates is observed, the cultures are discarded with the report "no growth in 48 hours." Such was the case in the first attempts to isolate the observed but not cultured stomach bacteria: overgrowth by commensal bacterial flora or no growth at all.

Sometimes, luck, or fate, intervenes. One day some cultures of stomach biopsy material were placed in the incubator as usual. But it was just before the Easter holiday, and the technician responsible for examining them took a few days off, and the culture plates were left unattended for several days. Lo and behold, when the plates were examined after an extended incubation, there were these mysterious-looking colonies. The same curved rod-shaped bacteria observed in the biopsy specimens were seen under the microscope when smears were made from the colonies. A prolonged incubation period was a necessary but unknown requirement for growing the organism.

We now know that the organism, *Helicobacter pylori,* has some demanding growth requirements in the laboratory, what clinical microbiologists call "fastidious." In the lab, they must be grown on nutrient-rich culture media supplemented with whole animal blood. They require oxygen, but it must be in reduced tension, only about 2-5% as opposed to the nearly 20% of room air (the requirement for reduced amounts of oxygen is called microaerophilic), and they need elevated levels of CO_2 (capnophilic). Also, on primary isolation from stomach material, the colonies take 5-7 days to grow, and even then, the colonies are small. They are translucent in appearance.

Now that the organism had been retrieved and described in laboratory culture, the next step was demonstrating that it could cause gastritis and peptic ulcers. It sounds simple enough, but there is one fundamental problem: common laboratory animals like mice and rats aren't infected by the organism. Dr. Marshall had treated several patients diagnosed with peptic ulcers with a regimen of antibiotics, not only getting them through an ulcer episode but also curing their ailment. With such promising results and no susceptible laboratory animals, the next move seemed obvious: give the organism to an uninfected human, see if the disease occurred, then try to cure it with antibiotics. But medical ethics being what they are, only one person could be infected: himself.

There was one slight hitch. Dr. Marshall was married, and he and his wife had four children. His wife, Adrienne, was a highly literate scientist and knew her husband's work well. In mulling it over, Dr. Marshall knew he would have to make a request of his wife. After pondering it for a while, he figured asking her forgiveness would be more fruitful than seeking her permission. So, after a biopsy showing he was organism free, it was down the hatch.

It didn't take long for his question to be answered. In a few days, he was overwhelmed by severe stomach pain, nausea, and vomiting. He looked and felt like death warmed over. There was no hiding this from his wife, so he fessed up. In addition to Dr. Marshall's health, her concern was for that of her children and their friends and acquaintances—this journey into the arena of scientific experimentation needed to cease. After a biopsy showed the presence of the organisms in his stomach tissue, Dr. Marshall took a regimen of antibiotics and was bug and symptoms free in a few days. His findings were revolutionary.

News of an event like that travels fast. At five o'clock one morning, an American writer called Dr. Warren, the pathologist, and asked him about the experiment. Dr. Warren, given to some hyperbole, told him it was true, adding that Dr. Marshall nearly died. It turned out the writer was not from a major reputable newspaper; he wrote for the "Star," a popular American tabloid usually seen in supermarket checkout stands and given to stories about such things as alien babies. But the word was out about the cause and cure of peptic ulcers. The trouble was that it wasn't accepted within the medical community.

Major breakthroughs in the field of medicine are rare, and when they occur, the news of their discovery follows a pattern. Major research centers using collaborative efforts by leading authorities issue press releases, hold news conferences, and experts not affiliated with the studies are interviewed and offer their support. In discovering *Helicobacter pylori* as the primary cause of gastritis, peptic ulcers, and stomach cancer, the leading investigators were two previously unknown individuals from Perth, Australia, with the worldwide announcement of the research first appearing in The Star supermarket tabloid. To say there was reluctance to accept the conclusions of the research is a tremendous understatement. Drs. Marshall and Warren had great trouble publishing their work in professional peer-reviewed journals and were often denied speaking engagements at international gastroenterology conferences. There reportedly were times when Dr. Marshall got up to speak, and attendees made a show of walking out of the venue. Radically changing accepted dogma is a challenging task.

In Australia, the acceptance of the work was easier, especially when the clinical success was so overwhelming. Eventually, researchers worldwide confirmed the nascent work done in Australia. It is now universally accepted that *Helicobacter pylori* is a prominent inhabitant of the human stomach worldwide, often causing gastritis, peptic ulcers, and occasionally stomach cancer. For their epic discovery, Drs. Barry Marshall and Robin Warren were awarded the Nobel Prize for Physiology and Medicine in 2005.

Helicobacter pylori is a crafty little creature. There is good evidence that it once colonized most humans, often causing debilitating, sometimes fatal, disease. Bacteria were first observed as causes of human illness in the 1880s, but *H.* pylori wasn't described as a potential pathogen until 1982. So, for 100 years, it was hiding in plain sight. The primary reason for the oversight is the organism's habitat within the body, the stomach and the upper small intestine (duodenum). These organs are awash in hydrochloric acid and digestive enzymes. Acid effectively kills bacteria, so to have an organism not just surviving but flourishing in this area seemed preposterous. But the bug is equipped with unique factors that make this remarkable feat possible.

Neutralizing the acid within the stomach is the top priority for *Helicobacter.* One of the breakdown products of protein is urea, a carbon with two amino groups attached. *Helicobacter* has a powerful enzyme, urease, that takes apart urea, yielding ammonia and carbon dioxide. The ammonia produced neutralizes acid, much to the benefit of the organism. The bug can also degrade short peptides with the same effect.

The physical features of *Helicobacter* give it an advantage in its environment. It has a spiral shape, allowing it to slither into nooks and crannies. It also has three powerful flagella, propelling it at great speed and enabling the bug to escape engulfment by neutrophils.

At some point, though, the organism must attach itself to cells lining the stomach. To do this, the organism has over a half dozen adhesins that allow the bug to attach itself to the cells lining the stomach, the extracellular matrix surrounding these cells, and the layer of mucin covering the stomach lining. By attaching to these surfaces, the toxic materials of the bacterium can be more easily transferred into the infected cells. In this infusion of toxins into host cells, the greatest damage of the organism to the stomach lining is seen.

Helicobacter has several toxins that can damage human cells, but two predominate. One is called cytotoxin-associated gene A, or CagA. The other is vacuolating cytotoxin A or VacA. CagA and VacA make a formidable one-two punch when both are present.

Helicobacter contains a secretion system used to inject toxin into a cell lining the stomach or duodenum. It acts similarly to the one found in *Salmonella*: the organism attaches to the human cell, a spike is formed outside the bacterium, the spike penetrates the host cell, and the toxin is injected into the cell. CagA is introduced into gastric and duodenal epithelial cells in this way. VacA attaches itself to the outside of the host cell, then enters. Once inside the human cells, the toxins begin their mischief.

CagA binds to and disrupts the actin cytoskeleton of cells. It also interferes with the junctions between cells. The affected cells round up and lose their form. Signaling inside the cell is altered, and the cell is greatly discomposed. VacA creates channels in the host cell membrane, so material from inside the cell flows out. It also can initiate apoptosis in the affected cell.

The net result of the activity of the *Helicobacter* toxins is the release of substances from the cell that the organism needs to survive. An important one is urea, which the bacterium can metabolize to neutralize stomach acid. Another is iron, an essential element for microbial growth.

The inflammation or erosion of the cells lining the stomach and duodenum is a condition known as gastritis. When *Helicobacter* invades and colonizes the stomach, gastritis results. The symptoms experienced are highly variable. Some individuals, like Dr. Marshall, become violently ill. Others have mild discomfort, and many have little or no symptoms. Some afflicted patients develop peptic ulcers, and a small percentage will develop stomach cancer. Once *Helicobacter* colonizes the stomach and settles in, it'll be there for life. The immune system is not able to clear it. Thankfully, though, antimicrobial agents that do a very good job of eliminating the pathogen are available.

There is clearly a wide display of symptoms in people whom *Helicobacter pylori* has infected. The reason why some are barely ill while others are severely affected can be summed up in two words...it depends. *Helicobacter* is extremely variable in its genetic makeup. In fact, just like fingerprints and snowflakes, no two strains infecting people are alike. Even in members of the same family who presumably infected each other, there are subtle differences in the genetic constitution of each person's bacterial strain. The organism's genome is subject to copying errors. Some people have strains with CagA and VacA toxins, some with only one, and others with neither. The molecular arrangement of the toxins can also vary, as can the attachment molecules' structure and the urease enzyme's strength.

People vary as well. Some have more acidic stomach fluid depending on their genetic makeup and diet. Our immune systems also show variability, with the power of cytokines differing among people. Neutrophils have a significant role to play in ulcer formation. Neutrophils are attracted by interleukin 8. In some people, the attraction of IL-8 is much stronger than in others, so the number and strength of neutrophils vary from one person to another.

Several organisms cause the illness known as gastroenteritis. The most common are members of the genera *Salmonella, Shigella, Campylobacter,* and select types of *E. coli.* The infections caused by these differing organisms follow a similar pattern: The organism is ingested, attaches to a segment of the bowel, unleashes its pathogenic brew of virulent materials, and the infected person's immune system counteracts the invader. Typically, after several days or a week of illness, the pathogen is removed, and the patient returns to health. Occasionally the individual becomes a carrier of the organism, shedding it with no ill effects to themselves. But for the most part, the infection is soon over, and the bug is gone.

With infection by *Helicobacter*, things are different. Soon after it infects, the patient experiences gastritis. The severity varies. It may present as a mild "upset tummy" or be a severe case of nausea, vomiting, bloating, and loss of appetite. As in cases of gastroenteritis caused by other organisms, the immune system is alerted, and a challenge to the invading microbe is mounted. The difference with infection by *Helicobacter* is that the organism is not cleared. The organism repels the immune response, and it stays in residence in the stomach. With other GI infections in which organisms not eliminated achieve a carrier state, the infecting bug rarely causes reinfection. Without laboratory tests, the patient is unaware that they still are colonized by the bacteria. But *Helicobacter*, once established, usually causes recurrent symptoms for many years.

Helicobacter invades the cells and mucin layer lining the stomach. With its flagella and spiral form, it slithers through the mucosal layer at considerable speed, making it a difficult target for neutrophils and macrophages. When it adheres to the epithelial cells it is firmly attached, which also impedes the pursuing phagocytes. To clear it, the adaptive immune system must be engaged and vigorous. Most pathogenic organisms can thus be readily cleared, but through the eons, *Helicobacter* has adapted adroitly to its encounter with the cells and molecules designed to eliminate it.

Lymphocytes known as CD-4 T-helper cells play a big role in controlling infections. Among this group of lymphocytes, the Th_1 group predominates in the cause to eliminate *Helicobacter*. When active and engaged, the TH_1 lymphocytes release interferon-gamma, a powerful attractant and activator of macrophages. Ideally, the macrophages will swoop into the area and engulf the invading bacteria, helping to

612

end the infection. TH_2 lymphocytes also are involved, inducing B-lymphocytes to produce antibodies. Another set of CD4 T-helper lymphocytes, known as the TH_{17} group, serves to attract neutrophils, which add to the elimination of the organism. Of course, the toxicity of the macrophages and neutrophils is high, and the process must be strictly regulated. The CD4 lymphocytes carrying out this job are the regulatory T-cells, the T_{reg} cells. They can dampen the inflammatory process and ultimately help prevent tissue damage by macrophage and neutrophil "friendly fire."

Helicobacter notably disrupts the activity of the Th_1 lymphocytes. The crux of the lymphocytes' activity is its ability to detect the invading bacteria and then send chemical signals to other immune system cells, such as macrophages. That's why they are called "helper" cells. The bacterial toxin VacA interferes with this process by inhibiting the chemical signals sent to the lymphocyte's nucleus to unleash the genes responsible for cytokine and interferon production. The net effect of this VacA interference is a diminished number of substances, such as interferon-gamma, produced. Without that attraction signal, the number of macrophages entering the infected area is reduced, as is the overall immune response.

Once activated by encountering the microbial antigen they are programmed to detect, lymphocytes normally begin to reproduce, making many more copies of cytokine-producing cells directed at the invading organism. *Helicobacter* produces an enzyme, GGT, that arrests the proliferation of lymphocytes. A second enzyme, arginase, metabolizes the amino acid arginine. For the bacterium, arginase accomplishes two tasks. Arginine is necessary for lymphocyte reproduction, so when it is in short supply, the cells don't replicate as efficiently as they should. In addition, when the bacterial enzyme metabolizes arginine, ammonia is produced, assisting the bug in counteracting the amount of acid in its environment.

Not only are the lymphocytes inhibited in their quest to send chemical signals and to reproduce, but *Helicobacter* also induces their death by apoptosis.

The result of these bacterial actions directed against the T-helper Th_1 cells is a standoff. The lymphocytes keep coming and are not entirely destroyed, but their activity is much less robust than needed. *Helicobacter* is able to persist.

Neutrophils, in addition to macrophages, play a major role in ridding us of invading bacteria. The eradication of *Helicobacter* from our stomach lining is no exception. To be involved, neutrophils must be attracted to the area, and a major factor in their migration is the activity of another CD4 lymphocyte, the Th_{17} cells. They're called Th_{17} cells because, when activated, they release the cytokine interleukin-17 (IL17), a powerful attractant for neutrophils. When lots of neutrophils swarm into an infected area, they gobble up the invading microbe, helping end the infection. However, *Helicobacter* has another trick it employs to help ensure its survival. It produces a molecule, IDO, that down-regulates the production of IL-17 by Th_{17} cells. That means fewer neutrophils than needed enter the infected area, giving the bacterium the advantage.

The T-helper lymphocytes must be tightly regulated lest they become overreactive and initiate tissue damage. Another T-helper CD4 lymphocyte carries out the control of the group, the one called the regulatory T-cell, usually abbreviated T_{reg}. The T_{reg} cells send down-regulating chemical signals to active CD4 lymphocytes, such as the Th_1, Th_2, and Th_{17} varieties, slowing down their activity. Without this control, there could be an overabundance of an immune response leading to tissue damage. *Helicobacter* has achieved the ability to encourage the conversion of naïve T-cells (those not yet directed to become a specific type of cell) to become T_{reg} cells. This overabundance of regulatory cells further dampens the immune response, favoring the bacterium.

Helicobacter pylori has been an uninvited companion of humans for thousands of years. An unusual bacterial predator, it doesn't cause an overwhelming, life-threatening disease in most people. In many, it persists unnoticed for the life of the infected person. Just how serious the infection can become depends upon several factors, including the organism's and the infected person's genetics. Worldwide, most individuals become infected as children, and their immune responses differ subtly from adults. As the infected child matures, the bacterium adapts until a balanced, steady-state existence is formed between the organism and host. Situations that disrupt that balance can lead to the emergence of significant diseases, including peptic ulcers and cancer. Stress is one factor that can diminish the immune response's activity, so perhaps the adage that high stress exacerbates peptic ulcers was on the mark.

Helicobacter is a carcinogen. Indeed, not everyone infected by it develops cancer, but some do. Two types of cancer predominate, adenocarcinoma and lymphoma. Besides the presence of the correct strain of the organism, many factors contribute, such as salt in the diet, genetic predisposition, other bacteria colonizing the stomach once *Helicobacter* raises the pH, and the amount of ulceration induced by the organism's activity and the immune system's response.

With the disruptive and long-term effects of the organism on the components of the immune system, there is reason to believe that *Helicobacter* infection can be associated with auto-immune diseases. Such associations are difficult to prove, and the mere presence of the organism in an afflicted patient is not proof of cause. But studies are ongoing.

Like most bacteria, *Helicobacter* can be treated relatively easily with antibiotics and antimicrobial substances. The Centers for Disease Control in the U.S. recommends that infections without symptoms do not need to be treated. In cases that require therapy, CDC suggests a multi-drug regimen. Reducing stomach acid with a proton-pump inhibitor (such as Prilosec or Nexium) heightens the activity of the antibiotics. Drugs like metronidazole (Flagyl), tetracycline, clarithromycin, and amoxicillin used in various combinations have proven effective. Also very useful are over-the-counter preparations containing bismuth salts (such as Pepto-Bismol).

There is reason to speculate that infection with *Helicobacter* is BENEFICIAL for some people. The organism is very good at reducing the degree of stomach acid. For some, removing the organism results in the over-production of acid in the stomach, potentially aggravating acid reflux disease. If the organism is present and no symptoms result from its being there, it may be best to leave well enough alone.

Of course, to treat *Helicobacter* in the stomach, you have to know it's there. Inserting a tube into the stomach and snipping off a bit of stomach lining for biopsy, analyzing for the presence of urease, culture, or PCR is one way, but it's a little drastic. Other less invasive tests are helpful. One that can be performed easily is to have the patient swallow a potion that contains urea that contains either carbon-13 or carbon-14, which can be detected by laboratory analysis. After swallowing the urea, the patient blows into a balloon. The content of the balloon is measured for the carbon type in the urea. Urea is broken down by urease to ammonia and CO_2. If the labeled CO_2 from the urea is found in the balloon, it is evidence of the presence of *Helicobacter pylori* in the stomach. The presence of the organism or parts of it in a stool specimen and the detection of antibodies to the organism in the blood are also useful tests when properly indicated and applied.

There are many fascinating details about *Helicobacter pylori*. It causes a range of disease states, from acute to chronic gastritis, peptic ulcers, mucosa-associated lymphoid tissue (MALT) lymphoma, and gastric cancer. The severity of some conditions can vary widely. Gastric cancer is the third leading cause of cancer deaths worldwide, and *H. pylori* is responsible for three-quarters of them. Peptic ulcers and gastric cancer cause over a million deaths yearly. Much has been learned since its discovery, including the means to diagnose and eradicate the bug. Hopefully, proper diagnosis and treatment can one day reach those who desperately need it.

Chapter 39
Consumption

Macrophage seeking
Malevolent red snappers.
The dreaded white plague.

Patrick Brunty was born in Northern Ireland on St. Patrick's Day, 1777, to a family of poor, illiterate farm workers. At an early age, Patrick showed academic prowess, and when he came of age, he was awarded a scholarship to Cambridge. Perhaps he felt his Irish heritage would be disparaged, so he changed his last name to Brontë, being particular about the insertion of the umlaut over the ë to lend it a touch of class. Little did he realize at the time that the name Brontë would become one of the most famous names in 19th-century English literature.

Patrick married Maria Branwell in 1812. They went on to have six children, five girls and a boy. After becoming an Anglican minister, Patrick accepted a post in the poor industrial community of Haworth in 1820. Theirs was apparently a happy family, with the father Patrick the primary educator of his children. Unfortunately, tragedy stalked the house. Wife and mother Maria, a bright, cheerful, well-educated woman, died of cancer at the age of 38. Her sister Elizabeth came to live with the family. Then the two eldest daughters, Maria and Elizabeth, died at ages 11 and 10, respectively. The three remaining daughters, Charlotte, Emily, and Anne, became very talented writers of high notoriety, their works greatly influencing English literature. But they too would experience early deaths, Anne at age 29, Emily at 30, and Charlotte at 38. Their brother Patrick also died early, at age 31. The father, Patrick, outlived his wife and all his children.

What struck most of the Brontë family was a disease that has been with human beings for as long as there have been human beings. Ancient writings from several different cultures refer to it, and examinations of skeletons of early ages attest to its presence. But with the advent of the industrial revolution in the early 19th century and its attendant overcrowding, poor ventilation, poor nutrition, and lack of sanitation, the disease tuberculosis exploded in numbers, killing millions indiscriminately.

TB has had several names throughout the ages, some associated with two of its major symptoms, weight loss and hemorrhage. The Greeks referred to it as phthisis (pronounced "thigh-sis"), from their word for "wasting away," *phthinein*. A more modern term was "consumption" because the disease " consumed " the patient. Another common name was "the white plague," owing to the facial pallor due to anemia. The term tuberculosis, from tubercle, was first used in the early 1800s when it was discovered that the disease is not confined to the lungs but can infect other tissues. The nodules formed on infected tissues resembled "tubers" (fleshy outgrowths); "-cle" meaning miniature.

The organisms that cause TB are members of a genus with an enormous number of species, *Mycobacterium*. It's an odd sort of bacterium with a peculiar name. The prefix *Myco* refers to fungus or toadstool, clearly having nothing to do with bacteria. The reason for the term is that when grown on artificial media in the laboratory, the colonies the organism forms resemble those formed by some fungi. In nature, there are close to two hundred species of *Mycobacteria* that inhabit many and varied habitats, often in dirt and water. Most have nothing to do with infectious diseases.

But one group of *Mycobacterium* many millennia ago became associated with humans and animals and has since become entirely dependent on them for their existence. The main species of this group that infects humans is *Mycobacterium tuberculosis*. A half dozen other closely related species can infect animals and cause the same symptoms in humans, but they are rare. We often use the term *Mycobacterium tuberculosis* complex to include these other species.

Mycobacterium is a unique, disparate group, different from other bacteria in several ways. The chief difference lies in their cell wall, which contains several distinct features. Nearly all bacteria have the substance peptidoglycan in their cell walls. It is a complicated structure combining carbohydrates (glycan)

618

and peptides, short strands of amino acids (peptido). Peptidoglycan (PG) is a strong mesh-like structure that gives the bug its shape and keeps it from coming apart because of the internal pressure of the cell. The PG layer of mycobacteria is like that of typical bacteria but with a few tweaks. Those minor variations allow it to connect to the "secret weapon" of mycobacteria, a thick, wax-like substance called mycolic acid. Gram-negative organisms like *E. coli* have lipids in their cell wall, but mycobacteria take the lipid content to a much higher level. This thick layer on top of the bacterium's cell wall serves several functions. For one, it enables the organism to stay alive inside the cell designed to kill it. It also prevents the entry of substances that may harm it, such as antibiotics.

TB is a respiratory infection, so it would be easy to liken it to the viruses that infect by the same route. But TB is much different than viruses like influenza and coronavirus. It's a bacterium and therefore much larger and heavier than the viruses. Also, TB doesn't infect the upper airway like the throat, larynx, or trachea. Its target is the lungs themselves. So, TB is much harder to "catch" than the viruses are. Typically, one must inhabit the same confined space as the infected person who is actively coughing and expectorating aerosols containing the organism. Spread of the infection occurs almost exclusively indoors, mainly in smaller confined rooms. After the expulsion of the organism from an infected individual in the form of an aerosol, the moisture surrounding the organism evaporates, leaving the organism suspended and wafting in the air. The more organisms in a room and the longer people congregate there, the greater the chance of its spread to an uninfected person.

Even when the organism within the aerosol is inhaled, a vital protective mechanism is in place to repel it. The mucus in the respiratory tract traps them, and the constantly beating cilia on the epithelial lining expel them. When functioning properly, it is a very efficient system. But, of course, this elegant scheme can break down when overburdened by environmental factors, like lots of dust, grit, smoke, and other assaults. This can open the door for some of the inhaled TB germs to make their way straight to the lungs.

Once the organism gets to the alveoli and surrounding tissues of the lungs, it encounters the pulmonary macrophages, cells tasked with keeping the lungs' inner workings free of foreign material, both microbes and inanimate substances. We each have billions of these cells constantly employed in healthy lung tissue, and they are very good at their job. Unlike our other vital organs, the lungs are exposed to the environment, and keeping them sterile is a full-time job.

Most bacteria that enter the lung tissue are harmless commensal organisms that are dealt with in quick order. The macrophage engulfs them within a phagosome, a lysosome combines with the phagosome within the macrophage, and toxic granules kill the organism. Some pathogenic bacteria have devised mechanisms to avoid the engulfment by the macrophages. Most notable is the organism *Streptococcus pneumoniae,* which, as its name suggests, is a common cause of pneumonia. It has a thick capsule of carbohydrate designed to make the job of engulfment by the macrophage more difficult, giving it time to set up an infectious process. Other organisms that cause pneumonia have similar weapons.

Mycobacterium tuberculosis (MTB) is different. Instead of avoiding the macrophages designed to kill them, MTB seeks them out, and its heavy lipid, wax-like outer membrane makes it very easy for the macrophages to engulf them. But once inside, within the phagosome, the bacterium gets the upper hand. Normally, the lysosome fuses with the phagosome and the organism's death results. But for MTB the result is altogether different. The lipid layer of the organism prevents the fusion of the lysosome with the phagosome. In fact, the phagosome itself unravels, releasing the organism into the cytoplasm of the macrophage, where it can multiply unfettered. Instead of being a killing machine, the macrophage is now an incubator for cultivating more *Mycobacteria.*

In addition to killing the invading organism, the macrophage sends chemical signals alerting other immune system components that trouble is afoot. Chief among these are interferon-gamma (IFN-γ) and tumor necrosis factor-alpha (TNF-α), which attract other macrophages into the area. Inside the infected initial macrophage, the organism is multiplying,

620

eventually killing the host cell. The freed organisms can now infect the attracted macrophages with the same fate as the initial one, multiplying with impunity. This sequence of events continues until many new organisms are produced.

Meanwhile, other members of the immune system are alerted, chiefly T-helper cells and other macrophages. They close ranks around the growing number of *Mycobacteria* inside the macrophages, forming a cellular capsule around it. *Mycobacterium* is not motile, so they stay in a confined location. This surrounding group of cells, along with the fibrin and other matrix material accompanying it, is called a granuloma, since the macrophages involved contain granules. The suffix "oma" refers to its resemblance to a tumor. Other entities can lead to the formation of granulomas: other bacteria, fungi, parasites, and even some human tissue that gets in the wrong place. But granulomas are characteristic of TB and are a very helpful diagnostic tool.

In tuberculosis the center of the granuloma becomes necrotic and assumes a dull white appearance, something like soft cheese. The Latin word for cheese is *caseus*, and granulomas with this type of necrotic center are referred to as caseating granulomas.

Mycobacterium tuberculosis is a very slow-growing organism. Some bacteria can reproduce every twenty minutes in the proper culture media. MTB takes around twenty hours. Being non-motile, it depends on the immediate environment for its nutrients, and since it is stuck in the middle of the granuloma there isn't much available. So it enters a state of quiescence, still alive but not doing much. This is the best outcome for the afflicted patient, having the bacterium in the latent state. As long as there are plenty of active CD4 lymphocytes this latent state persists, usually for many years.

Problems arise when the person's immune system breaks down. There are many causes for such a reduction in the immune response, some more impactful than others. Malnutrition, other diseases both physical and mental, medical therapies that affect immune status, continued exposure to harmful environmental conditions, and genetic alterations in some of our immune constituents play a large part. Getting infected by the organism isn't a sentence of overt tuberculosis. Other conditions play a significant role.

The major problem in tuberculosis is the formation of a cavity in the lung. When confined to an individual granuloma, that organism isn't very damaging. It assumes a latent stage and transmission to other individuals is not a concern. If the granuloma breaks down, however, the organisms leak out into nearby bronchial airspace and begin to proliferate wildly with the abundance of oxygen present in the lung. A cavity forms within the area. While the number of bacteria in a granuloma is in the low hundreds, the number in a cavity is in the tens of millions. Tissue destruction occurs, and at this point the prognosis is poor.

Sometimes the organism can enter the bloodstream and be carried throughout the body, potentially infecting several organs outside the lungs. The lungs, too, can be infected over again in multiple locations. When first observed in the early 1700s, the small growths throughout the organs were described as resembling millet seeds, and the term applied was miliary TB. Multiple organs, including the bones, can be infected, and it is a grave medical situation.

Because of its means of infection, inside macrophages and sequestered in granulomas, the humoral defenses of antibody and complement have little effect on the course of illness. Antibody is produced, but it is inconsistent. A little is made against the organism's cell wall, but more against the interior components and proteins, which, by its nature, gives an inconsistent pattern. The overwhelming immune response to infection by *Mycobacterium tuberculosis* is the cellular response led by macrophages and T-cells. Fortunately, we have a test to utilize this activity to aid in identifying those infected.

The tubercle bacillus was first grown in culture and identified in the laboratory of German researcher Robert Koch in the 1880s. It was a monumental achievement, and Dr. Koch received the Nobel Prize for his work in 1905. Shortly after the discovery of the organism, a skin test was devised using organisms that were killed, purified, and injected into the skin. People who had the organism in their body gave a reaction of swelling and induration (hardening) at the site of the injection. The original preparation was very crude, and it was improved upon by several workers, most notably French investigator Charles Mantoux in 1907. Even his better version needed revision and standardization, and it wasn't until the 1930s that a reliable preparation was available. It goes by several names, including the Mantoux test, PPD (for purified protein derivative), and tuberculin. The material is injected into the dermal layer of the skin, usually between the crook of the elbow and the wrist. If the person being tested harbors the organism, the injection site becomes swollen and hard after two or three days. (Redness doesn't count).

When injected into the skin, the material from the organism is internalized by macrophages in the area. Inside the macrophages it is processed, and small parts of the material are placed upon an MHC molecule, prominently displayed, and transported to the macrophage's surface. T-cells that have been previously activated by the presence of the organism in the body recognize the microbe's antigens being displayed by the macrophage, proliferate at the site, and the tissue damage ensuing results in the creation of the hardened area at the site of the injection. It takes about 2-3 days for this to take place. Done properly, the TB skin test is usually very reliable.

Another way of detecting T-cells that have been activated by *Mycobacterium tuberculosis* is to draw a blood sample and expose the lymphocytes in the sample to antigens of the organism. The T-cells' first response is to elicit interferon-gamma, which can be detected by chemical analysis. The blood must be tested shortly after being drawn to ensure the lymphocytes remain alive. The main advantage over the skin test is that no follow-up visit is necessary. For the skin test the tested individual must return within 2-3 days to have the test read. Both tests are subject to false positives and negatives, but, in the big scheme of things, they are very useful tools in determining the presence or absence of *Mycobacterium tuberculosis* within the tested person.

In developed countries, most people don't need to be routinely tested for the presence of TB. Healthcare workers who may have been exposed, laboratory workers, arrivals from countries where the disease is endemic, and anyone known to have been around someone diagnosed with tuberculosis are routinely tested.

The unique properties of the organism make laboratory work challenging. The bug is slow growing, has a very peculiar cell wall making it hard to stain, and it infects deep in lung tissue, not the upper respiratory tract. Specimen quality is very important. Applying routine laboratory techniques is insufficient to detect the organism; specialized procedures are required.

A representative specimen is critical to all laboratory testing. For pulmonary tuberculosis, the easiest specimen to obtain and the least expensive is the expectorated sputum sample. That's sputum, from deep in the lung, not saliva. Merely spitting into a specimen cup is inadequate if all that comes out is colorless, foamy saliva. What's needed is the gunky stuff from down below. Often the best way to obtain this better material is when the patient first wakes in the morning; sputum tends to accumulate during sleep. Sometimes a fine mist of an aerosol can be breathed in to loosen the material and help cough it up. If this doesn't work, a tube can sometimes be inserted down the trachea and material aspirated.

The routine stain applied to clinical material to observe bacteria is the Gram stain. Mycobacteria don't stain very well with this technique, however, often giving a speckled appearance or no staining at all. Particular to mycobacteria, though, is the fact that their cell walls make them resistant to the penetration of organic solvents as well as acid. This fact has given rise to the term "acid-fast," and they are collectively referred to as acid-fast bacilli. A staining technique known as the Ziehl-Neelsen stain is routinely done in clinical laboratories to detect the presence of mycobacteria. The bacteria do not divide evenly side by side or end to end like other organisms; they just sort of randomly snap off the mother bug. Since they stain red from carbo-fuchsin application, lab folks call them "red snappers."

Most mycobacteria grow very slowly; the TB bacillus takes around three weeks to show a colony on culture media.

Other bacteria in the sample, if it was collected through the mouth, grow much faster and will destroy the culture media before the mycobacteria have a chance to grow. To compensate for this, a sputum sample can be treated with two ingredients, one to digest and homogenize the sample by neutralizing the mucus, and another to kill the competing bacteria while sparing the mycobacteria. For the former, n-acetyl-cysteine is usually used (NAC), and for the latter, sodium hydroxide (NaOH) is commonly used since it doesn't kill mycobacteria at the concentration employed.

The smear and culture for mycobacteria, usually just called AFB for acid-fast bacilli, is not perfect but still can be very helpful in both establishing a diagnosis of active TB, and ensuring that a patient is not infectious during the early stages of therapy. Smear and culture are of no use in diagnosing patients with latent TB because they are not shedding organisms. That's where skin testing and interferon-gamma tests come in.

About 90% of people infected by *Mycobacterium tuberculosis* do not show signs of TB. Their cellular response to the infection is sufficient to keep the organism at bay. Some people, though, are overwhelmed by the infection. Also, changes in immune status, such as those which occur with malnutrition, immunosuppressive medications, exposure to noxious chemical aerosols, or infection with human immunodeficiency virus (HIV), can lead to the emergence of tuberculosis.

The most common symptoms of active TB are not universal but, when present, can point strongly to the diagnosis. One is unexplained weight loss over a month or two time period. Another is continuing night sweats, and a third is blood in the sputum. These are not unique to TB, but they certainly lead the physician to look in TB's direction. X-rays are also very distinctive in most cases.

Throughout human history the diagnosis of TB was close to a death sentence. Certainly there were attempts at treatment, but folk remedies and other such pursuits were futile. A new approach to treatment that often proved successful was introduced in Europe in the early to mid-1800s, the sanatorium.

For a long time, it had been the practice of wealthier people to go to health spas, seeking rest, relaxation, and more than a little pampering. Sometimes mineral springs were involved. This type of environment inspired the creation of sanatoria, and they began to multiply toward the end of the 1800s and early 1900s when the cause of TB became known. (The words saniTARium and sanaTORium are today often used interchangeably. But the clinics for treating TB were referred to as sanatoriums. The Latin root of the word is *sanitorius*, meaning "health-giving." The root for sanitarium is *sanitas*, meaning health. Changing a few vowels was done to distinguish the two).

In the era before antibiotics, sanatoriums offered the best treatment available when used correctly. Perhaps most importantly, they were located in remote areas, thus isolating infected people and preventing disease spread. While it is impossible to prove, the treatment of tuberculosis with fresh air, good nutrition, sunshine, and rest has a lot going for it.

Most TB patients contract their infection by being indoors with poor ventilation and particulate matter in the air. Fresh air, with open windows and doors with screens, minimizes the amount of extraneous matter entering the lungs, allowing the pulmonary macrophages to concentrate on fighting the infection.

Proper nutrition, including protein, vitamins, and fluids, provides the foundation for the immune system to react energetically to the infectious process and, just as important, to the rebuilding process. TB damages lung tissue: it needs to be repaired efficiently.

Vitamin D activates the genes responsible for releasing cathelicidin, an anti-microbial compound found in macrophages. Cathelicidin attacks the membrane of bacteria such as *Mycobacterium tuberculosis* and attracts T-cells and macrophages to the infected site. For a long time, it was known that cod liver oil was helpful in treating TB in some patients. This is because it is rich in vitamin D. For patients who were deficient in vitamin D, supplements like cod liver oil boosted the immune response.

Vitamin D is activated by sunlight. Having enough vitamin D in the body (over 30 nanograms/ml) and having it activated by sunlight is a good thing. Sunlight quickly dries out

626

the droplet nuclei of expectorated respiratory material, and the UV portion kills the bacteria.

Rest and lack of exertion remove the strain on the lungs, allowing them to heal faster. *Mycobacterium tuberculosis* is a strict aerobe, requiring oxygen for growth. Most infections occur in the upper lobes of the lungs. Reclining reduces oxygen tension in the upper lobes, presumably slowing the organism's growth.

With the introduction of anti-microbial agents to treat TB in the late 1940s and early 1950s, sanatoriums were suddenly out of favor. And it's no wonder. Patients had to leave their homes and live for many months in a remote place that was, for all intents and purposes, like a prison. They were confined to bed the entire time, with only reading material for entertainment. The mental strain was considerable. But there were undoubtedly many successes in the treatment of TB in the sanatoriums, though it is impossible to assess just how many recovered there versus how they would have done if treated at home.

Albert Schatz made one of the greatest scientific discoveries of all time. He was born in the northeastern United States in 1920 to a family of farmers who had emigrated from Europe. He planned on becoming a farmer as well, and to edify his knowledge of the subject he entered one of the top agricultural schools of the country at the time, Rutgers University in New Jersey. It just so happened that one of the pre-eminent researchers in soil microbiology, Selman Waksman, was doing research at Rutgers. Albert, who graduated at the top of his class, was attracted to the work the Waksman team was doing.

This was the 1940s, and with the war raging, Albert was drafted into the U.S. military. Because of his laboratory experience, he was assigned to a medical laboratory unit in Florida. There he became acquainted with human pathogens and their cultivation. After injuring his back, he was discharged from the military and returned to pursue his doctorate at Rutgers. Upon returning, he found that the laboratory was vigorously searching for new antibiotics. The university's expertise was soil microbes, and after the discovery of penicillin, it was felt that that was a fruitful avenue of research. In fact, the Waksman team had discovered three antibiotics from soil bacteria that killed Gram-negative bacteria, something penicillin didn't do. Unfortunately, they were too toxic for human use, but the door was open for further inquiry.

The genus *Mycobacterium* is soil-dwelling. While *M. tuberculosis* is confined to humans, its soil relatives live out their existence in environments shared with other soil microbes. Researchers at the Mayo Clinic in Minnesota suggested to Selman Waksman that, given his research department's expertise in soil bacteriology, it might be worth trying to find an antibiotic from a soil bacterium that interfered with the growth of *Mycobacterium tuberculosis*. Given the danger of working with the organism in the laboratory, Dr. Waksman opposed the idea. But Albert Schatz was intrigued and volunteered to take on the project for his graduate studies.

Albert was given some laboratory supplies and relegated to the basement, where he spent the better part of a year. Often sleeping on a wooden laboratory bench and equipped with a few amenities, he spent most of his time down there. But it paid off. Working with two women assistants, Doris Jones, and Elizabeth Bugie, the team was able to report in 1943 that a substance isolated from the soil bacterium *Streptomyces griseus* killed both Gram-negative and Gram-positive bacteria and, in fact, seemed to be effective against a strain of *Mycobacterium tuberculosis.* Subsequent testing in mice bore these results out, and the new antibiotic was sent to the Mayo Clinic for testing in humans. It proved a phenomenal success. A new era of antibiotic treatment for tuberculosis had begun. The antibiotic was called streptomycin.

The chemical company Merck, with facilities in both the U.S. and England, put its full resources into the development of streptomycin, and by the dawn of the 1950s it was the treatment of choice for TB. But there were problems. For one, streptomycin must be administered parenterally, that is intravenous or intramuscular; it cannot be taken orally. And unlike the treatment for other bacterial infections like strep throat or urinary tract infection, treatment for TB takes several months, so patients had to be hospitalized or in constant contact with doctors and nurses. Also, streptomycin can display adverse side effects like dizziness and unsteady feeling, hives on various body parts, and nausea and diarrhea. These are more apparent when the drug is administered over many months. Worst of all, the organism MTB can develop resistance during therapy. But all in all, the introduction of streptomycin lent hope to many for whom death was likely.

A notorious side story to the development of streptomycin was the behind-the-scenes intrigue of the people involved. Selman Waksman was the laboratory director in which the discovery was made. He was a widely recognized authority on the subject of soil bacteria. Albert Schatz, at the time of the discovery, was a graduate student working under the direction of Dr. Waksman. It was Schatz who camped out in the lab basement, inches away from a deadly bacterium for months on end. It was his relentless effort that brought the discovery to fruition, and his name was first on the first paper published on the matter. But all credit went to Dr. Waksman, who would receive the Nobel Prize for the discovery. Albert Schatz's name was never mentioned or acknowledged. Nor were the names of the two women who assisted him with the research. Not only that, but Dr. Waksman had also persuaded Albert to forego all royalties for the discovery, those in turn going to a foundation at Rutgers University and ultimately benefitting Dr. Waksman. Litigation ensued, and the entire affair became a messy blight on one of the most important discoveries of human history.

Streptomycin attacks the protein synthesis of bacteria by attaching itself to a portion of the bacterial ribosome. The main bacterial ribosomes are designated as 30S and 50S. It is the 30S ribosome to which streptomycin binds, disrupting the construction of growing proteins. Because of its chemical structure, streptomycin is classified as an amino-glycoside. It was the first of this class discovered. The group is used today mainly in treating infections caused by Gram-negative bacteria. The aminoglycosides do not by themselves enter the cytoplasm of bacteria. They must be actively transported in, and this transportation step leads to most of the resistance seen in the group.

With the end of World War II and the progress made in developing the first antibiotics, sulfa, penicillin, and streptomycin, much effort was put into finding new drugs. The realization that the first anti-microbial discovered, sulfadiazine, had been formulated many years before its application to infectious diseases prompted the search for similar previously created but unappreciated compounds. Two were found to combat TB: Para-aminosalicylic acid and Isoniazid. To make it easier to say, the names were reduced to letters, PAS and INH. (INH refers to the drug's chemical name, **I**so**N**icotinic acid **H**ydrazide). In the early 1950s, these two, along with streptomycin, were the standard treatment for TB. Unfortunately, resistance to each developed rather readily in the slow-growing bacteria, but it was found that cure rates were much higher when they were used in combination, a practice that continues today.

Other antibiotics were discovered through the years, including rifampin and ethambutol. A standard course of treatment for active TB today uses four drugs in combination, rifampin, isoniazid, pyrazinamide, and ethambutol, commonly referred to as RIPE. Other situations, such as positive skin test without symptoms or those at high risk, have different regimens.

However, a major problem has been encountered worldwide with the development of drug-resistant strains. Some TB bacteria are multi-drug resistant (MDR), defined as resistance to both rifampin and isoniazid. Extremely drug-resistant strains (XDR) are resistant to those two plus two others. Some choices of drugs remain, but they are less effective. An important reason for the emergence of these drug-resistant strains is the partial treatment of the disease. Some patients take their medication for abbreviated periods, either through neglect, fear of side effects, or non-availability of the drugs. This allows the bug to develop resistance, as those strains are given time to multiply when the drug is discontinued. These resistant strains can then be spread to others, with the initial infection due to a resistant strain.

There are several words that best describe the vaccine for tuberculosis: confusing, bewildering, perplexing, baffling, disconcerting, complicated. Sometimes exasperating applies. Even the name of the vaccine is unusual, just the three letters BCG, which don't suggest the targeted disease like most vaccine names do. The vaccine has been in use for a hundred years, but many questions remain about the extent of its effectiveness.

In the early 1900s, it was known that tuberculosis was caused by the bacterial organism *Mycobacterium tuberculosis*. It was also known that cattle had a similar disease, and the organism could be found on the cow's udder. Two French researchers working at the Pasteur Institute in Lille, France wondered if the phenomenon observed in smallpox could apply here– could a strain of tubercle bacilli infecting cows be used to vaccinate humans with minimal side effects? In 1908 Albert Calmette and Camille Guerin began passing a bovine isolate of TB on successive culture plates. In 1913 they felt it was ready for human trials, but World War I intervened. The vaccine had to wait until 1921. It was called "Bacille Calmette-Guerin," BCG.

During the 1920s BCG was mainly given to infants by the oral route. It proved to be safe. The questions were about its effectiveness. Those questions persist today.

Putting a huge damper on the use of BCG was the infamous "Lubeck Disaster." In Lubeck, Germany in 1930, infants were routinely administered the BCG vaccine by the oral route. Tragically, the vaccine material was contaminated with viable pathogenic *Mycobacterium tuberculosis* in the laboratory in which the vaccine was prepared. Seventy-three infants died, and another 135 were sickened but recovered. The tragedy cast a pall over the use of BCG. An investigation showed the means by which the vaccine strain was contaminated with viable virulent organisms, but questions remained. Indeed, many today who question vaccination in general point to the Lubeck Disaster.

Eventually, the BCG vaccine came to be used again, but there have always been questions about its effectiveness in preventing tuberculosis. Studies have varied significantly in their conclusions. There are several reasons for the confusion:

BCG doesn't prevent most people from contracting *Mycobacterium tuberculosis*. The best that can be hoped for is the disease won't progress as rapidly.

There are over two hundred species of mycobacteria, most of which live in the soil. There is some evidence that exposure to a wide range of mycobacteria will prime the cellular immune system to be more effective in combating *Mycobacterium tuberculosis* should it infect. Perhaps some people, because of where they live, have already acquired a low level of resistance to TB regardless of BCG administration.

There are four strains of BCG bacteria in use in the world today. Comparing one strain's effectiveness against another can be tricky. Also, immunity to TB depends on cellular immunity, with lymphocytes and cytokines playing a significant role. The genetics of people within a population can render some groups more susceptible to TB than others in a different geographic location, confounding conclusions about a vaccine that is only partially effective in subduing the disease.

Infestation with parasites can alter a person's immune responses. In areas of the world with a greater likelihood of TB, there is often a greater number of people infested with parasites. The net effect on the immune system and its response to infection by *Mycobacterium tuberculosis* is difficult to quantify when the parasite burden is high.

These and other questions abound. Each country of the world makes its own decision about the recommendation of vaccination against tuberculosis with BCG. The United States has never recommended its use. Other countries do. There is no doubt that BCG has saved millions of lives and prevented untold misery. One thing that always must be remembered, BCG is a live vaccine, and anyone receiving it will test positive with a tuberculin skin or blood test.

In the U.S. and other developed countries tuberculosis is no longer endemic. Most of the cases that are diagnosed originate in other countries. Diagnostic tools and therapy, along with vigorous public health intervention, help keep it under control. But worldwide, it remains a scourge. Well over a million deaths are recorded yearly, and millions more have their lives severely impacted by the disease.

Leprosy. The infectious disease leprosy has, of course, been known since ancient times, with frequent mention of it in the Christian Bible, both Old and New Testaments. The word "leper" has become a metaphor in the English language, meaning much more than the victim of a well-differentiated infectious disease. Leprosy is a very painful malady with severe neurologic damage and disfigurement. It is a chronic ailment, taking years of absolute misery to run its course. Leprosy doesn't kill; it leaves its victim in a state of ill health for decades. Of course, there is also the social dimension of the disease, with aversion, shunning, and loneliness in addition to the chronic symptoms. In many ways, leprosy is as bad as it gets.

Because of the stigma of the word leprosy, the name of the disease was officially changed to Hansen's Disease in honor of the Norwegian physician Gerhard Hansen, who recognized the condition as infectious. He first reported that bacteria were associated as a probable cause in 1873, a remarkable achievement considering the technology of the time. But most workers today still refer to the original term, leprosy.

Fortunately, leprosy in the developed world is extremely rare. Doctors, even infectious disease specialists, may never see a case of it during an entire career. But unfortunately, the disease is not extinct, and thousands of cases are seen each year around the world.

When the average person hears of an individual with a case of leprosy there is a tendency to think the worst: severe disfigurement. But people with the disease display an extensive range of symptoms. Some show only a few signs of skin lesions that don't multiply over time; they remain static and are more of a nuisance than a threat. This level is known as the tuberculoid type. Others, at the other end of the spectrum, experience the very worst symptoms and are severely afflicted. This type is called lepromatous. And there are three conditions in between these two extremes. In the less serious type, tuberculoid, there are a few skin lesions, and a biopsy shows numerous granulomas with plentiful T-cells but no organisms. There are multiple lesions in the more severe lepromatous type, with few granulomas and numerous bacteria observable on smears. Clearly, given that it's the same species and strain of bacteria, there is a marked difference in the immune response of one individual to another.

As we all know, the level of illness experienced by different people can differ significantly. Some people infected by influenza or coronavirus have only mild symptoms, or none at all, while others infected by the same virus become violently ill and require advanced medical treatment. Between these two extremes are most of us who are very ill for a few days or a week, then recover on our own. With tuberculosis, many who are infected develop well-formed granulomas to contain the organism and don't even know they have been infected until a skin test tells them. Others, of course, develop a life-threatening infection that needs prompt, vigorous medical treatment.

Most of our innate and acquired immune responses depend upon chemical signals to alert our immune system and direct its response. Cytokines are at the heart of this response. But not all cytokines are created equal. Like any protein in the body, they are manufactured at the direction of our DNA and protein transcription at the ribosomes. One alteration in the DNA, substituting one amino acid for another, may significantly alter the structure of a cytokine, or cytokine receptor, so that it functions at a lower, or higher, rate than the typical form. Such alterations in the structure of critical cytokines play a vital role in determining the outcome of infection by *Mycobacterium leprae*.

An important regulator of the lymphoid immune response is the cytokine lymphotoxin-alpha. Related to tumor necrosis factor-alpha, it has several functions, including the growth and attraction of lymphocytes. It has been shown that a single amino-acid substitution on lymphotoxin-alpha can significantly influence the course of leprosy. Other genetic alterations, such as in the receptor for vitamin D, the structure of tumor necrosis factor-alpha, interferon-gamma, and interleukin-10, can all play a role in determining the course of the disease.

634

Other factors may play a role as well. Adequate nutrition is of course very important. Also, co-infection with other organisms, such as parasites, which can alter the immune system's effectiveness, may increase the risk of the more severe form of leprosy.

Mycobacterium leprae is related to *Mycobacterium tuberculosis*. Thousands of years ago they diverged, but both remain pathogens for humans. *M. tuberculosis* has about 4,000 functional genes; *M. leprae* has about 3,000. So the latter has changed more by the deletion of genetic material than by the acquisition. That helps explains why the organism has a prolonged replication rate (2-3 weeks as opposed to about 20 hours for *M. tuberculosis*), and why it can't be cultured in the laboratory like other mycobacteria. But the two organisms invade the human body by similar mechanisms, the adherence to and penetration of monocytes.

Just how one acquires the organism *Mycobacterium leprae* is something of a mystery. Two possibilities predominate, from nasal secretions or from sloughed-off skin. The organism reaches very high numbers in nasal secretions, and the infection likely spreads from there by drainage and/or blowing of the nose, but it's hard to prove. Perhaps both.

Once the organism enters the body it is encountered by macrophages, which it willingly enters by a mechanism like that of *M. tuberculosis*. Just as with that organism, macrophages are unable to kill the intruder but instead carry it around the body. While it can invade several types of tissues, it has a strong predilection for the Schwann cells that envelop peripheral nerves and manufacture the myelin sheath that protects the nerve axon. By entering and disrupting the myelin production of the Schwann cells, the nervous system is compromised.

The organism can also enter the dermal layers of the skin, resulting in the formation of lesions. Just how many and where they are depends on the effectiveness of the immune response. In less severe cases (tuberculoid) the lesions are sparse, with no organisms detectable after a skin scraping. In severe cases (lepromatous), many lesions with many bacteria are observable.

Like tuberculosis, the immune response to leprosy is primarily cellular, with T-lymphocytes and macrophages surrounding the pathogen, walling it off, and holding it prisoner. The organism isn't killed, just held in a state of latency. But without that vigorous cellular response, the situation can rapidly get out of control. T-helper cells, that is, CD-4 lymphocytes, are critical to the success of the immune mission. And that's where leprosy can take a tragic turn for the worst.

T-helper cells of the CD-4 class are divided into different groups, the most prevalent being the T-helper-1 and T-helper-2 types. That's Th_1 and Th_2. The former controls intracellular pathogens, like *Mycobacterium leprae*, while the latter takes care of pathogens that attack outside the cells. For some reason, perhaps an alteration in the genomic make-up of the host or a product of the organism, the T-helper cells in leprosy shift from the Th_1 type to the Th_2. This allows the pathogen to establish its infectious state, as it doesn't have to deal with those pesky T-helper cells.

Leprosy is no longer a disease people in developed countries worry about, but it is of concern in underdeveloped areas. It is not extinct, nor will it be any time soon. Like its relative *Mycobacterium tuberculosis,* it is not eliminated by the immune system's reaction, merely kept at bay. It is treatable with antibiotics and good nutrition and needn't be perceived as the scourge it once was.

Other Mycobacteria. *Mycobacterium tuberculosis* and *M. leprae* are the human pathogenic types of the genus *Mycobacterium,* but other species can cause disease when given the opportunity. They are not frank pathogens and are easily controlled by our immune system in nearly all encounters. However, as with many organisms, if the immune system is compromised, they can take advantage of the opportunity and create an infection. Collectively, they are known as the "non-tuberculous mycobacteria."

The most notorious and potentially dangerous of these is the *Mycobacterium avium-intracellulare* complex, or MAC. Every one of us encounters one or more of the group regularly, but we are unaware of it because our immune system promptly rids us of the organisms. People with ultra-low counts of CD-4 lymphocytes are at particular risk. Mainly they cause pulmonary infection, but occasionally other organs can be infected. The group is especially resistant to common antibiotics, and the drugs of choice are often somewhat toxic. Depending on the patient's underlying condition, the infection can be difficult to treat successfully.

Several other species of mycobacteria are normally just part of the environment but can infect given the appropriate circumstances. Some produce pigments, and some grow rather quickly (3-4 days versus 3-4 weeks). A good microbiology lab is essential for their isolation and identification and guidance to appropriate antimicrobial therapy.

Chapter 40
Infection by Deception

From invertebrate
To unsuspecting victim.
Spiral predator.

Science prides itself on being orderly. Chemical names, abbreviations, atomic number and molecular weight, all arranged neatly on the periodic table of the elements. Every living thing given a scientific name, first the genus, followed by the species. Proper names assigned to every bone, muscle, and visceral organ of the body. The discipline of science demands exactitude since communication between workers is vital to advancing knowledge.

But the naming of infectious diseases takes a rather different course. Some diseases have names that have been around since ancient times, others more recent. Quite a few have more than one name. More recently, some diseases are nearly always referred to by an acronym rather than the proper name. It's hardly a neat and orderly process, but somehow it works.

Diseases that have been well recognized for centuries carry their traditional name with them. Rabies, tetanus, malaria, smallpox. They are often assigned a more scientific term, but the common name is usually employed. Variola is usually referred to as smallpox, rubeola as measles.

Often the species of the microorganism responsible for the disease is discovered well after the ailment has been described, and the bug is assigned the name of the disease. Examples are *Clostridium botulinum, Bordetella pertussis, Corynebacterium diphtheriae, Neisseria meningitidis,* and *Neisseria gonorrhoeae.* (One great mistake here was an organism thought to cause influenza was given the name *Haemophilus influenzae.* It turned out it doesn't actually cause the disease. Oops). Sometimes it's the other way around, when the organism is known, but the disease description follows. *Clostridium difficile* was known before the disease it caused came to be known as C diff (more properly pseudomembranous colitis). The genus *Campylobacter* was just an obscure organism many years before its role in the common intestinal disorder campylobacteriosis was described.

Oftentimes several different organisms can cause the same disease. Pneumonia, meningitis, urinary tract infection (UTI), upper respiratory tract infection (URI), gastroenteritis, and athlete's foot all can be caused by several organisms. Sometimes, the species name of the organism shown to be the cause is used as an adjective, such as pneumococcal pneumonia or meningococcal meningitis. That's a lot easier to say than pneumonia caused by *Streptococcus pneumoniae,* or meningitis caused by *Neisseria meningitidis.*

Some diseases have rather expansive names like acquired immune deficiency syndrome or severe acute respiratory syndrome. It's much easier to simply reduce it to a few letters, such as AIDS or SARS. Occasionally it is the organism's name that becomes reduced. Methicillin-resistant *Staphylococcus aureus* becomes MRSA and extended spectrum beta-lactamase producing *Enterobacteriaceae* becomes ESBL.

The name of the place where a disease or its causative organism was first described was, at one time, a convenient way to assign a name. Rocky Mountain spotted fever, Legionnaire's disease (described after its discovery at a convention of the American Legion at a Philadelphia hotel in 1976), Norwalk agent (now Norovirus), and Ebola (a river in Africa) are examples. This usually occurred when the causative organism and the disease course wasn't well established.

One of the more well-known infectious diseases named for the place of discovery is Lyme Disease, first described in the communities of Lyme and Old Lyme, Connecticut. This is a convenient name as it is simple to say, but it is most unjust for the good folks residing in the beautiful areas in southeastern Connecticut. (There are actually three communities, Lyme, Old Lyme, and East Lyme. The disease was first described in the area of the first two). The disease certainly did not originate there; it is found in many parts of the world. It was the perspicacity of two mothers, a local physician, and some state public health officials that brought to light the nature of the disease and its cause. The workers in Lyme, Connecticut, in the

1970s deserve many accolades for describing the disease, not the infamy of its name.

In 2015 the World Health Organization issued guidelines for naming newly discovered diseases, eliminating the use of geographic locations. But for those already established, the name usually persists.

There are three essential participants in the cycle of Lyme disease: (1) ticks of the genus *Ixodes*, (2) the causative organism *Borrelia burgdorferi*, and (3) the host animal. From the organism's perspective, the much-preferred animal host is the white-footed mouse or a chipmunk. It can infect the rodent, make many copies of itself in its tissues, and end up in the bloodstream. When another tick comes along and takes a blood meal, the organism can then be passed onto another animal host, perpetuating the bacterial species. While the rodent is infected, it is not sickened. The bacteria and the small creature get along quite well, with no ill effects to either. The bug has just enough control over the little animal's immune system to allow it to replicate without damaging the host. A "good" parasite does not want to damage the host. It needs the animal to stay relatively healthy so it can escape and get on to the next one. The relationship between *Borrelia burgdorferi* and the white-footed mouse and chipmunks is just such a compatible arrangement.

Trouble arises when the organism makes its way into a host, like a human, with an immune system that is in some ways different than the primary host. In this case the host (the human) is sickened. The bacterium has enough control over the host's immune system to allow itself to persist, but at the expense of creating numerous detrimental immune reactions. The organism does not reach high enough numbers in the bloodstream to enable it to be sucked up by a second biting tick, and humans don't get that many tick bites. For the organism, infecting a human is a dead end.

Ticks can bite some animals but not spread the disease. An important mammal in the chain is the white-tailed deer. While not seriously sickened by the bacterium, deer are large animals that many ticks can bite. They also can roam over wide geographic locations, taking their tick passengers with them.

Those ticks can then mate, produce eggs in new areas, and begin a cycle of infection with nearby rodents, which can spread the bacteria to other ticks. When deer populations increase, so do tick populations, broadening the possibilities for disease expansion.

There are two types of ticks, hard and soft. The obvious difference is a solid plate, called a scutum, covering the back of the former. They live in different places, with hard ticks dwelling in open fields on grasses and brush, while soft ticks usually live in enclosed areas like animal burrows. Both can spread disease, but the hard ticks are responsible for most of them.

The name tick comes from several European languages, meaning "touch." The word tickle has the same roots. Ticks are eight-legged and are classified with spiders in the class *Arachnida*. There are 14 genera of hard body ticks, but the ones responsible for spreading infectious diseases to humans are members of the genus *Ixodes*. The name *Ixodes* is from the Greek word for "bird-lime," a sticky substance applied to tree branches to trap birds, much like fly-paper traps flies.

There are many species of *Ixodes*, but only a few are associated with Lyme disease, and it varies with location. In the eastern U.S. it is *Ixodes scapularis*; western U.S., *Ixodes pacificus*; in Europe, *Ixodes ricinus*; in China, most likely it is *Ixodes persulcatus*. Environmental factors play a major role in the occurrence of Lyme disease, as there are many parts of the story, not the least of which is the number of mice and other suitable animals in a locality. Sometimes reforestation, returning farmland to a natural setting, enhances the population of mice, deer, and other animals in an area. If humans frequent this area for recreation or work, and ticks are present, the disease frequency increases. This is most likely what happened in Old Lyme, Connecticut, when the disease was first described.

Ticks go through three distinct stages after hatching from eggs: larva, nymph, and adult. We can think of it in people terms as toddlers, teenagers, and adults. Each stage requires blood from an animal for its survival. Unlike mosquitoes, where only the females take blood meals, both male and female ticks feed on blood. The female adults take a whole lot more since they make eggs and need to nourish them.

Ticks don't fly like mosquitoes, so they have another method of finding a suitable host. After hatching, larvae crawl to the end of a blade of grass or piece of shrubbery. With their hind legs they hang onto the vegetation. Their front legs have little barbs on them, and they sit there all day waving them around, waiting for an animal to come by. They are on a quest to find a suitable animal to suck its blood, and the process has the appropriate name "questing." When a little animal wanders by, they "grab" onto the unsuspecting animal and hop aboard. Then they crawl over the host's body, looking for just the right spot to attach. With humans that would be soft folds in the skin. The armpits and neck are prime locations, but there are several others. Nymphs, larvae, and adults all follow the same pattern.

Mosquitoes are in and out quickly. They land, insert their needle-like proboscis, take their blood, then fly away, the whole process taking just a few seconds. Ticks, on the other hand, need several days to get their blood meal, so they have evolved special means to allow that to happen.

They must stay attached, so a firm grip is essential. The mouthparts by which they attach have a barb on them that allows them to stick.

They must operate surreptitiously so the host animal won't try to remove them, and to that end they have two elegant properties. For one, they insert an anesthetic into the bite, making it painless. They also have the means to inhibit the local immune response to their presence. Think about getting a thorn in your finger; what happens after a day or two? Red, swollen, and painful. The same thing would happen around the attached tick, but they can circumvent the inflammatory response to their presence. Unfortunately for us, that immune mitigation works in favor of any pathogenic organisms they are carrying. Ticks also must ensure that the blood they are removing doesn't clot, so an anti-coagulant is a must.

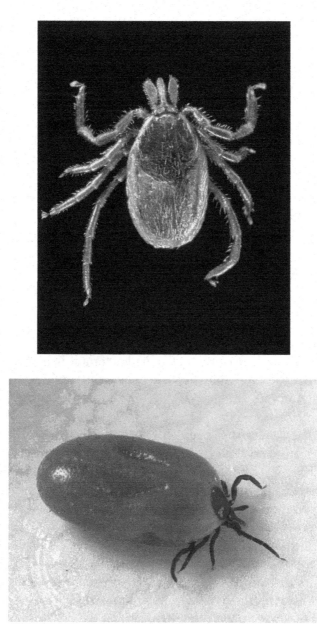

Top, Ixodes pacificus. Bottom, Ixodes scapularis
Engorged with blood. (PHIL)

Ixodes feeds on blood at all three stages, larva, nymph, and adult. It doesn't matter to them what kind of blood they obtain; bird blood is just as good as mammal blood. Some species also feed on reptiles. The Lyme disease-causing bacterium they may carry, *Borrelia burgdorferi*, does have a preference, and it is the mammalian species in which they can propagate and move about with impunity. Field mice and chipmunks fill the bill. In other species they can enter and set up an infection, but usually they meet their end if in the wrong host. Of course, they are merely passengers and go where their tick host takes them.

Borrelia burgdorferi does not survive over winter in *Ixodes* eggs, so the larvae are not infected and cannot inject the bacteria when they take their blood meal. If the blood of the animal they are feeding on is infected, they will pick up a load of bacteria with their blood. The larva usually doesn't need to feed again that season, but the bacteria have a way of staying alive in the young tick, even when it molts and becomes a nymph. When the nymph feeds, the bacteria it is harboring can then infect the new animal host. The same applies when the nymphs molt into adults.

The causative agent of Lyme disease is *Borrelia burgdorferi*. The genus is named for Amadee Borrel, a French microbiologist who worked to distinguish the groups of spirochetes. The species is named for Willy Burgdorfer who discovered the Lyme disease bacterium in 1982.

Borrelia burgdorferi differs significantly from other pathogenic bacteria. The most obvious distinguishing characteristic is their spiral, corkscrew-like shape. Flagella are little hairs that project from bacteria and beat rapidly to propel the organism through its environment. *Borrelia* has flagella, but they are internal, running up the inside of the bug from one end to the other. This is where they get the power to move so strongly in their corkscrew fashion.

The cell walls of *Borrelia* are like Gran-negative organisms, but with one great exception: they don't have lipopolysaccharide, commonly known as endotoxin, which is present in nearly all Gram-negative bacteria. Instead, they have a wide array of different lipoproteins in their cell wall. This makes them unusual among bacteria, and the immune system must adapt over time to recognize these many differing lipoprotein antigens.

Another feature of their cell wall is that they don't have the enzymes to recycle the wall's main component, peptidoglycan. Rather than being conserved and incorporated into other growing bacteria, *Borrelia* peptidoglycan flies off in every direction. This is significant in disease as the immune system is primed to detect and react to peptidoglycan as a foreign invader, whether it is attached to an organism or not.

Of particular note in *Borrelia burgdorferi* is its genetic makeup. Like all bacteria, it has one long strand of DNA that codes for its necessary structures and metabolism. The genes on this strand are highly conserved, and one strain of the organism looks just like another. But the organism can accumulate many smaller plasmids, usually round strands of DNA independent from the main chromosome. Over 20 different plasmids have been detected in *Borrelia burgdorferi*. In contrast to the main chromosome the plasmids are highly variable, both in their presence or absence within the organism and in their content. As a result, there are myriad strains of the organism in nature. Which one ends up in a human patient is a matter of chance.

Borrelia burgdorferi is unique among pathogenic bacteria because it does not produce toxins or penetrate host cells. It causes damage through its genetic variability and the immune system's response to it.

For *Borrelia burgdorferi* the animals it finds itself in differ radically, one being an insect and the other a mammal. Accommodations must be made. The organism is not free living, so it can't use its own enzymes to generate food. It must obtain all its nutrients from the animal in which it resides, whether insect, mammal, bird, or reptile.

When residing in its tick reservoir, the organism shuts down its own metabolism. It expresses a protein on its outer coat, allowing it to adhere to the tick's midgut. It can't do much else but just sit there, almost like it's in hibernation. When the tick feeds, though, everything changes. The blood that comes rushing in sends a signal to the organism's genome to shut down the protein production that allows it to stick to the wall of the tick's tummy and make its way to the tick's salivary glands. They then begin producing the proteins that will allow it to proliferate in its new mammalian host. First among these are the internal flagella, and the substances that will enable it to avoid the attack of complement.

Once inside the new mammalian host, the tick's invasive properties greatly aid the bacteria. There is the absence of pain, anti-coagulation, and the reduction of a localized inflammatory response, primarily neutrophils and complement. After entering the skin, the bacteria begin proliferating and moving every which way with their very active flagella. With their spiral shape and powerful flagella, they are no match for the cumbersome neutrophils and macrophages trying to capture them, and they disseminate quite far. They also produce a substance that acts very much like interleukin-10, an anti-inflammatory cytokine that slows down neutrophil induction.

The immune system catches up with them within a few days, and inflammation develops. The tell-tale sign is usually a distinctive rash described as a "bullseye," with a solid inner round red area, immediately surrounded by normal colored skin, then another round red circle. It is technically called erythema migrans, with erythema meaning redness and migrans meaning moving. They can be anywhere from a few inches to a foot around. It's all rather bizarre, really, but nonetheless distinctive. Sometimes the rash is not in the traditional bullseye shape but just a rash. It forms due to the innate immune system's effort to capture and kill the invading bacteria. Antibiotic treatment is usually very effective when applied at this first sign of trouble.

If only it were that simple: bullseye rash, antibiotics, end of story. Unfortunately, life sometimes throws us curveballs. Some people don't develop the distinctive rash; if they do, it is on their back where they can't see it. Some get the normal course of antibiotics and go on to develop significant symptoms anyway. A lot depends on the individual involved and the strain of bacteria. There are many variations.

Because of its robust motility, *Borrelia burgdorferi* can easily make its way into the blood vessels and lymph channels, allowing it to spread to every area of the body. The bugs can theoretically go anywhere, but they have a particular fondness for joints, the heart, and the central nervous system. They don't produce toxins and they don't penetrate cells. Instead, they firmly attach themselves to protein components of the extracellular matrix. That's the complex of tough fibers outside cells that support tissues and allow cells to communicate. The chief proteins of this matrix are decorin (a small protein associated with collagen), integrins, fibronectin, and others. *Borrelia burgdorferi* has proteins that allow for firm attachment to each one of these.

One would think that a bacterium just sitting outside a cell and attached to a protein would be a sitting duck for the immune system. But the organism has the means of allowing itself to survive. For one, it contains a protein known as CD47, commonly known as the "Don't eat me" protein. It is a protein expressed on human cells when they need to survive and cannot have macrophages eliminate them. *Borrelia burgdorferi* expresses the same one, avoiding macrophage engulfment.

Complement is the great enemy of bacteria, either acting alone or in concert with neutrophils. *Borrelia* is very good at circumventing the activity of complement, both early and late in the infection. An important regulator of the active C3b portion of complement is Factor H. The organism contains at least five proteins that bind Factor H, which then binds to the C3b molecule inactivating it. The effectiveness of complement is greatly lessened.

Disguise is another weapon the organism is very good at. All invading microorganisms have on their surface substances, either protein or carbohydrate, that are unique to them and foreign to the host animal. Known as PAMPs, or pathogen associated molecular patterns, they are prime targets for the cells of the immune system. Building antibody and T-cell responses to these microbial surface substances allows the host, through its adaptive immune response, to quickly rid itself of the pathogen.

The most common PAMP for Gram-negative bacteria is lipo-polysaccharide, or LPS. It is highly antigenic as several human proteins can detect its presence and signal a robust immune response. The problem with *Borrelia burgdorferi* is that it doesn't contain LPS, and the usual detection means are rendered useless. It does have nearly a hundred different alternative lipoproteins in its cell wall. These cell wall lipoproteins stimulate the innate immune system to produce cytokines, especially tumor necrosis factor and interleukins 6 and 8. Interferon is also produced. The abundant production of these cytokines creates most Lyme disease symptoms.

The deceptive technique the organism has mastered is routinely switching the lipo-proteins in its cell wall. One day one lipoprotein is present, a few days later another, and on and on as the bug is adept at changing them out. Antibody and T-cell response to one is useless with the subsequent iterations, allowing the organism to escape the ravages of the adaptive immune system. The main reason for this protein switching ability resides in a bacterial protein known as Vls-E. Its genes reside near the end of a plasmid designated Pp28-1. Located nearby the Vls-E gene are 15 other genes that code for similar but notably different lipoproteins. This arrangement allows the organism to mix and match genetic material, giving many combinations and resulting in lipoprotein differences.

These well-developed characteristics of rapid motility, complement avoidance, "don't eat me" protein, adhesin to the extra-cellular matrix, and ever-changing surface lipoproteins make for a very persistent bacterium. In nature, infected mice never get rid of it. Once infected, always infected. Fortunately for the mice, the organism doesn't do them any great harm. They live in a relatively benign co-existence. Unfortunately, that doesn't apply to human's relationship with the spirochete. Our immune response is sufficiently different from that of mice, so many infected people have severe symptoms. The symptoms in humans are not the result of direct injury by the organism; they produce no toxins and do not enter cells. But they persist for long periods of time, and the activity of our immune system in trying to get rid of them causes the symptoms.

One pernicious protein of the Lyme bacterium is a cell wall lipoprotein known as Arp. That stands for "arthritis related protein." The organism can infect a great many tissues, but it has a predilection for joints. Perhaps those tissues offer more receptors for its attachment proteins, or it can hide better there. Whatever the reason, arthritis is a hallmark of the disease, with

648

about 60% of infected persons displaying symptoms. Arp is an essential part of arthritis pathology, as tests in mice with organisms lacking Arp don't develop joint inflammation. Just what Arp does is not known, but it seems that it acts as a signal to the immune system to produce an abundance of inflammatory substances and thus induce joint inflammation and pain. It also seems that various forms of VlsE, the cell wall lipoprotein, act as a shield to protect Arp from an immune response.

Lyme disease was unknown in the 1970s, but it is currently recognized as the most common insect-borne disease in the United States, with over 300,000 cases annually. It is a very complex organism and disease progression with many novel and unpredictable facets. *Borrelia burgdorferi's* ability to elude and modulate the immune system, its many different surface proteins, its capacity to invade many different tissues of the body, and its potential to shut down much of its activities and exist in a near-hibernating state make for a disease with many presentations and outcomes. Lyme Disease can be one of the easiest infectious diseases to diagnose, and it can also be one of the most challenging and exasperating.

A few simple facts can lead to a quick, accurate diagnosis: history of a tick bite in an area where the disease is known to be endemic, and the tell-tale rash appearing a few weeks afterward. If the patient sees a physician at this stage, is prescribed an appropriate antibiotic, and complies with taking it for the prescribed duration, most Lyme Disease cases are cured. That's most, not all. A few people develop chronic symptoms despite compliance with appropriate early therapy.

Where things can get complicated is when early diagnosis is missed. The spirochetes will end up in many different parts of the body, and many different symptoms can be displayed. With many bacterial infections the isolation of the causative organism confirms the diagnosis. Appropriate samples from the patient are sent to the clinical laboratory, and direct observation under the microscope or bacterial culture, or both, are enough to confirm the diagnosis. This can't be done with borreliosis. The organism is too small in number in the blood to be seen under the microscope and does not grow in routine bacterial culture. Also, it hides out in obscure locations throughout the body, so getting an appropriate sample is not possible.

Lyme disease diagnosis depends entirely on looking for antibodies our body produces to the organism. This is complicated, especially for a resourceful organism like *Borrelia burgdorferi*. The bug is notorious for changing its surface material, so the antibodies produced can be non-specific. Other unrelated organisms may have just happened to produce a similar antigen, so the antibody to it may appear just like the one made to *Borrelia*, confusing the diagnosis. Lyme disease symptoms frequently mimic those of other diseases, so if the patient does not relate a travel history that would tip off a physician as to a possible infection, other avenues of illness and their causes may be explored needlessly.

The most common symptom of Lyme Disease other than the rash is arthritis. It was the unusual occurrence of arthritis among children in Connecticut in the 1970s that prompted researchers at Yale University to pursue investigations into the then-unknown disease. The knee is most commonly affected, but it can also involve other joints. Typically, there is redness, swelling, and pain. It is not the live organism burrowing through the joint that causes the symptoms, but the immune system's reaction to the organism, or, more likely, parts of the organism, that produce the reaction. As noted, *Borrelia burgdorferi* does not recycle the components of its cell wall known as peptidoglycan. It all is cast off like so much microbial rubbish. Peptidoglycan is immunogenic; the immune system reacts to it, and if it is concentrated in joint tissue, there will be an immune reaction that results in swelling and pain. The treatment of choice is often cortico-steroids to tamp down the immune response.

Another symptom of Lyme disease that appears in some patients involves the heart. Lyme carditis, when it occurs, happens quite early in the disease, just a few weeks after the tick bite. The bacterium likes to settle on extra-cellular matrix proteins, with the protein decorin being one of its favorite targets. Heart tissue contains a lot of decorin, and in some, but not all, patients, there is a notable adhesion of the organism to this protein. The result is a disruption of the electrical signals from the heart's upper chambers to the lower, often referred to as a heart block. Patients experience palpitations, shortness of breath, light-headedness, and sometimes chest pain. A few experience cardiac arrest.

Lyme carditis is not very common in Lyme disease patients, perhaps one in a hundred. The reason is unclear, but there may be a genetic difference in the structure of the decorin in these individuals, and the organism attaches more strongly. Without a known history of tick exposure, the diagnosis can be most troublesome, as it occurs early in the progression of the disease when antibody formation is not complete, and the serology studies can be misleading.

Lyme disease can also affect the central nervous system, giving symptoms such as numbness, double vision, and facial palsy. Sometimes more severe symptoms such as meningitis or encephalitis occur. The organism doesn't penetrate and navigate through human cells, but it is very good at traversing the junctions between them. They can thus penetrate the blood-brain barrier, and trouble ensues.

In the United States, most cases of Lyme disease go undetected and unreported. The Centers for Disease Control gets reports of about 30,000 cases annually, but they feel there are probably ten times that many cases. Early detection and treatment are key; most cases disappear after a couple of weeks of antibiotics such as doxycycline or amoxicillin. But as shown, Lyme disease can be the great imitator, with symptoms resembling those of other ailments and confusing diagnoses. A significant percentage of patients, probably around 10-15%, suffer long-term consequences of the disease. Just why is subject to speculation, but some reasons may be the organism's ability to hide itself and change its surface proteins, the mass production of bacterial by-products such as the cell wall component peptidoglycan that are immunogenic, the bacterium's ability to enter a quiet, non-metabolic state rendering it tolerant to antibiotics, the great variation in the different strains of organisms that can infect humans, and differences in the genetic make-up of the human hosts. These are not mutually exclusive, so several can apply in a single case.

Syphilis

Syphilis is one of the most historically impactful infectious diseases on human society. As in Lyme disease, the agent is a bacterial spirochete, one that goes by the name *Treponema pallidum*. (The name treponema comes from two Latin words, *trepein*, meaning "to turn," and *nema*, which means "thread;" pallidum is from the Latin word *paleo*, meaning "pale"). Today it is found worldwide, but just how it got there is a matter of some debate. There is an argument, based mainly on the evidence of the examination of skeletons, that it was endemic in Europe for many years. Another theory states that syphilis, as we know it today, was not present in Europe before the 1490s when the voyages of Christopher Columbus and his crews brought it back from the New World. Without laboratory testing or even the knowledge of the nature of its spread available at the time, speculation about the disease's origins will no doubt continue. What is known is that at the end of the 15th century and early 16th, syphilis burst on the scene in spectacular fashion and assumed great prominence in world affairs, affecting disciplines from philosophy, science, religion, politics, and art.

The Latin word for plague or contagion is *lues*. Lues venereum was the medical name assigned to the disease by French author and scientist Jean Fernelius when he wrote a review of the disease in the 1500s. The adjective luetic is still sometimes used. The disease received its common name from a character in a play written in 1530 by Girolamo Fracastoro. It was an updated version of an ancient Greek tale about a shepherd named Syphilus and his run-ins with Apollo and the bad karma that came of it. Somehow the name seemed to fit the great pestilence of the time.

No one would ever confuse Lyme disease with syphilis, but there are some general similarities. Most infectious agents enter us by inhalation or ingestion, but these two enter by penetrating the skin or genitalia. Both are caused by bacterial spirochetes, each having a half-dozen to a dozen spirals. They are both members of the same bacterial family, *Spirochaetaceae*. Both infections are often characterized by the formation of a rash, the pathognomonic bullseye of Lyme disease, and the diffuse secondary rash of syphilis. Both can have some devastating long-term symptoms affecting different areas of the body. Syphilis has historically been given the moniker "The Great Imitator" because its long-term symptoms can be confused with so many other ailments. The same might be said of Lyme disease. Both diseases are diagnosed by serologic studies, not bacterial culture or direct observation. Of course, one great difference is that *Borrelia burgdorferi* infects many animals, while *Treponema pallidum* only infects humans.

Syphilis is well known to come in stages. The first is the appearance of a genital sore, or chancre, a couple of weeks after exposure. The chancre isn't tender and painful, but it's usually unmistakable, although sometimes it is not detected. It subsides after about a month, only to be followed several weeks later by the second stage, the rash. The rash today is much different from that seen in the early 1500s. In those tumultuous days, the rash was cataclysmal. Massive, foul-smelling, bleeding sores all over the body that often became secondarily infected with pyogenic bacteria. One theory of the time held that this new disease resulted from the combination of gonorrhea with leprosy. It was termed the great pox. Today the rash is much more subdued, usually non-itchy red spots on several parts of the body. It can last up to a few weeks, then unceremoniously disappears. This reduction of serious symptoms is a great example of survival of the fittest, the fittest in this case being organisms that caused a much-lessened set of symptoms, allowing the infected human to pass the bug along to another person. In the more virulent infectious form, the bacterial agent died with its infected host.

Unfortunately, even though the primary chancre and secondary rash dissipate, the spirochete doesn't. The organism can stay alive someplace in the body. Sometimes, but not always, syphilis enters the third stage, called the latent stage, which itself can be divided into early and late stages. Early latent occurs in the first year following infection, and the late phase over one year.

Treponema pallidum is a sly invader, using several tricks to avoid the immune system's attack on it. For one, it is very slow to divide, taking over thirty hours per division, much longer than most other bacteria, making it more of a stealth invader. Also, it is unique in having very few surface proteins, so there are fewer targets for antibodies and immune cells. And, like its cousin *Borrelia,* it can vary the few surface antigens it contains, making itself a moving target.

The fact that we still have syphilis with us in the world today is most regrettable. There is no vaccine against it, but it has never been able to mount resistance to penicillin or other antibiotics. A proper course of antibiotic treatment eliminates the organism, especially if given at the first sign of disease. If every person in the world infected with syphilis could be treated effectively, then the organism would become extinct since there is no animal reservoir.

Treponema pallidum (PHIL)

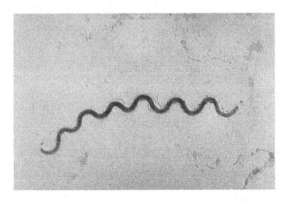

Leptospirosis (Weil's Disease)

Another spirochetal disease of significance is Leptospirosis, commonly called Weil's disease after Adolf Weil, who described the organism in 1886. Like Lyme disease, the spirochete causing leptospirosis is mainly a disease of non-human animals. There is some evidence that leptospirosis is the most common bacterial infection of animals worldwide. It is widespread in rodents.

The usual spot of attachment of the organism is the animal's kidneys. Once attached there, the bacterium doesn't make most animals sick. It is constantly being expelled in the host animal's urine, making it able to infect other animals, usually by consumption of contaminated plant material or water. The most common means of human infection is invasion through abrased skin when exposed to water contaminated by rodent urine.

There are over 60 recognized species of *Leptospira*. Some are highly pathogenic for humans. In humans, the organ most affected is the liver. Pathogenic strains adhere to the junctions between liver cells, causing their disruption and the release of bile. Jaundice results.

Pathogenic leptospires have some unique characteristics that make them virulent. After entering the body the organism enters the bloodstream. Monocytes and macrophages readily pick the bugs up, but the bacterium can survive inside them. The phagocytic cell releases numerous cytokines, sometimes leading to severe illness.

Leptospires have lipo-polysaccharide in their cell walls, which is usually recognized by immune system cells. But the organism sequesters its LPS, so the Toll-like receptor programmed to detect it is stymied. Also, the organism has several proteins that can inactivate key members of the complement system.

With these immune-modulating properties, pathogenic leptospires travel around the bloodstream of the infected individual with impunity. Some strains can attach to the endothelial cells of blood vessels, wreaking havoc with the body's coagulation system. That and the damage to the liver can make for a dire medical situation.

Section Four

*Concern for man and his fate must always form the chief interest of
all technical endeavors. Never forget this in the midst of your diagrams and equations.*
–Albert Einstein

Chapter 41
Beating 'em To the Punch

Eschewing toxins,
Employing natural methods.
Elegant vaccine.

The threat of infectious diseases isn't what it used to be. Certainly, we have enormous problems with microorganisms, and we always will. The pandemic of the novel coronavirus that began in late 2019 was a stark reminder of the unremitting ferocity of infectious diseases. But anyone born after the 1960s in the developed world can never appreciate the fearful impact of many diseases we now see as historical relics. Smallpox, diphtheria, typhoid, polio, tetanus, whooping cough. These are things you read about in history books. But to have held a child or other loved one in your arms as they lay suffering and dying of such a disease, with nothing on this earth to save them, is the most heart-wrenching experience of the human spirit. Infectious diseases know no boundaries. Anyone and everyone are susceptible. There is no escape from the illness or the anguish it brings.

To our great good fortune, we have curtailed these and other diseases. Smallpox is now extinct. Polio types 2 and 3 are gone as well. Diphtheria, the strangler, is not seen in the developed world. When we get a cut on our body, we don't immediately fear the onset of one of the most horrible things a human can experience: tetanus. When a stray dog bites us, we don't feel the panic of the possible onset of rabies and the horror that goes with it. These and other infectious diseases have been removed from our experience and consciousness by a medical marvel that started at the dawn of the 19th century: vaccination.

The concept of vaccination is simple. Our bodies are equipped with a vast and exquisite array of cells and chemicals designed by nature to help keep us free from invading organisms. But these defense mechanisms take time. Before our immune system can effectively respond to organisms that have acquired the means to circumvent the complex scheme organized against them, it may be too late, and the microbe has its way with us. With vaccination, we introduce the microbe (or a piece of it) into our body, but under our terms. We don't give it a chance to develop a foothold. If it does enter, our immune system is primed and ready to answer the challenge.

Our acquired immunity is the most effective deterrence against an invading microbe. The innate system works well but is designed to rebuff the initial challenge and hold it at bay. The actual removal and protection from infectious diseases come from our antibodies and cells that have acquired specific chemical receptors for specific chemical components of the invading organism. We don't even know we were challenged when it all works well.

Acquired immunity occurs as the result of a process. We have millions of lymphocytes circulating, both B and T types. Each B cell, and many T cells, have a unique chemical receptor on their surface. Their job is to wander around, bumping into things until they encounter a peptide or carbohydrate that fits into their receptor. They then get a signal to proliferate. The B cells start to crank out antibodies, and the T cells produce an antibody-like substance that sticks to their surface. That, crudely put, is the foundation of humoral and cellular immunity.

These B and T cells don't work on their own, however. They don't just bump into a complete organism and get turned on. The antibody-generating substance, or antigen, must be presented to them in a very orderly fashion. The presenting chemical is called the major histocompatibility complex, or MHC.

After infection, the offending organism is internalized into a cell, either a phagocyte such as a macrophage or dendritic cell or into a "non-professional" cell such as an epi- or endothelial cell. The host cell's digestive enzymes then digest the bug. Little pieces of the organism are then mounted up a ridge emanating from the MHC molecule. There are two types of MHCs, class I and class II. The MHC I receives peptides from organisms generated in the cell's cytoplasm, primarily viruses. MHC I is found in just about every cell in the body. The MHC II receives antigens from organisms that end up in intracellular vesicles, primarily bacteria, parasites, and fungi. MHC II is found only in macrophages and some T-lymphocytes. After being loaded with a microbial peptide, the MHC complex, whether I or II, makes its way to the cell's surface, there displaying the offending little piece of microbe or toxin. Eventually, a lymphocyte, either B or T, will come along, recognize the displayed antigen, and get activated.

The B cells begin to manufacture antibodies directed explicitly to the offending microbe's antigen and begin to proliferate prodigiously, thus creating many antibodies. The T cells don't produce antibodies. Depending on their type, their job is to destroy or help destroy the cell displaying the microbial antigen. They also proliferate extensively. If the T lymphocyte is of the CD8 type, it can directly kill the cell containing the microbe and displaying the antigen. Thus, the nickname is killer lymphocyte. If it is of the CD4 type, it works in harmony with other cells to facilitate the cell's destruction. That has earned them the nickname T-helper cell.

The first type of acquired immunity is called humoral immunity since the antibodies circulate throughout the body. The second type is called cellular immunity since it is centered in cells. The most effective vaccines induce both humoral and cellular immunity.

Several different types of vaccines are used. The first one developed, that used against variola, employed a strain of virus similar to the dangerous virus but not nearly as virulent.

Another type of vaccine is prepared by killing the organism, be it a virus or bacteria, and injecting it into a person. Influenza and injectable polio vaccines work this way.

Some organisms hurt us not by their direct invasion but by making a toxin that damages our tissues. A vaccine can be made not against the organism itself but against the toxin. The toxin is altered, leaving the antigenic portion intact but negating its ability to attach to its active site on our cells. Diphtheria and tetanus anti-toxins are this type of vaccine.

A very good vaccine preparation can be made by taking a strain of a virulent organism and altering (attenuating) it so that it loses its ability to cause damage during infection but still can stimulate the immune system to build an acquired defense against it. Oral polio, measles, mumps, and rubella vaccines are of this type.

Some organisms, particularly encapsulated bacteria, are resistant to the innate immune system by the nature of their carbohydrate capsule surrounding the cell. The capsule rebuffs complement and neutrophils, the main initial resistance force against such bacteria. Purifying and injecting the capsule material into a person triggers an acquired immune response, but it is only of the B-lymphocyte type and, therefore, short-lived. If the capsular material is conjugated onto a carrier protein such as the altered diphtheria toxin, a T-cell response is mounted in addition to the B-cell one, giving much longer protection. Vaccines against a cause of pneumonia, *Streptococcus pneumoniae*, use this principle.

A new vaccine modality was introduced shortly after the beginning of the Covid pandemic in late 2019 and early 2020. With highly technical and sophisticated techniques, the entire genome of the novel coronavirus was determined within weeks of its bursting upon the scene. The human cell receptor for the virus was determined to be angiotensin-converting enzyme 2, ACE2, which is found in multiple human tissues. The chemical structure of the virus's protein that attaches to ACE2 was determined; it is referred to as the "spike antigen." Like something out of a science fiction novel, researchers constructed a messenger RNA strand that would enter the ribosomes of human cells and code for the viral spike protein. Humans were made to make a viral protein, which as a foreign protein, is antigenic. This introduced a revolutionary form of vaccine production, messenger RNA, or mRNA. The Covid pandemic lent a sense of urgency to the program, and a new vaccine was made in less than a year. How this novel approach to vaccine production proceeds is of great interest.

Sometimes injecting a killed organism can make us ill. Not as sick as the viable wild-type organism attacking us, but some component of their structure is illness provoking. This is especially true of Gram-negative bacteria, which all have the endotoxin lipid-A in their cell wall. Injection of toxic lipid-A is illness provoking, as agents such as TNFα and IL-1β are released from the cells encountering it. In turn, these cytokines stimulate the release of other chemical agents. They all serve to give us fever and muscle aches. A solution to this is not to inject whole, dead Gram-negative bacteria but only antigenic pieces of the organism that result in a good level of protective acquired immunity.

Pertussis (whooping cough) vaccine is a good example of this. Initially, whole, dead *Bordetella pertussis* organisms were injected. Even though relatively few in number, the vaccine still commonly induced a mild fever and some muscle aches because of the lipid-A in the bacterial cell wall. Children often became febrile and more than a little fussy after their pertussis vaccination. But modern preparations use only parts of the pertussis organism, such as their attachment fimbriae or a modified toxin. This is known as the acellular preparation. Since it doesn't contain the entire bacterium and its endotoxin, acute toxic reactions are avoided. Unfortunately, there is some evidence that the immunity induced by this method doesn't last as long as the whole cell preparation. (Pertussis vaccine is usually administered to children in combination with diphtheria and tetanus vaccines, abbreviated DPT. When the acellular pertussis preparation is used the abbreviation is DTaP, the lowercase "a" standing for acellular).

The most effective and long-lasting vaccines are those in which an attenuated organism is administered alive. The microorganism can enter cells and engage in many metabolic activities that arouse immunity, but it cannot make us sick because it lacks a critical component. Unfortunately, attenuated organisms that can be guaranteed safe and effective are very few and far between. Sometimes hundreds of passes through cells or animals are needed, often taking years, with no guarantee of success. One recent scientific breakthrough that enables researchers to exploit the principle of a live attenuated organism while avoiding the risk is genetic engineering. Some viruses are well known to invade human cells but are incapable of inducing human disease. They enter a cell and go about their metabolic activities, but the body's innate immune system shuts them down very soon, before the full release of defense chemicals that make us sick and before the organism can proliferate beyond its initial stages. Such viruses are often pathogens of non-human animals or even of plants. When a critical gene from a pathogen is spliced onto such a virus's genome and injected into or consumed by a human, the individual gene product is immunogenic but not pathogenic. The result can be the development of acquired immunity against the target pathogenic strain from which the gene was taken. The vaccine against the Ebola virus uses this principle. The vaccine for malaria uses a piece of the circumsporozoite, the parasitic form which enters the liver. It is attached to an attenuated liver virus, hepatitis B.

For a vaccine to work most effectively, various adaptive immune system cells must be engaged. To help the process along, an unrelated substance known to enhance immune response can be administered along with the vaccine. These substances are called adjuvants, from the Latin word *juvare,* meaning "helper." Adjuvants are non-toxic, but they have the ability to attract the correct immune cells to the site of vaccine injection. The more engaged immune cells picking up vaccine material and transporting it to the nearest lymph tissue, the greater the chance for a high immune response to the vaccine and hence the pathogen.

Vaccines have remarkably reduced human and animal suffering and loss of life, but, alas, nothing is perfect. That's especially true when it comes to the practice of medicine. We never say "never" or "always." By the nature of their profession, epidemiologists and physicians think in terms of "very often" or "most likely." When we are injected with an organism, alive or dead, or a piece of one, there is no guarantee that the various components of our immune system will recognize it and form a perfectly orchestrated defense against it. Some vaccines may be only 80-90% effective. The older we get, the less the likelihood of vaccine effectiveness. For instance, most people in their 20s and 30s will develop a strong antibody response to the yearly influenza vaccine, about 90-95% (but not 100%). For people in their 50s, the antibody response is only seen in around 80% of vaccinees. For those over 70, the antibody response is only detected in about 70% of them. Better than nothing, but certainly no guarantee of immunity to that year's influenza strain. (A big reason why younger people who interact with older people should get their flu shot is to protect against infecting the more vulnerable older person whose vaccination may not have been effective).

This lack of universal immunity after vaccination is a big reason to vaccinate as many people as possible against a specific pathogen. Herd immunity is a somewhat abrasive term (none of us like to think of ourselves as part of the "herd"), but it says a lot. For an organism to spread by a communicable means, having most of the population already immune to it is the end of it. Without vulnerable individuals readily available for new transmission, the organism, and the disease it brings, will soon die out. The rate of immune individuals needed to thwart an infectious disease completely varies with the disease but usually, around 85-90% will do the trick. It sounds simple, but since not all vaccination attempts are successful, that level of immunity requires a very high level of community compliance.

Smallpox was the first (and let's hope not the last) infectious disease to be eradicated mainly by vaccination. In retrospect, smallpox would be the obvious one. The disease was so horrific that any means available to do away with it would be acceptable, even a procedure like variolation in the 18th century, wherein some of those vaccinated died of the inoculation. There is no animal carrier, so there was no need to vaccinate or cull large numbers of animals. Also, the disease has no carrier state, so if you have smallpox it shows up without any mystery. The ultimate end of the disease came from an epidemiologic tool known as "ring vaccination." When the disease had become rare, any report of its recurrence usually reached public health authorities, who would travel to the affected area as quickly as possible. The workers were already immune to the disease so they could work with impunity. Starting with those in immediate contact with the victim, they would vaccinate. Next, they would vaccinate those a little further away and work their way out. A relevant fact about variola is that even after exposure to the virus, you can still be successfully vaccinated with the vaccinia virus up to about 4-5 days post-exposure. By applying ring vaccination, those most likely to have been exposed are made immune, and the spread of the disease is much lessened.

The last person to have acquired smallpox in the wild was a cook who lived in Somalia, Ali Maow Maalin, in 1977. He had the variola minor strain. The last known case of variola major was reported in India two years earlier. (It is the policy of the World Health Organization to wait three full years before declaring a disease eradicated. The WHO did so for smallpox in 1980).

The eradication of smallpox, in the final years by the incredible work of Dr. D.A. Henderson and his international team, was one of humankind's great achievements. The knowledge gained in the last two centuries about our immune system and how it works has been astounding. The scientists of early times, such as Edward Jenner, knew nothing of microbes, antibodies, killer lymphocytes, or anything else about the immune system. We now know the structure and function of many molecules involved in the defense of our bodies, and we learn much more every day. It's been, and will continue to be, an amazing journey.

Summary of some common vaccines

Vaccine Type	Example
Live, related, less pathogenic microbe	Vaccinia virus for smallpox
Altered toxins	Diphtheria, tetanus
Killed entire microbe	Polio, influenza, pertussis
Multiple bacterial capsule types; toxoid carrier	Pneumococcus, Haemophilus
Live, attenuated virus	Measles, mumps, rubella, polio, rotavirus
Live, attenuated bacteria	BCG, (Tuberculosis)
Messenger RNA coding for microbe antigen (mRNA)	Coronavirus
Individual bacterial antigens	Pertussis
Microbial antigen attached to unrelated carrier virus	Ebola, coronavirus, malaria

Chapter 42
Hitting Them Where They Live

Poisons enemies,
They can poison our allies.
Indiscriminate.

Antibiotics aren't new. Microbes have been producing them for millions of years to help themselves gain an ecological advantage. And antibiotic resistance isn't new either. The target microbes have been producing the means to avoid destruction by the chemical substances directed against them for just as long. Humans just happened to discover this world of microbial biochemical warfare in the 1940s. It's still a little new to us, but the biological processes have been firmly developed.

Because of the variability of microbes, antibiotics don't work against all bacteria all the time. The number of different types of bacteria susceptible to a given agent is called the spectrum: An antibiotic that can kill a wide range of organisms is called a broad spectrum; one whose range of activity is confined to a few species is called a narrow spectrum. Choosing a proper antibiotic to treat an infection often depends on knowing which microbe is causing a disease. When known, it is best to use a narrow-spectrum drug to prevent collateral damage to our helpful microbes. A broad-spectrum drug is usually used if the infectious agent is not known, as is often the case early in an infection before laboratory tests are available. Sometimes, when the infection is serious, and the infectious organism isn't known, it is necessary to administer an "antibiotic cocktail," several broad-spectrum drugs at once, hoping that at least one will do the job. When laboratory results are known, then a more appropriate choice is made.

Antibiotics are poisons. They are designed by nature to kill. Fortunately for us, bacteria possess structures and enzymes different from ours, which are the targets of antibiotics. Substances like bleach kill bacteria, but clearly, giving an intravenous administration of bleach is a very bad idea. We want something that will kill bacteria but not harm us too much. Antibiotics meet the need.

Unfortunately, antibiotics are not specific in their killing. The organism harming us may be susceptible to it, but so are many other microbes that beneficially colonize our bodies. Antibiotics kill them too. An obvious example is using a drug like amoxicillin, a variation of penicillin, to treat an infection. Lactobacilli and other organisms in a woman's vagina are susceptible to amoxicillin and are killed by it, just like the target pathogen somewhere else in the body. That leaves the vagina open to colonization and infection by organisms not susceptible to amoxicillin. One that frequently jumps in is the yeast *Candida albicans,* which produces a painful irritation. Sometimes, curing one infection can lead to another.

There are several sites in bacteria for antibiotics to work. The most apparent structure that most bacteria possess and we don't is their cell wall. Like us, bacteria have a soft membrane surrounding the cell, but on top of that, bacteria have a rigid structure designed to hold the organism together. Bacteria are so small and have so much stuff packed inside they have very high internal pressure. They need their cell wall to prevent leakage and lysis.

There are two main types of bacterial cell walls, one found in Gram-positive bacteria and the other in Gram-negatives, but both have a common structural component: peptidoglycan, also known as murein. The word peptidoglycan comes from its two components: "glycan" because it has carbohydrates, and "peptido" from the presence of amino acids. Structurally it resembles a tightly woven net, with the carbohydrates, N-acetylglucosamine and N-acetylmuramic acid (NAG and NAM), forming a long string that circles the organism. In fact, lots of these NAG-NAM strings are circling the organism. By themselves, they aren't worth much; the real strength of the structure comes from the bridges of amino acids that connect each NAG-NAM strand. We might think of it as a chain-link fence, with the "poles" being NAG-NAM strings and the "fencing" in between being the amino acids linking the strings. Altogether, they make for one very effective structure.

Enzymes stitch together all this complicated latticework of molecules. Enzymes, made inside the cell, migrate to the edge of the cell to make it all happen. They dutifully pick up one molecule and attach it to another, creating a successful cell wall that will protect the organism from harm. Ordinarily, the process is done quickly and efficiently; when going strong, some bacterial cells can reproduce in only twenty minutes. A vital part of the bacterial cell wall is the network of amino acids stitched together between the strings of NAM and NAG carbohydrates. Break them apart, and the whole structure crumbles.

Most amino acids in nature are of the levo, or "L," also called the "left-handed" type. But bacteria contain at least one amino acid in their cell walls of the "D," or dextro, also known as the "right-handed" type. This key D- amino acid is D-alanine, which plays an important role. It connects the amino acid chain with the NAM component of the growing cell wall. If it fails, it's like having a weak link on a chain; the structural integrity is compromised. By having an unusual amino acid in their cell wall, bacteria can avoid the occasional destructive power of enzymes that only work on L-amino acids. But it also leaves them vulnerable to a particular type of antibiotic.

The term lactam is a combination of two words, lactone and amide. The "lact" part means "one," referring to the cyclic structure of the molecule, with the ring form looking like a single unit. The "am" part comes from amide, a side group found in all lactams. Lactams are a common organic molecular class, and they can have from three to six carbons. All are ring forms. The five and six-carbon rings are very stable; those with only three or four carbons are quite unstable. Specific enzymes must put them together to stabilize them. Lactams are given a general name by their number of carbons: alpha for 3, beta for 4, gamma for 5, and delta for 6. The beta-lactam (β-lactam), or four-carbon ring, is of vital importance in the field of antibiotics.

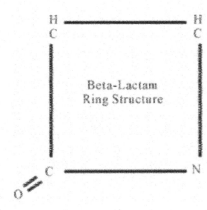

Beta-Lactam
Ring Structure

The beta-lactam ring contains four carbons, plus an amino group. It forms the nucleus of some of the world's most important antibiotics, the penicillins, cephalosporins, and carbapenems.

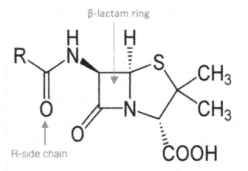

β-lactam ring

R-side chain

The basic structure of penicillin, showing the 4-sided beta-lactam ring. Alterations to the side chains can yield different antibiotics.

The heart of penicillin is the β-lactam ring. For the bacterial enzyme that constructs the amino acid mesh of peptidoglycan, the β-lactam ring mimics D-alanine. It's a case of mistaken identity. When the enzyme that puts D-alanine into the growing cell wall encounters the β-lactam structure, it picks it up instead. This gums up the whole works; it's like picking up bricks made of straw and putting them into the foundation of a building. The peptide cross linkage falters, and the cell wall is not complete. The result is the rupture and death of the bacterial cell.

A minute amount of penicillin is enough to wreak havoc on very many target bacteria. Less than 0.01 microgram of penicillin per milliliter of culture broth is enough to kill hundreds of millions of bacteria. Clearly, there is something more going on than the disruption of cell wall synthesis.

Bacteria have a built-in "self-destruct" system. When they grow in an environment with a high supply of nutrients, they grow rapidly but run the risk of the entire population depleting the nutritional resources surrounding them and all of them dying. They can do two things to get at least some of them to survive. Those that produce toxins do so when the population concentration is high, with the hope that the toxin can create more nutrients for them to exploit. They also can initiate a programmed death of many population members to ensure that at least some of them can survive and enter a new environment at some time. This latter maneuver is termed autolysis, a term adapted from the Greek words *autos*, or "self," and *lusis*, or "loosening." Bacteria have a system known as quorum sensing, consisting of a series of chemicals released and received that alert them that their population in a restricted area has reached very high numbers. When the threshold is reached, a series of reactions bring about the self-destruction of many individual cells.

β-lactam antibiotics like penicillin can initiate this autolytic system, probably because of the release of many little pieces of the cell wall. β-lactam antibiotics are extremely valuable, then, not only because they attack an anatomical structure in the invading microbe that we humans don't have, but they initiate a killing spree far greater than we would expect by direct contact.

The key to exploiting an anti-bacterial substance made in a fungus for use in humans is manipulating and altering the side chains attached to the central β-lactam ring. Simple "mold juice," or an extract of material generated by the growing fungus, is ineffective and sometimes dangerous. The medical breakthrough for penicillin was the chemical removal of a protein side chain made by the mold and attached to the β-lactam ring. After painstaking and meticulous procedures, researchers could isolate the active part of the substance in relatively pure form and inject it with impunity into a patient. The chemical work on penicillin didn't stop there. Many researchers found that various substances could be added to the basic ring, creating antibiotics of the penicillin class that were still active but with different properties.

Two main objectives were achieved by this chemical manipulation of the basic drug: the pharmacological properties could be altered, as could the bacteriological spectrum. With the pharmacological properties, drugs could be administered orally instead of intravenously, and fewer doses could be used. On the bacteriological spectrum side, adding certain side chains to the basic molecule enabled the creation of antibiotics with a broader or narrower spectrum of activity. The first alterations of penicillin allowed it to be given orally as opposed to an intravenous route (penicillin G is IM/IV only, and penicillin V is given orally). Ampicillin is a penicillin active against a broader range of Gram-negative organisms than the original penicillin.

The basic antibiotic, as it comes out of the microbe that produced it, represents what is known as the class of antibiotic. Penicillin is a class of antibiotic. There are many variations on the basic drug developed in the labs of pharmaceutical companies. Penicillin, amoxicillin, piperacillin, methicillin, oxacillin, and many more medications built by adding chemical side chains around the basic β-lactam structure of penicillin are members of the penicillin class. Each has its own characteristics and niche of activity.

Unfortunately, the lactam ring's unusual shape makes it vulnerable to chemical attack. Not long after penicillin's widespread use began in the late 1940s, doctors noticed some organisms that should be susceptible to it were resistant. This was especially true of *Staphylococcus aureus*, an often-aggressive Gram-positive coccus. Within the first few years of penicillin's release, Staph infections responded favorably to treatment, but as time went on, more anecdotal evidence emerged that the organism had developed resistance to the therapy. The reason for this was soon made clear: the organism had produced an enzyme that inactivated penicillin. Studies showed that the inactivation resulted from an enzyme that directly damaged the β-lactam portion of the drug, rendering it ineffective. The enzyme was initially given the name

670

penicillinase since its discovery involved penicillin, but a better term is β-lactamase since the β-lactam ring is the target of the enzyme. β-lactams are not stable molecules; they only have four carbons and an amide group attached. The enzyme of *Staphylococcus aureus* introduces a hydrogen ion from water into the ring, thus making it unstable and ensuring its breakdown. The process is known as hydrolysis.

During the early 1950s, the problem worsened as more and more isolates of Staph contained the resistance enzyme. Natural selection was in play: those strains of Staph susceptible to penicillin were killed by it, while those resistant lived to fight another day. Also, by several genetic mechanisms, surviving organisms could pass on their genes coding for resistance to other strains of Staph, and the problem kept getting larger, especially in healthcare centers.

The solution to the penicillin-resistant strains of *Staphylococcus aureus* came as a new side attachment to the traditional penicillin molecule. It was a benzene ring containing two methyl groups, and because of the latter, the antibiotic was named methicillin. On a two-dimensional diagram, the presence of the methyl-containing benzene ring doesn't look like much. But in its three-dimensional arrangement, it is very good at blocking the attachment of the β-lactamase enzyme produced by the staphylococcal organism. The discovery of methicillin spawned a new line of research that created a line of similar drugs, with names like oxacillin, cloxacillin, dicloxacillin, nafcillin, and several others. They had different pharmaceutical properties, but they all served the same purpose: they were penicillins effective against strains of *Staphylococcus aureus* that produced penicillinase. They were given the collective name penicillinase-resistant penicillins.

An adage has it that "Out of small acorns, giant oak trees grow." In 1961 in Japan, a scientific paper was published in a remote journal reporting the isolation of *Staphylococcus aureus* strains resistant to methicillin. The organisms were given the moniker "methicillin-resistant *Staphylococcus aureus*," or MRSA for short. Little did the researchers know at the time that MRSA would grow to be an enormous problem in healthcare for years to come, a problem we still haven't satisfactorily solved.

The appearance of MRSA marked a sea change in infectious diseases. Whereas the traditional resistance mechanism of *Staph. aureus* was to produce an enzyme that destroyed the β-lactam portion of the antibiotic, MRSA used a completely different mechanism. The transpeptidase that inserted D-alanine and mistakenly picked up β-lactam instead was replaced by an entirely different enzyme, which inserted D-lactate into the growing cell wall instead of D-alanine. It wants nothing to do with a β-lactam ring. So, the target protein of penicillin was replaced, making the antibiotic virtually useless.

For several decades, clinical isolates of MRSA were centered in hospitals and other healthcare facilities. Even if one contracted MRSA in the community, the source could invariably be traced back to a hospitalized patient. That all changed around the year 2000 when new strains of community-associated MRSA strains began to appear. Like the original reports in the early 1960s that were few and scattered, so were those of these new strains. But they didn't remain remote for long. Community-associated MRSA (CA-MRSA) became a major worldwide problem in just a few years.

Not only were they resistant to β-lactam antibiotics, but they also contained a powerful virulence factor, the Panton-Valentine leukocidin (PVL). PVL wasn't new; it was discovered in the 1930s. But it was only infrequently encountered clinically. Most strains of Staph possess enzymes that destroy red blood cells and some epithelial tissue. The PVL enzyme does that but also destroys neutrophils, the first line of defense of the innate immune system. Killing protective white blood cells gives the organism a head start in the infectious process. PVL's incorporation into these newly evolved CA-MRSA strains made for organisms that were much more potentially deadly and resistant to common antibiotics. What's more, they found their way into hospitals and other healthcare facilities, infecting patients already compromised by other diseases. We have several antibiotics which are effective against them, but early detection is essential for adequate treatment.

(One of the worst names in medicine is methicillin-resistant *Staphylococcus aureus* or MRSA. Methicillin had a lot of problems as an antibiotic, not the least of which was that it

672

could only be administered intravenously, and it wasn't very soluble in water. It isn't even made anymore, let alone used clinically. But it was the only penicillinase-resistant penicillin available at the time of the discovery of the resistance mechanism, and the name stuck. A far better name is β-lactam-resistant *S. aureus* since the organism is resistant to all members of the β-lactam classes of drugs, not just methicillin).

From the early days of antibiotic research, it was apparent that penicillin was ineffective against most Gram-negative rods. Some Gram-negative organisms, such as *Neisseria gonorrhoeae,* could be successfully treated, but common infectious agents, like *E. coli, Klebsiella,* and *Salmonella,* could not. Pharmaceutical companies did a magnificent job of altering the side chains of penicillin to make them work against these and other organisms. The first used was ampicillin, produced in the early 1950s. Ampicillin was effective against many, but not all, Gram-negative rods. It was used extensively in treating both serious and less serious infections. Later came piperacillin, which had an even broader spectrum of activity, including the difficult-to-treat *Pseudomonas aeruginosa.*

Just as the production of penicillinase and acquisition of β-lactam resistance in *Staph. aureus* began remotely, so did ampicillin resistance in Gram-negative rods. The first published paper on the subject appeared in 1963, with the report of an isolate of *Escherichia coli* that was resistant. Up until that point, all *E. coli* strains treated had been susceptible.

Most strains of *E. coli* and other Gram-negative rods naturally produce an enzyme that destroys penicillin. Unlike the enzyme produced by *Staphylococcus,* which is released into the environment, the one produced by the Gram-negative rods remains confined to the bacterial cell. It is a protein that resides between the cell membrane and the cell wall, an area known as the periplasmic space. It isn't there all the time. When the organism encounters a molecule of β-lactam, a sequence of chemical reactions enables the organism's genes to make the β-lactamase protein. There is a bit of a delay between the encounter with penicillin and the placement of the β-lactamase.

In the early days of ampicillin usage, the antibiotic worked beautifully against all strains of *E. coli* and several other Gram-negative rods. The resistance to ampicillin observed in the early 1960s wasn't a new enzyme acquired to attack ampicillin specifically. It was the same enzyme the organism always had, but it had mutated to enable it to combat ampicillin as well as penicillin. Like the emergence of strains of *Staphylococcus aureus* that were resistant to methicillin, there likewise appeared more and more strains of *E. coli* and other Gram-negative rods resistant to ampicillin, so that today more than half of all isolates of *E. coli* in hospitals are ampicillin resistant. The genetic material responsible for antibiotic resistance can spread from one organism to another, even to a different genus and species, and it can mutate to facilitate resistance to other antibiotics.

(Today, the antibiotic amoxicillin is often used instead of ampicillin because of its enhanced pharmaceutical properties. But ampicillin and amoxicillin share the same bacterial spectrum).

Following the remarkable work on penicillin, the floodgates of research on antibiotic discovery opened. In the early 1950s, new drugs were discovered and brought to market almost yearly. Amazing progress was being made in the fight against infectious diseases. Most of the work was done in advanced research facilities, heavily financed by the newly emerging pharmaceutical companies. But one of the most important of these discoveries came from a most unusual place, by an unheralded worker. The place was the island of Sardinia off the west coast of Italy, and the scientist's name was Giuseppe Brotzu.

Dr. Brotzu was a professor of hygiene at the University of Cagliari in Sardinia. Today we call such a position the director of the Department of Public Health. He was a brilliant scientist, well-trained in his field, and by all accounts, an excellent teacher. He was also a very private man, rather astute, seemingly aloof. His low-key personality and his remote location kept him out of public view. But he discovered the most widely prescribed antibiotic in history, the cephalosporins.

In Sardinia during World War II, two serious diseases predominated: malaria and typhoid fever. Dr. Brotzu, in his position as a learned epidemiologist, was chiefly responsible for the eventual eradication of malaria. Treating areas infested by mosquitoes to reduce their number while at the same time treating and isolating patients ill with disease broke the cycle of transmission and eliminated the disease.

As impressive as his work against malaria was, his lasting legacy was his work involving typhoid. Not the disease itself but a discovery of immense importance that accompanied his studies. Dr. Brotzu supervised the laboratory that tested raw sewage for the presence of typhoid bacilli, and he compiled data on its occurrence and geographic locations. A most unusual observation captured his attention. In the spot where one drainage pipe emptied into the sea, the people swimming there rarely got typhoid. He surmised that something in the water killed the organism and kept the swimmers safe. He also noticed the presence of a fungus on some of the culture plates that had an inhibitory effect on the organism's growth on culture plates, giving a "halo effect" around some of the fungal colonies where bacteria were unable to grow. He hypothesized that this fungus, known then as *Cephalosporium acremonium*, produced a substance responsible for the effect. His resources were limited, but the experiments he conducted confirmed his theory. He had discovered a fungus that produced an antibiotic like that made by *Penicillium*. But this one attacked and killed Gram-negative organisms in addition to Gram-positives.

Dr. Brotzu realized the enormity of his discovery. But it was 1943 in war-torn Italy. He knew a few organizations in his country that encouraged and financially supported research, but they weren't interested. "They didn't even answer," he once remarked. But luck intervened. A young American medical officer was touring his facilities in 1945 and learned of his discovery. He was familiar with the work being done at Oxford on antibiotics, and with his contacts there, he got the fungal strain sent to the Oxford lab for further testing. This fungus was even more challenging to work with than *Penicillium* because it produces not just one but three antibiotics. But after 18 years of arduous work, the first drug of its kind was ready for manufacture and release in 1962. Its name was Cephalothin; the Eli Lilly company marketed it as Keflin.

Like the penicillins, the cephalosporins are β-lactams, but the ring adjacent to the β-lactam is a six-carbon ring rather than the five-membered one found in penicillin. Still, the mode of operation is the same: disruption of the transpeptidase responsible for the insertion of amino acids cross-linking the growing peptidoglycan chain in the cell wall. The built-in advantage of cephalosporins over penicillins is their broader spectrum. Also, its chemical structure lends itself well to chemical manipulation, yielding a larger number of chemically modified antibiotics, which can improve their pharmacological properties and spectrum of activity.

The first major improvement in cephalosporins was the introduction of cefazolin in the early 1970s. The name can be pronounced two ways, cef-AZ-o-lin or cef-a-ZO-lin. Even though it is off-patent, many still refer to it by its trade name, Ancef. Whatever you call it, cefazolin was a marked improvement over the original formulation of Cephalothin because of its ease of administration and very good coverage of *Staphylococcus aureus*, including those strains that produce penicillinase. Cefazolin is still one of the most prescribed antibiotics in the world, both for treating infections and as a pre-operative medication to prevent infections during surgery.

Following the introduction of cefazolin, pharmaceutical companies introduced new formulations of cephalosporins at a furious pace. Many were "me-too" drugs, variations on a theme designed to capture market share as much as anything else. But several significant new drugs were introduced, which expanded the spectrum of activity of the cephalosporin class. Each new group was assigned a "generation." Cephalothin and cefazolin represent the first generation, cefuroxime the second. The biggest breakthrough came with what is commonly called the third-generation cephalosporins. This group, represented by antibiotics such as cefotaxime, ceftazidime, and ceftriaxone, markedly expanded the group's activity spectrum, targeting several significant organisms not responsive to the earlier generations. We are now up to the fifth generation of cephalosporins with antibiotics designed in the lab to target

676

methicillin-resistant *Staphylococcus aureus*. With their many varieties, cephalosporins are the most heavily prescribed antibiotics in the world. That's quite a way from the samples of raw sewage collected by Giuseppe Brotzu in Sardinia in 1943.

Medical students have been known to remark that the most challenging part of their pharmacology class is memorizing the numerous cephalosporins and their assigned generation and application. They have a point. There are dozens of cephalosporins, and most begin with cefa- or cepha-. At first glance, it is a tremendously complicated endeavor, but it becomes relatively straightforward in practice. Generally, it is best to use a first-generation drug, either cefazolin, given IV, or cephalexin, an oral preparation. There are a few isolated uses for the second-generation members, usually cefuroxime or the closely related cephamycin class drug cefotetan, but the third-generation drugs do the bulk of the work in serious infections. This would include cefotaxime, ceftazidime, ceftriaxone, and a few others. The fourth-generation drug, cefepime, is a little more active than the third-generation formulations, but only a little. The fifth-generation drugs are specifically formulated to combat methicillin-resistant *Staphylococcus aureus*.

A beta-lactam antibiotic that is rarely used is aztreonam, the only clinically useful member of the class known as the monobactams. It works only against aerobic Gram-negative rods.

Bacterial resistance to cephalosporins has grown exponentially since the first β-lactamase produced by Gram-negative rods was discovered in the early 1960s. Mutation after mutation of numerous enzymes has taken place in bacteria, so we now know hundreds of enzymes capable of destroying the β-lactam antibiotics, penicillins and cephalosporins. The genes coding for these enzymes are readily passed from one organism to another, and antibiotic resistance is growing, especially in the healthcare environment. Drug resistance is usually not confined to the β-lactams, which adds greatly to the problem.

To combat this growing resistance, a third type of β-lactam antibiotic was discovered and marketed. Known as the carbapenems, the drug differs from penicillins and cephalosporins in several ways. The chain adjacent to the β-lactam ring has a carbon at the top instead of a sulfur, thus the part called "carba-." They also contain a carbon linkage known as a penem, hence the second part of the name. But the molecule's core, the β-lactam ring, is the same.

The carbapenems do not originate in a fungus like the penicillins and cephalosporins. They come from a soil bacterium, *Streptomyces cattleya*. First isolated in 1976, the initial drug was called thienamycin, and it was amazing. It could kill an extensive range of bacteria, both Gram-positives and Gram-negatives, including the notoriously resistant *Pseudomonas aeruginosa*. But the antibiotic was most difficult to work with, and it took several years to isolate. Even then, thienamycin is unstable in water and breaks down quickly. However, scientists from several drug companies worked on it and came up with a few stable varieties while giving the same incredible spectrum of activity. Not only that, the carbapenems are resistant to the activity of the many enzymes that were able to destroy the advanced penicillins and cephalosporins, the so-called extended spectrum β-lactamases, or ESBLs. The carbapenems, such as imipenem and meropenem, were the go-to drug for antibiotic-resistant organisms. For some time, they have been considered the "antibiotics of last resort."

But even they have come to meet their match. In the early part of the 21st century, reports started emerging of carbapenemases, which are bacterial enzymes that destroy carbapenems. As in previous situations, their appearance was slow initially, but then it picked up momentum. Natural selection is a powerful force: kill off susceptible bacteria, and the antibiotic-resistant ones emerge to take their place.

As with the β-lactamases, there is not just a single resistance gene and enzyme, but a considerable variety. They have abbreviated names like KPC, NDM, VIP, CYM-10, OXA-48, and others. The genes coding for the carbapenemases are located on mobile genetic units and can spread relatively easily among different organisms. This occurs mainly in the healthcare environment, but a few reports of community-dwelling strains exist. When an organism acquires a gene making it resistant to the carbapenems, it is also resistant to the other β-lactam antibiotics, the penicillins and the cephalosporins. From the organisms' perspective, it's like "upgrading their software," going from an older model of β-lactamase to the latest version. As the genes become more common, not just the carbapenems can drive their further prevalence, but penicillins and cephalosporins as well. No one knows where this will take us in the next few decades, but if history is a helpful guide, it doesn't look good. Ampicillin resistance in *E. coli* was a rare event in the early 1960s. Today, over half of all hospital strains of *E. coli* are ampicillin resistant.

The β-lactams, of course, aren't the only class of antibiotics. In the "golden era" of antibiotic development in the 1950s, many were discovered, modified, tested, and released for medical use. When one looks at a tabular list of antibiotics available, it appears to be a never-ending supply. There are a couple hundred of them. But when we break it down to the antibiotic classes produced by one microorganism against another, we see that the list is short. After the β-lactams, there are only nine classes of antibiotics available for use in humans. All these classes have several members, which were constructed after chemical manipulation. But the classes of antibiotics are limited. And no new ones have been discovered in the last four decades. It seems the well is dry. Chemists will continue to probe to create new varieties, but the hope of finding a new class of antibiotic, e.g., penicillins or tetracyclines, is, it seems, remote.

Like the β-lactams, the glycopeptides attack the formation of the bacterial cell wall. Unlike the β-lactams, they aren't susceptible to the action of β-lactamases. The most used glycopeptide in the U.S. is vancomycin. There are several other members of the class, notably teicoplanin. Another variety is telavancin, technically a lipo-glycopeptide because of an added side chain. Others are oritavancin and dalbavancin. All members of the class are used almost exclusively against Gram-positive organisms because they are very large and don't penetrate the cell wall of the Gram-negatives.

Approved for clinical use in the United States in 1955, vancomycin was for years considered a second or third-tier antibiotic, used only in severe, complicated situations. That all changed with the emergence of MRSA, as it became the first drug of choice for severe cases. It still is today. When given orally, vancomycin is not absorbed from the intestinal tract, making it a reasonably good choice for treating problematic *Clostridium difficile* intestinal infections. All the glycopeptides are potentially toxic to patients and must be monitored carefully.

Another class of antibiotics that attack the bacterial cell wall is bacitracin. It is actually a mixture of several compounds collectively known as polypeptides. It was named after the patient in which it was first used, Margaret Treacy. Bacitracin prevents the transport of essential building blocks from the internal part of the cell to the outside. It is only effective against Gram-positive organisms can only be used topically; it cannot be injected or swallowed. Its most common use is in combination with other antibiotics in a skin ointment to prevent bacterial infection after damage to the skin.

Like all living cells, bacteria have a cell membrane. Theirs reside just below the cell wall. Two classes of antibiotics can attack the bacterial cell membrane while not at the same time attacking ours. There are two polymyxins used clinically. Polymyxin B is used topically, often in combination with other antibiotics. Polymyxin E, also known as colistin, is administered IV for systemic use. It is usually considered a back-up drug, employed in cases where an organism is resistant to the front-line antibiotics. The polymyxins go after the cell membranes of Gram-negatives.

Daptomycin, the only member of its class of lipopeptides, is active against Gram-positives, especially *Staphylococcus aureus*.

Bacteria manufacture proteins from the chemical code in their DNA, as our cells do. The code is copied onto a strand of RNA that then carries the message to ribosomes for protein production. There is a difference, though, in the construction of the bacterial ribosomes compared to ours, and that lays the foundation for the activity of several antibiotic classes. Known collectively as "protein synthesis inhibitors," the antibiotics of the classes tetracyclines, aminoglycosides, macrolides, lincosamides, and chloramphenicol are active in this area.

Ribosomes have two parts, each of a different size. In bacteria, the two sections are designated the 30S and 50S ribosomes. (Both the 30S and 50S sections are themselves made up of two parts, one being mostly protein, the other mostly RNA). When messenger RNA is initiated, the two ribosome sections come together and work to transcribe the genetic code. The general system is the same in bacterial and human cells.

Several antibiotics can attach themselves to sections of the bacterial ribosome and disrupt the synthesis of the protein coded along the messenger RNA. They either physically connect to a section of the ribosome to block the process before it is complete, or prevent the messenger RNA attachment.

The aminoglycosides were discovered very early in the search for antibiotics. Streptomycin was the first, and there was great excitement with its discovery. It was effective against *Mycobacterium tuberculosis* as well as a range of Gram-negative bacteria. Other members of the aminoglycoside class followed, and they represent an important weapon in the fight against invading bacteria. The aminoglycosides attach to a spot on the bacterial 30S ribosome, position 1408. By doing so, the progression of messenger RNA during translation is halted, and the bacterial proteins are not manufactured. We have different ribosomes, so the antibiotic does not attach to and disrupt our protein synthesis.

But the microbes have found a way to fight back. Bacteria have developed enzymes that alter the antibiotic before it reaches the ribosome's target site. Instead of destroying the antibiotic, the bacterial enzymes add a side group of simple organic compounds, impairing the antibiotic's ability to attach to the bacterial ribosome. The genes coding for these resistance enzymes can be passed from one organism to another, spreading aminoglycoside resistance among bacterial species and strains.

The aminoglycosides cannot be taken orally, so their route of administration is either intravenous or topical. They also don't penetrate some areas of the body, such as the central nervous system, so there are limitations in their use. Toxicity, especially to the kidneys and ears, has been a problem since their introduction, although in the latest versions, it is reduced. Still, they have been an extremely valuable addition to the antibiotic regimen. Aminoglycosides are used primarily against serious Gram-negative infections and in treating streptococcal heart valve infections (endocarditis) in hospitalized patients. In the community, they are an important part of antibiotic creams (e.g., Neosporin) and antibacterial eye drops. Today, in hospital settings, three drugs of the class predominate, gentamicin, tobramycin, and amikacin. All are made by different organisms but target the same bacterial ribosomal site. Bacterial resistance to one does not necessarily confer resistance to the others. But, like with all antibiotics, resistance levels are growing.

The class of antibiotics known as the tetracyclines was discovered a little after the aminoglycosides in the early 1950s. They resemble the latter in several ways. Produced by soil bacteria, they attach to the 30S ribosome preventing the affected bacteria from making protein. Their target site is different, however. They attach to the point where the messenger RNA hooks up to begin translation. Tetracyclines attach to the same point as the bacterial messenger RNA, so the process is stopped in its tracks.

Unfortunately, the attachment of tetracyclines to the 30S ribosome is reversible. Therefore, the antibiotic action is bacteriostatic, meaning the organism is slowed to a standstill rather than overtly killed. Usually, this is not a problem as the body's immune defenses can take over, but sometimes it results in relapses or treatment failure. When available, a bactericidal (killing) antibiotic is preferable.

The tetracyclines have several important characteristics in their favor, the most important of which is their great range of activity. Not only do they attack both Gram-positive and Gram-negative organisms, but they also are effective in treating intracellular organisms and some spirochetes. There are even some parasites that are affected. The drug can be given orally and intravenously, so it is used very commonly in the outpatient setting, treating ailments such as respiratory and genitourinary tract infections, skin infections, and specific conditions such as Lyme disease and brucellosis.

As the name suggests, tetracycline consists of four adjacent rings. The initial drug had to be administered four times a day. In the late 1960s, modifications resulted in antibiotics that were both intermediate-acting and long-acting. The long-acting drugs, doxycycline and minocycline, only had to be given once daily. Today, the most prescribed member of the tetracycline class is doxycycline (sometimes referred to by its original trade name, Vibramycin). A recent modification to the tetracycline multi-ring structure was adding a glycyl group to a minocycline molecule. The resulting antibiotic, known as tigecycline, has even broader activity and is not as susceptible to antibiotic resistance mechanisms affecting other tetracyclines. Tigecycline is known as a unique class of antibiotic known as the glycylcyclines, but it could just as easily be called a "third-generation tetracycline." Unfortunately, it is also bacteriostatic, not bactericidal.

Bacterial resistance to tetracycline comes in several forms. In one, the pores in the cell wall through which the drug must travel to get inside the bacterial cell can be altered, so the antibiotic is unable to enter the bacterial cell. In another, enzymes known as an "efflux pump" expel the antibiotic from the cell after it enters. The most common resistance mechanism is the ribosomal resistance protein, which binds to the tetracycline molecule and tears it away from its binding site. Organisms can share the genes for each of these mechanisms, and antibiotic resistance is not uncommon, especially in the hospital setting.

It was observed in the early 1950s that farm animals receiving tetracycline often grew larger than those that didn't. That's just plain weird. Antibiotics affect bacteria, not mammals and birds, yet the evidence of weight gain in animals was indisputable. For decades, the reasons for this were unclear; farmers just kept putting small quantities of tetracycline, and a few other antibiotics, in animal feed and growing bigger animals. It seemed like a no-brainer. But evidence has mounted that microbes in humans, as well as animals, have a direct impact on weight regulation. Which microbes, and in what way, is the subject of vigorous investigation. But it seems there is a direct correlation between the reduction of the gut microbiota and weight gain in some individuals. Putting antibiotics in animal feed also pushes the emergence of antibiotic-resistant bacteria, whose resistance genes can be spread to other microbes. Maybe putting antibiotics in animal feed wasn't such a good idea after all.

The other side of the bacterial ribosome, the 50S subunit, is the target of four other antibiotic classes. Specifically, the 23S portion of the 50S unit is the point of action. That is where the growing protein chain occurs, with the continual addition of individual amino acids by transfer RNA. Although chemically unrelated, the macrolides and lincosamides attach to and inhibit this area, stopping the synthesis of bacterial proteins dead in their tracks. Chloramphenicol also binds to the 50S ribosome but at a different site, accomplishing the same thing.

The first macrolide developed was erythromycin, found in 1951 and derived from a soil bacterium found in the Philippines. It has a very unusual biochemical shape, a 14-membered ring with two strange-looking carbohydrates as side chains. It is effective against a wide range of bacteria, both Gram-positive and Gram-negative, but because of its size and unusual properties, it has trouble entering quite a few Gram-negative organisms. Erythromycin has some pharmacologic problems; mainly, it accelerates bowel motility in many people, giving diarrhea and nausea, and it needs to be administered four times a day. A chemical modification of it, azithromycin, is currently the most prescribed macrolide, and with the catchy name "Z-pack," it's easy to remember. Given just once a day with reduced intestinal problems, it is usually worth the extra cost.

The lincosamides were first marketed in 1962, having been simultaneously discovered from two sources, soil bacteria from Lincoln, Nebraska, and Caracas, Venezuela. The original formulation, lincomycin, has been replaced by a closely related compound, clindamycin. It is used regularly in clinical practice, especially against Gram-positive pathogens and infections caused by anaerobic organisms.

Chloramphenicol should be the perfect antibiotic. It affects both Gram-negative organisms and Gram-positives, can be administered orally and intravenously, penetrates well into all body tissues, and can be easily made synthetically and inexpensively. But it has one fatal flaw (literally): in some individuals, perhaps one in 25,000, it causes an irreversible suppression of the bone marrow, aplastic anemia. This was noted shortly after its release in 1949. It has been relegated to back-up status, used only in dire emergencies involving multi-drug resistant organisms and with an ominous clinical outlook.

Unlike the other antibiotics that interfere with bacterial 50S ribosomes, the pleuromutilin class comes from a soil fungus, not bacteria. It was discovered in the early 1950s from a fungus called *Pleurotus mutilis*, hence the name pleuromutilin. (The fungus is now called *Omphalina mutila*). The antibiotic was neglected for over 50 years, but technology developed after the turn of the century enabled scientists to synthesize the drug and make it safe to administer to humans. Two antibiotics of the class used in humans are Lefamulin (trade name Xenleta), which is used to treat community-acquired pneumonia, and Retapulin (Altabax, Altargo), an ointment for skin infections, mainly impetigo caused by *Streptococcus pyogenes* and *Staphylococcus aureus*).

In addition to the antibiotics, that is, substances produced by one microorganism that are destructive to another microorganism, several non-biological antimicrobials are available. These are chemicals produced in a laboratory that can kill microbes. They do not originate in an organism like a fungus or a bacterium. Since they do the same work as antibiotics they are often referred to as such, even though there is a technical difference.

The first ones available, of course, were the sulfa drugs, which interfere with an organism's ability to manufacture folic acid, also known as vitamin B9. The sulfas by themselves are rarely used today, but adding a second compound to the mix, trimethoprim, has resulted in a commonly used antimicrobial.

Both sulfa and trimethoprim interfere with the organism's ability to manufacture the nucleic acid thymidine. Sulfa and trimethoprim are each picked up by bacterial enzymes in the construction process more vigorously than the intended substances, and the process aborts, leaving no folic acid and, hence, no thymidine.

The name trimethoprim/sulfamethoxazole is pretty hard to say. Even "trimeth/sulfa" doesn't exactly roll off the tongue, so the original trade names Septra and Bactrim are usually used, even though the medication has long been off-patent. Trimethoprim/sulfamethoxazole was approved by the U.S. Food and Drug Administration many years ago for treating uncomplicated urinary tract infections involving Gram-negative rods. In that regard, it has become a second-tier player. Bacterial resistance to it has long been a problem. But the drug has assumed new importance in recent years with the emergence of two new infections, one common and the other rare. Community-associated methicillin-resistant *Staphylococcus aureus* (MRSA), if confined to a simple skin lesion, usually responds quite well to it. A much less common infection usually found in patients with AIDS is a lung infection caused by the yeast *Pneumocystis jirovecii*, a potentially fatal infection in that patient population. It is often administered in that setting prophylactically. The FDA never approved the drug for either of these infections, so it is used off-label.

For a very long time, the drug used to treat malaria was quinine, which was and still is quite effective, but it has some drawbacks. After World War II, much research was given to developing synthetic compounds that could be produced and administered cheaply. One of the most successful of these was chloroquine, which became a standard of treatment for many years. In the early 1960s researchers discovered that certain compounds produced during the manufacture of chloroquine had anti-bacterial properties. After working with these compounds, called quinolones, an anti-bacterial compound called nalidixic acid became available. Active only against Gram-negative rods, it was used only to treat uncomplicated urinary tract infections. Since bacterial resistance developed rather readily and other, better agents were available, nalidixic acid (also known by its trade name Negram) virtually disappeared. It was revived in the late 1980s when researchers fiddled around with the core molecule and found that adding a fluorine atom at a key location and some other changes gave a much better drug, and the fluoroquinolones were born. Since their introduction, they have become one of the most prescribed antimicrobial drugs in the world.

The quinolones affect the DNA of the bacterial cell. The DNA in prokaryotes is not enclosed in a nuclear membrane like ours but twists and coils throughout the cell. There are enzymes called gyrases and topoisomerases that control the unwinding and re-winding of the DNA, and it is this process that is impacted by the quinolones. The killing is rapid and very effective.

The first fluoroquinolone introduced for humans was ciprofloxacin, usually called Cipro, its trade name. Others have followed, and all end with the suffix –oxacin. Several are available today, differing in pharmacologic properties but virtually identical in their spectrum of activity.

It's easy to see why fluoroquinolones are used so much. They can be administered both orally and intravenously, are effective against a wide range of organisms, and penetrate well into most human tissue. But they aren't perfect. It was noticed shortly after their introduction that some people develop very painful joints and tendons. Some people develop central nervous system symptoms. Fluoroquinolones should not be used in young children except for serious infections.

Because the fluoroquinolones are made synthetically in the laboratory and did not evolve in nature, there was some hope initially that bacteria would not have the genetic and chemical means to develop resistance very easily. Unfortunately, this hope has proven to be false, as resistance, especially in the healthcare setting, has been significant, and is rising. In some medical centers, up to 30% of Gram-negative bacteria causing infections are resistant to the entire group.

Another class of antimicrobial agents prepared entirely synthetically in the laboratory are oxazolinodones. Only one agent is available for treating humans in this class, linezolid.

The oxazolinodones were first produced by the DuPont company in the 1970s for treating plant pathogens, but with a lot of work, linezolid was approved to treat human infections in the year 2000. Linezolid is used exclusively to treat Gram-positive infections, primarily methicillin-resistant *Staphylococcus aureus* (MRSA) and certain species of the genus *Enterococcus*, a relative of the streptococci, that are resistant to the antibiotic vancomycin. Linezolid attaches to the 50S ribosome of bacteria and apparently prevents the combination of the 50S and 30S segments, therefore shutting down protein synthesis. The most important side effect is the suppression of blood cell production in the bone marrow, primarily blood platelets. Fortunately, unlike chloramphenicol, the suppression is reversible once the patient is taken off the medication. Linezolid is usually used as a backup drug when a more common one cannot be. A more recent addition to the oxazolinodones is tedizolid. Other promising oxazolidinones are under development, including some that can be used in the treatment of tuberculosis.

There are around 210 antibiotics approved by the FDA for use in the United States, quite a formidable number. But that number is really misleading. There are only a few more than a dozen classes of antibiotics in existence, and some of those have very limited use. It is not unusual to see a new antibiotic released and marketed as a new "class" of antibiotic, but it is simply a modification of an existing one. No new antibiotic or antimicrobic classes have been discovered in years; all recent additions have been chemical modifications of existing ones. It seems the well is very close to running dry. That makes the emergence of antibiotic resistance by bacteria much more concerning. The subject of resistance is complex and difficult to predict, but there surely is a pattern of an increasing number of resistant strains that make treatment decisions difficult. Often, the outcomes are tragic.

Some bacteria are adept at acquiring resistance to antibiotics. Others are not. When Alexander Fleming made his famous discovery of the inhibition of bacterial growth by the mold *Penicillium*, he was using the bacterium *Staphylococcus aureus*. Today, over 90% of the clinical isolates of that organism are resistant to penicillin. On the other hand, another Gram-positive bacterium, *Streptococcus pyogenes*, the cause of strep throat and some other very serious infections, has never developed penicillin resistance and is 100% susceptible. A similar theme emerges throughout the spectrum of infecting bacteria and antimicrobial agents to combat them. Some species of bacteria are very good at acquiring resistance to the antibiotic, while others remain susceptible. When we discuss antibiotics on a macro level, we must speak generally. Antibiotics are a long way from losing their effectiveness against many infecting species.

Bacterial antibiotic resistance today is most troublesome in two main areas: the staphylococci and the Gram-negative rods. Unfortunately, these are some of the most likely culprits to cause us great harm. There are certainly others, but Staph and GNRs head the list. With Staph, the most worrisome is, of course, methicillin-resistant strains (again, this is perhaps the worst named term in all biology; it should be β-lactam antibiotic-resistant strains). The common occurrence of these strains necessitates using potentially toxic antibiotics over an extended period rather than a less toxic one (e.g., nafcillin) that causes less collateral damage. In the case of Gram-negative rods, serious infections may cause sepsis, which can rapidly result in serious consequences. The initial antibiotic administered to treat an infection is usually selected empirically (from the Greek *empeirikos*, "by experience"). It won't be effective if the infecting bacterial strain is resistant to it. By the time the proper drug is selected, the patient may have gone beyond the point of no return.

One of the most useful services the clinical microbiology laboratory renders to healthcare is determining and reporting the susceptibility and resistance of bacteria to anti-microbial agents. Isolating and identifying the infectious agent is important, but it's only half the battle. Knowing the appropriate medication to use to clear the infection is vital. To this end is the anti-microbial susceptibility test.

The susceptibility test is straightforward. Make dilutions of the drug to be tested, put an equal amount of the infecting organism into each dilution, and see how much of the drug is required to inhibit the organism's growth. The amount of the drug in the test tube where the organism fails to grow is called the minimum inhibitory concentration, or MIC. For instance, if a strain of *E. coli* isolated from an infection is able to grow in 1 microgram per milliliter of an antibiotic, but not in the tube containing 2 micrograms, the MIC is reported as 2 mcg/ml. If it is not able to grow in the smallest dilution of the series, the MIC is reported as less than or equal to the smallest amount tested. If it grows in all the dilutions, the MIC is reported greater than the highest dilution tested.

The amount of antibiotic that appears in the bloodstream after administration is known. Each drug will have a peak and trough. In selecting the appropriate antibiotic for use, it is important to correlate the MIC with the level of drug usually achievable in the blood. If the MIC indicates that the drug can treat the infection under usual circumstances, the lab attaches the interpretation of "susceptible," abbreviated "S." If not, the interpretation is "resistant," or "R." This system works most of the time, but careful attention to detail is required. Not all antibiotics enter all spaces of the body in the same concentrations they achieve in the blood. What may work in a urinary tract infection may not apply to a central nervous system infection. The S and R interpretations apply to usually achievable serum levels of the antimicrobic.

Usually, it is enough for an antimicrobial agent to arrest the growth of the invading bacteria. The drug slows it down so the immune system can finish the job. But for some infections, the antimicrobial used must be able to kill the infecting bacteria, not just inhibit their growth. In these situations, the lab can determine the minimum bactericidal concentration or MBC. Just because growth is not observed in a test tube doesn't mean that all the organisms are dead. A sample from the tubes showing no growth is transferred to antibiotic-free media and incubated overnight. The culture plate showing no growth from the lowest dilution represents the MBC.

The term "antibiotic stewardship" is a good one, encompassing the judicious use of antibiotics. This includes, of course, their use in hospitals and healthcare settings, but also agriculture and industry. Several bacterial genes coding for antibiotic resistance in human pathogens have been found to have originated in organisms that do not cause disease and are not intimately associated with humans. But their genes were passed along to human pathogens somewhere along the way, and the chain continued. Clearly, it's important that new chains of antimicrobial resistance are not allowed to happen, or at least minimized. This means that antibiotics only be used when absolutely necessary, with the correct drug selected for the job, and not used in excess.

That's easier said than done. Ask any primary care physician, and they will likely tell you that one of their biggest headaches is trying to convince their patient that an antibiotic will not cure their infection or condition. Sometimes an antibiotic is prescribed to make the patient happy. Some people don't take all their antibiotics when prescribed, put the excess away in the medicine cabinet, then haul it out and "self-prescribe" when they feel sick. In some countries, antibiotics are available without a prescription; in others, they are sold on the black market. All of this adds to the problem of antibiotic resistance.

Hospitals keep track of the level of antibiotic resistance in their institutions by a tabulation known as an antibiogram. It is simply the number of antibiotic susceptible strains isolated over a defined period, usually a year, computed as a percentage of that organism's total number of isolates. For instance, if a hospital had 1,000 strains of *Escherichia coli* isolated from individual patients during the year from various sources such as urine, blood, and others, and 850 of them were susceptible to ciprofloxacin, the figure posted would be 85, for 85% of strains susceptible. These numbers are recorded and tracked through the years, and the results are worrying. The number of resistant strains doesn't usually show a marked increase, but an increase nonetheless. The number susceptible may go from 85% one year to 83% the next, then 80%. And on and on. It's like that for many antibiotics. Just where it all ends up is unknown, but the trend is unmistakable. The clock is ticking.

Chapter 43
Gut Check

Vital to health, yet
Underappreciated.
Gut microbiome.

Gut is a word that has many uses. We can gut a fish. A courageous person has a lot of guts. A coward can be described as gutless. We can hate someone's guts. When things are not going well, we try to gut it out. Facing a difficult situation may be a gut check. An offensive remark can seem like a punch in the gut. Sometimes we act on a gut feeling. Difficult decisions can be gut-wrenching. The inner parts of a device can be described as its guts. Fire can gut a building. Laying out our emotions is spilling one's guts. Sometimes we need to explore the fundamentals of something, to get to the guts of the matter.

It's somewhat unfortunate that the word gut is often used so cavalierly, minimizing its importance. It is a vital set of organs, for many reasons. The digestion, manufacture, and absorption of nutrients, immune system development, and warding off microbial predators are important parts of the digestive system's function. There are others. Like all our vital organs, a properly functioning digestive system is essential for good health.

In anatomy, the gut is an informal word describing part of our intestinal tract. While the alimentary canal runs from the mouth to the anus, the word gut commonly refers to the intestines. The word comes from several sources, mostly meaning "flow through a channel." In ancient times the abdominal viscera were thought to be the center of emotions.

The intestines are conveniently divided into sections. After the stomach is the small intestine, consisting of the duodenum, jejunum, and ileum. We're lucky we only use the word duodenum, not the original Latin name, *intestinum duodenum digitorum,* "intestine of twelve fingers length." Place your hands side by side on a flat surface. The length across the fingers, plus two fingers more, is the length of the duodenum, hence the name from the Latin *duodeni,* meaning "twelve."

Seriously. The name jejunum comes from the Latin *jejunus*, meaning "empty," on the assumption that the jejunum is empty after death. The name ileum is also from the Latin, *ilium*, meaning "flank" or "groin," indicating its location near the hip bone (ilium).

Most of our digestion and absorption occurs in the small intestine. The pancreas and the liver's bile duct empty here, aiding the process. In most adults, the small intestine is about ten feet in length, but that doesn't tell the whole story. The internal lining has innumerable nooks and crannies, looking something like a car's air filter. Surface area is a key feature.

The small intestine is not a hospitable place for bacteria. A few transiently survive, so the small bowel is not sterile, but it is nothing like the large intestine. Most of our digestion and nutrient absorption happens in the small intestine. If it is occupied by too many bacteria, the bugs will help themselves to the nutrients, robbing the infected individual. Acid from the stomach, bile, and digestive enzymes keep the bacterial count low. Some people, for a variety of reasons, get an overgrowth of bacteria in their small intestine, a condition called small intestinal bacterial overgrowth, SIBO. One pathogenic organism, *Helicobacter pylori,* can infect the duodenum, causing peptic ulcers and sometimes cancer, because it can survive in an acidic environment (Chapter 38). A few organisms that cause gastroenteritis, most notably *Shigella* and enterohemorrhagic *E. coli,* can multiply in the small intestine to achieve high numbers, but they don't invade there; they attack in the large intestine (Chapter 13). Some parasites infest the small intestine partly because of the nutrient-rich environment. *Ascaris* and hookworm are among them (Chapter 20). *Giardia lamblia* infests the duodenum (Chapter 19). Norovirus, the cause of acute nausea, vomiting, and diarrhea, targets cells in the small intestine.

The large intestine is also conveniently divided into sections. The opening to the large intestine is the cecum, a pouch about two and a half inches long. Attached to the cecum is the appendix. (To find the location of the cecum and appendix, trace a line from your naval to your right hip bone crest. The appendix is located two-thirds the distance, closer to the hip bone. It's called McBurney's point). After the cecum is the colon, which is divided into three sections, ascending, transverse, and descending. The sigmoid colon is the terminal section of the descending segment (*sigmoid*, because it somewhat resembles the letter S). The rectum is the final colon segment.

Unlike the small intestine, the colon is replete with microorganisms. Billions of them. The vast majority are bacteria, but procaryotes, yeast, archaea, and viruses are also present. (Archaea look like bacteria but are a distinct group. They aren't known to cause human disease, but their metabolism sometimes resembles that of bacteria).

The word biome refers to a geographic area inhabited by a wide variety of life forms that have in common their ability to flourish in the same environment. In nature, the main plant life in an area assigns the biome a name, e.g., grassland, coniferous forest. Many living creatures are found in a biome, ranging from enormous trees to microscopic organisms. Often, a biome's inhabitants interact in a way beneficial to both. Sometimes the activity of one organism is detrimental to another. It's an ongoing, dynamic environment.

The organisms in our bowel form a biome, and given their size, it is called a microbiome. All organisms that live in the gut can thrive under moist conditions at 98°F (37°C). They each have the means to obtain nutrition from the material in the colon, and most do not need oxygen to replicate.

As soon as we are born, our gut microbiome forms and begins to grow. In babies from a vaginal delivery, organisms inhabiting the birth canal initially predominate. In those delivered by Caesarian section, it is the microbes from skin flora. As we age, our microbiome matures with us, vastly expanding in the numbers and species of bacteria. People differ in the content of their gut microbiomes. The genes of humans are 99.9% identical. But the collective genes of different gut microbiomes show considerable variation between people, even in members of the same family and household. Age, gender, diet, and lifestyle choices are all influential.

Historically, microscopic organisms of the gut were regarded as insignificant commensal freeloaders. If they didn't invade a human and cause damage, they were ignored by microbiologists or considered a nuisance when an intestinal pathogen was sought in laboratory tests. Most bowel bacteria flora cannot be grown on laboratory culture plates, so it wasn't possible to easily work with them. The characterization of non-pathogenic fecal bacterial flora was, for a long time, regarded as an esoteric, academic exercise.

Technology developed in the early 21st century radically altered that paradigm. Identifying and enumerating most of the nearly thousand organisms in each person's colon is now possible using genetic microarray sampling. Each bacterial species has its own unique molecular configuration on one part of their ribosomes, the 16S section. Routine testing can now be done to enumerate which and how many 16S ribosomes are present in each person's stool sample, giving an accurate overview of the bacterial species present and their proportionate numbers. Comparisons of the gut microbiome can be made between healthy and unhealthy people, and the presence or absence of key microbes can be evaluated. The science is in its infancy, but some facts seem evident.

In the clinical microbiology laboratory, technologists employ nutrients to grow bacteria. The nutrients are called media, and the growth of large numbers of bacteria is called a culture. The nutrients used to grow the bugs are called culture media. Two main types of culture media are used, liquid and solid. Liquid culture media is a broth made from nutrients known to support the growth of the microorganisms sought. A common one is trypticase soy broth, made by enzymatic digestion of soybean meal. There are many others. Solid culture media is prepared by adding a small amount of the hardening substance agar to the broth. Assorted ingredients can be added to further enrich the media. Whole blood and blood products are often used. When organisms grow on the culture media they form colonies, and the bacteria forming them can be identified.

We might think of the human colon as an enormous microorganism culture medium. Nutrients are supplied by the human host. Those microbes that are able to metabolize the nutrients provided will flourish and grow, while those unable to will wither and die out. Sometimes lab workers impart their culture media with noxious substances such as antibiotics to select for the desired microorganism. Bugs susceptible to that agent will not grow, allowing the antibiotic-resistant pathogen to grow unobstructed and be identified. The same principle is at work in the colon: if the human host consumes a noxious substance, bacteria resistant to it will flourish while those susceptible will not.

Many bacteria interact with other organisms. Some produce an antibiotic that inhibits or kills other bacteria. Some bacteria produce substances enabling other organisms to grow. Occasionally, an organism unable to grow on laboratory culture media will grow on it if another organism grows and produces a needed nutrient. The dependent bacteria grow around the other as small satellite colonies.

Bacteria can be infected by viruses. This makes for an interesting situation in the establishment and maintenance of the bacterial flora in the gut. Viruses that invade bacteria are called bacteriophages. That's usually shortened to "phages". Usually, the phages are specific to unique species of bacteria. Which bacteriophages are present in the gut, which bacteria they invade and kill, and the overall effect on the gut microbiome is sometimes important. A person may have an imbalance in their colon's bacterial flora, but if it is due to a phage that attacks and kills an important strain of bacteria it's difficult to evaluate and correct.

When microbes metabolize a substrate they often release a by-product. Lab workers can use the presence of the by-product to aid in identifying the organism. A good example is the fermentation of the carbohydrate lactose, the sugar found in milk. Generally, non-infectious bacteria like *E. coli* and *Enterobacter* ferment lactose, resulting in acid formation. The acidic environment can be easily detected with common dyes. Pathogenic organisms like *Salmonella* and *Shigella* don't ferment lactose, so no acid is produced. There are many other by-products of bacterial metabolism. In the gut microbiome, most are inconsequential and pass out of the colon. But some can have a direct effect on other bacteria. Some can affect human cells.

The life and death dynamics observed on laboratory culture media are constantly at play in our gut microbiome. Some organisms thrive on the nutrients provided, while others succumb for a lack of proper nutrition or the presence of a substance that poisons them. Organisms can affect other members of the biome, either to their betterment or detriment. It's a constantly changing, dynamic system.

A critical factor determining the gut microbiome's dynamics is the diet of the human host. The adage "We are what we eat" could be altered a little to read "THEY are what we eat." Some bacteria are saccharolytic; they thrive on sugars. Others are proteolytic, doing their best feeding on proteins. Some bacteria can metabolize cellulose and create energy from it. Just like a lab tech putting varied ingredients into a culture medium to try to grow a select organism, food products assimilated into the gut will do the same. Potentially toxic substances can select for some species by killing their rivals.

It's difficult to draw firm conclusions about the content of the gut microbiome on human health. Genetic arrays are now available that can compare the bacterial populations of a large number of individuals. If there is a preponderance of a condition or symptom among individuals who share similar gut microbiome profiles, then it is reasonable to conclude that there is a possibility of cause and effect. Altering the bacterial flora of some individuals, then seeing a change in the condition or illness along with a difference in the microbiome profile, is also good evidence. In such cases, it is not yet possible to precisely pinpoint which microbe(s) is involved, but usually, such a precise answer is not needed.

There are some cases in which the nature of an infectious condition can be directly attributed to diet and specific microbes. As discussed in Chapter 36, the oral bacterium *Streptococcus mutans* is a ravenous metabolizer of sucrose (white sugar). When a person's diet is high in the continued use of sucrose, *S.*

mutans attaches to tooth enamel and creates a significant acid environment to which other acid-loving microbes are attracted. The bacteria combine to form a biofilm (dental plaque), leading to tooth enamel erosion and dental caries. Eliminating sucrose from the diet has a demonstrable effect on the reduction of tooth decay.

As discussed in Chapter 15, *Clostridium difficile* is usually a passive inhabitant of the colon. Many people harbor the organism with no ill effects. But when antibiotics are administered, the bacterial flora of the colon undergoes change. Some organisms die off, and the balance of the gut microbiome is thrown off-kilter, a situation called dysbiosis (disrupted biome). *Clostridium difficile* is a spore former, and bacterial spores are not affected by antibiotics, so they survive. Normally, the spores are eliminated during bowel motility, but the spores remain if there is bowel stasis (constipation). The antibiotic suppresses the bacterial flora that normally competes with *Clostridium difficile*, so the spores germinate and have an ecologic advantage because of reduced competitors. The previously docile commensal turns into a viscous pathogen.

These are but two examples of food products or chemicals that can radically alter bacterial ecology with resultant disease. Similar situations are at play in the gut microbiome.

Because of the gut microbiome's variables and complexity, it is impossible to draw firm conclusions as in the case of the association of *Streptococcus mutans* and sucrose and dental caries, and *Clostridium difficile* and antibiotic administration with enteric colitis. But sometimes there is considerable circumstantial evidence, which can be compelling. Here are some observations that have been made about the association between the gut microbiome and health. There are many others:

As mentioned in Chapter 40, soon after the discovery and application of antibiotics farmers noticed that when they were administered to their livestock the animals grew heavier. If a few animals in a herd or flock are ill and need antibiotic treatment, it is often easier to put the medication in the feed for all since singling out the ill ones would be difficult. Also,

698

treating the entire group might prevent healthy animals from becoming sick. The practice became widespread when it became apparent that giving livestock a steady supply of antibiotics yielded larger animals. Tetracycline was the antibiotic most used, but there were others. It seems most likely that the reason for the animal's weight gain was the disruption of their gut microbiomes. Just how is subject to speculation, but it has been shown that some intestinal organisms influence the production of leptin, a hormone that regulates appetite and general energy maintenance. Leptin acts on the hypothalamus in the brain. Abnormal levels can affect fat storage and behavioral changes. Some intestinal bacteria are instrumental in the production of leptin. If their numbers are decreased, there may be a deficit in leptin production, perhaps influencing weight gain.

While coincidence is not evidence of causation, there has been a significant increase in obesity rates in humans since the introduction of and widespread use of antibiotics. Also, some preservatives used in processed foods are designed to inhibit bacterial growth. The use of antimicrobial agents along with the consumption of foods incompatible with the health of the gut microbiome may be in part responsible for the profound rise in the number of obese people.

Some vitamins are synthesized by bacteria in the colon. An important one that doesn't get much notoriety but is nevertheless important is vitamin K2. For a long time, it was felt that the K vitamins were useful just in the coagulation of blood (the designation "K" comes from the German word *koagulation*). Like its cousin K1, vitamin K2 does that, but recent research has shown it to be very important in the maintenance of calcium. Two areas where this is important are bone integrity and the prevention of calcification of blood vessel lesions, lessening the chance of sclerosis. Keeping the colon's bacteria active in vitamin K2 production helps in this area.

Gut microbes also manufacture vitamins B5 and B12, pantothenic acid and cobalamin, respectively. The former is important in fat metabolism, the latter in the integrity of the nervous and circulatory systems. A healthy gut microbiome helps ensure a plentiful supply of both.

When bacteria metabolize a nutrient, they often create a by-product. We're all familiar with the by-product of yeast fermentation, ethyl alcohol. Many bacteria in the colon produce by-products known as short-chain fatty acids. There are many depending on the bacterial species, including butyrate, propionate, acetate, pentanoate, hexanoate, and valerate. Each of these can be utilized by the human host as an energy source, water absorption, regulation of blood flow through tissues, epithelial cell replacement, or as an aid in a metabolic process. Compromising the colon's bacterial flora may decrease the amount of short-chain fatty acids and their nutritional and metabolic benefit.

All of our internal organs are sterile. When a microbe enters, the immune system becomes active, utilizing multiple weapons to expel the invader. The colon, though, harbors not just a few but billions of microbes, both to our benefit and theirs. Immune tolerance is key to this peaceful coexistence. Just how this comes about is the subject of intensive investigation, but a few facts are known.

Mice can be raised in special environments to be germ-free. The germ-free state is called gnotobiotic, from two Greek words *gnostos,* meaning "known," and *bios,* meaning "life." When the immune system of germ-free animals is closely examined, it is found to be significantly deficient. Macrophages and several types of lymphocytes are very slow to respond to infectious challenges. But after the germ-free mice are infused with a gut microbiome from other mice, their immune responses are close to normal. Clearly, the bacteria implanted in the colon influence the performance of immune cells.

The lining of the interior surface of the colon is called the mucosa. A thin layer of mucus overlays the epithelial cells. The epithelial cells have tight junctions. Intimately associated with the epithelial cells is an underlying network of connective tissue called the lamina propria. The lamina propria contains a large number of cells of the immune system, including macrophages, dendritic cells, and T-lymphocytes. It is especially rich in the number of antibody-producing cells it harbors, the plasma cells.

Most of the antibodies produced are of the IgA or secretory type. IgA is unique among the antibodies, in that it can enter and pass through epithelial cells. If on its journey through the epithelial cells and mucin it should encounter an antigen of a microbe, it attaches to it and neutralizes the microbe. IgA antibodies don't bind complement, so there is only negligible inflammation. There are two types of IgA antibodies, one group that binds proteins on the microbes, and another that binds carbohydrates. The immune cells in the lamina propria produce a steady stream of a wide variety of IgA antibodies, helping to prevent the bacteria in the gut from becoming overly aggressive.

This arrangement of mucus, tight junctions, and immune cell repositories combine to prevent the entry of gut bacteria into the sterile areas in the bowel lining. Bacteria in the gut can get trapped in the mucin, can't penetrate the tight junctions of the epithelial cells, or can be bound by the IgA antibodies secreted by the plasma cells in the lamina propria. But there is also chemical cross-talk between the bacteria and the cells in the intestinal wall, including cells of the immune system. Some bacteria stimulate an immune response, while others suppress it. It's like a "good-cop bad-cop" affair. This activity seems to have the net effect of "training" the immune cells to become active. But if we disrupt the balance of the gut microbiome, the training of the immune cells becomes disharmonious. Sometimes this can lead to problems somewhere else in the body.

The mucus lining the colon is predominantly carbohydrate. Some gut bacteria are saccharolytic, meaning they metabolize carbohydrates. If the saccharolytic bacteria reach excessive numbers, the integrity of the colon's protective layer can be in jeopardy. This may allow for the penetration of some bacteria and their potentially hazardous by-products into the colon's lining, with subsequent entrance into the general circulation. Chronic inflammation and exacerbation of medical conditions may result.

One of the best studied bacteria of the gut microbiome is *Bacteroides thetaiotaomicron* (theta-iota-omicron; some lab techs call it the sorority bug. Most call it B. theta). There are nearly a thousand species of bacteria in the human gut microbiome; B. theta comprises about 6% of the bacterial volume. It's a major player. A significant attribute of B. theta is its ability to efficiently stimulate or suppress its genes in response to chemical signals it receives.

The mucosal layer of the large intestine is vital to health. B. theta interacts with the cells producing the mucus layer, and sends chemical signals to the epithelial cells of the colon, telling them to produce more or less mucin. Amazingly, this bacterium functions like a gland. B. theta conducts this type of chemical messaging with several metabolic systems in the colon.

Humans have around 22,000 non-redundant genes on our chromosomes. Collectively, the microbes of our gut microbiota have about 3.3 million genes, 150 times as many. The microbes in our colon can metabolize nutrients we can't. That often works to our benefit. In some cases, microbial metabolism is essential for good health. Some people get overwhelming life-altering infections with intractable *Clostridium difficile.* Despite aggressive antibiotic therapy, the infection becomes chronic. The therapy that has the best outcome in these patients is fecal microbiota transplantation, FMT. FMT demonstrates very well the importance of a well-balanced gut microbiome in all aspects of our health, including enhancing our immune system and the freedom from infectious diseases.

Humans and the microorganisms we harbor evolved together. For thousands of years, intimate molecular relationships have developed, including the robust functioning of our immune system. Keeping the gut microbiome functioning properly is vital. Most important is a diet with abundant vegetables, fruits, and grains, the kind of things people ate thousands of years ago. Modern research and commercial enterprise have developed live colon bacteria (probiotics) and packaged nutrients (prebiotics) to assist with establishing and maintaining the proper bowel flora, which may help in some cases. The organisms in our gut are part of us for our entire lives, just like our organs and tissues. It's good to keep in mind that if our gut microbiota ain't happy, ain't nobody happy. We're eating for two.

Afterword

Countries worldwide have holidays commemorating those who have given their lives for their country. The United States marks Memorial Day (the last Monday of May) and Veteran's Day (November 11th). In Germany it is Volkstrauertag (the Sunday closest to November 16th), Australia has Anzac Day (April 25), and the Netherlands observes Dodenherdenking (May 4). Taking time to reflect on and give honor to those who made sacrifices for their fellow citizens is respectful and fitting.

It would be equally respectful to give a thought of thanksgiving to those who sacrificed immensely for the health of all of us who live free of some of the most ravaging diseases. Some infectious diseases are just as destructive as the horrors of war. All people can be affected by infectious diseases, not just soldiers.

Florence Nightingale and her band of 38 nurses sailed off to the Crimean War in the 1850s, experiencing immeasurable horrors and agonies. Howard Ricketts camped out in an army tent in Montana, assiduously dissecting ticks trying to find the agent of Rocky Mountain Spotted Fever. He later died in Mexico at age 39 from a related disease, typhus. Carlos Chagas spent years working from an abandoned boxcar in the steamy Amazon jungle, treating the poor. It led him to the discovery of the disease American trypanosomiasis. Denis Burkitt spent much of his professional life in Africa, going on his "10,000-mile safari," treating the sick in remote locations and taking copious notes on his observations. His work was instrumental in the discovery of the Epstein-Barr virus.

There are so many more. Today's researchers are no less dedicated in their quest to alleviate disease and suffering from infectious diseases. We owe them all, past and present, our deepest gratitude.

Many of the infectious diseases reviewed in this work are known to many of us only through history and textbooks. Occasionally one will make the news, only to be replaced shortly after that by the next breaking story. But the only human infectious disease to be declared extinct is smallpox. All the others still infect. Not very much in the developed world, but in the underdeveloped.

Recent data collected by the World Health Organization and other agencies report that the yearly death rate worldwide for measles was 126,000. Most of those deaths were in young children. For tuberculosis the worldwide death rate recently was 1,600,000. There are still around nine million cases of typhoid fever every year, with over 100,000 deaths. For malaria it's 247 million cases with 620,000 deaths, the dead being mostly children and pregnant women. With cholera it's difficult to say because there are so many unreported cases, but it's at least 2.9 million cases and nearly 100,000 deaths. The list goes on. Many diseases aren't highly fatal, but they are extremely debilitating.

We've greatly curtailed these horrible ailments in the developed world. We mustn't forget the underdeveloped.

The Covid pandemic was a stark reminder of the ferocity of infectious diseases. The first reports of it were merely rumors emanating from The People's Republic of China in December 2019. In just three months, most of the world was in lock-down mode, overwhelmed by the virus. Infectious diseases will always be with us, despite the spectacular scientific advances achieved.

Here are a few things to ponder going forward:

Temperatures around the earth are warming, directly affecting the worldwide ecology of insects and the animals they parasitize. Mosquitoes, ticks, lice, fleas, and others can harbor and transmit numerous infectious pathogens, which often jump from one species to another. Human travel has always influenced the spread of infectious diseases, now more than ever.

Survival of the fittest is an inviolable fact of nature. When an antibiotic is administered, the organisms susceptible to it will wither and die, but they are often replaced by drug-resistant ones. The genes for resistance can be spread among the microbial population, broadening the reach of drug-resistant organisms. Since the introduction of antibiotics in the 1940s, there has been an inexorable progression of drug resistance. The proper metaphor is more trickle than flood, but it continues unabated. The ultimate result may be "pan-resistant" microbes, bugs resistant to all available antimicrobial agents.

The idea of using microbes as weapons is not new. Historical attempts were crude and rarely successful. Technology available today makes creating highly virulent viruses and bacteria a matter of routine. Both intentional and accidental release of severe pathogens can easily disrupt world affairs.

Infectious diseases are ubiquitous and unrelenting. We must always be on our guard. Expect the unexpected.

References and Further Study

Textbooks.   There are many fine textbooks on the subjects of infectious diseases, immunology, and anatomy and physiology.

The book used for research in the area of infectious diseases was Mandell, Douglas, and Bennett's *Principles and Practice of Infectious Diseases*, 9th edition. It is a highly technical two-volume work written primarily for professionals in the field.

For research on the immune system, the volume consulted the most was *Janeway's Immunobiology* by Kenneth Murphy, Casey Weaver, and Leslie Berg, 10th edition. It is also very technical and written for advanced students and professionals in the field.

Some chapters use descriptions and terms of anatomy and physiology. The chief source for that material was *Principles of Anatomy and Physiology* by Gerard Tortora and Bryan Derrickson, 16th edition.

Each of these textbooks requires a solid foundation in the field. The book *Immune* by Philipp Dettmer is a much lighter read, published in 2021. For the novice, it gives a comprehensive overview of the immune system.

While not a textbook per se, *Wikipedia* serves as a highly valued reference on many subjects.

There are some very informative videos of immune system activity on *Khan Academy's* website.

The scientific articles cited here are open source. Access to a medical library is not needed.

Chapter 1.   Because of her immense influence and remarkable personal story, many books have been written about Florence Nightingale. The source used for this work was *Florence Nightingale* by Mark Bostridge, published in 2008. It runs over 600 pages and is full of thoroughly researched details on the life of Ms. Nightingale.

The diagnosis of Ms. Nightingale's ailment following her experience in the Crimean War is, of course, speculative, but the article by Barbara Dossey, *Florence Nightingale: her Crimean fever and chronic illness*, published in the Journal of Holistic Nursing on June 16, 1998 is compelling in ascribing it to brucellosis.

Chapter 2.   Like Florence Nightingale, Louis Pasteur is an immensely important figure in the history of medicine, and much has been written about him and his work. In Chapter 2, the subject of the discovery of Pasteurization is discussed. The chief references were *The Life of Pasteur* by Rene Vallery-Radot, published in 1919. Also used was *Biography: Louis Pasteur: A controversial figure In a debate on scientific ethics* by B. Lee Ligon, published in Seminars in Pediatric Infectious Diseases, April 2002.

Chapter 3.   Smallpox history is presented in *History of Smallpox and Its Spread in Human Populations,* by Catherine Theves, Eric Crubezy, and Phillippe Biagini in ASM Journals/ Microbiology Spectrum, July 2016.

707

The origin of smallpox from animal viruses is addressed in a paper from Russia, *The Origin of the Variola Virus*, by Igor Babkin and Irina Babkina. It was published in the March 10, 2015 edition of the Journal *Viruses*.

The story of Lady Mary Wortley Montegu and her influence on variolation is most elegantly portrayed in Wikipedia. Many references are cited. Two of the most informative are books, *Lady Mary Wortley Montagu* by Isobel Grundy, published in 1999, and *The Life of Lady Mary Wortley Montagu* by Robert Halsband, published in 1956.

The chief reference for the tale of variolation in the U.S. was the book *The Fever of 1721* by Stephen Coss, published in 2016.

Edward Jenner's biographical information can be found on The Jenner Institute website. Another highly informative source is the article *Edward Jenner and the history of smallpox and vaccination* by Stefan Riedel, in Baylor University Medical Center Proceedings, January 2005.

A description of cowpox can be found in the article *Chasing Jenner's Vaccine: Revisiting Cowpox Virus Classification* by Darin Carroll et al, published in PLoSONE, August 8, 2011.

Most of the information about Variola pathophysiology is found in Mandell's *Principles and Practice of Infectious Diseases*, 9th edition.

Chapter 4.   The history of theriac is summarized in a May 26, 2012 article in the medical journal The Lancet. Entitled *The theriac in antiquity,* it was appropriately written by three Greek authors, Demetrios Karaberopoulos, Marianna Karamanou, and George Androutsos.

The history of the discovery and application of quinine is found in an article from Cambridge University Library, *Products of the Empire: Cinchona: a short history*. Wikipedia has an extensive review under the title *Quinine.*

The story of William Henry Perkin and the discovery of aniline dyes is reviewed in Open Mind BBVA, July 13, 2018, *Mauve: the History of the Colour that Revolutionized the World.*

Paul Ehrlich accomplished a great deal in his illustrious career. His work on the development of Salvarsan is reviewed in *Paul Ehrlich,* on the website of The Science History Institute.

The fascinating story of the sled-dog relay carrying diphtheria antiserum to Nome Alaska in 1925 is described in detail in the January 13, 2021 edition of Sports Illustrated, *Doggone It, If They Could Do It…,* by Jon Wertheim.

Wikipedia has a good review of Gerhard Domagk and his discovery of sulfanilamide.

The tragic story of the death of Calvin Coolidge Jr. is ably told in an article at the Shapell Manuscript Foundation, *Calvin Coolidge Jr.'s Death,* by Benjamin Shapell and Sara Willen, July 6th, 2017. The experience of Franklin Roosevelt Jr. with a near-fatal streptococcal infection and the cure by sulfa is found in an issue of Time magazine published on December 28, 1936, *Prontosil.*

The origin of the U.S. Food and Drug Administration resulting from the tragic use of a sulfa elixir is found in the book *The U.S. Healthcare System: Origins, Organizations, and Opportunities,* by Joel Shalowitz, page 398.

There are many references on the discovery of penicillin. The article by Jonathan Wood, published July 16, 2010, in the Oxford News Blog, is very descriptive. It's entitled *Penicillin: the Oxford story.*

The book *Miracle Cure* by William Rosen gives a comprehensive history of the discovery of antibiotics.

Chapter 5.   Much of the information for this chapter on the travails of Mary Mallon comes from the book *Fever,* by Mary Beth Keane, published in 2013.

The basics of epidemiology and hospital infection control can be found on the CDC's website under the heading Infection Control Basics.

Chapter 6.   There are many very good textbooks on the agents of infectious diseases. The one used for this chapter was Mandell's *Principles and Practice of Infectious Disease,* 9th edition.

Chapter 7.   A review of the physiology and function of neutrophils can be found in the article *Neutrophils: Molecules, Functions, and Pathophysiological Aspects,* published in the May 1, 2000 edition of Laboratory Investigation. Five authors contributed; Veronique Witco-Sarsat was the senior author.

Chapter 8.   Two references do an in-depth job describing the complement system and its function. One is from Frontiers in Immunology, published June 2, 2015. Written by French authors Nicolas Merle, Sarah Elizabeth Church, Veronique Fremeaux-Bacchi, and Lubka Roumenina, it is entitled *Complement system part I–molecular mechanisms of activation and regulation.*

The reference book *Janeway's Immunobiology,* 10th edition, Chapter 2, is also very descriptive.

Chapter 9.   Monocytes, macrophages, dendritic cells, and The Mononuclear Phagocyte System (formerly known as the Reticuloendothelial System, RES) are discussed in detail in the March 2015 edition of Annual Review of Immunology. The article, *Macrophages: Development and Tissue Specialization,* was written by Chen Varol, Alexander Mildner, and Steffen Jung.

Chapter 10.   An extensive biography of Alois Alzheimer appears in the June 2006 edition of the International Journal of Biological Sciences. It is titled *Alois Alzheimer: A Hundred Years after the Discovery of the Eponymous Disorder;* the lead author is Antonio Tagarelli.

The American Parkinson Disease Association has a detailed biography of James Parkinson on its website. It was written by Peter Beidler.

The role of microglial cells in Alzheimer's Disease is explored in an article in Frontiers in Aging Neuroscience, June 30, 2022. The title is *The Role of Microglia in Alzheimer's Disease From the Perspective of Immune Inflammation and Iron Metabolism.* Seven authors from China collaborated; the lead author is Hui-Zui Long.

Microglial cells' role in Parkinson's Disease is thoroughly discussed in an August 30, 2018, article in Frontiers in Cellular Neuroscience, *Microglial Implication in Parkinson's Disease: Loss of Beneficial Physiological Roles or Gain of Inflammatory Functions?* The lead author is Cynthia Lecours.

Atherosclerosis is a complex disease. The contribution of macrophages to the disorder is eloquently discussed in *Macrophages in atherosclerosis: a dynamic balance.* It was published in the October 13, 2013 edition of Nature Reviews Immunology. The authors are Kathryn Moore, Frederick Sheedy, and Edward Fisher. All were at the New York School of Medicine at the time of publication.

Septic shock is a very dangerous medical event. *The role of monocytes in the progression of sepsis* is a detailed paper written by Elena Sukhacheva. It was published on August 26, 2020 in Clinical Laboratory International.

The International Osteoporosis Foundation has a comprehensive review of osteoclasts and their role in osteoporosis. Under the heading *Pathophysiology,* there is a discussion of the biological causes of osteoporosis.

The etiology of inflammatory bowel disease is complex, and the activity of macrophages in the various disorders is integral. A review of macrophages and their involvement in IBD is found in the article *Roles of Macrophages in the Development and Treatment of Gut Inflammation.* It was written by Chinese authors Xuebing Han, Sujuan Ding, Hongmei Jiang, and Gang Liu. It was published in the March 2nd, 2021 edition of Frontiers in Cell and Developmental Biology.

A review of the role of macrophages in the disease rheumatoid arthritis is elegantly presented in the paper *Rheumatoid arthritis macrophages are primed for inflammation and display bioenergenic and functional alterations.* Eight researchers are listed, with Megan Hanlon form Dublin, Ireland the lead author. The article was published in the journal Rheumatology. It was published July 5, 2023.

The involvement of macrophages in the disease lupus is presented in a paper titled *Macrophage Polarization and Plasticity in Systemic Lupus Erythematosus,* published in the December 20, 2021 edition of Frontiers in Immunology. The authors are Miriame Mohamed Ahamada, Yang Jia, and Xiaochuan Wu

Chapter 11. A thorough discussion of lymphocytes and their function is presented in the textbooks listed above, *Janeway's Immunobiology* and Mandell's *Principles and Practice of Infectious Diseases.*

Chapter 12. The topics in chapter 12 are reviewed in Mandell's *Principles and Practice of Infectious Diseases.*

Chapter 13. A detailed biography of Theodor Escherich is presented in a paper published in Clinical Infectious Diseases, published October 15, 2007. Entitled *Theodor Escherich: The First Pediatric Infectious Physician?* It was written by Stanford Schulman, Herbert Friedmann, and Ronald Simms.

Bacterial genetics is discussed in great detail in the book Medical Microbiology, 4th edition, Chapter 5. It was written by Randall Holmes and Michael Jobling.

Shigellosis, enterohemorrhagic, enterotoxigenic, aggregative, invasive, and urinary tract *E. coli* is discussed at length and detail in Mandell's *Principles and Practice of Infectious Diseases.*

Chapter 14. Salmonella infections are reviewed in the article *Salmonella: A review on pathogenesis, epidemiology and antibiotic resistance.* It appeared in the June 9, 2015 online edition of Frontiers in Life Science. Malaysian researcher Shu-Kee Eng was the lead author.

The subject of typhoid fever is discussed in detail in *Salmonella enterica Serovar Typhi and the Pathogenesis of Typhoid Fever.* It was published in the September 2014 edition of Annual Review of Microbiology. The authors are Gordon Dougan and Stephen Baker.

The intentional *Salmonella* attack in Oregon is documented in an article in Wikipedia entitled *1984 Rajneeshee bioterror attack.*

Chapter 15. A detailed description of C diff infection can be found in Mandell's *Principles and Practice of Infectious Diseases.* A description of the activity of the toxins is elegantly presented in the article *Toxins A and B from Clostridium difficile Differ with Respect to Enzymatic Potencies, Cellular Substrate Specificities, and Surface Binding to Cultured Cells.* The lead author is Esteban Chaves-Olarte. It was published in the Journal of Clinical Investigation, October, 1997.

Chapter 16. The pathogenicity of *Brucella* explained in detail in an article that appeared in the June 6, 2015 edition of The American Journal of Pathology. It is titled *Pathogenesis and Immunobiology of Brucellosis; Review of Brucella–Host Interactions.* The lead author is Paul de Figuerido.

A review article written by Eric Daniel Avila-Calderon et al. shares much information on *Brucella* vaccines. Titled *A History of the Development of Brucella Vaccines,* it is published in the 2013 edition of BioMed Research International.

Listeria Pathogenesis and Molecular Virulence Determinants is a thorough reference on infections caused by *Listeria.* Written by Jose

Vazquez-Boland et al., it is published in Clinical Microbiology Reviews, the July, 2001 edition.

Chapter 17. A discussion of the disease tetanus and the action of its toxin can be found in Mandell's textbook *Principles and Practice of Infectious Diseases.* Another valuable reference is the article *Tetanus: a Review of the Literature,* written by T.M. Cook, R.T. Protheroe, and J.M. Handel. It was published in the 87th volume of the British Journal of Anaesthesia, 2001.

Peter Cornelis Wever and Leo van Bergen wrote an in depth and fascinating article, *Prevention of tetanus during the First World War.* It was published by group.bmj.com in November 2012.

Botulinum Neurotoxins: Biology, Pharmacology, and Toxicology is a review article published in the April 2017 edition of Pharmacological Reviews. It was written by Marco Pirazzini et al.

A description of diphtheria toxin is found in an article written by Randall Holmes, *Biology and Molecular Epidemiology of Diphtheria Toxin and the tox Gene.* It was published as a supplement in the Journal of Infectious Diseases, volume 181, 2000.

The toxins of pertussis are discussed in *Pertussis toxin and adenylate cyclase toxin: key virulence factors of Bordetella pertussis and cell biology tools,* by Nicholas Carbonetti. It was published in Future Microbiology, March 2010.

Very good pertussis vaccine reviews can be found in two articles. One is *Historical Review of Pertussis and the Classical Vaccine,* by James Cherry. It was published as a supplement in the 1996 edition of The Journal of Infectious Diseases, volume 174. The other is published in the journal Vaccines, the June 8, 2020 edition. Titled *Acellular Pertussis Vaccine Components: Today and Tomorrow,* it was written by Kaylan Dewan et al.

The biography of Filippo Pacini is covered in Wikipedia under the title *Filippo Pacini.* That of John Snow is portrayed in the article *John Snow and the Broad Street Pump,* from the UCLA Department of Epidemiology.

Cholera is reviewed in Mandell's *Principles and practice of Infectious Diseases.*

Chapter 18. The story of the typhus hoax in World War II Poland is recounted in an article published in the September 22nd 2015 edition of Atlas Obscura. Titled *How a Fake Typhus Epidemic Saved a Polish City From the Nazis,* it was written by Matt Soniak.

The University of Chicago Library has an extensive collection of material on Howard Taylor Ricketts. An article with the title *Howard Taylor Ricketts* summarizes his life and scientific contributions.

The biography of Stanislaus von Prowazek can be found online at Encyclopedia.com, under the title *Prowazek (Provazek) Stanislaus von Lanov.*

The history of typhus and warfare is summarized in Wikipedia under the title *Typhus.*

712

The pathophysiology of the disease is discussed in detail in Mandell's *Principles and Practice of Infectious Diseases,* 9th edition.

Chapter 19. The disease giardiasis is thoroughly discussed in *Biology of Giardia lamblia,* written by Rodney Adam. It was published in the July 2001 edition of Clinical Microbiology Reviews.

Chapter 20. The ability of helminths to alter the immune response is reviewed in a paper written by Rick Maizels, Hermelijn Smits, and Henry McSorley. Titled *Modulation of Host Immunity by Helminths: The Expanding Repertoire of Parasite Effector Molecules,* it was published in Immunity, November 20, 2018.

There are several very good parasitology texts. *Principles and Practice of Clinical Parasitology,* edited by Stephen Gillespie and Richard Pearson, gives a good overview of many species of parasites.

Chapter 21. A thorough discussion of the "kissing bugs," triatomines, is included in the article *Triatomines: Trypanosomiasis, Bacteria, and Viruses Potential vectors?* Published in Frontiers Cellular and Infection Microbiology, November 16, 2018, the senior author is Caroline Barreto Viera.

The biology of *Trypanosoma cruzi* is discussed at length in a January/March 2012 issue of the Brazilian journal Infectio. Written in English, the title is *Biology of Trypanosoma cruzi: An Update.* The lead author is Andre Vianna Martins.

A biography of Carlos Chagas is found in the article *Prophet in his own country: Carlos Chagas and the Nobel Prize.* Written by Rachel Lewinsohn, it is published in the fall, 2003 edition of Perspectives in Biology and Medicine.

Chapter 22. *History of the discovery of the malarial parasites and their vectors* goes into great detail on the subject. It was written by Francis Cox, and published in the volume 3, 2010 edition of Cox Parasites and Vectors.

The life cycle of malarial parasites is portrayed very nicely with vivid photos and illustrations on the website *Malaria Site, life cycle.*

The relationship between malarial parasites and the immune response to them is discussed at length in the article *The immunological balance between host and parasite in malaria.* It was published in the volume 40, 2016 edition of FEMS Microbiology reviews. Katrien Deroost is the senior author.

The details of the malarial parasites' excursion through the liver are reviewed in *The silent path to thousands of merozoites: the Plasmodium liver stage.* Written by Miguel Prudencio, Ana Rodriguez, and Maria Mota, it was published in the journal Nature Reviews/ Microbiology, volume 4, 2006.

Anti-malarial drugs are discussed in the article *The past, present and future of anti-malarial medicines,* published in Malaria Journal, volume 18, 2019. It was written by Edwin Tse, Marat Korsik, and Matthew Todd.

The malarial vaccine is discussed in Wikipedia under the title *Malaria vaccine.*

Chapter 23.   An in-depth discussion of the discovery of Ebola virus is found in the book *No Time To Lose, a life in pursuit of deadly viruses,* by Peter Piot.

An overall view of the hemorrhagic fever viruses is presented in *Hemorrhagic fever viruses: Pathogenesis, therapeutics, and emerging and re-emerging potential.* The article was written by authors from Brazil, with Lizdany Florez-Alvarez the lead author. It was published in the October 25, 2022 edition of Frontiers in Microbiology.

The pathogenicity of Ebola virus is discussed in *Molecular mechanisms of Ebola virus pathogenesis: focus on cells death,* in the journal Nature. L. Falasca was the lead author. It appeared in the May 29, 2015 edition.

A review article in volume 78, 2001 of Current Microbiology explores Dengue fever.   It is titled *Current Understanding of the Pathogenesis of Dengue Virus Infection,* and the senior author is Puneet Bhatt.

The compelling story of Walter Reed and his work on yellow fever is reviewed in an article on the website of The Army Historical Foundation. Written by Patrick Feng, it is entitled *Major Walter Reed And The Eradication Of Yellow Fever.*

The Yellow Fever Vaccine: A History, by J. Gordon Frierson, was published in the Yale Journal of Biology and Medicine, volume 83, published in 2010.

Detailed reviews of Yellow fever, West Nile, and Zika virus can be found in Mandell's *Principles and Practice of Infectious Diseases,* 9th edition.

The unique immune system of bats is discussed in the article *Accelerated viral dynamics in bat cell lines with implications for zoonotic emergence,* published in eLife, February 3, 2020. The lead author is Cara Brook.

Chapter 24.   A detailed analysis of retroviruses with emphasis on HIV is contained in *Molecular Biology and Diversification of Human Retroviruses,* written by Morgan Meissner, Nathaniel Talledge, and Louis Mansky. It was published in the June 2, 2022 edition of Frontiers in Virology. Mandell's *Principles and Practice of Infectious Disease* has an extensive description of the virus and its means of infecting.

Recommended treatment options for HIV infection can be found on the website of the Centers for Disease Control and Prevention.

Chapter 25.   The association between the introduction of sanitation and on onset of the polio pandemic is addressed in *How modern sanitation gave us polio.* Written by Allison Guy, it appears on the website Next Nature. It was published January 7, 2014.

An article published in Current Topics in Microbiology and Immunology in February, 2005 summarizes the life cycle of the polio virus. It is entitled *Poliovirus, Pathogenesis of Poliomyelitis, and Apoptosis.* The lead author is B. Blondel.

The book *Polio: An American Story,* by David Oshinsky is a thorough look at the disease.

A thorough description of the "iron lung" is given in a Science Museum article published October 14, 2018. It is titled *The Iron Lung.*

A biography of the remarkable woman Sister Elizabeth Kenny was published in the 1983, volume 9 edition of Australian Dictionary of Biography. Written by Ross Patrick, it is titled *Kenny, Elizabeth (1880-1952).*

The story of the development of polio vaccines is recounted in the journal Science, volume 288, June 2, 2000. Written by Stuart Blume and Ingrid Geesink, it is titled *A Brief History of Polio Vaccines.*

Chapter 26.   The website of The Texas State Cemetery has a biography for author Fred Gipson. It is titled *Frederick Benjamin Gipson.*

A detailed account of the history of rabies may be found in the article *The history of rabies in the Western Hemisphere.* Nine authors are listed, with Andres Velasco-Villa being the lead. It was published in the October 2017 edition of Antiviral Research.

A detailed description of the pathophysiology of rabies can be found in a paper published in the September 3, 2008 edition of Future Virology. Bernhard Dietzschold is the lead author of *Concepts in the pathogenesis of rabies.*

The compelling story of the development of the rabies vaccine by Louis Pasteur is recounted in the article *Louis Pasteur, monster slayer.* Written by Maya Prabhu, it appears on the website VaccinesWork. It was published Mach 23, 2022.

The discovery of the parasite *Toxoplasma gondii* is recounted in an article in the July 1 edition of International Journal for Parasitology, written by J.P. Dubey. It is titled *History of the discovery of the life cycle of Toxoplasma gondii.*

The life cycle of *Toxoplasma* is described in the textbook *Principles and Practice of Clinical Parasitology,* edited by Stephen Gillespie.

The immunomodulation ability of *Toxoplasma* is discussed in detail in *A Toxoplasma dense granule protein, GRA24, modulates the early immune response to infection by promoting a direct and sustained host p38 MAPK activation.* Lead author is Laurence Braun. It was published in the International Journal of Experimental Medicine, volume 210, 2013.

The subject of the role of *Toxoplasma* in behavior is discussed in the paper *Toxoplasma gondii infection, from predation to schizophrenia: can animal behaviour help us understand human behaviour?* From The Journal of Experimental Biology, volume 216, it was published in 2013. Joanne Webster is the lead author.

Another paper on the subject of altered mental status potentially caused by *Toxoplasma* is *The Machiavelli Microbe* by Sam Kean. It appears in the Summer 2015 edition of Science History Institute.

Chapter 27.   An article detailing the life of Rhazes appears in the Annals of Saudi Medicine, volume 27, 2007. Written by Samir Amr and Abdulghani Tbakhi, it is titled *Abu Bakr Muhammad Zakariya Al Razi (Rhazes): Philosopher, Physician and Alchemist.*

The work of Peter Panum in the investigation of measles is eloquently reviewed by Kathryne Dycus in the article *Peter Panum and the "geography of disease."* It is published in the journal Hektoen International, summer 2021.

A description of rinderpest and its eradication appears on the website of HFHA, Healthy Farms Healthy Agriculture. Titled *Rinderpest's Reign of Terror,* it was written by Katie Loberti, and is dated September 8, 2020.

A study published in February of 1938 gives a thorough recounting of the disease measles. *A Historical, Epidemiological and AEtiological Study of Measles (Morbilli; Rubeola).* Written by J.A.H. Brincker, it appears in Proceedings of the Royal Society of Medicine.

A detailed description of measles infection and pathogenesis is presented in a paper published in the July 28, 2016 edition of the journal Virus, titled *Measles Virus Host Invasion and Pathogenesis.* Five authors are listed; Brigitta Laksono is the lead author.

The development of the measles vaccine is recounted in an article by Jeffrey Baker that appeared in the journal Pediatrics, November 3, 2011. Its title is *The First Measles Vaccine.*

Chapter 28.   *The History of Plague—Part 1. The Three Great Pandemics,* by John Firth, appears on the website of JMVH, volume 20.

The discovery of the agent of bubonic plague, *Yersinia pestis,* is recounted in an article from the website of Antimicrobe.org. Titled *Discovery of Yersinia pestis,* it was written by Rebecca Maki.

The means by which *Yersinia pestis* causes infection is discussed in the article *Interaction between Yersinia pestis and the Host Immune System.* It was written by Chinese researchers Bei Li and Ruifu Yang, and appeared in the May 2008 edition of Infection and Immunity.

The story of the involvement of *Yersinia enterocolitica* in cases of pseudo appendicitis from chocolate milk appears in the January 12, 1978 edition of the New England Journal of Medicine. The lead author is R. E. Black.

Chapter 29.   The accidental release of viable anthrax spores from a Russian factory in 1979 is summarized in an article by Michael Fishbein titled *Anthrax—From Russia with Love.* It appears on the website MedicineNet.

The activity of anthrax toxins is discussed in *The Ins and Outs of Anthrax Toxin,* written by Swiss researchers Sarah Friebe, F. Gisou van der

Goot, and Jerome Burgi. It appeared in the journal Toxins in the March 10, 2016 edition.

Anthrax Pathogenesis, an article written by Mahtab Moayeri et al., was published in volume 69, 2015 edition of Annual Reviews of Microbiology. It relates a detailed look at the subject.

Chapter 30. *The Biology of Influenza Viruses*, by Nicole Bouvier and Peter Palese, was published in the Journal Vaccine, September 12, 2008.

Influenza Pathogenesis: The Effect of Host Factors on Severity of Disease, by Anshu Gounder and Adrianus Boon, was published in the Journal of Immunology, volume 202, 2019.

Innate immunity to influenza virus infection was written by Akiko Iwasaki and Padmini Pillai. It is published in Natural Reviews Immunology, May, 2014.

The activity of influenza protein PB1-F2 is discussed in *The influenza A virus protein PB1-F2,* by Zsuzsanna Varga and Peter Palese. The article is published in the November/December 2011 edition of Virulence.

A thorough discussion of influenza vaccines is found in *History and evolution of influenza control through vaccination: from the first monovalent vaccine to universal vaccines.* The senior author is I. Barberis. The article is published in Journal of Preventive Medicine and Hygiene, volume 57, 2016.

Chapter 31. Each of the Herpes viruses are discussed in detail in Mandell's *Principles and Practice of Infectious Diseases,* 9th edition. Descriptions of anatomy are given in Tortora's *Principles of Anatomy and Physiology,* 16th edition.

A thorough discussion of the Herpes virus family is in the book *Cell Biology of Herpes Viruses,* edited by Klaus Osterrieder, 2017.

A detailed description of Herpes Simplex viruses is presented in *Herpes Simplex Virus Cell Entry Mechanisms: An Update.* Krishnuraju Madavaraju is the lead author of the paper published in the January 18, 2021 edition of journal Frontiers in Cellular and Infection Microbiology.

Manipulation of the Innate Immune Response by Varicella Zoster Virus, was published in the January 24, 2020 edition of Frontiers in Immunology. Chelsea Gerada is the lead author.

Epstein-Barr Virus: Diseases Linked to Infection and Transformation was written by Hem Jha, Yonggang Pei, and Erie Robertson. It was published in Frontiers in Microbiology, October 25, 2016.

The website of Cancer Research UK has an interesting presentation on the discovery of the Epstein-Barr Virus. It is titled *50 years of Epstein-Barr virus.*

The Royal Society Publishing has an obituary on its website of Denis Burkitt written by Michael Anthony Epstein. It is titled *Denis Parsons Burkitt, 28 February 1911-23 March 1993.*

Cytomegalovirus is discussed in detail in *The life cycle and pathogenesis of human cytomegalovirus infection: lessons from proteomics,* by Pierre Jean Beltran and Ileana Cristea. It was published in the December 2014 edition of Expert Reviews of Proteomics.

Pathogenesis of human cytomegalovirus in the immunocompromised host is an article written by Paul Griffiths and Matthew Reeves. It was published in the December 2021 edition of Nature Reviews Microbiology.

Herpes virus 6 (roseola) is discussed in *Latency, Integration, and Reactivation of Human Herpesvirus-6,* which was published in the July 24, 2017 edition of the journal Viruses. It was written by Shara Pantry and Peter Medveczky.

The possible involvement of roseola virus in multiple sclerosis is discussed in the article *Type of Herpes Virus Tied to Multiple Sclerosis,* which appeared in the January 10, 2020 edition of The Scientist. It was written by Katarina Zimmer.

A detailed review of Kaposi Sarcoma Virus appears in the paper *Kaposi Sarcoma Pathogenesis: A Triad of Viral Infection, Oncogenesis, and Chronic Inflammation.* It was published in Translational Biomedicine, volume 1, 2010. Janet Douglas was the senior author.

Chapter 32. *The Early History of Coccidioidomycosis: 1892-1945* was written by Jan Hirschmann, and published in the May 1, 2007 edition of Clinical Infectious Diseases.

Coccidioides immitis and posadasii; A review of their biology, genomics, pathogenesis, and host immunity was published in the volume 9, 2018 edition of the journal Virulence. The authors are Theo Kirkland and Joshua Fierer.

Chapter 33. The article *Candida albicans pathogenicity mechanisms,* written by Francois Mayer, Duncan Wilson, and Bernhard Hube, gives a detailed description of the organism. It was published in the February 15, 2013 edition of the journal Virulence.

Another comprehensive review of the organism is the article *Candida albicans Pathogenesis: Fitting within the Host-Microbe Damage Response Framework,* which was published in the October 2016 edition of Infection and Immunity. The lead author is Mary Ann Jabra-Rizk.

Chapter 34. *Neisseria meningitidis: Biology, Microbiology, and Epidemiology,* an article written by Nadine Rouphael and David Stephens, was published in the journal Methods in Molecular Biology, volume 799, 2012.

Mechanism of meningeal invasion by Neisseria meningitidis was published in the March/April edition of the journal Virulence. Mathieu Coureuil is the lead author.

Chapter 35. Much is yet to be learned about Coronaviruses. A start is the article *Pathophysiology of COVID-19: Critical Role of Hemostasis.* The senior author is Sonia Aparecida de Andrade. The article was published in Frontiers in Cellular and Infection Microbiology, June 3, 2022.

Another provocative article is *SARS-CoV-2-mediated evasion strategies for antiviral interferon pathways.* Written by Korean authors Soo-Jin Oh and Sarah Shin, it was published in the Journal of Microbiology, volume 60, 2022.

Chapter 36. Mandell's *Principles and Practices of Infectious Diseases,* 9th edition, contains detailed information about the pyogenic pathogens Staph. and Strep.

Chapter 37. In the 12 September 2019 edition of Frontiers in Immunology, there is an article on the immunomodulation of RSV. Written by Jonatan Carvajal et al., it is titled *Host Components Contributing to Respiratory Syncytial Virus Pathogenesis.*

Recommendations for the RSV vaccines can be found on the website of the Centers for Disease Control and Prevention.

The affect rubella virus has on the developing fetus is discussed in detail in the article *Investigating the Molecular Basis of Rubella Virus-Induced Teratogenesis: A Literature Review.* Written by Mariam Goubran, it is published in the University of Saskatchewan Undergraduate Research Journal, Volume 4, 2017.

Insights into virulence factors determining the pathogenicity of Cronobacter sakazakii, written by Niharika Singh, Gunjan Goel, and Mamta Raghav, is published in the July 2015 edition of the journal Virulence.

Chapter 38. An autobiography by Barry Marshall appears on the website of The Nobel Prize. It is titled *Barry J. Marshall, Biographical.*

The history of the discovery of *Helicobacter pylori* and its role in disease is recounted in *Discovery by Jaworski of Helicobacter pylori and its Pathogenic Role in Peptic Ulcer, Gastritis, and Gastric Cancer.* Published in the Journal of Physiology and Pharmacology, 2003, volume 54, it was written by J. W. Konturek.

The interaction of *Helicobacter pylori* and the immune system is discussed in the article *Helicobacter pylori and T Helper Cells: Mechanisms of Immune Escape and Tolerance.* The lead author is Tiziana Larussa. It was published in volume 2015 of the Journal of Immunology Research.

Testing for *Helicobacter pylori* is reviewed in *Diagnosis of Helicobacter pylori infection: Current options and developments.* Written by Yao-Kuang Wang et al., it is published in the World Journal of Gastroenterology, October 28, 2015.

Chapter 39. The story of the Bronte family and their encounters with tuberculosis is recounted in an article published in The Yorkshire Post March 22nd, 2019. Titled *This is why the Bronte sisters died so young,* it was written by Grace Newton.

History of Tuberculosis. Part 1 –Phthisis, consumption, and the White Plague, by John Frith, is published in the June 2014 edition of The Journal of Military and Veterans' Health.

Tuberculosis: A Review of Current Trends discusses several aspects of the disease, including pathophysiology, diagnosis, and treatment. The lead author is A. Sanyaolu. It is published in the May 6, 2019 edition of Epidemiology International Journal.

Mandell's *Principles and Practice of Infectious Disease,* 9th edition, covers the topic of tuberculosis in great detail.

The story of the discovery of streptomycin is told by the researcher at the center of it, Albert Schatz, in his article *The True Story of the Discovery of Streptomycin.* It is published in the August, 1993 edition of the journal Actinomycetes.

The importance of Vitamin D in mitigating infection by *Mycobacterium tuberculosis* is reviewed in the article *The vitamin D–antimicrobial pathway and its role in protection against infection.* Written by Adrian Gombart, it is published in the November 2009 edition of Future Microbiology.

The Leprosy Mission International has a website that addresses many aspects of the disease, including its history.

The article *Nerve Growth Factor and Pathogenesis of Leprosy: Review and Update* is published in the May 7, 2018 edition of Frontiers in Immunology. The lead author is Tinara Leila de Souza Aarao.

Chapter 40. The biology of *Ixodes scapularis* is discussed in the article *Insights into the development of Ixodes scapularis: a resource for research on a medically important tick species.* Written by Katherine Kocan, Jose de la Fuente, and Lisa Coburn, it is published in the journal BMC, Parasites and Vectors, November 14, 2015.

The June 2021 edition of Frontiers in Medicine has an article that thoroughly discusses Lyme disease. Titled *Report of the Pathogenesis and Pathophysiology of Lyme Disease Subcommittee of the HHS Tick Borne Disease Working Group,* the senior author is Sam Donta.

A paper on *Borrelia burgdorferi* appears in the February 2017 edition of Frontiers in Immunology. Titled *Borrelia burgdorferi Keeps Moving and Carries On: A Review of Borrelial Dissemination and Invasion,* it was written by Jenny Hyde.

A detailed discussion of the immune modulation of Lyme Disease is contained in the paper *Borrelia burgdorferi Pathogenesis and the Immune Response.* Written by Mary Petzke, it is published in Clinics in Laboratory Medicine, August 2015.

A discussion of Lyme disease neurological symptoms and diagnosis is presented on the website verywell health. The article, titled *An overview of Lyme Neuroborreliosis,* was written by James Myhre and Dennis Sifris. It is dated March 30, 2020.

The article *The pathogenesis of syphilis: the Great Mimicker, revisited* describes the disease in great detail. Authored by Rosana Peeling and Edward Hook, it is published in the December 2005 edition of The Journal of Pathology.

Weil's disease (leptospirosis) is eloquently reviewed in Paul Levett's article in the April 2001 edition of Clinical Microbiology Reviews. It's titled *Leptospirosis.*

Chapter 41. *A guide to vaccinology: from basic principles to new developments* summarizes the types of available vaccines as well as their history. The article was written by Andrew Pollard and Else Bijker, and it is published in Nature Reviews/Immunology, the February 2021 edition.

Chapter 42. The online version of Merck Manual has a detailed description of all the classes of antibiotics. Written by Brian Wirth, there are two versions, professional and consumer. The professional version is titled *Overview of Antibacterial Drugs.*

Chapter 43. *The gut microbiome in health and in disease* is a comprehensive article published in Current Opinion in Gastroenterology, the January 2015 edition. It was written by Andrew Shreiner, John Kao, and Vincent Young.

A detailed review of the gut microbiome and its effects is *Microbiota in health and diseases.* The lead author is Kaijian Hou. The article is published in the April 2022 edition of Signal Transduction and Targeted Therapy.

The book *Missing Microbes* by Martin Blaser discusses the effects of antibiotics on gut dysbiosis and health.